Infections of Leisure

FOURTH EDITION

Infections of Leisure

FOURTH EDITION

EDITED BY

David Schlossberg

Professor
Temple University School of Medicine
and
Medical Director
Tuberculosis Control Program
Philadelphia Department of Public Health
Philadelphia, Pennsylvania

ASM PRESS

WASHINGTON, DC

Address editorial correspondence to ASM Press, 1752 N St. NW, Washington, DC 20036-2904, USA

Send orders to ASM Press, P.O. Box 605, Herndon, VA 20172, USA
Phone: (800) 546-2416 or (703) 661-1593
Fax: (703) 661-1501
E-mail: books@asmusa.org
Online: estore.asm.org

Library of Congress Cataloging-in-Publication Data

Infections of leisure / edited by David Schlossberg.—4th ed.
   p. ; cm.
 Includes bibliographical references and index.
 ISBN 978-1-55581-484-7 (pbk.)
   1. Communicable diseases—Popular works.   2. Leisure—Health aspects—Popular works.   3. Zoonoses—Popular works.   I. Schlossberg, David.
   [DNLM: 1. Infection—etiology.   2. Disease Vectors.   3. Leisure Activities.   4. Zoonoses.   WC 195 I438 2009]

RC113.I54 2009
616.9'0471—dc22

                                                    2009007559

To Dr. Burke A. Cunha, prolific writer, masterful teacher and clinician, and valued friend. As a member of the American Osler Society, he exemplifies Osler's dictum to "serve the art of Medicine as it should be served."

CONTENTS

CONTRIBUTORS

Frederick J. Angulo
Enteric Diseases Epidemiology Branch, Division of Foodborne, Bacterial and Mycotic Diseases, Centers for Disease Control and Prevention, 1600 Clifton Rd., MS A38, Atlanta, Georgia 30333

Bertha S. Ayi
Mercy Infectious Disease and Epidemiology Center, 801 5th St., Sioux City, Iowa 51103

Buddha Basnyat
Nepal International Clinic, Himalayan Rescue Association, and Patan Hospital, Lal Durbar, GPO Box 3596, Kathmandu, Nepal

Jesse D. Blanton
Poxvirus and Rabies Branch, National Center for Zoonotic, Vector-Borne, and Enteric Diseases, Centers for Disease Control and Prevention, Atlanta, Georgia 30333

Bruno B. Chomel
Department of Population Health and Reproduction, School of Veterinary Medicine, University of California, Davis, Davis, California 95616

Mark A. Clemence
Department of Internal Medicine, Wheaton Franciscan Medical Group, Hales Corners, Wisconsin 53130

C. Glenn Cobbs
Division of Infectious Diseases, University of Alabama at Birmingham, Birmingham, Alabama 35294-0006

Julie M. Collins
Department of Medicine, Temple University Hospital, Philadelphia, Pennsylvania 19140

Thomas A. Cumbo
Private practice in infectious disease medicine, 17 Limestone Ct., Suite 3, Williamsville, New York 14221

Burke A. Cunha
Infectious Disease Division, Winthrop-University Hospital, Mineola, New York 11501, and State University of New York School of Medicine, Stony Brook, New York

John R. Dunn
Communicable and Environmental Disease Services, Tennessee Department of Health, 425 5th Ave. North, Cordell Hull Building, 1st Floor, Nashville, Tennessee 37047

David Dworzack
Department of Medical Microbiology and Immunology and Section of Infectious Diseases, Department of Internal Medicine, Creighton University Medical Center, Omaha, Nebraska 68131

Robert Edelman
Center for Vaccine Development, Division of Geographic Medicine, Department of Medicine, and Division of Infectious Diseases and Tropical Pediatrics, Department of Pediatrics, University of Maryland School of Medicine, 685 West Baltimore St., Room 480, Baltimore, Maryland 21201

James G. Fox
Division of Comparative Medicine, Massachusetts Institute of Technology, 77 Massachusetts Avenue, Bldg. 16-825C, Cambridge, Massachusetts 02139

Mark Gendreau
Department of Emergency Medicine, Lahey Clinic, Burlington, Massachusetts 01805

Ellie J. C. Goldstein
R. M. Alden Research Laboratory, Santa Monica, California 90404, and UCLA School of Medicine, Los Angeles, California 90024

Craig E. Greene
Department of Small Animal Medicine, College of Veterinary Medicine, University of Georgia, Athens, Georgia 30602

Jeffrey K. Griffiths
Graduate Programs in Public Health, Department of Public Health and Family Medicine, and Department of Medicine, Tufts University School of Medicine, 136 Harrison Ave., Boston, Massachusetts 02111

Richard L. Guerrant
Center for Global Health and Division of Infectious Diseases and International Health, University of Virginia School of Medicine, Charlottesville, Virginia 22908

Geeta Gupta
Division of Infectious Diseases, University of California Irvine Medical Center, Route 81, Bldg. 53, Rm. 215, 101 The City Dr. S., Orange, California 92868

Richard F. Jacobs
Department of Pediatrics, University of Arkansas for Medical Sciences, Arkansas Children's Hospital Research Institute, and Pediatric Infectious Diseases, Arkansas Children's Hospital, 800 Marshall St., Little Rock, Arkansas 72202-3591

Diane H. Johnson
Infectious Disease Division, Winthrop-University Hospital, Mineola, New York 11501, and State University of New York School of Medicine, Stony Brook, New York

Vivek Kak
W. A. Foote Hospital, 1100 E. Michigan Ave., #305, Jackson, Michigan 49201

John W. Krebs
Rickettsial Zoonosis Branch, National Center for Zoonotic, Vector-Borne, and Enteric Diseases, Centers for Disease Control and Prevention, Atlanta, Georgia 30333

Matthew E. Levison
Drexel University College of Medicine and Drexel University School of Public Health, Philadelphia, Pennsylvania 19102

Bennett Lorber
Section of Infectious Diseases, Department of Medicine, Temple University School of Medicine and Hospital, Philadelphia, Pennsylvania 19140

Alexandra Mangili
Division of Geographic Medicine and Infectious Disease, Tufts Medical Center, Boston, Massachusetts 02111

Arezou Minooee
Department of Internal Medicine, University of California Irvine Medical Center, Bldg. 200, Suite 720, 101 The City Dr. S., Orange, California 92868

Mukesh Patel
Division of Infectious Diseases, University of Alabama at Birmingham, Birmingham, Alabama 35294-0006

Leland S. Rickman (deceased)
Epidemiology Unit, Division of Infectious Diseases, University of California, San Diego, San Diego, California 92103

Gordon E. Schutze
Section of Retrovirology and Baylor International Pediatric AIDS Initiative, Baylor College of Medicine, Texas Children's Hospital, Houston, Texas 77030

Martin S. Wolfe
Traveler's Medical Service of Washington, DC, and George Washington University Medical School, Washington, DC 20037

Jonathan M. Zenilman
Division of Infectious Diseases, Johns Hopkins Bayview Medical Center, 4940 Eastern Ave., Baltimore, Maryland 21224

PREFACE

The fourth edition of *Infections of Leisure* continues to identify and organize the infectious risks associated with our leisure time activities. Time away from work or school affords us the chance to travel, swim, sail, climb, camp, hike, garden, and taste exotic foods. We continue to pamper our (sometimes unusual) pets and to play increasingly challenging sports. However, all these activities expose us to an expanding list of pathogenic microbes, some of which are entirely new and others of which are increasingly resistant to current therapy. For this new edition, every chapter has been thoroughly updated, and three new chapters have been added: "Infectious Risks of Air Travel" (chapter 16), "Perils of the Petting Zoo" (chapter 17), and "Infections on Cruise Ships" (chapter 18). All the activities described herein carry risks with their attendant pleasures, and, as in the previous editions, the risks are outlined and discussed in a convenient, user-friendly, and accessible format. A new feature has been added to this edition: at the completion of each chapter a list of "Practical Tips" highlights salient points of prevention and management of infections discussed in the chapter. We hope this edition continues to provide a practical resource for this diverse, fascinating, and challenging group of infectious diseases.

I am deeply grateful to Jeffrey Holtmeier and Kenneth April of ASM Press for their professionalism, wisdom, and friendship.

PREFACE TO THE FIRST EDITION

Many of us spend our leisure time hiking, sailing, snorkeling, and camping. We like to sample new foods, pamper our pets, and travel to magical places. All these pursuits enrich our lives but carry attendant risks. This book details the infections that complicate exposure to vacation climates, pets, recreational activities, and exotic cuisine.

There are many infectious disorders that fit this category, and they frequently overlap. Thus, touring a tropical paradise affords one the opportunity to eat poisoned food, swim in contaminated waters, and sustain serious injury from marine life. The great outdoors adds arthropod-borne infection and polluted water to the dangers of zoonoses. Clearly, risks are multiple, and a comprehensive guide is necessary. This book attempts to organize the wealth of information about these interesting and varied infections in a convenient and accessible format.

AT THE SHORE

Mark A. Clemence and Richard L. Guerrant

I

FISH AND SHELLFISH INTOXICATIONS

Introduction

In the United States, the consumption of seafood in 2007 alone totaled more than 4.2 billion lb, or 14.8 lb per person per year (327). An increase in the consumption of seafood is occurring, with a resultant increase in the number of cases of fish- and shellfish-related food poisonings. Contaminated seafood was the leading cause of food-borne illness outbreaks, according to the Center for Science in the Public Interest, with seafood causing 340 outbreaks with 5,133 cases of food-borne illness in the United States between 1990 and 2001 (69a). In addition, improved reporting of cases due to a greater awareness by the public and health care personnel of the association between seafood consumption and illness has also contributed to this observed increase (205, 206, 385). Food-borne diseases associated with fish and shellfish can be categorized into allergic, infectious, and toxin-mediated

etiologies (385). The Centers for Disease Control (CDC) and the U.S. Department of Health and Human Services reported on all types of food-borne illness in the United States from 1988 to 1992. Bacterial causes were involved in more than 79% of confirmed outbreaks, whereas chemical poisonings from fish and shellfish toxins were responsible for 12.3% of outbreaks of confirmed etiology (91).

Vertebrate fish intoxication can be divided into three groups, as follows: (i) ichthyosarcotoxic fish contain toxin in their viscera, mucous membranes, skin, or musculature; (ii) ichthyo-otoxic fish contain toxin in their gonads; and (iii) ichthyohemotoxic fish contain toxin in their blood. At least nine types of ichthyosarcotoxism are known, among which ciguatera, scombroid, and puffer fish poisoning are the most common (205).

The term "shellfish" includes crustaceans, which are mobile animals that have a hard articulated exoskeleton, and mollusks, which have hard shells and are sedentary or have limited locomotion. Crustacean species include lobsters, shrimp, crabs, scampi, and crawfish. Mollusks can be divided into the bivalves, which have two shells joined by a hinge, and the gastropods, which have a whorled snail-like shell. The bivalves include oysters, mus-

Mark A. Clemence, Department of Internal Medicine, Wheaton Franciscan Medical Group, Hales Corners, WI 53130. *Richard L. Guerrant,* Center for Global Health and Division of Infectious Diseases and International Health, University of Virginia School of Medicine, Charlottesville, VA 22908.

#1

sels, clams, and scallops. Gastropods of commercial importance include whelks and periwinkles. With the exception of scallops, which reside in deeper waters, all mollusks grow in and are harvested from nearshore coastal waters (465). Ingestion of shellfish containing toxins produced by dinoflagellates may induce dramatic and sometimes fatal illness (Table 1).

Dinoflagellates and Red Tides

Dinoflagellates, or plankton, are unicellular plant-like organisms with a worldwide distribution which serve as an important element of the food chain in marine animals. During blooms, these organisms may achieve concentrations high enough to impart a reddish or yellow discoloration to the sea due to the local production of neurotoxins and pigmented proteins, hence the name "red tide" (391). Of the 15 species of toxic dinoflagellates known to inhabit the waters surrounding the United States, 4 are related to human poisoning and 6 are associated with the formation of red tides (385).

The association of red tides with human illness has been known since ancient times, with the earliest description being from the Bible (Exodus 7:20–21): "And all the water that was in the Nile was turned to blood. And the fish that were in the Nile died, and the Nile became foul, so that the Egyptians could not drink water from the Nile." North American Indians were aware of red tides and their association with poisoning due to mussel ingestion (68). In 1793, George Vancouver described what may be the first description of poisoning due to shellfish ingestion, which affected sailors exploring passages off the mainland coast of what is now British Columbia; several men became ill after eating roasted mussels, and death occurred in one of them within 5 h (449). Walker, in 1884, described several people who became ill after eating oysters in Florida, possibly related to a red tide (456).

Red tides can be caused by nontoxigenic dinoflagellates, and shellfish may become poisonous even in the absence of a red tide (205). Vectors of shellfish poisoning are mainly filter feeders that ingest large quantities of these dinoflagellates, many of which are toxigenic. The continuous filtration can result in the accumulation of large quantities of toxin within the digestive glands of the shellfish or, in the case of the Alaskan butter clam, the siphon (177).

Paralytic Fish Poisoning

Paralytic shellfish poisoning (PSP) results from the ingestion of marine mollusks containing potent neurotoxins, with the best known being saxitoxin, named after the Alaskan butter clam, *Saxidomus*. Several other toxins are known, each of which shares the ability to invoke a variety of biological effects, including occasionally severe and sometimes fatal impairment in sensory, cerebellar, and motor functions.

From 1973 to 1987, state health departments reported 19 outbreaks of PSP (mean size of outbreak, eight persons) to CDC's Food-Borne Disease Outbreak Surveillance System (81), which accounted for 1.1% of all outbreaks of food-borne disease in the United States from 1972 to 1977 and 1.0% of outbreaks from 1978 to 1982 (391). The implicated mollusks included mussels, oysters, clams, scallops, and cockles. Puffer fish were the cause of 13 cases of PSP in Florida in 2002 (94). Worldwide, it was estimated that more than 1,600 cases occurred in 1974 alone, with more than 300 deaths (A. Prakash, presented at the First International Conference on Toxic Dinoflagellate Blooms, Wakefield, MA, 1975). In 1990, two outbreaks occurred in the United States, with one involving six people who ingested mussels harvested off the Nantucket coast in Massachusetts and the other involving four people, with one fatality, in Alaska (7, 81). The incidences of PSP in Old Harbor and Kodiak, AK, have been estimated at 15 and 1.5 cases per 1,000 persons per year, respectively (154). The case fatality ratio is about 8 to 9%, usually secondary to respiratory failure (291). No deaths, however, were re-

TABLE 1 Fish and shellfish poisoning

Disease	Source	Toxin	Mechanism	Epidemiology	Clinical data	Mortality	Treatment
Shellfish poisoning							
Paralytic shellfish[a]	Alaskan butter clam (*Saxidomus giganteus*), mussels, oysters, scallops, cockles	Saxitoxin (heat stable)	Like tetrodotoxin; blocks Na+ channels	Low temp; >30°N or S; 10 outbreaks with 63 cases from 1971–1977 in New England, Southwest, Alaska	0.5–3 h; paresthesias or dysesthesias of mouth and extremities; 14% with N/V/D[e]	8–9% (usually within 12–24 h)	Supportive
Neurotoxic shellfish[b]	May be aerosolized in the surf	Brevetoxins (heat and acid stable) A, B, C (polycyclic ethers)	Probably via altering Na conductance	Gulf coasts of Florida and Texas	<3 h; paresthesias; temp reversal; cerebellar and GI[f] symptoms	Rare	Supportive; B2 agonists; cholinergic antagonists; Ca^{2+} channel blockers
Amnesic shellfish (neurovisceral toxic syndrome)	*Nitzschia pungens* diatoms in mussels	Domoic acid (heat stable)	Neuroexcitatory like glutamic acid; causes hippocampal necrosis	Atlantic, Pacific, and Indian Oceans	0.25–38 h ($\bar{x}$ = 5.5 h); N/V, GI bleeding; HA[h]; memory loss	3%	
Diarrheic shellfish	Shellfish with dinoflagellate *Dinophysis fortii* or *D. acuminata*	Okadaic acid	Blocks phosphatase that degrades A/G kinase products	Japan and The Netherlands	5–6 h (range, 0.5–30 h); N/V/D with abdominal cramps		

(Table continues)

TABLE 1 *(continued)*

Disease	Source	Toxin	Mechanism	Epidemiology	Clinical data	Mortality	Treatment
Fish poisoning (ichthyosarcotoxic)							
Puffer fish[c]	Puffer fish, shellfish, salamanders, frogs, newts	Tetrodotoxin (heat stable, nonprotein)	Blocks Na channels; axonal transmission	Japan, New Jersey, Long Island	10–45 min (<3 h); paresthesias; weakness; paralysis; hypotension; bradycardia; respiratory paralysis	59% (in first 24 h)	Supportive
Ciguatera[d]	Larger (>5-lb) carnivorous reef fish (barracuda, herring, jacks, grouper, snapper, moray eels, etc.)	Ciguatoxins and maitotoxin (heat-stable tasteless polyether)	Blocks C^{2+} regulation of Na$^+$ channels (opens voltage-dependent Na$^+$ channels)	<35°N and S; subtropical/tropical (Florida, Hawaii, S. Pacific); most common marine food poisoning in United States	2–30 h ↑ or ↓ BP[g]; N/V/D with abdominal pain; temp reversal; teeth "loose"	<12% (rare)	Symptomatic (mannitol; opiates are dangerous)
Scombroid fish	Tuna, mackerel, skipjack, bonito, albacore, bluefish, mahimahi	Histamine (heat stable) from bacterial decarboxylation of histidine	Histamine reaction	Common worldwide, especially coastal United States	Minutes–hours ($\bar{x}$ = 30 min); flush; HA, dizziness, burning	Rare	Antihistamine (intravenous cimetidine)

[a]Primary causes are red tides and dinoflagellates such as *Protogonyaulax catenella* and *P. tamarensis.*
[b]Primary causes are red tides and unarmored dinoflagellates such as *P. brevis.*
[c]Tetraodontidae; also known as fugu.
[d]The primary cause is the dinoflagellate *Gambierdiscus toxicus.*
[e]N/V/D, nausea, vomiting, diarrhea.
[f]GI, gastrointestinal
[g]BP, blood pressure.
[h]HA, headache.

ported for 10 outbreaks involving 63 cases reported to the CDC from 1971 to 1977 (2). In one analysis of two outbreaks of PSP in Alaska, those residents who knew nothing about PSP reported the same frequency of symptoms as those who knew about the potential lethal effects of PSP (154).

The effects of PSP are harmful not only to humans but also to fish, birds, and other wildlife that rely on aquatic sources of food. The ecological consequences can be devastating. One of the earliest signs of a toxic bloom is the sudden and unexplained death of large numbers of fish and wildlife in the vicinity of a bloom. The American Indians were aware of these associations and avoided fish and shellfish ingestion during such times (68). These ecological effects may persist for months following the onset of an outbreak and require a year or more for affected shellfish to become safe for human consumption (177). Economic consequences can be equally devastating as the shellfish industry becomes paralyzed during this period. Widespread reporting by the news media and strict adherence to public safety measures lead to a significant depression of demand for fish and shellfish not only in affected areas but also in unaffected regional areas. It is estimated that the cost of surveillance and enforcement during outbreaks of PSP in the United States is about $1.2 million per year (177).

The dinoflagellates responsible for paralytic fish poisoning are widely distributed globally, but actual outbreaks usually occur endemically in specific geographic areas. Such blooms are usually unpredictable and can occur with rapid accumulation of toxic concentrations. Most cases of PSP occur in cold, temperate waters above 30°N and below 30°S (134, 205); however, tropical cases have been reported in Thailand (249), Singapore (426), India (232), Guatemala (375), Malaysia (227), New Guinea (177), the Solomon Islands (133), Mexico (9), and El Salvador (9). Most North American cases occur along the Pacific coast, from central California to Alaska and the Aleutian Islands, and on the East Coast, in the New England coastal area as well as Nova Scotia, New Brunswick, and Quebec, Canada (177). The majority of outbreaks are reported in coastal areas, but inland cases have occurred, occasionally in areas remote from the seas (391).

Along the West Coast, cases tend to occur from May to October, and on the East Coast, they occur from July to September (177). The Alaskan butter clam can be dangerous year-round (180). The period of toxicity usually lasts for a few days during each outbreak, but toxic levels may persist for many months. Factors favoring toxic blooms include warm water temperatures (usually when water temperatures reach 16°C), periods of high solar radiation, the attainment of optimal concentrations of trace vitamins and minerals, and periods of turbulence such as during hurricanes, dredging, and the transplantation of shellfish (177, 391). Afflicted shellfish can be found along open coasts, in bays, and in estuarine areas. The most important hydrographic factor is probably a thermocline-imposed barrier, i.e., areas where water temperatures are greater than 16°C (177). Occasionally, red tides may be precipitated by the lowering of salinity, such as at sites of river discharge or during periods of heavy rainfall.

Many types of molluscan shellfish may become toxic. The 19 outbreaks reported to the CDC during 1973 to 1987 were due to the ingestion of mussels, clams, oysters, scallops, and cockles. In Alaska, during 1976 through 1989, 55% of the 42 reported outbreaks were due to the ingestion of Alaskan butter clams. Other shellfish implicated in Alaskan outbreaks included mussels, cockles, steamer clams, sea snails, and razor clams (81). In addition to the ingestion of shellfish, cases of PSP have also been linked to the ingestion of mackerel, scads, and several species of crabs (177).

Mollusks become toxic when they ingest toxic dinoflagellates. The toxins accumulate in the digestive glands and can remain there for a long time. This toxic accumulation can occur even in the absence of the buildup of sufficient numbers of dinoflagellates to discolor the water. If placed in dinoflagellate-free sea-water, it can take up to 12 days for shellfish to become nontoxic. In the case of the Alaskan butter clam, toxins tend to accumulate in the siphon, from which they are eliminated very slowly (177). Scallops, on the other hand, do not accumulate toxins in the adductor muscle, which is the part usually ingested, although toxins may accumulate in the other tissues.

Several species of toxic dinoflagellates have been implicated in outbreaks of PSP. In North America, *Protogonyaulax catenella* is the principal dinoflagellate species responsible for outbreaks along the northwest Pacific coast of the continent, whereas *Protogonyaulax tamarensis* is responsible for most outbreaks along the north Atlantic coast in addition to some outbreaks on the Pacific coast (177, 385). In the tropics, *Pyrodinium bahamense* is responsible for most outbreaks (133, 227, 232, 375, 426). Each of these species is armored, ranging in size from 25 to 46 μm, and has a tendency to become highly bioluminescent during blooms (385). During the winter months, most toxic dinoflagellates exist as cysts in the sediment beneath the sea. Turbulent conditions can disperse these cysts; when water temperatures reach optimal conditions (16°C), blooming occurs by excystment and the formation of motile cells (177, 391).

There are 21 molecular forms of PSP toxins, of which saxitoxin is the primary toxin responsible for the biologic effects of PSP (362). Other toxins include neotoxin and the gonyautoxins, designated by roman numerals in the order of their discovery (391, 406). These toxins are pharmacologically similar to tetrodotoxin and are estimated to be 50 times more potent than curare and 1,000 times more potent than cyanide (362, 484). Saxitoxin is an alkaloid, nonprotein, low-molecular-weight, water-soluble toxin that is heat stable (426). Cooking does not inactivate it, and it tends to become concentrated in broth (81). It bears some resemblance to guanine and may undergo trimethylation to form a toxic acetylcholine-like compound (406). The toxic

effects result from binding of the toxin to either the cell membrane, a cation receptor, or both to inhibit sodium influx, thus blocking the action potential along neuronal axons or skeletal muscle (134, 205, 391, 406, 426). Higher concentrations may have a similar electrophysiologic effect on cardiac and smooth muscle (7). Evidence exists that under acidic conditions, as in the stomach or in pickling containers, nontoxic products may become converted to toxins (5, 232). Furthermore, shellfish may be capable of converting nontoxins to potent neurotoxins (5). Children may be more susceptible to the toxic effects (375). The lethal dose of saxitoxin has been estimated to be 0.3 to 1.0 mg; a single mussel may contain 30 to 50 mg (134). The safe level of toxin in shellfish has been defined as 80 μg/100 g of shellfish (75).

The symptoms of PSP usually begin within 30 min after the ingestion of toxic shellfish but can occur up to 3 h later. The incubation period appears to be related inversely to the amount of toxin ingested. Initially, there may be paresthesias and dysesthesias of the lips, tongue, and face, which subsequently can progress to involve the neck, arms, fingertips, legs, and toes. Gastrointestinal symptoms, usually nausea, vomiting, and diarrhea, were seen in only 14% of patients in one series (40). Many people have described a "feeling of floating" (289). Progression of symptoms is usually dependent on the dose of toxin ingested (391); more severe cases may be accompanied by weakness, ataxia, incoordination, and cranial nerve findings such as bulbar paresis, iridoplegia, dysphonia, and dysphagia (177, 205, 277, 426). Other associated symptoms include headache, salivation, intense thirst, and temporary blindness (177). High toxin intake can result in muscular paralysis and respiratory failure, which is the usual cause of death in fatal cases. The illness can be sufficiently severe to require hospitalization in 30 to 60% of affected patients (203). When it does occur, death usually ensues within 12 h (205, 426). If the patient survives 12 to 18 h, the prognosis for recovery is good (73). Recovery usually occurs within a week without complications (385); however, several patients in one outbreak described persistent headaches, memory loss, and fatigue lasting for several weeks (375).

The diagnosis is based on a history of recent shellfish ingestion in the appropriate clinical setting. Routine laboratory tests are usually nonspecific and not helpful in establishing the diagnosis (134). The MB fraction of creatine kinase may be elevated in the absence of myocardial damage (97). Diagnosis can be confirmed by a standard mouse bioassay method in which toxin concentrations of the suspect shellfish are calculated by determining the dilution of a shellfish homogenate required to kill a 20-g mouse in 5 to 7 min. The value can then be used to calculate an absolute concentration by comparison with a known control (5, 177). Drawbacks include a precision of ±20%, interference from sodium chloride, and the need to keep a constant supply of mice (419). Other techniques have been developed, such as a fluorimetric assay, an immunologic assay, a colorimetric assay, and high-pressure liquid chromatography (419). Efforts to isolate the toxin from gastric contents have been limited (426).

Treatment is largely supportive. Attempts should be made to remove unabsorbed toxin through gastric lavage or the administration of a cathartic or enema (134, 205, 299, 385). Mechanical ventilation may become necessary in the event of respiratory failure. Hemodialysis was used successfully in one patient (24). Atropine should be avoided because saxitoxin and its derivatives may be anticholinergic (385).

Neurotoxic Shellfish Poisoning

Ptychodiscus brevis (formerly *Gymnodinium breve*) is the dinoflagellate responsible for neurotoxic shellfish poisoning, a syndrome similar to PSP; however, the symptoms of neurotoxic shellfish poisoning are usually milder, and paralysis and respiratory failure do not occur (205). This dinoflagellate produces neurotoxins and is responsible for the formation of red

tides off the Gulf coasts of Florida and Texas; occasionally, sea currents can carry the organism to Florida's Atlantic coast (183, 205, 322). In 1987, a red tide due to *Ptychodiscus brevis* formed off the coast of North Carolina and was associated with an outbreak of neurotoxic shellfish poisoning involving 48 people (316). The source of this bloom was probably a red tide carried from Florida's southwest coast by Gulf Stream currents (432). Five cases were reported to the CDC from 1970 through 1974 (205).

Ptychodiscus brevis ranges in size from 20 to 40 micrometers in length and is about 13 micrometers in width. It has been referred to as a "naked organism" because it lacks the shell of polysaccharide plates which characterizes *Protogonyaulax* species and other dinoflagellates (415). The neurotoxins produced by the dinoflagellate probably do not accumulate in fish but do concentrate in filter-feeding shellfish in the vicinity of a bloom. Shellfish are not affected by the toxins, but humans become affected by ingestion of those shellfish containing high levels of neurotoxin. Shellfish which may become toxic include oysters, clams, coquinas, and other bivalve mollusks (21).

Five or more separate nonprotein toxins or toxin components are produced by *Ptychodiscus brevis*. These are termed "brevetoxins" and include brevetoxins A, B, C, and Gb-4. Brevetoxins A, B, and C are polycyclic ethers which have similar structures and may be interconvertible (385, 406). The toxins are lipid soluble, acid stable, and base labile; some are heat stable (22). They probably act by altering sodium conductance at or near sodium channels (372). Animal studies have demonstrated various and diverse biologic effects, including smooth muscle contraction through postganglionic parasympathetic acetylcholine release in dogs, inhibition of neuromuscular transmission in skeletal muscle, central nervous system stimulation with cardiovascular and respiratory impairment in dogs and cats, and norepinephrine release from nerve endings in rats (15, 22, 47, 254, 386). Brevetoxin B has been used as a model for a red tide pigment toxin (406).

Symptoms of neurotoxic shellfish poisoning usually begin within 3 h after ingestion of contaminated shellfish and include circumoral paresthesias which progress to involve the pharynx, trunk, and extremities (205, 385). Reversal of hot and cold temperature sensation, as in ciguatera fish poisoning (406), can occur, as well as cerebellar symptoms such as vertigo, ataxia, and incoordination (21, 205, 385). Gastrointestinal symptoms are common and include nausea, diarrhea, and abdominal and rectal pain. Bradycardia, headache, cramping of the lower extremities, and dilated pupils have been reported (21). Severe cases may be accompanied by convulsions, with subsequent need for respiratory support (385). Paralysis and respiratory failure are not seen. No deaths are known to have been reported (134, 385).

The diagnosis is based on clinical grounds in the appropriate setting. There is no known antidote, and treatment is supportive and symptomatic, including airway management and use of intravenous (i.v.) fluids, atropine, and pressors if required. Symptoms are self-limiting and usually resolve completely without sequelae in a few days (134, 205, 385). One patient in North Carolina required admission to an intensive care unit for severe symptoms of bilateral carpopedal tremor and myalgia, total body paresthesia, ataxia, and vertigo after the ingestion of 45 oysters. Recovery was complete in approximately 9 h (316).

The lack of an armored shell allows for aerosolization of the dinoflagellate during red tides by turbulent surf. This results in a unique syndrome seen along Florida's beaches characterized by respiratory and conjunctival irritation with the development of a nonproductive cough, shortness of breath, lacrimation, rhinorrhea, and sneezing. Asthmatics may develop a wheeze. The syndrome is reversible upon leaving the beach (134, 205). Beta-2 agonists, cholinergic antagonists, and calcium channel blockers may alleviate some of the respiratory symptoms (385).

Amnesic Shellfish Poisoning

In 1987, a previously unrecognized illness occurred among several hundred people who had ingested mussels harvested from cultivation beds located in three river estuaries on the eastern coast of Prince Edward Island, Canada (349, 431). The affected individuals developed an acute illness characterized by severe nausea, gastrointestinal bleeding, and a severe and protracted neurologic disorder which included disorientation, confusion, dizziness, seizures, coma, and a persistent memory loss. Many individuals required prolonged hospitalization, and several deaths were reported. This syndrome, also known as neurovisceral toxic syndrome, was subsequently linked to domoic acid, a toxin produced by the diatom *Nitzschia pungens* f. *multiseries*. A nontoxic form of the species, *N. pungens* f. *pungens,* is a common coastal diatom during the warmer months in the estuaries of Prince Edward Island and Galveston, TX, and is replaced by *N. pungens* f. *multiseries* when fall and winter storms occur (125, 161).

The implicated organism is widely distributed in the coastal waters of the Atlantic, Pacific, and Indian oceans, but not all strains have been shown to produce domoic acid. Gulf Coast oysters were recently shown to contain this toxin, indicating a potential for human poisoning in this area (125). Mussels from the Canadian outbreak were shown to have high concentrations of this toxin in their digestive tracts. During the outbreak, a substantial bloom of *Nitzschia pungens* was noted by marine biologists patrolling the area (418). A possible reason for this is that freshwater runoff from record-breaking storms that year may have stratified the ocean layers of the estuaries, thereby enhancing the nutrients at just the right time in the diatom's life cycle. Similar blooms have been recorded since the initial outbreak, but proper surveillance measures enacted for domoic acid after the initial outbreak have effectively protected the public as well as the shellfish industry. Shellfish can clear the toxin from their tissues once exposed to clean seawater free of the toxic diatom (360).

Domoic acid is a heat-stable neuroexcitatory amine similar to glutamic and kainic acids. It is about 2 to 3 times more potent than kainic acid and 30 to 100 times more potent than glutamic acid. Extracts of seaweed containing this toxin have been used in Japan as an ascaricidal agent for many years, although concentrations are significantly less than those causing illness, and no adverse effects have been documented (349). In rats, domoic acid stimulates kainic acid receptors in the hippocampus and can produce limbic seizures, memory and gait abnormalities, and degeneration of the hippocampus (349). Autopsy reports of victims of the Canadian outbreak revealed neuronal necrosis and astrocytosis in several areas of the brain, particularly the hippocampus and amygdala (431).

At least 107 individuals were involved in the outbreak. Symptoms began 15 min to 38 h (median, 5.5 h) after the ingestion of mussels (349). In approximate order of appearance, they included nausea and vomiting (76% of the patients), abdominal cramps (50%), gastric bleeding, diarrhea (42%), incapacitating headache (43%), dizziness, confusion, loss of short-term memory (25%), weakness, lethargy, somnolence, coma, and seizures. Eighteen percent of patients were hospitalized; death occurred in three (140, 349). The memory loss was anterograde in all but the most severe cases and persisted for at least 2 years in a few individuals. Cognitive functioning remained intact. Cardiovascular instability was also noted, presumably due to the early excitatory effects of domoic acid. Alternating hemiparesis and ophthalmoplegia were noted in two patients (431). Evidence suggests that elderly individuals may be more susceptible to the neurologic effects of domoic acid, possibly due to diminished renal function (349, 477).

Puffer Fish Poisoning

Ingestion of fish in the order Tetraodontoidea, which includes puffer fish (Fig. 1), porcupine fish, and the ocean sunfish, can result in an acute illness referred to as puffer fish poisoning or tetraodotoxication. This syndrome, although rare in the United States, is not all that uncommon in Japan, where 6,386 cases were reported in a 78-year period, with a mortality rate of 59% (405). Also known as *fugu-fugu* in Japan, puffer fish there is considered a delicacy and is specially prepared by trained individuals who require licenses to serve this popular dish, which can cost up to $400 for one meal in

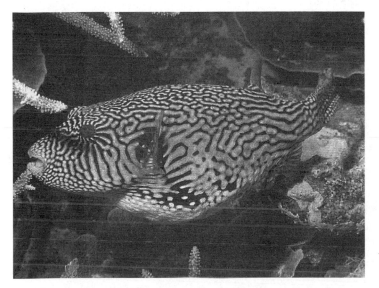

FIGURE 1 The puffer fish is considered a delicacy in Japan and must be prepared by specially trained chefs to avoid fugu poisoning. (Reproduced from *Reef: a Safari through the Coral World* [413a] with permission from the publisher.)

Japan (93). In spite of these precautions, about 50 cases of fugu poisoning occur annually in association with these specialty restaurants (180). Although personal importation of fugu into the United States is illegal, the Food and Drug Administration has permitted fugu to be imported and served in Japanese restaurants in the United States by certified fugu chefs on special occasions (93). Captain James Cook, on his second voyage, ate a piece of puffer fish liver and became acutely ill, requiring 4 days to recover (299). Species of fish in this family are widespread and are found in warm and temperate waters throughout the world; some species are eaten in New Jersey and Long Island (299). In April 1996, three cases of fugu poisoning occurred in three chefs in San Diego who shared prepackaged, ready-to-eat fugu illegally imported from Japan (93).

Tetrodotoxin is a heat-stable nonprotein toxin which is concentrated in the liver, ovaries, and intestine of infected fish. It is not unique to puffer fish and has been isolated from six different classes of animals, including shellfish, salamanders, and a newt found on the campus of Stamford University in Connecticut (150). Certain frogs and newts in Central and South America harbor this toxin, and their skins are used to manufacture poison darts (299).

Tetrodotoxin has its own receptor, located at or near the sodium channel of the external nerve axon cell membrane. Binding at this receptor inhibits nerve impulse propagation along preganglionic cholinergic, somatic motor, sensory, and sympathetic nerves in the central, peripheral, and autonomic nervous systems. Direct effects on the brainstem medulla can induce emesis or hyperemesis and respiratory depression. It is not a curare-like agent and does not act directly on the acetylcholine receptor at the motor endplate. Structurally, it resembles morphine, which may explain some of its narcotic activity. Primary pharmacologic effects include local anesthesia, hypotension, hypothermia, emesis, respiratory depression, and decreased systemic vascular resistance. High levels of toxin can inhibit impulse relay in skeletal or cardiac muscle (405).

Symptoms usually begin within 3 h (usually 10 to 45 min) of ingestion of affected fish. Symptoms include lethargy, weakness, paresthesias (including a numbness of the face and extremities), a floating sensation, emesis or hyperemesis, ataxia, salivation, and dysphagia (134). The extent of symptomatology varies with the amount of toxin ingested (180). Muscular weakness can progress to total paralysis, including respiratory paralysis. Hypotension, bradycardia, and fixed dilated pupils can occur in severe cases (134). Symptoms usually resolve over a period of days; the prognosis is good if the patient survives 18 to 24 h (49). Death occurs in about 60% of patients within the first 24 h (180).

The diagnosis is based on clinical grounds. Treatment consists of airway support and volume expansion with intravascular fluids, such as normal saline and possibly pressors. Attempts should be made to remove unabsorbed toxins through gastric lavage and emesis (405). Some evidence exists that gastric lavage with 2% sodium bicarbonate is effective if used within the first hour of intoxication (487). Atropine is useful in the management of bradycardia. The anticholinesterases edrophonium, physostigmine, neostigmine, and galanthamine, as well as veratrine-like agents and cysteine, may have some benefits, although none of these have been examined in large-scale studies. Apomorphine currently appears to have the best antiemetic properties (405). Other potential treatment options include hyperbaric oxygen, the narcotic antagonist naloxone, and possibly monoclonal neutralizing antibodies (405, 406).

Ciguatera Food Poisoning

Ciguatera is a distinct clinical syndrome that may follow the ingestion of certain tropical reef fishes which have acquired toxicity through the food chain. The name was give by Don Antonio Parra in Cuba in 1787 from the Spanish *cigua,* which refers to the poisonous turban shellfish (family Turbinidae) (175). Sailors with Captain Cook suffered from this malady during his voyages (109). Outbreaks of ciguatera occur in tropical and subtropical regions between the latitudes of 35°N and 35°S (207). Ciguatera is the most commonly reported food-borne illness of marine origin in the United States; overall, it accounted for 5.8% of all food-borne outbreaks from 1972 to 1977 and 7.4% of outbreaks from 1978 to 1982 (391). The CDC has reported that 90% of cases in the United States occur in Florida and Hawaii (205). In Miami alone, there were 43 outbreaks involving 129 cases reported from 1974 to 1976, which probably represented less than 10% of the actual cases due to the inability of the public and medical profession to recognize the illness; the actual incidence was estimated to be 50 cases/100,000 persons/year (262). In 1987, an outbreak occurred in North Carolina, involving 10 persons in what was probably the first case of ciguatera associated with consumption of fish harvested from mainland U.S. coastal waters outside of Florida (315). In 1995, an outbreak of ciguatera occurred in U.S. soldiers serving in Haiti who had eaten locally caught fish (354). A number of cases have been reported in nontropical areas, such as Vermont and Iowa, due to the retail sale of affected fish from Florida (307). In some areas of the world, the disease is so prevalent that only the largest outbreaks are reported. An epidemiologic analysis reported on more than 3,000 cases in the South Pacific (25). On one Pacific atoll, a 43% annual incidence was found during a routine survey of households during one such epidemic (391).

Gambierdiscus toxicus is the primary dinoflagellate responsible for the production of a number of closely related but distinct toxins responsible for the complex symptomatology of ciguatera (315). Other dinoflagellates, including *Prorocentrum lima,* may also be toxigenic (470, 485). These dinoflagellates adhere to dead coral, bottom-associated marine algae, and seaweed (391). Herbivorous fishes ingest the dinoflagellates, and the toxins are subsequently passed up the food chain to larger carnivorous reef fishes that concentrate the toxins in their tissues and result in human poisoning. Toxins are ultimately accumulated in viscera, although muscle tissue may also contain lethal

amounts. Contamination of reef fishes is more likely to occur during storms or other periods of turbulence (391). Larger fish are more likely to be contaminated (158, 185). Fish are unaffected by the toxins (180). More than 400 species of fish have been implicated in ciguatera, including anchovy, barracuda, filefish, herring, jacks, moray eels, oceanic bonito, parrotfish, porgy, seabass or grouper, red snapper, squirrelfish, surgeonfish, triggerfish, trunkfish, and wrasse (180). In Miami, the high incidence of ciguatera due to the ingestion of barracuda has resulted in the ban of the sale of this fish (386).

The toxins recovered from fish implicated in ciguatera include ciguatoxin(s), maitotoxin, lysophosphatidylcholine (maitotoxin-associated hemolysin), scaritoxin(s), palytoxin, and ciguatoxin-associated ATPase inhibitor (247, 406). The toxins are lipid soluble, colorless, odorless, and heat stable; thus, affected fish lack any unusual taste, odor, or appearance, and cooking does not inactivate the toxins (158). Ciguatoxin is a polyether compound that probably acts by competitive inhibition of calcium regulation of the sodium channel (158, 361). For this reason, calcium gluconate has been advocated in the treatment of ciguatera, although this has not been proven (391, 406). The toxin appears to act by opening voltage-dependent sodium channels in all cell membranes, with initial neural stimulation followed by conduction block, primarily in skeletal muscle and neuronal membranes and less so in cardiac muscle. Higher doses can result in phrenic nerve paralysis and respiratory arrest (158). Maitotoxin is cardiotoxic and is also the most potent marine toxin known. Its cardiotoxic effects are due to enhanced calcium influx through the cardiac membrane, with a resultant calcium-overloaded state. These effects are abolished by verapamil in a rat model (246). In ciguatera, maitotoxin can result in hypotension, whereas ciguatoxin has hypertensive effects; the former may be responsible for ciguatera shock, whereas the latter may play a role in the chronic hypertension seen in chronic ciguatera (406). Immune sensitization to polycyclic ethers occurs in ciguatera by a T-cell-dependent mechanism which results in serotonin release via abnormally released immunoglobulin E (IgE). Subsequently, hypotension can ensue in response to certain medications (e.g., paraldehyde), foods, and factors generated by shock (e.g., thromboxane A2). Morphine may form polycyclic ethers on epoxidation or endoperoxidation of the olefin moiety; this may account for the dramatic hypotension seen in some victims of ciguatera when opiates are administered (406).

The symptoms of ciguatera have an ethnic variation which may be due to differences in diet; persons of Philippine or Chinese extraction are more severely affected, Hawaiians are the least affected, and other groups are interposed between (406). Overall, 175 symptoms have been noted (406). The incubation period has been reported to be 2 to 30 h (25, 262, 315). Gastrointestinal symptoms such as watery diarrhea, nausea, vomiting, and abdominal pain tend to predominate early, followed by neurologic symptoms, although great variation exists (315, 385). Virtually all patients experience gastrointestinal symptoms during the course of their illness, which usually resolve in 24 to 48 h (134, 385). Myalgia and weakness, particularly of the lower extremities, may occur at any time. Intense generalized pruritus may occur, and women may even complain of pruritus of the vaginal vault (180). Bradycardia with hypotension occurs in 10 to 15% of cases (406); higher doses of toxin(s) may elicit a biphasic response where bradycardia and hypotension are followed by tachycardia and hypertension (313). Shock and respiratory failure may occur within minutes. Skin lesions and a distinct erythematous desquamative rash have occasionally been reported (134). Fever, lacrimation, severe muscle spasms, and dysuria may also occur (247, 385).

Initial neurologic symptoms usually consist of circumoral and distal paresthesias. Vertigo and ataxia are common and are accompanied by a wide variety of other neurologic manifestations, such as cranial nerve palsies, motor paralysis, blurred vision, and coma (385). Pregnant women may complain of bizarre seizure-like fetal activity (134). Temperature reversal is an unusual characteristic commonly seen in ciguatera and usually occurs in 2 to 5 days (406). Hot objects may seem cold, and cold objects can elicit an electric shock-like sensation. Serious thermal injury has been reported due to the individual's failure to recognize extreme heat as being such (391). In the Bahamas, natives may be seen holding beer cans wrapped in towels to keep their fingers from touching the cold metal (180). Teeth may seem painful or loose. Nightmares are quite common, whereas others may complain of auditory hallucinations and zoopsia (134, 470). All food may taste metallic (180).

Symptoms may wax and wane during any 24-h period and give a "pseudodiurnal periodicity" (158). Alcohol may exacerbate or induce the recurrence of symptoms in up to 28% of recovered patients (158). Other conditions that increase blood flow, such as increased temperature or physical exertion, can also exacerbate symptomatology (262, 315). Whereas gastrointestinal symptoms usually resolve in 24 to 48 h, neurologic, musculoskeletal, and cardiovascular symptoms may persist for months to years (134, 158, 385). Furthermore, recurrence of symptoms may intermittently appear for several months after recovery. The total duration of symptoms is usually several days to months, with neurologic symptoms and pruritus being the slowest to resolve (391). Sensitization is common, and immunity does not occur (134). Some individuals may never eat fish again, as exposure to even minuscule amounts of ciguatera toxins may reproduce dramatic symptoms (180, 391). Malignancy has developed in a few individuals (406). Death is rare and occurs in up to 12% of reported cases; no deaths occurred in 184 cases reported to the CDC in 1970 to 1974 (205).

The diagnosis is based on clinical grounds. Laboratory abnormalities, if present, are usually due to fluid and electrolyte disturbances secondary to gastrointestinal manifestations.

Elevated serum ammonia levels with abnormal prothrombin and partial thromboplastin times may reflect liver toxicity (406). When severe muscle spasms are present, there may be marked elevations of creatinine phosphokinase, serum glutamic oxaloacetic acid, and lactic acid dehydrogenase (247). Reversible T-wave changes on electrocardiograms have been reported (450). The toxins may be detected by a mouse bioassay which is subject to the same limitations as that for detection of saxitoxin and its derivatives in PSP (see above). Radioimmunoassay, often referred to as a "poke" or "stick" test, and chromatography have also been utilized to detect ciguatera toxins, though they are expensive and subject to other limitations as well (247, 391).

Treatment is primarily symptomatic and supportive. Attempts to remove toxin through emesis or gastric lavage with activated charcoal should be made if vomiting has not occurred. A cathartic may be administered to remove toxin from the lower intestinal tract (134, 205). i.v. mannitol provided rapid and dramatic relief in 24 patients with ciguatera in one study, with rapid recovery from shock and coma in 2 patients. The effect of mannitol on the course of ciguatera is unknown but may be due to competitive inhibition of the toxin(s) on the sodium channels or to the neutralization of toxin(s) (344). Atropine may be used to control symptomatic bradycardia (406). Calcium gluconate and dopamine infusions have been effective in the treatment of hypotension (406). Amitriptyline has been used successfully to alleviate paresthesias (50). Pruritus has responded to antihistamines and the avoidance of alcohol, excessive exercise, and high ambient temperatures (391, 406). Myalgia may respond to acetaminophen and indomethacin. Opiates and barbiturates should be avoided, as they may aggravate hypotension (406).

A ciguatera diet has been devised to be used in the treatment of affected patients (406). It consists of a diet high in protein, carbohydrates, and vitamins and the avoidance of fish, shellfish, seeds, nuts, mayonnaise, and their products. In addition, alcohol, marijuana, solvents, herbicides, insecticides, glues, epoxies, ethers, resins, and cosmetics should be avoided as well. These restrictions should be maintained for at least 3 to 6 months after complete resolution of symptoms, and probably for 12 months in the severely affected. Ingestion of fish weighing more than 2.3 kg (5 lb) or fish caught during red tides should be avoided by the general public, as these fish are more likely to contain ciguatera toxins (270).

Scombroid-Fish Poisoning

Scombroid-fish poisoning is an acute clinical syndrome characterized by symptoms of histamine toxicity resulting from the ingestion of spoiled fish (317). It represents the most common form of ichthyosarcotoxism in the world (23). In the United States, 30 to 153 cases of scombroid-fish poisoning were reported annually to the CDC from 1978 to 1982 in a total of 73 outbreaks; this accounted for 7.2% of all food-borne disease outbreaks (82, 134, 391). Among 697 outbreaks of food-borne disease caused by chemical agents from 1973 through 1987, scombroid-fish poisoning was responsible for 29% of the outbreaks and 27% of the cases (206). Half of the 18 outbreaks reported to the CDC in 1982 occurred in fish served in restaurants and cafeterias (391). In March 1998, 24 people on a Hollywood movie set became ill after eating trays of escobar, a trendy seafood that has caught on with many West Coast crowds (108). The escobar was traced to a Florida supplier who had also sent a shipment to a celebrity ski resort in Utah, where several other cases were reported. Tuna burgers were the cause of five outbreaks of scombroid-fish poisoning involving 18 people in North Carolina from July 1998 to February 1999 (32). Most cases in the United States are reported from coastal states and Hawaii, although cases have occurred in the Midwest (134, 391).

The disease is associated with ingestion of fish which belong to the families Scombroidea and Scomberesocidae, which include tuna, mackerel, skipjack, bonito, and albacore.

Nonscombroid fish, such as mahi-mahi, blue-fish, amberjack, herring, sardines, and an-chovies, as well as cheese, have also been implicated (138, 429). Scombroid fish are dis-tributed worldwide throughout temperate and tropical waters and have occasionally been found in polar waters (205).

Histamine has been identified as the toxin responsible for the symptoms of scombroid-fish poisoning (317). The affected fish do not contain high levels of histamine in their flesh at the time of capture; instead, they contain histidine. Histamine is produced during the process of spoilage by the enzymatic decar-boxylation of histidine by certain marine bac-teria, particularly *Morganella morganii, Klebsiella pneumoniae, Escherichia coli,* clostridia, *Achromo-bacter histamineum, Plesiomonas shigelloides, En-terobacter intermedium, Serratia marcescens, Serratia plymuthica, Serratia fonticola,* and *Hafnia alvei,* which are common surface bacteria on fish (138, 266, 278, 324, 429). This occurs opti-mally at temperatures between 20 and 30°C (205). Typically, this takes place when previ-ously refrigerated fish is allowed to warm for a period of time before it is prepared. Hista-mine is heat stable and not destroyed by cook-ing. It is also stable at freezing temperatures. Oral histamine administered in large doses is rapidly metabolized in the liver and intestinal mucosa, and symptoms, if present, are gener-ally mild. For this reason, the presence of an unknown synergistic substance(s) has been proposed to account for the high levels of his-tamine noted in individuals afflicted with scombroid-fish poisoning (138, 317).

Symptoms generally appear within several minutes to several hours of ingestion (median of 30 min), with a median duration of 4 h (205). Symptoms may persist for 12 to 24 h (134). The fish has occasionally been described as being sharp, peppery, or bitter but usually not as being unpleasant (391). Symptoms ini-tially appear as flushing and a hot sensation of the skin, dizziness, headache, a burning sen-sation in the mouth and throat, shortness of breath in the absence of bronchospasm, itch-ing with or without urticaria, and palpitations.

Gastrointestinal symptoms appear as diarrhea, nausea, and rarely vomiting. A sunburn-appearing skin rash with sharply demarcated borders may develop, as well as conjunctival injection. More severe symptoms include dif-ficulty swallowing, respiratory distress with bronchospasm, hypotension, tachycardia, and blurred vision (134, 138, 205, 391). People receiving isoniazid and other inhibitors of en-dogenous histaminase may have more severe symptoms (391). Deaths have occurred but are very rare.

The diagnosis is made on clinical grounds and is usually fairly evident, as the incubation period is relatively short and several people are usually affected at once. Many people are er-roneously diagnosed as having a "fish allergy" and are told to abstain from eating fish for the rest of their lives (134). Laboratory data are usually not helpful. Levels of histamine and its metabolite N-methylhistamine are elevated in urine samples at the time of onset of symptoms and may persist for more than 24 h, although this is not routinely checked (317). Laboratory confirmation of scombroid-fish poisoning is accomplished by measurement of histamine in suspect fish. The concentration may vary from one portion of the fish to another, so several areas must be sampled. The Food and Drug Administration has established the maximum safe level of histamine in tuna to be 450 μmol per 100 g of fresh tuna; fresh tuna contains levels of <9 μmol per 100 g (138, 317). In one recent outbreak in Tennessee, marlin was the implicated fish and contained levels of his-tamine of >2,500 μmol per 100 g (317).

Treatment is supportive and symptomatic. If the gastrointestinal symptoms are not severe, gastric lavage or catharsis may be employed to remove unabsorbed histamine (39). Depend-ing on the severity of symptoms, management can best be accomplished by the use of any one or a combination of agents such as epi-nephrine, oxygen, diphenhydramine, hydrox-yzine, and corticosteroids (406). Aminophyl-line may be used for the rare case of severe respiratory distress due to bronchospasm (134). i.v. cimetidine has been reported to provide rapid and complete resolution of symptoms in severe cases that did not respond to antihistamines (39). Caution must be exercised in the simultaneous use of H1 and H2 blockers to avoid hypotension (406).

Diarrheic Shellfish Poisoning

Diarrheic shellfish poisoning has not been reported in the United States to date but has been implicated in a number of short-lived outbreaks of acute onset of diarrhea following shellfish ingestion in other parts of the world, particularly Japan and The Netherlands. It is caused by the ingestion of okadaic acid and other toxins concentrated in shellfish that feed on the dinoflagellates that produce the toxins. Okadaic acid does not directly stimulate intestinal secretion but instead causes a significant increase in paracellular permeability (442). During the period of 1976 to 1982, more than 1,300 cases were diagnosed in Japan, while sporadic cases occurred in The Netherlands and Chile (472). In 1989, 150 people on the Adriatic coast of Italy were afflicted by this illness after the ingestion of contaminated mussels. This was the first case of diarrheic mussel poisoning observed in the Mediterranean area (44). Okadaic acid has been detected in Gulf of Mexico shellfish and phytoplankton (125).

Dinophysis fortii is the responsible toxin-producing dinoflagellate in Japan, whereas *Dinophysis acuminata* produces the toxin in outbreaks occurring in The Netherlands (177, 235). Mussels, clams, and scallops are the implicated shellfish causing human outbreaks (44). Outbreaks are associated with dinoflagellate blooms (235).

Symptoms usually begin about 5 to 6 h after shellfish ingestion, with a range of 30 min to 12 h (44, 235). Although usually mild, the severity of the illness is dependent on the amount of toxin ingested (235). The symptoms consist of diarrhea, abdominal cramps, nausea, and vomiting. No fatalities have been reported, and recovery generally occurs within 2 days. Treatment is supportive, as the symptoms are self-limited (61, 235).

PFIESTERIA PISCICIDA

Pfiesteria piscicida is an estuarine dinoflagellate first described in 1991 (160). This usually nontoxic organism feeds on aquatic organic material but can produce toxins that can kill fish. The toxin can induce the formation of open ulcerative lesions, hemorrhaging, and death of fish and shellfish. Beginning in autumn 1996, fish with "punched-out" skin lesions and erratic behavior caused by exposure to toxins produced by *P. piscicida* or *Pfiesteria*-like species were seen in the Pocomoke River and adjacent waterways on the eastern shore of Maryland. In August 1997, similar fish kills were again reported (166). That same month, 24 sportsmen, environmental workers, and commercial fishermen who had contact with the water reported illness (166). The human illness, known as "possible estuary-associated syndrome," has been a topic of much debate due to the lack of specific testing and possible implication of unrelated factors (92). Possible estuary-associated syndrome is not an infectious disease, and there have been no cases associated with eating fish or shellfish harvested from waters where *P. piscicida* has been found. Thirty-seven cases were reported to the CDC prior to 1998, and very few have been reported since then (370). The reason for the drop-off in cases since 1998 is likely due to the paucity of "fish events" due to *P. piscicida* since 1 June 1998 (92).

Symptoms were more likely to occur in those with the most exposure to the contaminated water. These included neuropsychiatric symptoms (including new or increased forgetfulness), severe respiratory distress (including asthma), headache, narcosis, severe stomach cramping, nausea with vomiting, and eye irritation with reddening and blurred vision (108, 160, 166). Neuropsychiatric symptoms tended to last the longest and completely resolved by 6 months, usually by 10 to 12 weeks.

The cause of *Pfiesteria* suddenly becoming toxic is unknown, but it has been linked to coastal chicken and hog farmers in Maryland and North Carolina (108).

THE VIBRIOS

Introduction

Prior to the 1960s, studies of vibrios as pathogens of human disease focused primarily on *Vibrio cholerae*, the etiologic agent of cholera. Pacini originally described a vibrio-like organism as the etiologic agent of Asiatic cholera in 1854 (217). The organism was not isolated until 32 years later by Koch, who called the bacillus *"Kommabacillus,"* referring to its curved shape. *V. cholerae* was the only currently recognized vibrio known to cause human disease until 1951, when Fujino described a bacterium resembling *V. cholerae* which was responsible for an epidemic of acute gastroenteritis in Japan involving 272 people, with 20 deaths. He named this organism *Pasteurella parahaemolyticus*, which was placed in the genus *Vibrio* in 1963. Two distinct biotypes were recognized at that time and were subsequently found to be separate species. In 1968, biotype 1 became known as *Vibrio parahaemolyticus*, whereas biotype 2 became known as *Vibrio alginolyticus* (226). Since then, 34 species of *Vibrio*, of which 13 are known to be pathogenic to humans (Table 2), have been recognized. Furthermore, several unnamed species were recently identified, so the list is likely to grow (217).

Pathogenic members of the genus *Vibrio* are gram-negative, curved, rod-shaped facultative anaerobes which are capable of both fermentative and respiratory metabolism. They are motile organisms which measure 1.5 to 3.0 μm in length and 0.5 to 0.8 μm in width. They contain a single sheathed polar flagellum in liquid medium and occasionally may display shorter lateral flagella on solid media. They are anaerogenic (with the exception of *Vibrio furnissii* and some strains of *Vibrio damsela*) and oxidase positive (except for *Vibrio metschnikovii*) and have the ability to reduce nitrate to nitrite. Most are susceptible to the vibriostatic effects of the compound O/129 (30).

The pathogenic vibrios can be divided into two groups based on the ability to grow in a saline environment (188). Nonhalophilic vibrios can grow in the presence or absence of sodium chloride and include *V. cholerae*, non-O1 *V. cholerae*, and *Vibrio mimicus*. Halophilic vibrios, on the other hand, require sodium chloride to support growth and survival and reach very high concentrations in waters of 5 to 8% salinity (217).

TABLE 2 Clinical presentations of pathogenic *Vibrio* infections in humans[a]

Pathogen	Symptom			
	Diarrhea (watery/dysentery)	Wound	Otitis	Sepsis
Nonhalophilic				
V. cholerae O1	+	±		
V. cholerae non-O1[b]	+/+	+	+	±
V. mimicus[b]	+/+		+	
Halophilic				
V. parahaemolyticus	+/+	+	±	±
V. hollisae (EF13)[b]	+/±			±
V. fluvialis (EF6)	+/+			
V. furnissii	+			
V. alginolyticus		+	+	
V. vulnificus (L+)[b]	±			++
V. damselae (EF5)		+		
V. metschnikovii (gp16)		+		±

[a]Single cases of *V. cincinnatiensis* and *V. carchariae* infection have been reported, with sepsis and shark bite would infections, respectively.
[b]Especially associated with oyster consumption.

Isolated vibrios can occasionally be confused with other bacteria of medical importance, such as *Enterobacteriaceae, Pseudomonas, Aeromonas,* and *Plesiomonas.* The *Enterobacteriaceae* are straight rather than curved and are oxidase negative, with peritrichous or circumferential flagella. *Pseudomonas* species, although oxidase positive, have an oxidative rather than fermentative metabolism. Species of *Aeromonas* and *Plesiomonas* do not require sodium chloride for growth and are able to grow in the presence of the vibriostatic compound O/129 (437).

Most standard laboratory media used for biochemical testing contain 0.5% sodium chloride and therefore support the growth of both halophilic and nonhalophilic vibrios. Isolation is usually accomplished through the use of selective or enrichment media. Alkaline peptone broth is the most suitable general enrichment medium for all pathogenic *Vibrio* species (141). A modified two-step method has been utilized successfully to prevent bacterial overgrowth by other bacteria in the peptone broth (369). Thiosulfate-citrate-bile salts-sucrose (TCBS) agar is the most widely used selective agar medium for isolation of pathogenic *Vibrio* species, but several newly described pathogens may fail to grow on this agar medium (186). Furthermore, individual variations in commercially available TCBS agars may affect recovery of the organisms (464).

Vibrios are aquatic organisms that can be found in a wide variety of environmental water sources, such as oceans, estuaries, lakes, and ponds. The highest concentrations are generally achieved in the marine waters along the East and Gulf Coasts, primarily in the summer months; lower concentrations exist along the West Coast. Their numbers fluctuate widely, with marked variation due to such variables as temperature, salinity, sediments, and the presence of certain marine organisms, particularly the copepods and other plankton, in which vibrios may play a role in salt retention by these species (107).

Water temperature appears to be the single most important variable affecting the growth and survival of vibrios. Pathogenic vibrios are usually isolated from waters where temperatures exceed 10°C for at least several consecutive weeks (41, 407). They are less frequently found in waters where temperatures exceed 30°C (401, 468). Variation occurs worldwide and among different species; for example, *V. cholerae* prefers temperatures between 20 and 35°C (217).

Individual *Vibrio* species have different optimal sodium chloride requirements, with a range of 5 to 30%, which accounts for the primary isolation of these organisms from marine and estuarine waters (41, 401, 439, 464). Although *V. cholerae,* non-O1 *V. cholerae,* and *V. mimicus* do not require sodium chloride for growth, they achieve larger numbers in its presence. *V. cholerae* has an optimal requirement of 2 to 20% salinity, whereas halophilic vibrios usually achieve optimal concentrations in sodium chloride concentrations of 5 to 8% (217). Pathogenic vibrios may be isolated from freshwater, where salinity is less than 5%, probably due to a complex interaction between high water temperatures and increased organic content which may compensate for the detrimental effects of low to absent salinity (298, 392, 407, 408). Evaporation of fresh and brackish waters during summer months may increase the sodium chloride content (369).

As temperatures drop below 10°C, the pathogenic vibrios rapidly disappear from the water but can persist throughout the winter in the sediment. This has been shown for *V. parahaemolyticus, V. cholerae,* and *V. alginolyticus* and may well hold true for all pathogenic vibrios (228, 229, 464, 468). As water temperatures increase during the spring and summer months, the organisms can then reemerge once again to reach high concentrations, accounting for as much as 26 to 40% of the total bacterial population in some areas (340).

By associating themselves with higher organisms such as shellfish, plankton, and fish, the vibrios may maintain large numbers and prolong their existence. Adsorption onto the chitinous component of plankton has been shown to significantly prolong the survival of some pathogenic vibrios, and it is possible that this represents a major means of prolonging survival for all pathogenic species (209, 210, 228, 234, 340, 392). Bivalve molluscan shellfish which filter feed on zooplankton may themselves become rapidly contaminated during periods of high bacterial counts. Improper storage of the shellfish may then allow proliferation of the pathogenic bacteria, with resultant outbreaks of food poisoning (121, 139, 233, 389). Crustacean shellfish and fish can also become contaminated during such periods of abundant vibrio growth (34, 209, 345, 392). *Vibrio* species have also been cultured from the teeth, skin, and gum lines of sharks (20, 63).

The spectrum of human disease due to the pathogenic vibrios is dependent mainly on the causative species and ranges from mild self-limiting gastroenteritis and soft tissue infections to severe necrotizing wound infections and fulminant bacteremia, primarily in patients with underlying diseases. Illness can result from a variety of means, such as ingestion of contaminated shellfish or exposure of open wounds to contaminated seawater. Raw oyster eaters, particularly those with liver disease, have been shown be at risk of developing vibrio illness (123). An increase in the incidence of vibrio-related illness is occurring due to a variety of reasons, including increased awareness by the public and the medical profession of *Vibrio* infections, improved biochemical and serologic means for the detection of vibrios, increased recreational exposure to coastal regions, increased foreign travel, increased seafood ingestion, and enhanced survival in immunocompromised individuals (123, 217).

Vibrio species have been isolated from virtually every geographic region within the United States, although most cases occur along coastal areas. Of 713 isolates obtained from various human anatomical sites and reported to the CDC, 75% belonged to one of three species, namely, *V. cholerae, V. parahaemolyticus,* and *Vibrio vulnificus,* with gastrointestinal symptoms predominating (141). Between 1974 and 1978 in a Chesapeake Bay community, 40 *Vibrio* isolates were recovered from 32 patients, with *V. parahaemolyticus, V. vulnificus,* and non-O1 *V. cholerae* accounting for 33 of the total isolates. Illnesses were mild and self-limiting, and no mortalities were reported (192). Over a 10-year period in a Gulf Coast community, 23 cases of *Vibrio* infections were reported, with *V. vulnificus, V. parahaemolyticus,* and non-O1 *V. cholerae* accounting for all but 2 cases, including gastroenteritis in 3 patients, wound infection in 14 patients, and bacteremia in 12 patients (45). The CDC estimates that 8,028 *Vibrio* infections and 57 *Vibrio*-related deaths occur annually in the United States (292).

V. cholerae

Seven cholera pandemics have been recorded since 1817, six of which began before the 20th century (378). The current, seventh one began in Sulawesi, Indonesia, in 1961 and then spread to Asia, Africa, the Middle East, Oceania, and parts of Europe, while sparing the Western Hemisphere (36, 475). No cases of domestically acquired cholera were reported in the United States after 1911 until 1973, when it was diagnosed in a resident of the Gulf Coast of Texas (460). In 1978, 11 people were involved in an outbreak of cholera following the ingestion of crabs gathered from a Louisiana coastal marsh (36), and in 1981, 16 oil workers were involved in a cholera outbreak on a Texas oil rig after eating rice cooked in water which had been contaminated by canal water containing sewage discharged from the rig (222). These and other similar cases account for a total of more than 65 cases of domestically acquired cholera reported to the CDC, most of which have been isolated incidents (420). Almost all of these cases were reported for the Gulf of Mexico region, but there has been at least one such case acquired from the Chesapeake Bay (272). All of the Gulf Coast isolates were of the El Tor biotype, serotype Inaba, which strongly suggests that this organism is endemic along the Gulf Coast. Since then, *V. cholerae* sero-group O1, including toxin-producing strains, has been isolated from U.S. coastal waters of the Gulf of Mexico and Chesapeake Bay throughout the year (106, 230). Numbers tend to be highest in the warmer summer months, and the vibrios are frequently associated with plankton and shellfish. Toxigenic and nontoxigenic strains of *V. cholerae* O1 have been cultured from shellfish harvested from U.S. commercial waters (62, 199, 374, 448). Pollution does not appear to be a necessary factor, as the organism can be found in waters with no evidence of human waste (374). Case-controlled studies of localized outbreaks of *V. cholerae* O1 in the United States have shown that the recent ingestion of raw or partially cooked seafood or contact with contaminated water is a significant risk factor (36, 222, 473). Contaminated imported food can be a source of localized outbreaks in the United States. In 1994, a cluster of cases occurred in Indiana and was traced to food imported from El Salvador (86).

In January 1991, toxin-producing strains of *V. cholerae* O1, biotype El Tor, serotype Inaba, appeared in several cities in Peru, which marked the first time in the 20th century that cholera was reported in South America (77, 85). As of January 1992, over 300,000 cases of cholera were reported in 14 countries in North and South America, with almost 4,000 deaths. U.S. citizens accounted for 17 of these cases, including 6 associated with travel to South America and 11 associated with the ingestion of crabs imported illegally from Ecuador. Between 1 January and 29 February 1992, 42 cases were identified in the United States among travelers to and from South America; 40 of these cases, including one death, were reported among passengers on the same airline flight from South America to the United States (420).

Over 70 different serotypes of *V. cholerae* exist, based on the somatic "O" antigen (463). These strains are phenotypically indistinguishable and share a common flagellar "H" antigen. *V. cholerae* serotype O1 is the strain as-

sociated with cholera. All others are referred to as noncholera vibrios, non-O1 *V. cholerae*, or nonagglutinable vibrios (NAG) due to their inability to agglutinate in O1 antiserum. Most strains of *V. cholerae* O1 produce an enterotoxin (cholera toxin) which is responsible for the severe fluid losses seen in cholera. Non-O1 *V. cholerae* strains do not produce cholera toxin but may produce toxins capable of eliciting an illness identical to cholera (312, 338, 482). *V. cholerae* can be divided into two biovars, classical and El Tor. Classical strains tend to be more virulent than the El Tor biotypes. El Tor strains were originally detected by their ability to lyse sheep erythrocytes, but this trait has not been shown to be consistent. They agglutinate chicken erythrocytes, are not sensitive to polymyxin B, and are Voges-Proskauer positive. Classical strains fail to lyse sheep erythrocytes or agglutinate chicken erythrocytes, are Voges-Proskauer negative, and are sensitive to polymyxin B. Biotypes may also be distinguished by phage susceptibility, a tool used mainly for epidemiologic purposes. Additionally, both biotypes can be classified further into one of three serotypes, i.e., Inaba, Ogawa, or Hikojima (437). The El Tor biotype initially appeared in regions in the Ganges Delta where cholera is endemic in 1969 and quickly became the dominant biotype for most of the world (29). The more severe classical strain reappeared in Bangladesh in 1982 and has become the dominant strain in that region (390). At the time of this writing, all biotypes in the Western Hemisphere have been of the El Tor biotype. The reasons for the persistence of El Tor strains include their greater ability to survive in the environment and a larger ratio of symptomatic cases to asymptomatic carriers (1:30 to 1:100 for El Tor and 1:2 to 1:4 for classical biotypes) (169).

Under adverse environmental conditions, *V. cholerae* O1 can enter a state of dormancy in which the organism remains viable and potentially pathogenic yet fails to grow on conventional culture medium. The presence of the organism under such conditions has been demonstrated clearly by fluorescence and immunologic techniques in the absence of a positive culture. It has been proposed that in this way, *V. cholerae* O1 may persist indefinitely and go undetected in waters such as those of the Gulf Coast, only to emerge periodically under more favorable conditions to cause disease. This may also explain the periods between epidemics in areas where cholera is endemic. This phenomenon has been referred to as "viable but nonculturable" (463).

In the United States, cases of cholera have usually occurred in the summer or fall months following the ingestion of raw or undercooked shellfish (194). Once in the intestinal tract, the organism may become adherent to the intestinal cell wall by means of a specialized pilus, where it may grow and produce enterotoxin (184, 195). Factors diminishing transit time, such as the ingestion of solid foods rather than liquids, may increase the chances of colonization and development of cholera (269). Furthermore, because the organism is less likely to survive in an acidic environment, the use of antacids or previous gastrectomy may increase one's chances of developing disease (396). Adherence of the organism to chitin particles in shellfish may also enhance survival in acidic environments (473). For some reason, persons with blood type O have been noted to be at a higher risk of cholera (409).

Cholera toxin is a heat-labile protein produced by most strains of *V. cholerae* O1. The molecule is composed of five B subunits arranged in a circle around an A1 and an A2 subunit. The B subunits are responsible for binding of the toxin to the receptor, ganglioside GM1, on cell membranes. The A1 subunit, bound to the complex by the A2 subunit, stimulates adenylate cyclase activity, causing increased levels of cyclic AMP and hypersecretion of chloride, with the result of massive losses of salt and water (146). Cholera victims may lose over 1 liter of fluid per h and up to 100% of their body weight in 4 to 7 days of diarrhea as a result of the toxin (130, 189). Cholera toxin is not the only factor capable of causing the severe diarrhea in cholera victims; an identical illness has been noted in

individuals infected with nontoxigenic variants of *V. cholerae* O1 (309, 314). Factors other than cholera toxin which have been proposed to play a role in producing illness include a heat-stable toxin similar to a toxin produced by *V. parahaemolyticus* (197), lecithinase (285), phospholipase (96), and prostaglandin E (351). *Escherichia coli* may produce a plasmid-mediated toxin that is very similar in structure and mode of action to cholera toxin (146).

The incubation period for cholera varies from 6 h to 5 days. The average is 2 days in areas of endemicity (62). Initial symptoms may include anorexia, abdominal cramping, and mild diarrhea. Vomiting without nausea typically begins within hours of the onset of diarrhea. Fever is usually absent or low-grade. Stools are initially brown in color and loose, but within hours they become watery and pale gray in appearance and lose all odor except for perhaps a "fishy" smell. Scattered flecks of mucus give the stools a "rice water" appearance. A feeling of relief, rather than tenesmus, accompanies each bowel movement. Peak stool losses occur at around 24 h of illness. Shock may occur within 12 h in untreated cases, with death ensuing in 18 h to 5 days. Gallbladder disease has been reported, including one case of acute cholecystitis in Alabama in which *V. cholerae* O1 was isolated from the gallbladder and bile. Serum vibriocidal antibodies were present as well (473). Chronic, asymptomatic gallbladder carriage has also been documented, especially for areas of the world where cholera is endemic and where the risk of exposure is great (164, 457). Extraintestinal infections are rare, but occasionally nontoxigenic strains may be isolated from wound infections (223, 473).

Cholera is fatal in fewer than 1% of properly recognized and treated cases, although the mortality rate can be as high as 50% if patients are left untreated (62, 309, 473). The mainstay of therapy consists of rapid and effective fluid and electrolyte replacement. Oral rehydration is effective for most patients who are able to tolerate this mode of therapy. Currently, oral rehydration salt packets are available, as well as a variety of other premixed rehydration solutions which have been shown to be effective in the treatment of cholera. In the event that vomiting is severe enough or the patient is too obtunded to tolerate enteral hydration, i.v. infusion of lactated Ringer's solution has been effective in initial rehydration, with oral therapy being initiated as soon as the patient is able to tolerate it. Normal saline is less effective because it lacks bicarbonate and potassium. The amount of fluids administered should be determined on the basis of dehydration at presentation as well as the rate of ongoing losses (420).

Antibiotics may decrease the duration of illness, the period of *Vibrio* excretion, and the amount of fluids needed for rehydration (309). Ciprofloxacin is the drug of choice in the treatment of cholera (156). It is given as a single dose of 1.0 g. Doxycycline may also be administered as a single dose of 300 mg. Trimethoprim-sulfamethoxazole is recommended for children and pregnant women. It should be noted that fluid rehydration is still considered the mainstay of therapy. Antispasmodics, antidiarrheal agents, and corticosteroids are not indicated in the treatment of cholera (420). Although a parenteral vaccine is currently available within the United States, it is not likely to be of benefit because of the low risk of infection in international travelers and the small number of cases acquired to date in the United States (74).

Non-O1 *V. cholerae*

Strains of *V. cholerae* that do not agglutinate in O1 antiserum, or non-O1 *V. cholerae* strains, are common inhabitants of both sewage-contaminated and sewage-free waters of bays, estuaries, brackish inland lakes, and seafood. Besides being environmental contaminants, the organisms have been isolated from domestic animals, waterfowl, and a variety of wildlife (121). Non-O1 species have even been implicated in enteric infections of horses, lambs, and bison in western Colorado (368). Most disease-associated isolates have been obtained from the coastal waters of Florida, the Gulf of Mexico, and the Chesapeake Bay, although isolates may be found all along the East Coast (384). Fewer isolates are noted along the West Coast, possibly due to colder water temperatures. Infections due to non-O1 strains have also been acquired from freshwater lakes distant from the sea (110, 320). Infections are more common during the warmer months of summer and fall.

The first reported case of human disease due to a non-O1 strain of *V. cholerae* acquired in the United States occurred in 1972 in Louisiana in an individual who developed profuse and prolonged diarrhea following the ingestion of raw oysters (120). Since then, this organism has increasingly been recognized as a cause of human illness in this country, usually occurring as cases of sporadic illness (194). In a Chesapeake Bay hospital over a 15-year period, 40 *Vibrio* isolates were obtained, of which 10 were strains of non-O1 *V. cholerae* (192). Similarly, in a Gulf Coast community over a 10-year period, 4 of 23 *Vibrio* isolates were non-O1 *V. cholerae* (45). Although diarrheal illness is the most common manifestation of disease due to non-O1 *V. cholerae* strains, 10% of cases are wound infections and an additional 10% are ear infections (309). Septicemia, meningitis, and acalculous cholecystitis have been reported (101, 240, 461). Unlike the strains which cause cholera, non-O1 species are rarely linked to epidemic disease (312). Isolated outbreaks of illness have usually occurred in association with a common contaminated food source. Three previous outbreaks of diarrheal illness linked to non-O1 *V. cholerae* in the Czech Republic, Sudan, and Australia were linked to food sources in two cases (potatoes and an asparagus salad) and polluted well water in the other (3, 114, 474). In 1992, an epidemic of cholera-like illness occurred in Madras, India, associated with an atypical strain of *V. cholerae* which was subsequently designated *V. cholerae* O139 (363). Infection with the strain has been described as identical to cholera, and imported cases have been described in the United States (88).

More than half of non-O1 *V. cholerae* isolates received by the CDC are from stool samples (309). Gastroenteritis is the most common

#14

manifestation of illness in the United States and is almost always due to the ingestion of raw oysters (123, 312, 384, 469). In the United States, the incubation period has generally been less than 48 h, but it was as long as 4 days in at least one foreign outbreak (473). The following symptoms were noted in one review of U.S. cases: diarrhea (100%), abdominal cramps (93%), fever (71%), and nausea and vomiting (21%) (312). Another review reported nausea and vomiting occurring more frequently (77% and 69%, respectively) (204). The diarrhea can be severe, with up to 30 watery stools per day, and up to 25% of patients have bloody diarrhea (309). In some cases, fluid losses may equal those seen for cholera (38). Illness generally lasted an average of 6.4 days in the cases reported in the United States (range, 2 to 12 days) but lasted less than 2 days in some overseas outbreaks (3, 114, 312).

Non-O1 strains of *V. cholerae* exert their pathogenic effects through a variety of extracellular toxins and hemolysins. Enterotoxins identical or nearly identical to cholera toxin have been detected (482). Although rare in the United States (312), up to 40% of isolates in India and Bangladesh may produce these toxins (38, 117). In fact, the severity of diarrheal illness seems to correlate with production of these toxins (117, 217). The lack of a cholera-like toxin in U.S. isolates indicates that other mechanisms are involved in their pathogenicity. Other factors which may be produced include enterotoxins other than the cholera-like toxins, including an enterotoxin that is also produced by *V. mimicus* and *Vibrio fluvialis* (13, 309, 333, 334), several hemolysins (481), including a hemolysin similar to the Kanagawa hemolysin produced by *V. parahaemolyticus* (196), and a Shiga-like toxin which may be responsible for the occasional bloody diarrhea (337).

Septicemia due to non-O1 strains of *V. cholerae* is a less frequent complication of infection. From 1977 through 1979, there were 70 isolates of *V. cholerae* reported to the CDC, 12 of which were obtained from the blood

(384). The case fatality rate for septicemia has been estimated at 61.5% based on previously reported cases in the United States (384). Predisposing factors include alcohol abuse, previous gastric surgery, advanced age, and chronic underlying conditions, such as hematologic malignancy, liver disease, immune deficiency, diabetes mellitus, peripheral vascular disease, and achlorhydria (123, 124, 217, 243, 309, 384). The source of the vibrio in many cases is raw oyster ingestion (123). In addition to septicemia and gastroenteritis, non-O1 *V. cholerae* has also been implicated in cases of wound infections (217, 309, 384), otitis media and otitis externa (147, 309, 434), prostatic abscess (384), cholecystitis (350), pneumonia (243), and meningitis (143, 240, 306), including one case of neonatal meningitis in an infant who drank milk from a bottle stored near live crabs (380). Extraintestinal infections are usually the result of contact with seawater (309).

Most cases of non-O1 *V. cholerae* infection are relatively mild cases of gastroenteritis which are usually self-limiting in nature; only a minority require hospitalization (3, 312). Treatment should consist of supportive care, with i.v. hydration in severe cases of gastroenteritis (188). Septicemic cases and severe localized infections such as meningitis should be treated with i.v. antibiotics. In cases of gastroenteritis, antibiotics may decrease the severity of illness and shorten its duration (188). Non-O1 *V. cholerae* strains are susceptible in vitro to a wide range of antibiotics, including tetracycline, trimethoprim-sulfamethoxazole, chloramphenicol, and nalidixic acid (311). Susceptibilities to ampicillin and gentamicin are variable (311).

V. parahaemolyticus

V. parahaemolyticus has a worldwide distribution in both tropical and temperate inshore coastal and estuarine waters. Isolates have been obtained from water, sediment, suspended particulates, plankton, fish, and shellfish in a marine environment (309). Although it is halophilic, the organism can occasionally be isolated from freshwater areas, possibly through association with the chitin of plankton and shellfish or sediments, which may allow it to survive in areas of lower salinity (226). Most cases of illness occur in summer, when warmer water temperatures favor growth of the organism. During winter, the organism can be isolated from sediment (463). *V. parahaemolyticus* has been isolated from nearly every coastal state in the United States and is frequently found in Canadian waters as well (226). Outbreaks of diarrheal illness are the most common form of disease caused by this organism, and disease usually follows the ingestion of raw or improperly cooked seafood, particularly crabs, shrimp, lobsters, and raw oysters. Most U.S. outbreaks have been caused by gross mishandling of seafood, such as improper refrigeration, insufficient cooking, cross-contamination, and recontamination (374). Incubation of the organism in seafood can reduce the generation time to as short as 12 min (149). Previously thought to be a rare strain of *V. parahaemolyticus* and not described in the United States until 1982 (259, 336), a urease-positive strain of *V. parahaemolyticus* representing a new serovar has been established as the predominant cause of *V. parahaemolyticus*-associated gastroenteritis on the West Coast of the United States and Mexico (1, 239).

In Japan, over 70% of food-borne diarrheal illness is caused by *V. parahaemolyticus* (374). First described as a pathogen in the United States in 1971 following the ingestion of improperly cooked crabs in Maryland (304), the organism has increasingly been recognized as a cause of sporadic cases of diarrheal illness, usually in association with food-borne outbreaks (38). During the years 1973 to 1998, 40 outbreaks of *V. parahaemolyticus* disease were reported to the CDC, with most cases occurring in the warmer months (116). In a Chesapeake Bay hospital over a 15-year period, *V. parahaemolyticus* was the most common *Vibrio* species identified and accounted for 16 of 40 isolates obtained from 32 patients (192). During an outbreak of *Vibrio* gastro-

enteritis among attendees at a scientific congress in New Orleans, *V. parahaemolyticus* accounted for 35 of the 51 stool specimens yielding a *Vibrio* species (282). In 1997, the largest reported outbreak of confirmed *V. parahaemolyticus* infections occurred in North America (89). A total of 209 cases were identified, with one fatality. The outbreak was associated with raw oysters harvested from California, Oregon, Washington, and British Columbia. Extraintestinal manifestations may also occur, sometimes including fatal septicemia.

The incubation period has ranged from 4 to 96 h (28). In a review of eight *V. parahaemolyticus* outbreaks in the United States (28), the clinical manifestations included diarrhea (98%), abdominal cramps (82%), nausea (71%), vomiting (52%), headache (42%), fever (27%), and chills (24%). The illness was self-limited in most cases, with a median duration of 3 days. Fever rarely exceeds 38.9°C. Abdominal pain can be severe (149). The diarrhea is acute in onset and usually watery and mild, although it can rarely be severe enough to cause dehydration, hypotension, and acidosis (287, 297). A dysentery-like illness with fecal leukocytes, superficial ulcerations of the colonic mucosa, and blood and mucus in the stool has been described in India and Bangladesh (38, 43, 159). This form of disease has rarely been encountered in the United States (43, 309). The incubation period for dysentery-like disease is shorter (as short as 2.5 h), although the duration of illness approximates that of the more common form of illness (473).

The ability to cause human disease has been associated with a heat-stable enterotoxin capable of lysing erythrocytes on Wagatsuma agar (226). Strains producing this thermostable direct hemolysin (TDH) are known as "Kanagawa positive," named after the prefecture in Japan where it was first studied (198, 309). The observation that over 95% of clinical isolates and <1% of environmental isolates are Kanagawa positive has suggested that TDH is the toxin associated with pathogenicity (226, 309). In several studies involving animal mod

15

els, purified TDH was able to produce clinical and histopathologic effects similar to those seen in disease due to *V. parahaemolyticus* (303, 335, 491). In one report from the Pacific Northwest, only 6 of 13 clinical isolates from patients with diarrhea or wound infections due to *V. parahaemolyticus* were Kanagawa positive (239). The ability of Kanagawa-negative strains lacking TDH to produce diarrheal illness has led to the discovery of other enterotoxins (190, 437). In addition to several hemolysins with unclarified or potential roles in pathogenicity, including a Shiga-like toxin (190, 226), a TDH-related hemolysin has been suggested to be an important virulence factor in TDH-negative clinical isolates (403). The presence of specific intestinal adherence factors may contribute to the pathogenicity of some strains (172).

In rare instances, *V. parahaemolyticus* can result in extraintestinal infections. A history of trauma or insult to the infected anatomical site can be elicited in the majority of cases (217). Wound infections or cellulitis can develop as a primary focus of infection or can result from secondary hematogenous seeding (271). Although less common than stool isolates, wound isolates can constitute a significant number of *V. parahaemolyticus* isolates. Five of 16 *V. parahaemolyticus* isolates collected over a 15-year period in the Chesapeake Bay region were acquired from wounds (192). Vascular thrombosis and gangrene have been reported (257). In some instances, *V. parahaemolyticus* and another *Vibrio* species may be isolated concurrently (353). Ocular (416, 422) and ear (192, 309) infections can occur, as well as pneumonia (490) and osteomyelitis (376).

Most cases of *V. parahaemolyticus* gastroenteritis are self-limited and resolve in a matter of days. Rarely are cases severe enough to require vigorous fluid support. Mortality is unusual and has been estimated to be 0.04% in Japan (38). From 1981 to 1988, there were four fatalities due to *V. parahaemolyticus* in Florida. All patients were bacteremic and had either cirrhosis or an underlying malignancy (243). In view of the fact that most cases of

infection due to *V. parahaemolyticus* are cases of gastroenteritis, methods to avoid such illness include the proper handling of seafood. Heating at 60°C for 15 min kills *V. parahaemolyticus*. In addition, storage at temperatures at or below 4°C inhibits growth of the organism (447). Persons susceptible to septicemia, such as those with liver disease or any other immunosuppressive condition, should probably avoid raw seafood ingestion (123, 192).

V. vulnificus

Beginning in 1964, the CDC began receiving extraintestinal isolates that were thought to be variants of *V. parahaemolyticus* but were shown to be different by means of a variety of biochemical tests, including the ability to ferment lactose (38). After this organism was referred to initially as the "halophilic lactose-positive marine vibrio," the name *Beneckea vulnifica* was proposed, although not widely accepted (366, 437). The virulence of this particular species was first recognized in 1976 by a review of clinical isolates reported to the CDC which revealed that 53% of the isolates were recovered from blood (193). The name *Vibrio vulnificus* was formally recognized in 1979 (142). This organism has been found in seawater, sediments, zooplankton, and shellfish (188). In two separate studies, over 50% of oysters sampled during selected months (425) and 11% of crabs harvested during summer months (119) yielded *V. vulnificus*. Water temperature seems to be an important factor; organisms are rarely isolated from waters with temperatures lower than 17°C (194). Almost all cases of infection have been reported between the months of May and October (374). Cases have been reported along the coasts of both the Pacific and Atlantic oceans (as far north as Cape Cod), Hawaii, and the Gulf of Mexico and occasionally in such inland areas as New Mexico, Oklahoma, Kentucky, and the Great Salt Lake (4, 6, 35, 45, 192, 330, 414). In a Gulf Coast community over a 10-year period, 12 of 23 *Vibrio* isolates obtained were *V. vulnificus,* of which 9 were wound isolates (45). Similarly, in a Chesapeake Bay hospital over a 15-year period, 10 of 40 *Vibrio* isolates were *V. vulnificus,* of which 7 were obtained from wounds (192). The organism can proliferate in seafood at room temperature but is killed by storage at or near freezing temperatures or by cooking seafood at boiling temperatures (339). *V. vulnificus* has been isolated in oysters that have been refrigerated for 4 days (219).

V. vulnificus is one of the most invasive and rapidly lethal human pathogens ever described. Two major syndromes can result from infection with this organism (221). Primary septicemia typically follows the ingestion of raw oysters by individuals with liver disease. This syndrome can have a rapidly fatal course in up to 60% of cases (423). The other major presentation is that of wound infections, which may occur by either primary inoculation or secondary hematogenous spread in a bacteremic individual. Antibiotics, vigorous debridement, and occasionally amputation are necessary to control the massive necrosis and systemic spread which can occur (236). Unlike other vibrioses, gastroenteritis is not a major hallmark of infection with this species, and although gastrointestinal symptoms may accompany other forms of illness, the relationship is unclear (217, 220). In one epidemiologic study of *V. vulnificus* infections in Florida from 1981 to 1987, 7 patients out of a total of 62 (11%) had gastrointestinal symptoms as their only manifestation of disease (245). Stool specimens yielded *V. vulnificus,* and blood cultures were negative. The diarrhea was described as watery, profuse, and accompanied by vomiting and abdominal pain. Six patients (86%) were hospitalized for a median of 6 days. Medications that reduce gastric acidity may be a factor in the development of gastroenteritis (220). Of 62 cases reported in Florida between 1981 and 1987, 38 were primary septicemia (62%), 17 were wound infections (27%), and the remaining 7 were the gastrointestinal illness referred to above (11%) (245). Other infections due to *V. vulnificus* include pneumonia (113, 238), endocarditis (443), osteomyelitis (452), ocular infections (126), and meningitis (193). One reported case of endometritis due to *V. vulnificus* occurred in a female who had engaged in sexual intercourse in seawater (438).

The severity of infections due to *V. vulnificus* is dependent on host as well as bacterial factors. The presence of an acidic polysaccharide capsule correlates strongly with virulence (479). This capsule may confer resistance to phagocytosis and bactericidal activity of human serum (252, 308, 488). Strains may shift between encapsulated and unencapsulated forms at a very low frequency by poorly understood mechanisms. Growth of both encapsulated and unencapsulated phenotypes is enhanced significantly by the presence of iron (479). The organism is able to use transferrin-bound iron for growth if the transferrin is 100% iron saturated (normal human serum is 30% saturated). Iron in hemoglobin and hemoglobin-haptoglobin complexes may also be utilized (308). *V. vulnificus* also produces siderophores, which are low-molecular-weight chelators that bind available iron (404). Mouse studies have shown that passage of the organism through the animal may enhance virulence significantly, which suggests that the reintroduction of strains shed by infected individuals may increase the potential pathogenicity of environmental or food-borne strains if reintroduced to the environment by infected individuals (237). Various toxins and enzymes may be produced by the organism. They include mucinase, protease, lipase, DNase, chondroitin sulfatase, hyaluronidase, cytolysin, and collagenase (168, 341, 410). The contribution to virulence by each of these factors has not yet been determined fully. An anticytolysin antibody has been detected in the sera of individuals with invasive disease, suggesting that this toxin may play a major role in invasive forms of disease (167).

Individuals susceptible to primary septicemia are most commonly those with liver disease, particularly alcoholic cirrhosis. Adults with liver disease who eat raw oysters are 80 times more likely to develop illness with *V. vulnificus* than those without liver disease and 200 times more likely to die from *V. vulnificus* infections (95). This is due in part to shunting of blood around the liver, thereby bypassing the hepatic reticuloendothelial system and subsequent clearing by hepatic macrophages. Additionally, these individuals may also have deficiencies in leukocyte chemotaxis and complement that can impair host defenses (188). Patients with hepatic disease commonly have high serum iron levels due to liberation of iron stores from damaged hepatocytes (478). In addition, other conditions leading to increased serum levels of iron, such as thalassemia major and hemochromatosis, can also contribute to primary septicemia (217). Alcoholics without liver disease are at risk for primary septicemia, probably due in part to saturated transferrin levels (56). Other conditions predisposing individuals to primary septicemia include hematopoietic disorders, chronic renal insufficiency, dyspeptic disease or a history of gastric resection, the use of immunosuppressive drugs, and diabetes mellitus (383). Primary septicemia occasionally occurs in previously healthy persons (245).

There is little doubt that the gastrointestinal tract is the portal of entry in primary septicemia. The organism can survive between pH 3.6 and 12.5 when incubated at 37°C for 1 h and grows best between pH 7 and 9 (347). Therefore, the organism is capable of surviving passage through the stomach. Most commonly, this occurs following the ingestion of raw oysters. An epidemiologic study of oyster eaters in Florida between 1981 and 1988 estimated the age-standardized annual incidence of any *Vibrio* illness per million persons as 95.4 for raw oyster eaters with liver disease, 9.2 for raw oyster eaters without liver disease, and 2.2 for eaters of nonraw oysters (123). Although these estimates were based on the chances of developing any *Vibrio* illness, the risk was shown to be greatest for *V. vulnificus.* Other types of raw fish or shellfish may cause septicemia, and on previous occasions, illness followed ingestion of deep-fried fish, grilled crab, boiled shrimp, and broiled grouper (135, 245). *V. vulnificus* invades the gastrointestinal

mucosa at the level of the proximal small bowel and moves into the systemic circulation to produce sepsis (346, 355). On occasion, the organism may penetrate the intestinal wall into the ascitic fluid of cirrhotics to produce peritonitis (346).

The mean incubation period is 16 h, although it has been as long as 2 weeks (37, 423). Chief symptoms associated with septicemia include fever (94%), chills (91%), and nausea (58%) (217). Diarrhea occurs in less than half of patients with primary septicemia (221, 245). Approximately one-third of patients become hypotensive within 12 h of admission (191). Signs and symptoms of disseminated intravascular coagulation and septic shock may appear (191). Thrombocytopenia and leukopenia are common, although leukocytosis can appear less frequently (309). Arthritis and arthralgias may develop, and the organism has been cultured from affected joints (37, 221). Other associated clinical characteristics may include the rapid development of anemia, adult respiratory distress syndrome, and heart block (188).

Over 70% of patients with primary septicemia develop skin lesions, usually within the first 36 h of illness (309, 414). Lesions are more common on the trunk and extremities and frequently begin as tender erythematous or ecchymotic areas which may progress to bullae or vesicles that develop into necrotic ulcers (430, 437). They may occasionally appear as ecthyma gangrenosa-like lesions, erythema multiforme, cellulitis, and papular or maculopapular eruptions (217, 466). Similar lesions have been reported for individuals who had bacteremia due to *Pseudomonas aeruginosa, Aeromonas hydrophila,* and *Yersinia enterocolitica* (414). Gangrene of a limb can develop as a result of major vessel occlusion (430). Histological examination reveals cellulitis with subcutaneous tissue necrosis and septal panniculitis characterized by paucity of an inflammatory infiltrate in the dermis (430). Necrotizing vasculitis and subepidermal bullae can be seen, as well as gram-negative coccobacilli.

Gram stain and culture of vesicular or bullous fluid may yield the organisms, which have been described as resembling seagulls (135).

Localized wound infections with *V. vulnificus* may occur in otherwise healthy people after an open wound comes in contact with seawater or seafood contaminated with the organism. A typical scenario is the development of a wound infection following injuries sustained while peeling shrimp, cleaning crabs, or shucking oysters (188, 245, 309). Infection may also follow exposure of a preexisting wound to seawater. Approximately one-third to one-half of cases of wound infections due to *V. vulnificus* occur in patients who have underlying illnesses, such as alcohol abuse, congestive heart failure, stasis ulcers, arthritis, liver disease, diabetes mellitus, and malignancy (37, 221, 423). Initially, the wound may appear trivial, but in a matter of hours it characteristically becomes edematous and erythematous, with development of lymphadenopathy and lymphangitis. Intense pain may develop at the wound site. Patients are frequently ill with fever and chills (37, 423). Anorexia, nausea, and vomiting may occur, although less frequently than in primary septicemia (37, 221). Occasionally, more than one *Vibrio* species may be isolated from the wound (353). Unlike primary septicemia, wound infections usually remain localized, but bacteremia with secondary development of cutaneous infections can occasionally occur (383). Approximately one-third of individuals with localized wound infections have positive blood cultures (309). Individuals with underlying diseases (rarely healthy persons) may develop progressive cellulitis, myositis, or fasciitis (188). Leukocytosis is usually noted; thrombocytopenia and disseminated intravascular coagulation generally do not occur (383). Severe necrotizing fasciitis can occasionally occur, with gross purulence and easy separation of fascial planes. Findings of fascial necrosis separate this entity from cellulitis (148). The histopathology of wound infections is similar to that which occurs in primary septicemia, although it is generally not

as severe. Mortality ranges from 7 to 22% of cases, being higher for those individuals with underlying diseases, who are more likely to develop progressive soft tissue involvement and bacteremia (188).

Treatment of *V. vulnificus* infections consists of rapid recognition with prompt institution of antibiotics and supportive measures, along with management of adult respiratory distress syndrome, disseminated intravascular coagulation, and shock, if present (188, 309, 346). Surgical debridement of all necrotic tissue is recommended (200). Proximal amputation of infected limbs may be necessary in severe cases of wound infection (188). Tetracycline has been shown to be highly effective against *V. vulnificus* in a mouse model (48). Low efficacy was noted for ampicillin, cefotaxime, and cefazolin. Carbenicillin and gentamicin were not effective. Current antibiotic regimens consist of ceftazidime (2 g i.v. three times a day) and doxycycline (100 mg orally or i.v. twice a day) or doxycycline in combination with ciprofloxacin or an aminoglycoside (156). The data supporting the use of fluoroquinolones are limited; ciprofloxacin has been used effectively in the treatment of one case of infection due to *V. vulnificus,* but conclusive clinical studies are lacking (10, 293).

V. mimicus

In 1981, a new *Vibrio* species was detected by virtue of DNA and biochemical analysis. Previously thought to be a biochemical variant of *V. cholerae,* the new species differed in its inability to ferment sucrose and its negative Voges-Proskauer reaction. The name *V. mimicus* was proposed because of its similarity to *V. cholerae* (118). The organism is nonhalophilic and has been isolated from both saltwater and freshwater (100). A high percentage of strains (49%) are able to grow in 6% sodium chloride (141). Brackish water with an average salinity of 4.0% was found to be suitable for *V. mimicus.* It has been isolated from fish and shellfish (usually oysters) as well as from freshwater prawns (99, 248, 402). Unlike *V. chol-*

erae, it probably does not adhere to plankton samples in the environment (100). During the period from 1977 through 1981, the CDC received 21 clinical isolates of this organism, although the true incidence is unknown (402). Nineteen of the isolates were obtained from stool samples, and the other two were obtained from human ears. Clinical isolates have been obtained from the waters of the Gulf of Mexico, the Mid-Atlantic Coast, and the Chesapeake Bay (402). Among 40 *Vibrio* isolates collected over a 15-year period in a Chesapeake Bay hospital, 3 were identified as *V. mimicus;* all were isolated from stool samples (192). The organism has also been implicated along with *V. fluvialis* in a case of terminal ileitis (459).

Gastrointestinal illness is the predominant manifestation of disease and typically follows the ingestion of seafood, primarily raw oysters (402). In the largest reported review of illness due to *V. mimicus* in the United States, involving 21 cases, the median incubation period was shown to be 24 h, with a range of 3 to 72 h (402). Symptoms included diarrhea (94%); nausea, vomiting, and abdominal cramps (67%); fever (44%; occasionally up to 38.3°C); and headache (39%). Three of the 17 patients with diarrhea had bloody diarrhea (18%). The median leukocyte count was 13,400, with a median differential of 73% polymorphonuclear cells, 7% bands, 16% lymphocytes, and 4% monocytes. Electrolytes were all within normal limits. Diarrheal illness lasted a median of 6 days. Two cases were ear infections acquired from contact with seawater. Outbreaks of seafood-associated gastroenteritis caused by *V. mimicus* have been described in Japan (100).

Approximately 10% of clinical strains and 16% of all strains produce a heat-labile toxin that appears to be identical to cholera toxin (309). An enterotoxin similar to that described for non-O1 *V. cholerae* and *V. fluvialis* has been described (333).

Antimicrobial testing has shown that *V. mimicus* is susceptible to tetracycline, which may be the drug of choice for severe infec-

tions (402). The combination of trimethoprim and sulfamethoxazole, aminoglycosides, chloramphenicol, and ampicillin have been shown to be effective in vitro. Eighty-three percent of environmental isolates in one study were shown to be resistant to ampicillin, with intermediate sensitivity and no resistance to tetracycline in 17% of isolates (100).

V. fluvialis

V. fluvialis was first isolated in 1975 from the stool of a patient with diarrhea in Bahrain (151). In 1976 to 1977, it was responsible for an outbreak of diarrheal illness involving over 500 persons in Bangladesh (211). About one-half of the patients were children under 5 years of age. Originally referred to as group F by the Public Health Laboratory in Maidstone, England, and as enteric group EF-6 by the CDC, it was later named *V. fluvialis* (from the Latin for "river") in 1980 on the basis of its original isolation from river and estuarine waters (265, 473). This organism has marked biochemical similarities to *Aeromonas* species and can be distinguished by its ability to grow in 6 to 7% sodium chloride (in which *Aeromonas* species do not grow) and its inability to grow in the presence of the vibriostatic agent O/129 (in whose presence *Aeromonas* species grow) (473). Based on these similarities, it is probable that many clinical isolates previously reported as *Aeromonas* species may have actually been *V. fluvialis* (400). One-third of organisms labeled as *Aeromonas* in the past by the British Public Health Laboratories were found to actually be *V. fluvialis* on reexamination (265). In the United States, the organism has been isolated from water and sediment in New York Bay (400), from shellfish in Louisiana, and from water and shellfish in the Pacific Northwest and Hawaii (424). Almost all cases of infection due to *V. fluvialis* in the United States have been gastrointestinal illnesses. A history of seafood ingestion before the onset of illness was reported in most cases (244). In Florida between 1982 and 1988, 12 clinical isolates of *V. fluvialis* were recovered, 10 of which were obtained from stool samples,

1 of which was obtained from the drainage of a colostomy bag, and 1 of which was recovered from a wound (244). Over a 15-year period, one isolate was recovered from a stool sample in a Chesapeake Bay hospital (192). A fatality occurring in the United States due to *V. fluvialis*-related illness has been reported in the case of a Texas man who developed profuse diarrhea with electrolyte imbalance (424). Outbreaks of gastroenteritis linked to a common food source have been reported (433). Occasionally, wound infections can occur in association with injuries sustained near seawater (244, 424). The organism was recovered from purulent bile in one patient in Japan with acute suppurative cholangitis (489).

The median incubation period for gastrointestinal illness has been reported to be 39 h, with a range of 16 to 60 h and a median duration of illness of 6 days (range, 1 to 60 days) (244). In the Bangladeshi outbreak, reported clinical features included diarrhea (100%), vomiting (97%), abdominal pain (75%), moderate to severe dehydration (67%), and fever (35%) (211). Invasive disease probably occurs, as 75% of the patients in that outbreak had fecal leukocytes and blood in the stools. Secondary infection occurs rarely (241).

V. fluvialis is capable of stimulating fluid accumulation in rabbit ileal loops (400). An enterotoxin similar to that described for non-O1 *V. cholerae* and *V. mimicus* has been described (333). Other factors associated with toxicity may also be produced, with a variety of effects, including cytolytic activity against mammalian erythrocytes, lethal activity in mice, and nonhemolytic cytotoxicity (226, 276).

Severe cases of gastroenteritis should be treated with i.v. fluid and electrolyte replacement and antibiotics (437). *V. fluvialis* is sensitive to tetracycline, ampicillin, chloramphenicol, gentamicin, and the combination of trimethoprim and sulfamethoxazole (241).

Vibrio hollisae

V. hollisae was previously known as enteric group EF-13 until 1982, when it was shown to be a separate species by DNA hybridization studies (186). It was named after the researcher at the CDC who first identified it. *V. hollisae* grows inconsistently on TCBS agar and so may not be isolated routinely (310). Isolation may rely on recovery of colonies on blood agar plates (310). There are few ecological studies on *V. hollisae,* but it has been isolated from deep-sea invertebrates and healthy coastal fish (127, 331). Fifteen clinical isolates were received by the CDC from 1971 to 1981, of which 14 were stool isolates and 1 was a blood isolate (310). Cases occurred in states along the Atlantic and Gulf coasts, with three cases in Florida, four in Maryland, and one each in Virginia and Louisiana. In Florida in the years 1981 to 1988, 34 isolates of *V. hollisae* were identified from clinical cases, of which 28 were obtained from individuals with gastrointestinal illness, 4 were obtained from individuals with septicemia, and 2 were isolated from wounds (123). The risk of infection is most often associated with raw seafood ingestion, particularly ingestion of raw oysters, although cases of illness have followed ingestion of fried fish and fish preserved by drying and salting, which suggests that this organism may be resistant to some methods of cooking and preservation (123, 283, 310, 365).

In nine selected cases of gastrointestinal illness reported to the CDC, all patients had diarrhea and abdominal pain, five had vomiting, and five had fever (310). Diarrhea was bloody in one case. The median white blood cell count was 11,200 cells per μl. The median duration of illness was 1 day (range, 4 h to 13 days). Reported cases of septicemia include one fatal case occurring in an individual with hepatic cirrhosis (310) and another case occurring in a 65-year-old man who developed septicemia following consumption of a freshwater catfish and was successfully treated with tobramycin, cefamandole, and tetracycline (283).

Several toxins may be produced, including a hemolysin with potential virulence activity (486) and a heat-sensitive enterotoxin which has been associated with some virulent strains (251). *V. hollisae* possesses gene sequences homologous with those coding for the thermo-stable direct hemolysin in *V. parahaemolyticus* (332).

V. damsela

V. damsela, previously known as enteric group EF-5, was renamed in 1981 after the damsel-fish, in which it is an important pathogen (281). This organism is known to cause skin ulcerations and death in fish and has been iso-lated from seawater (281). Between 1971 and 1981, eight clinical isolates were reported to the CDC, of which seven were obtained from wounds (one was a urine isolate) (310). Cases occurred on the Atlantic, Pacific, and Gulf coasts and were reported in Florida, Louisiana, Hawaii, and the Bahamas. Typically, infection is the result of injuries sustained to the foot or leg while swimming or handling fish (103). Infection is usually seasonal and probably de-pendent on water temperature and possibly the interaction of *V. damsela* with certain fish species (103, 310, 394).

Lesions usually began as erythematous and indurated areas which may later exhibit a pu-rulent discharge (131, 310). Immunocompe-tent patients may require little more than local wound care, but severe necrotizing and oc-casional fatal infections have been described (103, 310). One fatal case involved a diabetic, alcoholic patient who had sustained a small laceration to his hand while cleaning catfish (103). The initial superficial wound evolved into an edematous and necrotizing process with bulla formation. He subsequently died of medical complications, including disseminated intravascular coagulation. Tissue damage may be toxin mediated (10, 131). *V. damsela* may produce an extracellular hemolytic toxin which has been shown to be lethal in mice (253). Of five *V. damsela* isolates tested, all were sensitive to gentamicin and chloram-phenicol, four were sensitive to tetracycline and cephalothin, and none were sensitive to sulfonamides, ampicillin, or penicillin (310).

V. alginolyticus

Originally classified as biotype 2 of *V. para-haemolyticus, V. alginolyticus* was found to be a separate and distinct species on the basis of several fermentative and biochemical proper-ties. It was renamed *Vibrio alginolyticus* in 1968 (387). This organism was not known to be pathogenic in humans until 1973, when six isolates from tissue specimens collected in 1969 thought to be *V. parahaemolyticus* were in actuality found to be *V. alginolyticus* (38). The ecological niche of this organism is prob-ably similar to that of *V. parahaemolyticus,* and it has been isolated from seawater, fish, shrimp, crabs, oysters, and clams (226). The numbers of this organism in seawater are gen-erally higher than those of *V. parahaemolyticus,* and it is associated with warm water temper-atures (226, 463). This organism fails to grow at temperatures of <8°C (38). In the United States, clinical isolates of *V. alginolyticus* have been obtained from waters along the Atlantic, Pacific, and Gulf coasts, as well as in Hawaii and the Chesapeake Bay (38, 45, 192).

Clinically, wound and ear infections rep-resent the majority of cases of illness due to this organism (38, 217). Wound infections al-most always follow exposure of open wounds to seawater (437). Frequently, a number of different organisms may be isolated, making the pathogenic role of *V. alginolyticus* uncer-tain (217). In one study in Western Australia, 56% of infected wounds contaminated with seawater yielded *V. alginolyticus* (359). In a similar study in Hawaii, the organism was iso-lated from 11% of traumatic marine injuries (352). In Florida in the years from 1981 to 1988, 14 clinical isolates of *V. alginolyticus* were reported, of which 11 were wound iso-lates (79%) (123). The incubation period is about 24 h (38, 359). Most wound infections are self-limiting and consist of mild cases of cellulitis with various amounts of a seropuru-lent exudate, but more severe cases with bac-teremia may be noted in immunocompro-mised individuals (38, 45, 216, 397). One fatal case of bacteremia involved a 37-year-old woman who was doused in seawater after an explosion on a recreational boat (136). The organism was isolated from burn wounds as well as blood. The organism may produce ex-tracellular protease and collagenase, although the role of these factors in the virulence of this organism has not yet been established (178, 309). Local wound care is probably sufficient for superficial wounds in immunocompetent individuals, but patients with impaired host defenses or severe or complicated infections should be treated with antibiotics. In vitro, *V. alginolyticus* is susceptible to tetracycline, the combination of trimethoprim and sulfamethoxazole, aminoglycosides, and chloramphenicol (261).

V. alginolyticus has a predisposition towards individuals with ear disorders (463). These infections are generally associated with swimming in seawater. Both otitis media and otitis externa have been reported (38, 397). This organism has rarely been associated with gastrointestinal illness, although cases have been reported (123, 258, 325). Conjunctivitis, pneumonia, osteomyelitis, and a case of an epidural abscess due to *V. alginolyticus* have been reported (226, 267, 342, 397). Peritonitis has been reported for an individual undergoing peritoneal dialysis who had changed his peritoneal dialysis fluid bag on the beach without taking adequate precautions (428).

V. furnissii

V. furnissii was originally classified as biovar II of *V. fluvialis*. This species differs from *V. fluvialis* in its aerogenicity (produces gas from glucose). In 1983, it was renamed *Vibrio furnissii* in honor of a researcher at the British Public Health Laboratories in Maidstone, England (55). The organism has been recovered from the marine environment (265). Most clinical isolates have been from Japan and other parts of the Orient (309). Illness related to this species consists of gastroenteritis, most likely due to ingestion of raw or undercooked seafood (55). Occasional outbreaks of gastroenteritis have been recorded, including one such episode on board a flight from Tokyo to Seattle involving 23 passengers (70, 72). Symptoms included diarrhea (91%), abdominal cramps (79%), nausea (65%), and vomiting (39%). Two patients required hospitalization, and one died. The organism was also recovered from the feces (along with *V. fluvialis*) of an infant with diarrhea and has also

been isolated from the stools of asymptomatic individuals (187, 260). *V. furnissii* is capable of producing an enterotoxin similar to that described for *V. fluvialis* and *V. mimicus* (333).

V. metschnikovii

Formerly known as enteric group 16, *V. metschnikovii* was first described in 1888 (264). In 1978, it was redefined on the basis of DNA homology studies (264, 437). Freshwater and marine isolates of this organism have been obtained from rivers, estuaries, sewage, cockles, lobsters, oysters, clams, and a bird that died of a cholera-like illness (264). Human disease involving this organism was not recognized until 1978, when it was recovered from the blood of an 82-year-old diabetic female in Chicago who presented to a hospital with septicemia due to an inflamed gallbladder (218). She was treated successfully with a cholecystectomy and antibiotic treatment with clindamycin and tobramycin. Although the organism has been isolated from the stools of asymptomatic individuals (437), diarrheal illness has been described in at least one instance (302). An extracellular cytolysin has been characterized, although its role in virulence is uncertain (301).

Vibrio cincinnatiensis

Only one case of human disease involving *V. cincinnatiensis* has been reported to date (42). A 70-year-old man with a history of alcohol abuse developed disorientation and questionable nuchal rigidity upon admission to a hospital. A spinal tap was performed which revealed a gram-negative bacillus; an identical isolate was obtained from his blood. Genetic and biochemical analysis revealed that this was a new *Vibrio* species which was subsequently named *Vibrio cincinnatiensis* (54). The patient was treated successfully with 9 days of moxalactam. There was no history of exposure to saltwater or ingestion of seafood.

Vibrio carchariae

First isolated from a brown shark that died in captivity in 1984, *V. carchariae* has been known to be a pathogen to fish (170). Named *Vibrio carchariae* from the Greek *carcharias,* meaning shark, this species had not been implicated as a human pathogen until a single report described the case of a wound infection occurring in an 11-year-old girl who was attacked by a shark off the South Carolina coast (348). She suffered extensive trauma to her left calf, requiring plastic surgery. A swab of the leg obtained on the day of the shark bite revealed the presence of *V. carchariae.* Minimal drainage occurred from the wound, which subsequently healed well. Antimicrobial testing showed it to be susceptible to cephalothin, cefamandole, cefoxitin, gentamicin, and the combination of trimethoprim and sulfamethoxazole. Resistance was noted to ampicillin and carbenicillin; amikacin sensitivity was intermediate.

MYCOBACTERIUM MARINUM

M. marinum was first isolated by Aronson in 1926 from saltwater fish that died in a Philadelphia aquarium (14). In 1942, Baker and Hagan isolated this mycobacterium from freshwater platyfish in Mexico, and they named it *Mycobacterium platypoecilus* (26). Human disease attributed to this organism was not recognized until 1951, when an epidemic of self-limiting skin granulomas occurred in a town in Sweden, involving 80 individuals; 75 were children, and lesions were mostly on the elbows (273). All five adult patients were avid swimmers, which suggested that a common swimming pool may have been involved. Tissue specimens from patients and cultures of the swimming pool yielded an atypical mycobacterium which the investigators termed *Mycobacterium balnei* (Latin for "of the bath"). In order to affirm the association between the organism and the clinical findings, the investigators inoculated themselves with the mycobacterium and were able to produce the lesions. In 1959, the previously reported mycobacterial isolates were found to represent the same species (104). *Mycobacterium marinum* became the officially recognized name because this was the earliest term proposed by Aronson. The first association of this organism with

tropical fish tanks was made in 1962 (421). Since then, *M. marinum* has become a well-recognized cutaneous pathogen with a strong association with an aquatic environment and water-related activities. The organism has been called a "leisure-time pathogen" and the disease referred to as a "hobby hazard" (144, 181). Manifestations of disease have also been referred to as "fish fancier's finger" and "swimming pool granuloma."

M. marinum belongs to Runyon group I (the photochromogens) of atypical mycobacteria, along with *Mycobacterium kansasii* and *Mycobacterium simiae.* These organisms are capable of producing a yellow carotene pigment when exposed to a strong light. *M. marinum* grows optimally on Lowenstein-Jensen medium, and unlike the case for other mycobacteria, growth occurs at 28 to 32°C rather than at 37°C. This is an important distinction, which may be responsible for the fact that most *M. marinum* infections do not invade beyond the superficial, cooler regions of the skin (102). Colonies may be visible in as early as 7 days, although rarely may take up to 2 months (8, 104, 256). Growth also occurs on blood agar, though not on MacConkey agar. The organisms are acid fast and appear as long, slender, occasionally beaded rods, but they may appear short and compact. Biochemical reactions include a negative response to niacin, neutral red, and arylsulfatase and a positive response to Tween 80 hydrolysis in 10 days (8, 104).

M. marinum is a pathogen of salt- and freshwater fish. It is widely distributed in the environment and may be isolated from contaminated water, the walls of swimming pools or aquariums, and dead or diseased fish (329). Affected fish may be cachectic and frequently show skin changes consisting of pigment changes, loss of scales, blood spots with eventual formation of ulcers, and fin and tail rot (453). Microscopically, miliary tubercles may be found in virtually every organ system. The disease is thought to spread among fish by the ingestion of infective material. In humans, the organism most commonly causes benign superficial cutaneous illness, although destructive tenosynovitis, osteomyelitis, septic arthritis, sclerokeratitis, and rarely, disseminated systemic illness have been reported (98, 102, 137, 163, 212, 224, 225, 242, 398, 455). The organism is usually acquired through abrasions, lacerations, or punctures sustained in an aquatic environment. Commonly associated activities include swimming, boating, fishing, handling of fish and shellfish, and the keeping of tropical fish tanks. Occasional nonaquatic exposures have been documented from an asphalt school yard, school desks, an electrical installation, rose thorns, and even a laboratory (104, 144, 224, 451). Cases have been reported along the Gulf, Pacific, and Atlantic coasts as far north as Oregon and Long Island (212). Inland cases also occur. An epidemic in Colorado involving 290 individuals was linked to community swimming pools (305).

The incubation period ranges from 2 weeks to 2 months (208). Superficial lesions appear, which usually range in number from one to six and appear as chronic, dusky, erythematous plaques or verrucoid papules or nodules in areas subject to trauma (201). More than 75% of reported cases involved the hand and upper extremity, usually the dominant right hand (208, 212). The lesions can appear as solitary granulomas or verrucous papules of 1 to 2.5 cm in diameter, which may ulcerate and drain purulent material. Most lesions are asymptomatic and cause only cosmetic inconvenience. Symptoms, if present, are mainly slight tenderness and discharge. Limitation in movement of the affected extremity may be noted. Lymphadenopathy occurs rarely (208). Occasionally, spread in a sporotrichoid fashion may occur. Rarely, disseminated cutaneous spread develops (60, 242). One such case involved a 16-month-old child who developed disseminated lesions after being bathed in a bathtub which her father had previously used to clean his fish tanks (242). The time lag between appearance of the lesion and its correct diagnosis ranges from a few weeks to a few years. Left untreated, 80% of the lesions may resolve completely in an average of 14 months, with

the longest reported case being 45 years (358, 455). Truncal cutaneous dissemination in an AIDS patient who kept tropical fish as a hobby has been described (371).

Histologically, the lesions of *M. marinum* change their appearance according to the age of the infection (60). Early lesions (2 to 3 months duration) show nonspecific inflammatory infiltrates in the upper corium. Multinucleated giant cells and epithelioid cell granulomas generally appear at 4 to 6 months of age, and typical tuberculoid structures appear in older lesions. All stages can be observed simultaneously. Staining of tissue specimens reveals the organism in only about 10% of cases. Ten or more slides of thick smears from homogenized tissues are often required for examination after preparation with auramine-rhodamine fluorochrome stain (98).

Deep tissue infections were first widely recognized in 1973 (467). Superficial lesions may invade deeper tissues by attempted self-excision, by intralesional cortisone injections, or by incomplete surgical excision that is not combined with appropriate antibiotics (212). Unlike superficial lesions, these infections are more destructive and more resistant to treatment. Tendon and synovial structures of the wrist and hand are affected in most cases. Diffuse edema at the site of infection is the most common finding (201). A slight fullness may be palpated at the site of the affected tendon sheath. Unlike the case in pyogenic infections, the dorsum of the hand does not swell and a throbbing pain does not occur. Joint limitation with subsequent development of draining sinus tracts may occur. Up to one-half of deep infections involving the hand and wrist may be associated with carpal tunnel syndrome (256). Systemic complaints, fever, and lymphadenopathy are usually absent. The erythrocyte sedimentation rate is usually normal, and X-ray findings are nonspecific (201). Factors associated with a poor prognosis include persistent pain, the presence of a draining sinus tract, and previous local injection of corticosteroids (98).

Diagnosis relies primarily on isolation of the organism by staining or culture. A thorough history should be obtained to include such informational items as hobbies and recreational interests. *M. marinum* rarely grows at temperatures utilized for the incubation of most other mycobacteria. If *M. marinum* is suspected, specimens should be incubated at 30°C on Lowenstein-Jensen medium (in addition to incubation at 37°C for the isolation of other mycobacteria) (104). Specific mycobacterial skin testing has been utilized, but with inconsistent results (208, 224). The differential diagnosis of *M. marinum* infections includes sporotrichosis, tularemia, nocardia, yaws, syphilis, leishmaniasis, common warts, coccidioidomycosis, blastomycosis, histoplasmosis, tuberculosis verrucosa cutis, sarcoidosis, gout, rheumatoid arthritis, iodine or bromine granuloma, and benign or malignant tumors (201). Although usually self-limiting, superficial infections should probably be treated with antimicrobial agents. Minocycline has long been considered the drug of choice, but clarithromycin and doxycycline have been equally efficacious (59, 156, 214, 279). Resistance to doxycycline has been described (275). *M. marinum* does not respond to many of the antimycobacterial agents. It is usually susceptible to rifampin, ethambutol, trimethoprim-sulfamethoxazole, and amikacin (129). Ciprofloxacin has shown good in vitro activity against *M. marinum* (105). In vitro susceptibility has also shown that gatifloxacin, levofloxacin, and moxifloxacin display activities similar to that of ciprofloxacin (51). Treatment should probably be continued for at least 6 to 12 weeks (129). Patients should be instructed not to pick at their lesions to reduce the risk of deeper tissue involvement (212). Deeper tissue involvement usually requires surgical intervention, which may include excision, tenosynovectomy, synovectomy, arthrodesis, or incision and drainage of infected bone or joints (212). Superficial lesions should not be excised or biopsied without the addition of appropriate drug therapy in order to decrease the risk of deeper tissue spread (212).

MARINE TRAUMA

Sharks

Shark attacks have been a popular focus of many books and movies, which often depict these creatures as ruthless savage predators randomly attacking swimmers or divers along beaches or other aquatic recreational areas. Attacks have been recorded in the United States for several hundred years. In the years between 1670 and 2003, there were 833 shark attacks reported in the United States, with 52 fatalities (64). During 2003 alone, 55 confirmed unprovoked attacks occurred, which was lower than the 63 unprovoked attacks reported in 2002, 68 attacks in 2001, and 79 attacks in 2000. Of the 350 species of sharks, only 32 have been implicated in the 30 to 100 shark attacks reported annually worldwide (16). In the United States, the most common offenders are the great white (Fig. 2), gray reef, blue, and mako sharks. Most shark attacks occur in temperate waters between the latitudes of 46°N and 47°S. Associated risk factors include murky, warm water (70°F), sewer outlets, late afternoon and early evening hours, recreational areas, deep channels or drop-offs, movement, and bright objects (16). The victim does not see the shark in most cases, although skin abrasions from "bumping" (due to the shark's skin denticles) may precede the bite. In more than 70% of reported attacks, the victim was bitten one or two times (57).

Sharks can range in length from 9 in. to 50 ft (the whale shark). The largest great white shark verified was 19.5 ft long (57). Sharks are extremely well adapted as predators in their environment, with exceptional sensory systems enabling them to detect electrical fields and motion, which may compensate for their poor color vision. Specialized telereceptors known as the ampullae of Lorenzini are exquisitely sensitive to vibration and low-frequency sound waves, allowing these animals to detect struggling creatures (16). Keen olfactory and gustatory chemoreceptors allow them to sense body fluids.

The shark's jaws consist of multirowed crescent-shaped sets of ripsaw teeth which are

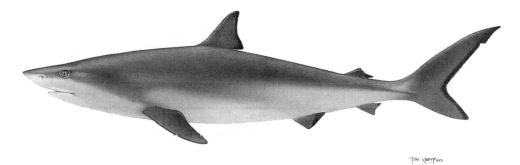

FIGURE 2 A number of shark species have been implicated in shark attacks in North American waters. Specialized sensory systems compensate for poor color vision by allowing a shark to detect motion as well as electrical fields of its prey. Ripsaw teeth are replaced every few months. (Courtesy of the U.S. Fish and Wildlife Service.)

replaced every few months. The biting force has been estimated at 18 tons per in²! The jaw opening of some sharks may be large enough to accommodate a horse's head (16).

Sharks usually feed slowly and purposefully, but they occasionally become frenzied, snapping at anything in sight, usually by an inciting event. Humans are usually mistaken for food (seals). Recent shark attacks in Northern California have been focused on surfers who entered migratory habitats of the elephant seal, which the shark feeds on (16). Possible explanations for the precipitation of a shark attack include anomalous behavior by the shark, the violation of courtship patterns, or territorial invasion (27).

Initial management of the shark attack victim consists of basic trauma management, including checking of the airway and breathing, bleeding control, and the management of hemorrhagic blood loss (16, 57). The immediate life threat is hypovolemic shock and occasionally primary pulmonary or cardiac injury. Bleeding is controlled with compression and occasionally ligation of vessels. Wounds should be irrigated, debrided, and packed open with primary closure. Tetanus toxoid (0.5 ml intramuscularly [i.m.]), tetanus immune globulin (250 to 400 U i.m.), and prophylactic penicillin, imipenem cilastatin, expanded-spectrum cephalosporin, chloramphenicol, or aminoglycoside have been indicated (16, 17, 57). Wounds are susceptible to contamination by both aerobes and anaerobes, including *Aeromonas, Vibrio,* and *Clostridium* (57). Buck and colleagues cultured the teeth of a great white shark caught off Long Island and isolated the following organisms: *V. alginolyticus, V. parahaemolyticus, V. fluvialis, Pseudomonas putrefaciens,* and *Staphylococcus* species (63). *V. carchariae,* a newly recognized human pathogen, was responsible for a wound infection following a shark bite off the South Carolina coast (348).

Measures to be taken to avoid a confrontation with a shark include avoidance of shark-infested waters or waters near sewage outlets or deep channels (especially at night or dusk), never swimming with open wounds or in isolated waters, and storing captured fish away from divers (16, 57). If confronted with such a situation, the swimmer should leave the water with slow, purposeful movements, facing the shark and avoiding the urge to flee rapidly. In deeper waters, the diver should seek refuge near a wall or other object offering protection from behind or find a confined area which the shark would have difficulty accessing. The shark may desist with blows to the snout, gills, or eyes.

Barracudas

Sphyraena barracuda, or the great barracuda, is the only species implicated in human attacks (16, 57). These fish may grow to 10 feet in length and weigh 100 pounds. They can be found in tropical and semitropical waters of the Atlantic (Brazil to Florida) and Pacific (Hawaii) oceans. Barracudas involved in attacks are usually solitary, although attacks have occurred by schools. Attacks are swift and ferocious and usually occur out of confusion in turbid waters or when fish are attracted by shiny objects. Their teeth are canine-like and sharp. The bite produces a V-shaped or straight laceration, often in rows. Treatment is analogous to that for shark bites.

Moray Eels

Moray eels (Fig. 3) are found in tropical, semitropical, and some temperate waters (16). They are fierce and muscular bottom dwellers that hide in crevices and under rocks and coral. Some species may grow to up to 15 ft in length. Divers usually confront these creatures while probing around rocks and coral with their hands. Most smaller species flee when confronted. If provoked or cornered, an eel may inflict a serious laceration with its viselike jaws and fang-like teeth.

Occasionally, an eel does not release its grip. Attempts to disarticulate the jaw or kill the animal may be necessary. An eel's skin is leathery and may not be cut easily. Treatment is similar to that for shark bites (16).

Other Marine Animals

Needlefish are long, streamlined surface fish found in tropical waters that may attain lengths of up to 2 m (16). They have a long sharp snout which has been reported to occasionally impale people, as this fish frequently jumps out of the water (274). Injuries have involved the chest, abdomen, neck, and head, with one case of a fatal brain injury (288). Sea lions, especially mating males or females and their pups, can occasionally be aggressive (19). Since sea lions are mammals, rabies prophylaxis should be considered (57).

Microbiology of Traumatic Marine Wounds

Most of the pathogenic bacteria in seawater are halophilic, heterotrophic, motile, gram-negative rods (17). The genus *Vibrio* represents one such group. The potential for a wound to become infected is based on several factors, including the size and extent of the wound and the colonization of the waters. Host factors tend to play a role as well, with immunosuppressed individuals being more likely to develop systemic spread. One study in Hawaii of acute marine infections revealed an 11% incidence of *V. alginolyticus* wound isolates, with most other bacteria comprising flora typical of cutaneous infections (352).

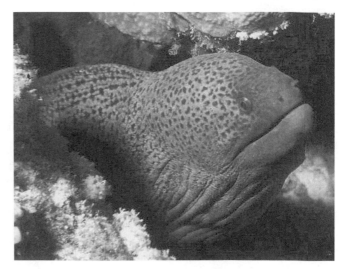

FIGURE 3 Moray eels usually flee when confronted. Fanglike teeth and viselike jaws allow them to inflict serious damage if confronted. (Reprinted from http://www.abc-kid.com/eel/index5.html.)

Minor wound infections may do well without antibiotics, but individuals with liver disease, immunosuppressed individuals, and those with iron overload states may benefit from oral ciprofloxacin or the combination of trimethoprim and sulfamethoxazole (17). Penicillin, ampicillin, cephalosporins, and erythromycin are not acceptable alternatives. Potentially serious or complicated wounds should probably be treated with i.v. antibiotics, including cefoperazone, cefotaxime, ceftazidime, gentamicin, chloramphenicol, and tobramycin. Fulminant infections may be treated with a combination of imipenem and cilastatin. A minor wound infection with a classic erysipeloid reaction *(Erysipelothrix rhusiopathiae)* may be treated with penicillin, erythromycin, or cephalexin (Table 3).

VERTEBRATE ENVENOMATIONS

Stingrays

Eleven species of stingrays are found in U.S. waters; of these, seven are found in the waters of the Atlantic Ocean and four are found in the Pacific Ocean (17). Stingrays are fre-

TABLE 3   Microorganisms associated with marine wound infections and recommended antimicrobial therapies[a]

Microorganism	Therapy	
	First choice	Alternative
Aeromonas hydrophila	TMP-SMX[b]	Gentamicin, tetracycline
Bacteroides fragilis	Metronidazole	Clindamycin
Chromobacterium violaceum	Treatment should be guided by clinical presentation and in vitro susceptibility testing (mezlocillin and aminoglycoside have been used, according to a case report)	
Citrobacter diversus	Imipenem	Ciprofloxacin (or others if susceptible in vitro)
Clostridium perfringens	Penicillin G	Clindamycin, metronidazole
Enterobacter cloacae	Cefotaxime, ceftriaxone, or ceftizoxime + aminoglycoside	Imipenem, aminoglycoside, TMP-SMX, ciprofloxacin
Erysipelothrix rhusiopathiae	Penicillin G or ampicillin	Cephalosporins (e.g., cephalexin)
Escherichia coli	TMP-SMX	Cephalosporin; ampicillin, quinolones, aminoglycoside
Mycobacterium marinum	Minocycline	Rifampin + ethambutol, rifampin + TMP-SMX
Providencia stuartii	Cefotaxime, ceftriaxone, or ceftizoxime + aminoglycoside	Imipenem, aminoglycoside, sulfatrimethoprim, ciprofloxacin
Pseudomonas aeruginosa	Aminoglycoside + antipseudomonal penicillin	Aminoglycoside + ceftazidime
Salmonella enterica serovar Enteritidis	Ceftriaxone	Ampicillin, ciprofloxacin, TMP-SMX
Staphylococcus aureus		
Methicillin sensitive	Semisynthetic penicillin	Vancomycin
Methicillin resistant	Vancomycin	TMP-SMX (?)
Streptococcus species	Penicillin G	Erythromycin, clindamycin
Vibrio species (see text)	Tetracycline ± aminoglycoside (if systemic spread is suspected)	TMP-SMX (possibly quinolone if susceptible in vitro)

[a] With rapid emergence of antimicrobial resistance, these empirical recommendations should be confirmed by in vitro susceptibility testing.

[b] TMP-SMX, trimethoprim-sulfamethoxazole.

quently implicated in cases of human envenomation, with at least 2,000 stingray injuries recorded in the United States annually (57). They may be subdivided into four categories, as follows (in ascending order of toxicity): the butterfly rays (gymnurid type), the eagle and bat rays (myliobatid type), the stingrays and whiprays (dasyatid type), and the round rays (urolophid type) (17). Stingrays are found in tropical, subtropical, and warm temperate waters in shallow intertidal areas, such as bays, lagoons, river mouths, and sandy areas between reefs. These marine animals, which may reach up to 50 to 60 ft^2 in size, are round, diamond, or kite-shaped objects with wide wing-like pectoral fins. They often lie on the surface bottom covered by sand, with only their eyes, spiracles, or parts of their elongated, whip-like tail exposed. Stingrays have one to four venomous stingers arranged on the dorsum of the tail. The stingers consist of dentine spines which are tapered and retroserrated so they may enter the skin easily but are extracted with difficulty and worsening of the laceration (17). Each spine is covered by an integumentary sheath which houses a venom gland in the ventrolateral groove along either side. The spine is covered by a layer of venom and mucus. The venom is a highly unstable and very heat-labile protein consisting of at least 10 amino acids, with toxic components such as serotonin, 5'-nucleotidase, and phosphodiesterase (17, 173). Envenomation usually occurs when an unwary swimmer steps on the stingray while wading in shallow waters. The stingray in turn strikes the individual by lashing its tail upward, forcing its spines into the victim. The lower extremities are involved in most cases, although any part of the body is susceptible.

Initial manifestations consist of intense localized pain with soft tissue edema and bleeding (17, 411). The pain may intensify and spread over a period of 30 to 90 min and then gradually diminish over the next 6 to 48 h. Minor wounds resemble cellulitis, but more severe wounds may appear dusky and cyanotic, with progression to rapid hemorrhage

and necrosis of fat and muscle. Secondary infection is common (57).

The venom affects the cardiovascular system and can cause peripheral vasoconstriction or dilatation and cardiac arrhythmias (411). Respiratory depression (via the medullary centers) and convulsions may also occur. Other symptoms include nausea, vomiting, generalized edema (with truncal wounds), limb paralysis, and hypotension (17).

Initial treatment should consist of irrigation with cool water or saline to produce local vasoconstriction and debridement with exploration to remove any sheath contents left in the wound (17, 57). X-rays should be obtained to identify any missed fragments. The wound should be soaked in hot water (113°F) for 30 to 90 min. The benefit of this probably has to do with the thermolabile nature of the protein. Narcotics and infiltration with 1 to 2% lidocaine without epinephrine may provide pain control. Regional-nerve anesthesia with 0.5% bupivacaine may be necessary (17). The wound should be packed open for primary closure or sutured loosely. Antibiotic prophylaxis is recommended. Steroids and antihistamines are without documented efficacy (57).

Scorpion Fish

Scorpion fish can be found in shallow reef waters of the Gulf of Mexico, the Florida Keys, and the coastlines of California and Hawaii (16). Members of this group are responsible for about 300 envenomations annually in the United States (381). Several hundred species are known to exist and can be divided into the following three genera, based on the structure of the venom glands: *Synanceja* (stonefish), *Scorpaena* (sculpin, scorpion fish, and bullrout), and *Pterois* (zebrafish, lionfish, and butterfly cod) (17, 57). Scorpion fish often hide under rocks, in coral crevices, or buried in the mud, blending in excellently with their surroundings due to their colorful and ornate camouflage. Stonefish are unattractive bottom dwellers which are regarded as the most lethal of these poisonous marine denizens. The potency of their venom is comparable to that of cobra venom. A small number of domestic envenomations occur in tropical fish hobbyists who carelessly handle illegally obtained scorpion fish (441). The venom organs consist of 12 to 13 dorsal, 2 pelvic, and 3 anal spines. The ornate pectoral spines are not venomous. Paired glands exist at the base of the anterolateral spines, and venom flows along grooves in these spines. Approximately 5 to 10 mg of venom may be found in each paired gland (17). When threatened, these fish erect the dorsal spines, flare out the armed gill covers, and protrude the pectoral and anal fins (18). Venom is injected in a manner analogous to that for a stingray envenomation. The potency of the venom varies according to the species. The pharmacology of scorpion fish venom is poorly understood (446). Wounds inflicted by lionfish are mild compared to those by scorpion fish, with stonefish wounds being the most severe (17).

Intense pain occurs immediately after the injury and radiates up the extremity (17, 57). If the injury is left untreated, the pain peaks in 60 to 90 min, often lasting 6 to 12 h or perhaps days. Stonefish envenomation may produce pain severe enough to precipitate delusions (18). The wounds initially appear ischemic and cyanotic, with surrounding areas of erythema, edema, and warmth (17). Progressive cellulitis and local induration may follow, occasionally with vesicle formation. Tissue necrosis with sloughing may occur within 48 h. Wounds may take months to heal, with occasional soft tissue fibrous defects or cutaneous granulomata persisting. Secondary infection or deep abscesses may occur. Systemic effects include paresthesias, skin rash, nausea, vomiting, arthralgias, fever, diarrhea, delirium, seizures, abdominal pain, hypertension, arrhythmias, limb paralysis, congestive heart failure, hypotension, and death. In the case of stonefish envenomation, dyspnea and circulatory collapse may occur within 1 h, with death ensuing within 6 h (57).

Initial treatment of scorpion fish injuries is analogous to that for stingray injuries, with proper irrigation and debridement to ensure removal of any persistent source of venom (17, 57). Inadequate debridement may predispose the injury to ulceration with tissue extension. Immersion in hot water (113°F) for 30 to 90 min may alleviate the pain, possibly secondary to toxin inactivation; longer durations may be needed for persistent pain. Wounds should be packed open for primary closure or sutured loosely to allow drainage. Antibiotic therapy is recommended for deep puncture wounds of the hand or foot because of the high incidence of tissue complications (17). Recommended antibiotics include expanded-spectrum cephalosporins, trimethoprim-sulfamethoxazole, chloramphenicol, tetracycline, aminoglycosides, and imipenem-cilastatin (17). Severe systemic reactions due to *Synanceja* species (and, less rarely, other scorpion fish) necessitate the use of i.v. stonefish equine antivenin. It is supplied in 2-ml ampules, with 1 ml capable of neutralizing 10 mg of dried venom. Antivenins are produced in Australia and India and may be acquired in the United States from the Health Services Department, Sea World in San Diego, and the Steinhart Aquarium in San Francisco. Physicians may alternatively locate antivenin by contacting an accredited regional poison center (17).

Sea Snakes

Sea snakes are probably the most abundant reptiles in the world. Fifty-two species are known, and all are venomous (18). At least seven species have been implicated in fatal envenomations (57). Sea snakes are marine-adapted serpents belonging to the family Hydrophidae and are close relatives of cobras and kraits. They are widely distributed in tropical and subtropical waters along the coasts of the Indian and Pacific oceans and the Gulf of California. There are no sea snakes in the Atlantic Ocean or the Caribbean Sea (18, 57). These reptiles have a flat tail which assists them in propulsion. They can travel with ease in both forward and reverse directions. Some species may attain lengths of up to 10 ft. These creatures can remain submerged in the water for hours by utilizing an air retention system to control buoyancy. Although they are usually docile, they may attack when provoked, especially during the mating season (18). Sea snakes have two to four maxillary fangs, each of which is associated with a pair of venom glands. Fangs of most species are too short to penetrate a diver's wet suit (17). Many envenomations are avoided by the fact that the fangs are easily dislodged. The venom is more potent than terrestrial snake venom, and its toxicity is derived primarily from potent neurotoxins (446). Neurotoxins may exert their effects through the inhibition of cholinesterase or by blocking presynaptic or postsynaptic impulses. Most sea snake venom contains only postsynaptic neurotoxin, which binds strongly to the acetylcholine receptor at the neuromuscular junction. The venom may contain other toxins, including hyaluronidase, phosphodiesterase, phospholipase A, and proteases (446). Phospholipase A and other myotoxins may cause muscle necrosis with myoglobin release (412). These myotoxic, hemolytic, neurotoxic, and vasoactive components constitute a serious medical emergency if envenomation occurs.

The bites are extremely small and characterized by multiple pinhead, hypodermic-like puncture wounds numbering from 1 to 20 (18). Initially, the pain is only minimal, without any local reaction. Neurologic symptoms occur within 2 to 3 h in most cases and always within 8 h of the bite. If no symptoms develop within 8 h, significant envenomation did not occur. Typical signs and symptoms include painful muscle movement, myoglobinuria, euphoria, trismus, malaise, anxiety, ascending paralysis, slurred speech, dysphagia, ptosis, and ophthalmoplegia. Death is rare and is usually due to more severe reactions, including myonecrosis, respiratory insufficiency, bulbar paralysis, and hepatic, cardiac, or renal failure (17, 19).

Diagnosis is based on several factors, such as location (sea snake bites only occur in the water), absence of pain (initial pain is unusual), the typical appearance of the fang bites (usually one to four), identification of the snake (it should be caught if possible), and the development of characteristic symptoms within 8 h (occasionally as early as 5 min) (16).

Treatment is similar to that for most terrestrial snake bites (17). Local suction without incision can be performed if used immediately with a plunger device. Incision and drainage are of no value if delayed for several minutes after the bite, and cryotherapy is contraindicated. The affected limb should be immobilized, with application of a proximal venous and lymphatic occlusive band or use of the pressure immobilization technique (a cloth pad is pressed directly over the wound by a circumferential elastic wrap at a pressure of ≤70 mm Hg) to minimize systemic toxicity. Antivenin is effective if used within 24 to 36 h and should be used quickly (445). The minimum initial dose of sea snake antivenin is 1 to 3 vials; up to 10 vials may be required. Polyvalent equine antivenin to *Enhydrina schistosa* (beaked sea snake) and *Notechis scutatus* (terrestrial tiger snake) neutralizes the bites of most sea snakes. Anaphylaxis and serum sickness may occur, and intradermal sensitivity testing with 0.02 ml of a 1:10 antivenin dilution should be done. *N. scutatus* antivenin is a second-choice alternative (17). Antivenin in the United States may be obtained from the sources listed in the section on scorpion fish.

Weeverfish

Weeverfish, also referred to as sea cats, sea dragons, adderpikes, and stangs, are found in the temperate waters of the Atlantic Ocean, Mediterranean Sea, and European coastal waters (19). Weeverfish are one of the most venomous fish found in these waters. They are small fish (<50 cm) that can be found buried in the mud or soft bottom with only their head exposed. They produce a venom located in glands associated with dorsal and opercular dentine spines which are capable of piercing a leather boot. Weeverfish are generally docile, yet if provoked, they may become extremely aggressive and strike. Victims are usually professional fisherman or wading swimmers.

The venom is a heat-labile protein substance which also contains 5-hydroxy-tryptamine, histamine, epinephrine, and norepinephrine (446). An intense burning pain is felt immediately following the sting (19). The pain often spreads throughout the entire limb, generally peaks in intensity within the first hour, and usually subsides within 24 h, although it may persist for days. The initial wound is pale and edematous and becomes erythematous, warm, and ecchymotic with increasing edema. It may take months to heal. Headache, delirium, fever, dyspnea, diaphoresis, nausea, vomiting, seizures, hypotension, and cardiac arrhythmias may occur (16).

Treatment is analogous to that for stingray envenomations. The pain is often poorly controlled, even with the liberal use of narcotics (16). An antivenin may be available soon (57). Weeverfish should never be handled when alive; they may survive for hours out of water (19).

Catfish

More than 1,000 species of freshwater and saltwater catfish exist (57). These fish are named for the sensory barbels surrounding the mouth. Catfish have long thin venom glands covered by an integumentary sheath located on lateral ridges along the dorsal and pectoral spines (321). Catfish may lock these fins in an extended position when excited, thereby inflicting a dramatic sting if mishandled. Fragments of tissue and spine may remain in the wound. The venom contains dermonecrotic, vasoconstrictive, and other bioactive agents (57). Immediate severe pain, throbbing, and weakness occur. The pain usually radiates locally and proximally and generally resolves in 30 to 60 min, occasionally lasting 48 h. Nausea, vomiting, respiratory distress, and mild hypotension may occur. Muscle fasciculations and local muscle spasms are common. The wound site may appear pale and bleed longer

than expected. Cyanosis at the puncture site may occur, followed by local tissue necrosis or skin sloughing. Swelling of the extremity, a serous discharge, slow wound healing, and local lymphadenopathy may persist for weeks to months (321). Secondary infections are common, and gangrene has been reported. Envenomation by the oriental catfish (*Plotosus lineatus*) may produce more marked systemic symptoms (57).

Treatment is analogous to that for stingray envenomations, although the venom is not as potent (16). X-rays should be obtained, as the radiopaque spines are frequently left in place. The wound should be thoroughly irrigated and debrided. Irrigation with permanganate, bicarbonate, acetic acid, or papain has not been shown to have any benefit. Tourniquets have no value (16). Updating of tetanus immunization, as with other marine puncture wounds, is essential. Antibiotics should be administered if the wound is dirty or complicated. Local wound care alone is probably adequate for properly treated clean wounds in healthy individuals (321).

INVERTEBRATE ENVENOMATIONS

Coelenterates

The phylum Cnidaria (formerly Coelenterata) is a massive group of marine invertebrates consisting of more than 9,000 species, among which at least 100 are hazardous to humans (17). Classes are Scyphozoa (true jellyfish), Hydrozoa (fire coral, Portuguese man-of-war, and Pacific blue bottle), and Anthozoa (sea anenomes and soft coral) (176). These species may contain millions of nematocysts (also known as "stinging capsules" or "nettle cells"), which are microscopic toxin-containing organs capable of injecting venom into their prey when triggered. Nematocysts are found along the outside of long streaming tentacles and near the mouth of the animal. Each nematocyst consists of a minute capsule (cnidoblast) that contains a spirally coiled thread with a barbed end. Specialized triggers (cnidocils) on the capsule are capable of force-fully ejecting the venomous barbs at pressures of up to 2 to 5 lb/in^2, enough to penetrate a surgical glove (57). This produces a severe "sting." The size of the barb and the potency of the venom vary between the different species. The cnidocil may be triggered by abrasion or freshwater contact. A single man-of-war envenomation may involve several hundred thousand nematocysts (16).

Human reactions to jellyfish toxin may be classified as systemic, local, chronic, or fatal (66). Local reactions include persistent or recurrent eruptions, eruptions distant to the site of envenomation, exaggerated local angioedema, papular urticaria, and contact dermatitis. Chronic reactions include keloid formation, pigmentation, fat atrophy, mononeuritis, autonomic nerve paralysis, gangrene, vascular spasm, and ataxia. Systemic reactions may include muscle cramps, nausea, vomiting, tachycardia, abdominal pain, and hypertension. Death may occur through cardiotoxic, central respiratory, or renal mechanisms. Anaphylaxis has been reported (440).

The potency and composition of the toxin vary between species. After injection of large doses of toxin into human skin, a perivascular mononuclear cell infiltrate appears within the dermis. A cell-mediated and humoral immune response then occurs. Lymphokines and prostaglandins account for some of the cutaneous manifestations of jellyfish envenomation (65). Serotonin, histamine, or histamine-releasing agents are responsible for much of the burning pain and urticaria. High-molecular-weight toxins may inhibit nerve activity through altered ionic permeability. These protein and tetramine fractions have direct and indirect effects on the autonomic nervous system and end organs, particularly the vascular, cardiac, and central nervous systems. A destabilizing effect on the cell membrane appears to be mediated by the calcium channel. Verapamil may block this effect (57).

Fire corals (Millepora) are not true corals. They are branching bottom dwellers which may attain heights of 1 to 2 meters. They de-velop upright, clavate, blade-like, or branching calcareous growths that form encrustations over rocks, shellfish, other coral, and man-made objects. The white to yellow-green lime carbonate exoskeleton may become razor sharp. The nematocyst-bearing tentacles protrude from numerous minute surface gastropores (18). These stings account for the majority of coelenterate envenomations. An intense burning pain, with central radiation and reactive regional lymphadenopathy, follows envenomation (17).

The Portuguese man-of-war *(Physalia physalis)* (Fig. 4) and the Pacific blue bottle *(Physalis utriculus)* are not true jellyfish; they are colonial hydroids (176). These open-sea surface creatures are widely distributed in the Atlantic *(Physalia physalis)* and Pacific *(Physalia utriculus)* oceans and are most commonly found in the semitropical Atlantic Ocean. They are composed of a large nitrogen- and carbon monoxide-filled sail, which may achieve lengths of up to 30 cm across. Numerous nematocyst-laden tentacles (up to 750,000 nematocysts per tentacle) stream downward from the sail, attaining lengths of up to 30 m *(Physalia physalis)*. The animal is carried along by wind and ocean currents. Fish and other objects may become entangled in the tentacles, which contract rhythmically in search of prey. Broken-off tentacle fragments may retain their potency for months (16).

Chironex fleckeri (the box jellyfish or sea wasp) is the most venomous sea creature known (16). Death may occur within 1 min of envenomation, and the overall mortality has been reported to be as high as 20%, although this number may be inflated, as evidenced by more recent studies (343). These creatures are found in the protected waters off the northern Australian coast. To date, there have been 55 confirmed deaths due to stings from these creatures (326). A less lethal variety is found in the waters of the Chesapeake Bay (57). Up to 10 ml of venom may be injected during a "sting." These creatures are small creatures (2 to 10 cm in diameter) capable of attaining speeds of up to 2 knots in steady winds with

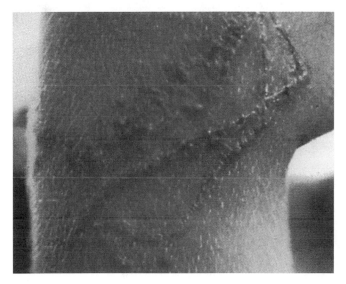

FIGURE 4 The sting of the Portuguese man-of-war is one of the most painful conditions known to afflict the skin. The wrapping of the tentacles typically results in linear circumferential stripes, which are caused by the deposition of urticariogenic and irritant substances, not by the force of the swing. (Reprinted from reference 459a with permission of the publisher.)

swift currents. Factors determining the severity of envenomation include the length and width of the wheal, the length of the contact, the thickness of the skin, the percentage of nematocysts discharged, and the "venom load," which is related to recent feeding (284). A sheep-derived antivenin is available and is given i.v. or i.m. (20,000 U, or one vial, i.v. over 5 min or three vials i.m.) (284). Verapamil is contraindicated (435).

Sea anenomes are sessile, multicolored, flower-like anthozoans which may attain diameters of up to one-half meter (16). They have fingerlike projections containing numerous modified nematocysts, referred to as sporocysts. They are usually encountered by skin divers and waders.

Irukandji syndrome may follow stings by the Cubozoa class of jellyfish (e.g., *Carukia barnesi*) (66). A small but transient sting initiates this reaction. A severe, boring pain may develop in the abdomen or sacrum, with gradual spread to the thighs and chest, where the sensation is described as cramping. Excruciating myalgia persists over the next 24 to 48 h. Other symptoms include tremor, anxiety, piloerection, hyperpnea, headache, nausea, vomiting, sweating, restlessness, tachycardia, blood-streaked sputum, and oliguria. A rapidly developing pulmonary edema leading to acute respiratory failure may develop (145). This syndrome, similar to excess catecholamine release, is assumed to represent a toxic reaction to the venom of the small jellyfish (66).

The person who has endured a coelenterate sting should immediately soak the area in 5% acetic acid (vinegar) (17). Isopropyl alcohol (40 to 70%) is a reasonable alternative, although some argue that this may cause further venom release. Other detoxicants of possible benefit include dilute ammonium hydroxide, sodium bicarbonate, olive oil, sugar, urine, and papain (unseasoned meat tenderizer). Fresh water should never be applied to the area, as this may trigger further nematocyst release. The area should be soaked for at least 30 min or until the pain disappears. The area should not be abraded or scrubbed. Any large tentacles or remaining fragments should be removed by a forceps with doubly-gloved hands. Once cleaned, shaving cream should be applied and the area shaved gently.

Anaphylaxis should always be anticipated. After decontamination, corticosteroids or topical anesthetics can be used. Antibiotics are usually not needed, but large open lesions should be cleaned daily and covered with a thin layer of nonsensitizing antiseptic ointment. Tetanus immunization should be current. Wounds should be checked by a physician for signs of infection 3 and 7 days after the injury.

Echinoderms

Sea urchins and starfish are found in this group of marine animals. Their venom contains many toxic substances, including steroid glycosides, serotonin, and acetylcholine-like substances. Certain sea urchins may produce potent neurotoxins (16).

Sea urchins are globular or flattened animals with a hard shell enclosing their vital organs (18). Regularly arranged spines and a triple-jawed seizing organ (pedicellaria) cover this shell. Spines may be venom bearing or non-venom-bearing. The pedicellariae are dispersed among the spines and may grab hold with their pincer-like jaws. They also contain venom glands that release toxic material when they contract. The venom inflicts intense burning stings (Fig. 5), which may progress to muscular paralysis, respiratory distress, and occasionally death if numerous spines are involved. Hot water may provide relief. The pedicellariae and embedded spines should be removed with care because they are easily fractured. Residual spines may form granulomas (17).

Starfish are simple, free-living, stellate echinoderms covered with simple thorny spines of calcium carbonate crystals held erect by muscle tissue (18). Glandular tissue interspersed throughout or located beneath the integument produces a slimy, venomous substance that causes a contact dermatitis. Envenomation occurs when the victim contacts the thorny spines, some of which may grow to 6 cm in length. Envenomation can rarely induce systemic symptoms, including paresthesias, vomiting, and muscular paralysis. The dermatitis may be treated with hot water and topical calamine with 0.5% menthol.

Mollusks

Cone shells are potentially lethal gastropods that possess a sophisticated venom apparatus (16). At least 18 to 400 species have been implicated in human fatalities. They are nocturnal feeders located in the Indo-Pacific area. A set of minute harpoon-like radular teeth may contain venom, which is injected from an extensible proboscis. The venom interferes with neuromuscular transmission in a manner analogous to that for curare. Initial symptoms include local ischemia, cyanosis, and numbness. More severe envenomations may induce paresthesias and generalized muscular paralysis with respiratory failure. Other symptoms in-

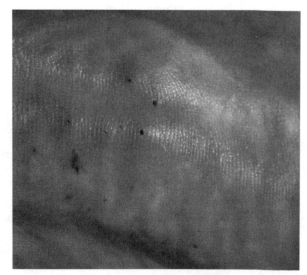

FIGURE 5 Wounds caused by a sea urchin. Sea urchins have spines that may be several inches long. When stepped upon by an unwary swimmer, the spines may be driven deep into the skin and break off, resulting in an extremely painful injury. Secondary infections are nearly inevitable if the spines are left in. (Reprinted from reference 459a with permission of the publisher.)

clude dysphagia, aphonia, weakness, diplopia, blurred vision, cerebral edema, disseminated intravascular coagulation, coma, and cardiovascular collapse. Death may occur in as little as 2 h. Therapy is largely supportive. Hot-water immersions may alleviate some of the pain.

Octopuses are cephalopods found in the warm waters of the intertidal zone (16). The Australian spotted *(Octopus maculosus)* and blue-ringed *(Octopus lunulatus)* octopuses have been implicated in human fatalities. The blue-ringed octopus is covered with poorly visible blue rings which become iridescent peacock blue when the organism is angered. Parrot-like and powerful chitinous jaws are capable of penetrating through the dermis of the skin and into the muscle tissue. Venom is injected into the victim, who is usually a naive swimmer playing with what seems to be a harmless creature. The toxin blocks nerve conduction, most likely by altering sodium conductance. Myocardial and respiratory depression is observed in animal models. Following the initial bite, an intense burning or throbbing with central radiation occurs. Within 30 min, marked local erythema, swelling, pruritus, and pain may occur. Severe envenomations include nausea, vomiting, paresthesias, blurred vision, aphonia, dysphagia, ataxia, myoclonus, flaccid paralysis, hypotension, and respiratory failure. Treatment is supportive, with wide excision of the involved area down to deep fascia. Closure may be primary or by a full-thickness skin graft. There is no effective antivenin available.

Dermatitis

Most cases of dermatitis in swimmers and beachgoers are the result of contact with the Coelenterata. In 1991, an outbreak of cercarial dermatitis was noted among 37 students frequenting a Delaware beach. In 1999, 63 confirmed cases of cercarial dermatitis were reported among 450 families swimming near a snail-infested beach near Quebec City (268). Cercarial dermatitis, or "swimmer's itch," is a cutaneous inflammation due to penetration of the skin by cercariae, which are the free-living

larval stages of bird schistosomes (76). Hosts include migratory waterbirds, including shore-birds, ducks, and geese. Adult worms are carried in the bloodstream and produce eggs that are passed in the feces. Once exposed to the water, the eggs hatch to produce miracidia, which infect mollusks. The parasite develops in the snail to produce cercariae, which penetrate the skin of birds to complete the cycle. Humans are accidental hosts. The cercariae are able to penetrate the skin but do not develop further.

This dermatologic entity has a worldwide distribution. Symptoms include reddening and itching of exposed skin in the water or immediately after emerging and delayed onset of pruritic raised papules, which may form vesicles. Previous exposure may elicit a more severe response upon reexposure. Treatment consists of antihistamines and topical antipruritic medications.

Cutaneous larva migrans is a dermatitis caused by invasion of the skin by larval nematodes (328). Most infections are due to the filariform larvae of the dog and cat hookworm, *Ancylostoma braziliense,* although several other larval nematodes may cause the disease, including *Ancylostoma caninum, Ancylostoma duodenale,* and *Necator americanus.* Adult *A. braziliense* inhabits the intestines of dogs and cats. It produces eggs which pass in the feces to hatch in the soil in 1 to 2 days. Within a week, they become infective filariform larvae. Humans are inadvertent hosts when the larvae penetrate the skin, although they usually do not penetrate further than the epidermis. The disease has a worldwide distribution and is much more common in tropical and semitropical areas. People who frequent beaches are at increased risk (hence the synonym "sandworm").

Symptoms develop within a few hours of penetration into the skin. An itching red papule develops, which may form a serpiginous track. The surrounding tissues become edematous and acutely inflamed. The tracks may become encrusted and secondarily infected. The pruritus may become extremely intense. Untreated, the larvae may persist in the skin for months. Treatment consists of thiabenda-zole administered orally or topically.

SWIMMER'S EAR

Swimmer's ear, or acute otitis externa, is the most common medical problem faced by swimmers (393). It begins not as an infection but as an eczema of the ear canal caused by retention of water in the ear following bath-ing, showering, or swimming (382). By the time medical attention is sought, the ear is usually secondarily infected. The normal ex-ternal auditory canal is sterile bacteriologically in up to 30% of the population, with the re-mainder harboring a mixed flora including *Staphylococcus albus, Staphylococcus epidermidis,* diphtheroids, and to a lesser extent, *Staphylo-coccus aureus* and viridans group streptococci (31, 417). In external otitis media, cultures usually reveal mixed floras, with gram-negative bacteria predominating in up to three-fourths of affected individuals under the age of 21 years. *Pseudomonas* species, the most common offending organisms, are isolated in up to one-half of cases (69). Other species in-clude *Proteus vulgaris, Escherichia coli, Staphylo-coccus aureus, Staphylococcus epidermidis,* strep-tococci, diphtheroids, *Enterobacter aerogenes, Klebsiella pneumoniae,* and *Citrobacter.* Approx-imately 40% of infected ears yield fungal iso-lates, with *Aspergillus* species representing the majority of such (393).

The pathogenesis of swimmer's ear is mul-tifactorial, with cerumen playing a major role. Cerumen imparts an acid reaction to the ex-ternal canal, lowering its pH to 5 and thereby inhibiting bacterial and fungal growth. In ad-dition, its lipid content provides a protective surface to the squamous epithelium and pilo-sebaceous elements of the canal. Cerumen therefore provides a chemical and mechanical barrier to infection. Excessive moisture in the external canal, which can occur during swim-ming, bathing, or excessive sweating, can lead to mechanical disruption of this barrier, with subsequent desquamation and maceration. In addition, the decrease in cerumen results in a raising of the pH to 7, which allows bacterial species to proliferate. As inflammation occurs, a purulent exudate forms which mixes with the dry skin, providing a wet environment suitable for bacterial growth.

The earliest symptom is usually itching, which often leads to manipulation (393). Trauma from cotton swabs or mechanical ob-jects inserted into the canal can exacerbate the condition. A purulent discharge develops, ac-companied by progressive tenderness and pain. Hearing loss may result from canal skin edema and accumulation of debris. The diagnosis can be confirmed by manipulation of the tragus and pinna, which elicits a severe painful re-action. Attempts at otoscopic visualization may be hampered by the pain as well as the accumulation of debris. Regional lymphad-enopathy and cellulitis of the external auricle can occasionally occur. Fungal otitis externa may be accompanied only by itching and a feeling of fullness. In these cases, hyphae may be visualized on microscopic examination, or in the case of *Aspergillus niger,* a grayish mem-brane may be noted in the external canal.

Initial treatment should begin with the rec-ognition and elimination of specific precipi-tating factors, such as swimming or manipu-lation of the ear, until the disorder is corrected (393). Pain control may be necessary during the first 24 to 48 h of treatment (399). Severe cases may require narcotic analgesics or even hospitalization for i.m. analgesics and i.v. an-tibiotics. Thorough irrigation and cleaning are essential to remove the purulent debris and al-low penetration by topical antibiotics. Various cleansing solutions have been utilized, includ-ing 3% acetic acid, 70% alcohol, 3% boric acid–70% alcohol solution, and Burow's so-lution (393). Cleansing and irrigation may be required on a daily basis. In cases where the debris is too thick, an expanding cellulose wick may be implanted within the canal to allow antibiotic penetration.

Topical antibiotics are usually adequate in all but the most severe cases, which may re-quire systemic agents. The most widely pre-scribed otic solutions contain the antibiotics neomycin and polymyxin, which are effective against most of the usual pathogens. Neomycin is effective against *Proteus* and *Staphylococcus* species; polymyxin is usually effective against *Pseudomonas*. Chloromycetin otic drops are available for less commonly encountered anaerobic infections. In the event of otitis externa due to *Aspergillus niger,* local application of amphotericin B, oxytetracycline and polymyxin, iodochlorhydroxyquin, and nystatin may be effective (393). Candidal infections may be treated with topical nystatin. Most otic preparations also contain an acidifying agent(s) and a topical steroid to reduce the inflammation.

Individuals prone to otitis externa who are frequently exposed to water may benefit from any of several commercially available ear plugs and other devices which prevent water from entering the canal. A recent comparison of seven different ear protectors used by a group of swimmers found the most effective plugs to be cotton wool coated in paraffin jelly (373). Prevention may be enhanced further by the use of acidifying drops and/or drying ear drops before and after swimming. Domeboro, Swim Ear, Aqua Ear, Ear Magic, and VoSol otic drops are several such agents (393). Alternatively, the user may make his or her own preparation by mixing white vinegar with 70% alcohol. Controversy exists with regard to swimming with tympanostomy tubes in place (215, 280, 296). While some experts advocate the use of protective ear plugs or avoidance of water immersion, others have recommended pre- and postexposure antibiotic otic drops. A third group utilizing data revealing that the incidence of otitis media was no greater in swimmers with tympanostomy tubes in place who swam without protection than those without tympanostomy tubes has recommended that no ear protection or instillation of pre- and postexposure antibiotic drops is necessary (155, 215, 263, 280, 480). Until this matter is clarified, it may be prudent to advocate some means of protection against infection in prone individuals who are frequently exposed to water (393).

VIRAL HEPATITIS AND OTHER VIRAL INFECTIONS ASSOCIATED WITH WATER AND SHELLFISH

Marine samples of water have been estimated to yield between 5×10^6 and 15×10^6 total viruses per ml (33). Even though the majority of these viruses are nonpathogenic in humans, viral agents associated with hepatitis and gastroenteritis are known to be present in and capable of producing disease through contaminated water (111, 112). Samples of water taken off the Texas Gulf Coast have revealed the presence of enteroviruses such as coxsackievirus, echovirus, poliovirus, and hepatitis A virus (152). These enteroviruses were detected in over 40% of waters deemed safe for recreational use by fecal coliform standards. Thirty-five percent of waters approved for shellfish harvesting yielded enteroviruses (152). Enteroviruses have been reported to survive 2 to 130 days in seawater in laboratory studies (294), and possibly up to 18 months (165). Temperature seems to be the most important factor, with many enteroviruses able to survive for months at temperatures below 10°C (153). Marine sediments also protect against virus inactivation, probably by reducing the rate of thermal inactivation (153).

Although controversy exists, swimming areas have been suggested to be involved in the spread of some common viral illnesses (67, 388). In Wisconsin, a statistically significant increase in the use of public beaches by children with documented enteroviral illness was noted compared to that by children without enteroviral illness (67, 115, 388). Several other reports have similarly suggested increased enteroviral infections in swimmers using public swimming areas (58, 67, 71, 388; J. W. Mosely, presented at the Discharge of Sewage from Sea Outfalls International Symposium, London, United Kingdom, 1974). A survey of oysters contaminated by enteroviruses in Japan found nearly identical viruses in sick children in the immediate area. It was suggested that water and oyster contamination ultimately depends on the prevalence of enteric viral infections in local inhabitants (483). In addition to

more common and less severe enteroviral illnesses, an outbreak of hepatitis A involving 20
campers in Louisiana was associated with
swimming in a contaminated swimming pool
(286).

Shellfish harvested from contaminated waters have been implicated in numerous outbreaks of food-borne illness (458). They
spread disease by virtue of their ability to filter
large amounts of water, retain filtered products
in the gills and alimentary tract, and accumulate them in the liver. Shellfish have the
ability to concentrate hepatitis A virus to up
to 15 times the level in the immediate water
(202). Commercially harvested waters are
monitored for contamination through the use
of bacterial counts. Although this method effectively decreases the incidence of illness related to contaminated shellfish, there is not a
reliable correlation between bacterial counts
and the presence of pathogenic viruses (152).
Several methods of detecting viruses or viral
particles have been investigated, although the
use of any one method of testing may not be
sufficient enough to provide accurate mea-
surements (483). Furthermore, viral testing has
proven to be costly and time-consuming
(174). Control measures have included the
regulation of drainage effluent into monitored
areas, supervision of drainage from commercial fishing boats, frequent testing of water and
shellfish from harvest areas for fecal coliforms
and other bacteria, closing of contaminated
waters, and removal of contaminated shellfish
from markets (174). Depuration measures in
which bacteria and viruses are removed by being bathed in rapidly circulating salt water
treated continuously by ultraviolet radiation
for up to 72 h have decreased the incidence
of food-borne outbreaks, although this process
is not infallible (132, 462). Outbreaks of viral
diseases have been attributed to depurated
shellfish (182). Prevention of illness additionally relies on public education, particularly in
regard to proper cooking of shellfish. It has
been shown that it takes up to 6 min of steam-
ing for the internal temperature of clams to

reach that of the immediate surrounding
(250). Clams open their shells in less than 1
min. Hepatitis A virus has been shown to be
inactivated by heating at 85°C for 1 min and
partially inactivated at 60°C for 60 min (290,
395). Recent evidence suggests that microwaving may be beneficial in inactivating hepatitis A virus; however, further studies are
needed (300).

Hepatitis A Virus

Hepatitis A was first linked to the ingestion of
raw shellfish in Sweden in 1956; 629 oyster-
associated cases were documented (377). The
first cases of hepatitis A linked to raw shellfish
consumption in the United States occurred in
1961; both clams and oysters were involved
(356). Hepatitis A virus caused <7% of the
224 recorded outbreaks of waterborne disease
in the United States between 1971 and 1978;
it caused none of the outbreaks recorded in
1981 (179, 364). During 1983 to 1988, the
incidence of reported cases of hepatitis A increased from 9.2 to 10.9 cases per 100,000
persons, which represented the first increase in
the frequency of hepatitis A in more than a
decade (79, 80, 83, 84). In 1988, 26,600 cases
of hepatitis A were reported in the United
States, 7.3% of which were associated with
food-borne or waterborne outbreaks (80, 84).
In August 1988, 61 persons developed hepatitis A after having ingested oysters illegally
harvested from coastal waters off Bay County
(78, 122, 123). That same year, the largest
documented epidemic to date occurred in
Shanghai, China, where more than 288,000
people developed hepatitis A after ingesting
raw or improperly cooked clams (174, 427).

Shellfish implicated in cases of hepatitis A
include oysters, clams, cockles, and mussels
(11). In addition, the illness has been traced to
contaminated lettuce, raspberries, ice-slush
beverages, and community water sources (78,
367, 379, 458). Sporadic cases also occur,
and the disease is probably underreported.
Restaurant-related outbreaks due to poor personal hygiene by infected food preparers have

#24

also been noted (11, 300). In many cases, a source for outbreaks is never determined (78, 300).

The incubation period ranges from 3 to 6 weeks. Presentation consists of a prodrome of fatigue, malaise, anorexia, nausea, and right upper quadrant discomfort. Dark urine subsequently develops, with liver enlargement and biochemical evidence of hepatitis. Icteric disease may be prolonged in adults, lasting 4 to 6 weeks; fulminant hepatic failure is rare, and chronic disease or a carrier state does not develop. Secondary cases in families may be seen. Attack rates vary, ranging from 10 to 97%, with higher rates associated with increasing dose and age (140, 458). A vaccine is currently available for use in patients over 2 years of age (87).

Norwalk Virus

Norwalk virus (norovirus) is the most common infectious cause of acute gastroenteritis following shellfish ingestion (140). Named after the town in Ohio where an outbreak of acute gastroenteritis occurred in 1968, this virus was not identified until 1972, by immuno-electron microscopy of bacterium-free stool isolates from the 1968 outbreak (128). The particles measured 27 nm long and were noted to be more visible when present in clusters covered with antibody. They were also noted to aggregate with convalescent- but not acute-phase sera from patients with gastroenteritis. A serum radioimmunoassay for IgM antibody to the Norwalk virus or the demonstration of a fourfold rise in titer, utilizing paired acute- and convalescent-phase sera, is more sensitive and specific than electron microscopy (140, 171, 231). Using similar methods, the Norwalk virus was identified as the cause of 42% of the 74 outbreaks of acute nonbacterial gastroenteritis investigated by the CDC between 1976 and 1980 (111, 112, 179, 231). Six additional outbreaks involving more than 820 persons were noted between 1981 and 1983 (111, 112). Drinking water and recreational water used for swimming were the vehicles of transmission in most of these earlier outbreaks. Contamination by human sewage was the most likely explanation, although this was never proven. Shellfish-associated Norwalk viral illness was first recognized in Australia in 1978, when 2,000 people developed acute gastroenteritis following raw oyster ingestion (323). Immuno-electron microscopy of 93 stool specimens revealed the 27-nm viral particle in 39% of those examined. An additional, as yet unclarified 22-nm viral particle was also identified in 50% of the specimens examined. In 1982, 103 well-documented outbreaks of oyster- and clam-associated illness involving 1,017 persons were attributed to the Norwalk virus in New York State in 1982 (318). Seroconversion to Norwalk virus antibody or a positive response for IgM antibody to the virus (or both) was noted in five of seven outbreaks; clams and oysters revealed Norwalk virus antibody by radioimmunoassay in four of six specimens examined, including clams and oysters from two of the outbreaks. Coliform tests of the waters from which the shellfish were harvested were well within acceptable limits. In 2002, 21 outbreaks of acute gastroenteritis due to Norwalk virus occurred on 17 cruise ships, demonstrating how easily Norwalk virus can be transmitted from person to person in a closed environment (90).

Incubation times have ranged from 24 to 48 h in most recorded outbreaks, with a duration of illness ranging from 2 to 60 h (mean, 12 to 60 h). Symptoms have consisted of nausea, vomiting, diarrhea, abdominal cramps, and headache, with vomiting being more prominent than diarrhea in children and diarrhea being more common than vomiting in adults. Fever, myalgia, chills, and upper respiratory complaints, such as a sore throat, cough, and runny nose, were also noted on occasion. The disease is rarely severe enough to require hospitalization, and no fatalities have been recorded. Secondary spread is quite common.

The antibody response is not entirely understood. Antibody prevalence appears to peak within the first 5 decades of life, reaching a prevalence in the United States of 50%. Children tend to acquire antibody earlier in less developed countries. Individuals exposed to the Norwalk agent in volunteer studies who do not become ill have been shown to not develop an antibody response. When immunity develops, it is specific towards the Norwalk virus and short-lived, lasting from 6 weeks to 2 months (128).

The mechanism by which the Norwalk virus causes diarrhea is not known. Related agents include the Hawaii, Snow Mountain, and Taunton agents, named after the places they were first described. Only the Snow Mountain agent has been associated with waterborne transmission. Illnesses caused by these Norwalk-like agents are indistinguishable from that due to the Norwalk agent. These other agents are antigenically distinct, and antibodies are not cross-protective (458).

Hepatitis E Virus

Hepatitis E virus is the only known cause of enterically transmitted non-A, non-B hepatitis. Hepatitis E virus is largely waterborne and has been responsible for epidemics of infectious hepatitis in parts of Asia, Indonesia, Africa, and Mexico (162). Previously known as enterically transmitted non-A, non-B hepatitis, illness due to hepatitis E virus was first documented in New Delhi, India, in 1955, when 29,000 cases of icteric hepatitis were identified following fecal contamination of the city's water supply (454). A similar epidemic occurred in 1975 in Ahmedabad, India, when the city's water supply became fecally contaminated as well (413). Both epidemics were thought to be due to hepatitis A virus until retrospectively analyzed paired serum samples from documented cases revealed in 1980 that neither hepatitis A nor B virus was responsible for the epidemics (471). It now appears that in developing countries, more than 50% of acute viral hepatitis cases are caused by agents other than hepatitis A or B virus (53). Numerous epidemics of hepatitis E have been reported in Pakistan, Bangladesh, Nepal, Burma, Borneo, Algeria, Somalia, Sudan, Ivory Coast, Mexico, China, Egypt, Ethiopia, and the former Soviet Union (162, 444). Imported cases have been reported in the United States (22a). One case acquired in San Jose, CA, has been described (255).

The incubation period appears to be 2 to 9 weeks, with an average of 6 weeks (53). Attack rates have been variable, with the highest rates noted in young to middle-aged adults (15 to 40 years old). The clinical presentation is that of a self-limiting disease resembling infection due to hepatitis A virus. Chronic liver disease or persistent viremia has not been reported. Mortality has been reported to be between 0.5 and 3.0% in the general population. Pregnant women in the third trimester of pregnancy have an unusually high mortality of up to 20%, for unknown reasons. In contrast, pregnant women infected with hepatitis A virus have a mortality rate ranging from 3 to 8%.

The diagnosis of infection due to hepatitis E virus has primarily been based on the identification of the virus in stool samples by immuno-electron microscopy. Hepatitis E virus is a spherical, nonenveloped virus 32 to 34 nm in size with a genome consisting of a single strand of polyadenylated RNA (52, 53). Identification of viral particles in clinical samples has been inconsistent, possibly due to proteolytic degradation or susceptibility to freezing and pelleting (53). Cynomolgus monkeys and, more recently, owl monkeys have been shown to be promising animal models of the serologic response to infection by hepatitis E virus (436). Radioimmunoassay or enzyme-linked immunoassay for hepatitis E virus antigen, using acute-phase or convalescent-phase IgM or IgG, has previously met with little success, possibly due to the lability of the virus (53). More recently, an enzyme-linked immunosorbent assay based on clonal recombinant hepatitis E virus antigen was developed to detect hepatitis E virus IgG and IgM antibodies (162). Preliminary results are encouraging.

Rotavirus and Small Round Virus

Rotavirus is a common viral pathogen responsible for a large percentage of childhood diarrheal illnesses. Rotavirus may be responsible for up to 50% of all cases of diarrhea in hospitalized children and 10 to 20% of cases of diarrhea in the community. By the third year of life, 90% of children have been exposed to rotavirus and develop antibody. Seventy percent of adults have antibody to rotavirus (476). Adult epidemics of diarrheal illness due to rotavirus in the absence of contact with children have been reported (46, 295). Waterborne transmission of rotavirus occurs and was first described in Africa in 1978 (364). In 1981, an outbreak of gastroenteritis due to waterborne transmission of rotavirus, involving 1,761 cases, occurred in Colorado (179).

Small round viruses are poorly understood uncultivable viruses which have been linked to shellfish-related epidemics of gastroenteritis (12, 157). They are morphologically distinct from other gastroenteritis viruses by electron microscopy and antigenically distinct from the Norwalk and Norwalk-like viruses. Asymptomatic individuals have been shown to shed the virus in some instances.

PRACTICAL TIPS

- When visiting coastal regions, be aware of environmental conditions and any current or recent restrictions that may be or have been in place, such as red tide warnings or sewage contamination.
- Recognize the signs and symptoms of seafood-related illnesses and be sure to obtain seafood only from a reputable source.
- Swim in marked areas and never dive alone.
- Enjoy the marine aquatic environment from a distance and do not disturb its natural features; leave it exactly as you find it so that others may admire its beauty as well.
- Plan ahead by identifying the nearest medical facility and keep a first aid kit handy; make sure to share any history of recent seafood ingestion or marine aquatic travel with any medical caregivers if injured or ill.

REFERENCES

1. **Abbott, S. L., C. Powers, C. A. Kaysner, Y. Takeda, M. Ishibashi, S. W. Joseph, and J. M. Janda.** 1989. Emergence of a restricted bioserovar of *Vibrio parahaemolyticus* as the predominant cause of vibrio-associated gastroenteritis on the West Coast of the United States and Mexico. *J. Clin. Microbiol.* **27:**2891–2893.
2. **Adams, W. N., and J. J. Miescier.** 1980. Commentary on AOAC method for paralytic shellfish poisoning. *J. Assoc. Off. Anal. Chem.* **63:**1336–1343.
3. **Aldova, E., K. Laznickova, and E. Stepankova.** 1968. Isolation of nonagglutinable vibrios from an enteritis outbreak in Czechoslovakia. *J. Infect. Dis.* **118:**25–31.
4. **Ali, M. B., and M. J. Raff.** 1990. Primary Vibrio vulnificus sepsis in Kentucky. *South. Med. J.* **83:**356–357.
5. **Anderson, D. M., J. J. Sullivan, and B. Reguera.** 1989. Paralytic shellfish poisoning in Northwest Spain: the toxicity of the dinoflagellate Gymnodinium catenatum. *Toxicon* **27:**665–674.
6. **Anonymous.** 1989. Case records of the Massachusetts General Hospital. Weekly clinicopathological exercises. Case 41-1989. A 65-year-old man with fever, bullae, erythema, and edema of the leg after wading in brackish water. *N. Engl. J. Med.* **321:**1029–1038.
7. **Anonymous.** 1991. Food safety. Paralytic shellfish poisoning. *Wkly. Epidemiol. Rec.* **66:**185–187.
8. **Anonymous.** 1988. Mycobacteria, p. 535–572. *In* E. W. Koneman, S. D. Allen, V. R. Dowell, Jr., W. M. Janda, H. M. Sommers, and W. C. Winn, Jr. (ed.), *Color Atlas and Textbook of Diagnostic Microbiology,* 3rd ed. J. B. Lippincott Co., Philadelphia, PA.
9. **Anonymous.** 1990. Paralytic shellfish poisoning (red tide). *Epidemiol. Bull.* **11:**9.
10. **Anonymous.** 1990. Shuck your oysters with care. *Lancet* **336:**215–216.
11. **Appleton, H.** 1990. Foodborne viruses. *Lancet* **336:**1362–1364.
12. **Appleton, H., and M. S. Pereira.** 1977. A possible virus etiology in outbreaks of food-poisoning from cockles. *Lancet* **i:**780.
13. **Arita, M., T. Takeda, T. Honda, and T. Miwatani.** 1986. Purification and characterization of *Vibrio cholerae* non-O1 heat-stable enterotoxin. *Infect. Immun.* **52:**45–49

14. **Aronson, J. D.** 1926. Spontaneous tuberculosis in saltwater fish. *J. Infect. Dis.* **39:**315–320.

15. **Asai, S., J. J. Krzanowski, and W. H. Anderson.** 1982. Effects of the toxin of red tide, Ptychodiscus brevis, on canine tracheal smooth muscle: a possible new asthma-triggering mechanism. *J. Allergy Clin. Immunol.* **69:**418–428.

16. **Auerbach, P. S.** 1984. Hazardous marine animals. *Emerg. Med. Clin. N. Am.* **2:**531–544.

17. **Auerbach, P. S.** 1991. Marine envenomations. *N. Engl. J. Med.* **325:**486–493.

18. **Auerbach, P. S., and B. Halstead.** 1982. Marine hazards: attacks and envenomations. *J. Emerg. Nurs.* **8:**115–122.

19. **Auerbach, P. S., and B. W. Halstead.** 1989. Hazardous aquatic life, p. 933–1028. *In* P. S. Auerbach and E. C. Geehr (ed.), *Management of Wilderness and Environmental Emergencies.* C. V. Mosby, St. Louis, MO.

20. **Auerbach, P. S., D. M. Yajko, and P. S. Nassos.** 1987. Bacteriology of the marine environment: implications for clinical therapy. *Ann. Emerg. Med.* **16:**643–649.

21. **Baden, D. G.** 1983. Marine food-borne dinoflagellate toxins. *Int. Rev. Cytol.* **82:**99–150.

22. **Baden, D. G., and T. J. Mende.** 1982. Toxicity of two toxins from the Florida red tide marine dinoflagellate Ptychodiscus brevis. *Toxicon* **20:**457–461.

22a.**Bader, T., K. Krawczynski, and M. Favorov.** 1991. Letter. *N. Engl. J. Med.* **325:**1659.

23. **Bagnis, R., F. Berglund, P. F. Elias, G. J. van Esch, B. W. Halstead, and K. Kojima.** 1970. Problems of toxicants in marine food products. I. Marine biotoxins. *Bull. W. H. O.* **42:**69–88.

24. **Bagnis, R., S. Chanteau, and S. Chungue.** 1980. Origins of ciguatera fish poisoning: a new dinoflagellate, Gambierdiscus toxicus adachi and fukoyo, definitely involved as a causal agent. *Toxicon* **18:**199–208.

25. **Bagnis, R., T. Kuberski, and S. Laugier.** 1979. Clinical observations on 3,009 cases of ciguatera (fish poisoning) in the South Pacific. *Am. J. Trop. Med. Hyg.* **28:**1067–1073.

26. **Baker, J. A., and W. A. Hagan.** 1942. Tuberculosis of Mexican platyfish (Platypoecilus maculatus). *J. Infect. Dis.* **70:**248–252.

27. **Baldridge, H. D., and J. Williams.** 1969. Shark attack: feeding or fighting? *Milit. Med.* **134:**130–133.

28. **Barker, W. H., Jr.** 1974. Vibrio parahaemolyticus outbreaks in the United States. *Lancet* **i:**551–554.

29. **Bart, K. J., Z. Huq, and M. Khan.** 1970. Seroepidemiologic studies during a simultaneous epidemic of infection with El Tor, Ogawa and classical Inaba Vibrio cholerae. *J. Infect. Dis.* **12**(Suppl.)**:**17–24.

30. **Baumann, L., A. L. Furniss, and J. V. Lee.** 1984. Genus I. Vibrio Pacini 1854, 411, p. 518–538. *In* N. R. Krieg and J. G. Holt (ed.), *Bergey's Manual of Systematic Bacteriology,* vol. 1. The Williams & Wilkins Co., Baltimore, MD.

31. **Becker, G. D., and G. J. Parell.** 1979. Otolaryngologic aspects of scuba diving. *Otolaryngol. Head Neck Surg.* **87:**569–572.

32. **Becker, K., K. Southwick, J. Reardon, R. Berg, and J. N. MacCormack.** 2001. Histamine poisoning associated with eating tuna burgers. *JAMA* **285:**1327–1330.

33. **Bergh, O., K. Y. Borsheim, G. Bratbak, and M. Heldal.** 1989. High abundance of viruses found in aquatic environments. *Nature* **340:**467–468.

34. **Binta, G. M., T. B. Tjaberg, P. N. Nyaga, and M. Vallard.** 1982. Market fish hygiene in Kenya. *J. Hyg.* **89:**47–52.

35. **Blake, P. A.** 1983. Vibrios on the half shell: what the walrus and the carpenter didn't know. *Ann. Intern. Med.* **99:**558–559.

36. **Blake, P. A., D. T. Allegra, J. D. Snyder, T. J. Barrett, L. McFarland, C. T. Caraway, J. C. Feeley, J. P. Craig, J. V. Lee, N. D. Puhr, and R. A. Feldman.** 1980. Cholera—a possible endemic focus in the United States. *N. Engl. J. Med.* **302:**305–309.

37. **Blake, P. A., M. H. Merson, and R. E. Weaver.** 1979. Disease caused by a marine vibrio: clinical characteristics and epidemiology. *N. Engl. J. Med.* **300:**1–5.

38. **Blake, P. A., R. E. Weaver, and D. G. Hollis.** 1980. Diseases of humans (other than cholera) caused by vibrios. *Ann. Rev. Microbiol.* **34:**341–367.

39. **Blakesley, M.** 1983. Scombroid poisoning: prompt resolution of symptoms with cimetidine. *Ann. Emerg. Med.* **12:**104–106.

40. **Blanc, M. H., A. Zwahlen, and M. Robert.** 1977. Symptoms of shellfish poisoning. *N. Engl. J. Med.* **196:**287–288.

41. **Bockemuhl, J., K. Roch, B. Wohlers, V. Aleksic, S. Aleksik, and R. Wokatsch.** 1986. Seasonal distribution of facultatively enteropathogenic vibrios (Vibrio cholerae, Vibrio mimicus, Vibrio parahaemolyticus) in the freshwater of the Elbe River at Hamburg. *J. Appl. Bacteriol.* **60:**435–442.

42. **Bode, R. B., P. R. Brayton, R. R. Colwell, F. M. Russo, and W. E. Bullock.** 1986. A new Vibrio species, Vibrio cincinnatiensis, causing meningitis: successful treatment in an adult. *Ann. Intern. Med.* **104:**55–56.

43. **Bolen, J., S. A. Zamiska, and W. B. Greenough.** 1974. Clinical features in enteritis due to

Vibrio parahaemolyticus. *Am. J. Med.* **57:**638–641.

44. **Bolleta, G., I. Bacchiocchi, G. Durante, and C. Maffei.** 1990. Letter. *Arch. Intern. Med.* **150:**2425.

45. **Bonner, J. R., A. S. Coker, C. R. Berryman, and H. M. Pollock.** 1983. Spectrum of vibrio infections in a Gulf Coast community. *Ann. Intern. Med.* **99:**464–469.

46. **Bonsdorff, C. H., T. Hovi, and P. Makela.** 1978. Rotavirus infections in adults in association with acute gastroenteritis. *J. Med. Virol.* **2:**21–28.

47. **Borison, H. L., S. Ellis, and L. E. McCarthy.** 1980. Central respiratory and circulatory effects of Gymnodinium breve toxin in anaesthetized cats. *Br. J. Pharmacol.* **70:**249–256.

48. **Bowdre, J. H., J. H. Hull, and D. M. Cochetto.** 1983. Antibiotic efficacy against Vibrio vulnificus in the mouse: superiority of tetracycline. *J. Pharmacol. Exp. Ther.* **225:**595–598.

49. **Bower, D., R. Hart, P. Matthews, and M. Howden.** 1981. Nonprotein neurotoxins. *Clin. Toxicol.* **18:**813–863.

50. **Bowman, P.** 1984. Amitriptylline and ciguatera. *Med. J. Aust.* **143:**802.

51. **Braback, M., K. Riesbeck, and A. Forsgren.** 2002. Susceptibilities of *Mycobacterium marinum* to gatifloxacin, gemifloxacin, levofloxacin, linezolid, moxifloxacin, telithromycin, and quinupristin-dalfopristin (Synercid) compared to its susceptibilities to reference macrolides and quinolones. *Antimicrob. Agents Chemother.* **46:**1114–1116.

52. **Bradley, D., A. Andjaparidze, and E. H. Cook.** 1988. Aetiological agent of enterically transmitted non-A, non-B hepatitis. *J. Gen. Virol.* **69:**731–738.

53. **Bradley, D. W.** 1990. Enterically-transmitted non-A, non-B hepatitis. *Br. Med. Bull.* **46:**442–461.

54. **Brayton, P. R., R. B. Bode, R. R. Colwell, M. T. MacDonnell, H. L. Hall, D. J. Grimes, P. A. West, and T. N. Bryant.** 1986. *Vibrio cincinnatiensis* sp. nov., a new human pathogen. *J. Clin. Microbiol.* **23:**104–108.

55. **Brenner, D. J., F. W. Hickman-Brenner, and J. V. Lee.** 1983. *Vibrio furnissii* (formerly aerogenic biogroup of *Vibrio fluvialis*), a new species isolated from human feces and the environment. *J. Clin. Microbiol.* **18:**816–824.

56. **Brennt, C. E., A. C. Wright, S. K. Dutta, and J. G. Morris, Jr.** 1991. Growth of Vibrio vulnificus in serum from alcoholics: association with high transferrin iron saturation. *J. Infect. Dis.* **164:**1030–1032.

57. **Brown, C. K., and S. M. Shepherd.** 1992. Marine trauma, envenomations, and intoxications. *Emerg. Med. Clin. N. Am.* **10:**385–408.

58. **Brown, J. M., E. A. Campbell, and A. D. Rickards.** 1987. Sewage pollution of bathing water. *Lancet* **ii:**1208–1209.

59. **Brown, J. W., III, and C. V. Sanders.** 1987. Mycobacterium marinum infections: a problem of recognition, not therapy? *Arch. Intern. Med.* **147:**817–818.

60. **Bruckner-Tuderman, L., and A. A. Blank.** 1985. Unusual cutaneous dissemination of a tropical fish tank granuloma *Cutis* **36:**405–408.

61. **Bryan, F. L., H. W. Anderson, and O. D. Cook.** 1987. *Procedures to Investigate Foodborne Illness*, 4th ed., p. 67. International Association of Milk, Food, and Environmental Sanitarians, Ames, IA.

62. **Bryant, R. G.** 1983. Food microbiology update. Emerging foodborne pathogens. *Appl. Biochem. Biotechnol.* **8:**437–454.

63. **Buck, J. D., S. Spotte, and J. J. Gadbaw, Jr.** 1984. Bacteriology of the teeth from a great white shark: potential medical implications for shark bite victims. *J. Clin. Microbiol.* **20:**849–851.

64. **Burgess, G.** 2004. *ISAF 2003 Worldwide Shark Attack Summary.* International Shark Attack File, Gainesville, FL. http://www.flmnh.ufl.edu/fish/Sharks/Statistics/2003attacksummary.htm.

65. **Burnett, J. W.** 1990. Some natural jellyfish toxins, p. 333–335. *In* S. Hall and G. Strichartz (ed.), *Marine Toxins: Origin, Structure, and Molecular Pharmacology.* American Chemical Society, Washington, DC.

66. **Burnett, J. W., and G. J. Calton.** 1987. Jellyfish envenomation syndromes updated. *Ann. Emerg. Med.* **16:**1000–1005.

67. **Cabelli, V. J., A. P. DuFour, and L. J. McCabe.** 1982. Swimming associated gastroenteritis and water quality. *Am. J. Epidemiol.* **115:**606–616.

68. **Carson, R. L.** 1961. *The Sea around Us*, p. 28–36. Oxford University Press, New York, NY.

69. **Cassissi, N., A. Cohn, and T. Davidson.** 1972. Diffuse otitis externa: clinical and microbiologic findings in the course of a multicenter study on a new otic solution. *Ann. Otol. Rhinol. Laryngol.* **86**(Suppl.)**:**39.

69a. **Center for Science in the Public Interest.** 2001. *Outbreak Alert! Closing the Gaps in Our Federal Food-Safety Net*, p. 1. Center for Science in the Public Interest, Washington, DC.

70. **Centers for Disease Control.** 1969. Follow-up outbreak of gastroenteritis during a tour of the orient—Alaska. *MMWR Morb. Mortal. Wkly. Rep.* **18:**168.

71. **Centers for Disease Control.** 1979. Gastroenteritis associated with lake swimming. *MMWR Morb. Mortal. Wkly. Rep.* **28:**413.

72. **Centers for Disease Control.** 1969. An outbreak of acute gastroenteritis during a tour of the orient—Alaska. *MMWR Morb. Mortal. Wkly. Rep.* **18**:150.

73. **Centers for Disease Control.** 1978. Paralytic shellfish poisoning—Washington. *MMWR Morb. Mortal. Wkly. Rep.* **27**:416–417.

74. **Centers for Disease Control.** 1988. ACIP: cholera vaccine. *MMWR Morb. Mortal. Wkly. Rep.* **37**:617–624.

75. **Centers for Disease Control.** 1983. Annual mussel quarantine—California. *MMWR Morb. Mortal. Wkly. Rep.* **32**:281.

76. **Centers for Disease Control.** 1992. Cercarial dermatitis outbreak in a state park—Delaware, 1991. *MMWR Morb. Mortal. Wkly. Rep.* **41**:225–228.

77. **Centers for Disease Control.** 1991. Cholera—Peru, 1991. *MMWR Morb. Mortal. Wkly. Rep.* **40**:108–110.

78. **Centers for Disease Control.** 1990. Foodborne hepatitis A—Alaska, Florida, North Carolina, Washington. *MMWR Morb. Mortal. Wkly. Rep.* **39**:228–232.

79. **Centers for Disease Control.** 1987. *Hepatitis Surveillance Report No. 51,* p. 10–17. U.S. Department of Health and Human Services, Atlanta, GA.

80. **Centers for Disease Control.** 1989. *Hepatitis Surveillance Report No. 52,* p. 19–21. U.S. Department of Health and Human Services, Atlanta, GA.

81. **Centers for Disease Control.** 1991. Paralytic shellfish poisoning—Massachusetts and Alaska, 1990. *MMWR Morb. Mortal. Wkly. Rep.* **40**:157–161. (Erratum, **40**:242.)

82. **Centers for Disease Control.** 1986. Restaurant-associated scombroid fish poisoning—Alabama, Tennessee. *MMWR Morb. Mortal. Wkly. Rep.* **35**:264–265.

83. **Centers for Disease Control.** 1987. Summary of notifiable diseases, United States. *MMWR Morb. Mortal. Wkly. Rep.* **36**:54.

84. **Centers for Disease Control.** 1989. Table III. Cases of specified notifiable diseases, United States. *MMWR Morb. Mortal. Wkly. Rep.* **37**:803.

85. **Centers for Disease Control.** 1991. Update: cholera outbreak—Peru, Ecuador, and Colombia. *MMWR Morb. Mortal. Wkly. Rep.* **40**:108–110.

86. **Centers for Disease Control and Prevention.** 1995. Cholera associated with food transported from El Salvador—Indiana, 1994. *MMWR Morb. Mortal. Wkly. Rep.* **44**:385–386.

87. **Centers for Disease Control and Prevention.** 1997. Hepatitis A vaccination programs in communities with high rates of hepatitis A. *MMWR Morb. Mortal. Wkly. Rep.* **46**:600–603.

88. **Centers for Disease Control and Prevention.** 1993. Imported cholera associated with a newly described toxigenic Vibrio cholerae O139 strain—California, 1993. *MMWR Morb. Mortal. Wkly. Rep.* **42**:501–503.

89. **Centers for Disease Control and Prevention.** 1998. Outbreak of Vibrio parahaemolyticus infections associated with eating raw oysters—Pacific Northwest, 1997. *MMWR Morb. Mortal. Wkly. Rep.* **47**:457–462.

90. **Centers for Disease Control and Prevention.** 2002. Outbreaks of gastroenteritis associated with noroviruses on cruise ships—United States, 2002. *MMWR Morb. Mortal. Wkly. Rep.* **51**:1112–1115.

91. **Centers for Disease Control and Prevention.** 1996. Surveillance for foodborne-disease outbreaks—United States, 1988–1992. *MMWR Morb. Mortal. Wkly. Rep.* **45**:1–66.

92. **Centers for Disease Control and Prevention.** 2000. Surveillance for possible estuary-associated syndrome—six states, 1998–1999. *MMWR Morb. Mortal. Wkly. Rep.* **49**:372–373.

93. **Centers for Disease Control and Prevention.** 1996. Tetrodotoxin poisoning associated with eating puffer fish transported from Japan—California, 1996. *MMWR Morb. Mortal. Wkly. Rep.* **45**:389–391.

94. **Centers for Disease Control and Prevention.** 2002. Update: neurologic illness associated with eating Florida pufferfish, 2002. *MMWR Morb. Mortal. Wkly. Rep.* **51**:414–416.

95. **Centers for Disease Control and Prevention.** 1993. Vibrio vulnificus infections associated with raw oyster consumption—Florida, 1981–1992. *MMWR Morb. Mortal. Wkly. Rep.* **42**:405–407.

96. **Chatterjee, G. C., and S. K. Das.** 1965. Purification and some properties of Vibrio El Tor phospholipase B. *Enzyme* **28**:346–354.

97. **Cheng, H.-S., S. O. Chua, J.-S. Hung, and K.-K. Yip.** 1991. Creatine kinase MB elevation in paralytic shellfish poisoning. *Chest* **99**:1032–1033.

98. **Chow, S. P., F. K. Ip, and J. H. K. Lau.** 1987. Mycobacterium marinum infection of the hand and wrist. *J. Bone Joint Surg.* **69A**:1161–1168.

99. **Chowdhury, M. A. R., K. M. S. Aziz, Z. Rahim, and B. A. Kay.** 1986. Toxigenicity and drug sensitivity of Vibrio mimicus isolated from fresh water prawns (Macrobrachium malcolmsonii) in Bangladesh. *J. Diarrhoeal Dis. Res.* **4**:37–40.

100. **Chowdhury, M. A. R., H. Yamanaka, S. Miyoshi, K. M. S. Aziz, and S. Shinoda.** 1989. Ecology of *Vibrio mimicus* in aquatic en-

vironments. *Appl. Environ. Microbiol.* **55**:2073–2078.

101. **Christenson, B., M. Soler, L. Nieves, and L. Souchet.** 1997. Septicemia due to a non-O:1, non-O:139 Vibrio cholerae. *Bol. Asoc. Med. P. R.* **89**:31–32.

102. **Clark, R. B., H. Spector, D. M. Friedman, K. J. Oldrati, C. L. Young, and S. C. Nelson.** 1990. Osteomyelitis and synovitis produced by *Mycobacterium marinum* in a fisherman. *J. Clin. Microbiol.* **28**:2570–2572.

103. **Coffey, J. A., R. L. Harris, M. L. Rutledge, M. W. Bradshaw, and T. W. Williams.** 1986. Vibrio damsela: another potentially virulent marine vibrio. *J. Infect. Dis.* **153**:800–802.

104. **Collins, C. H., J. M. Grange, W. C. Noble, and M. D. Yates.** 1985. Mycobacterium marinum infections in man. *J. Hyg. Camb.* **94**:135–149.

105. **Collins, C. H., and H. C. Uttley.** 1988. In-vitro activity of seventeen antimicrobial compounds against seven species of mycobacteria. *J. Antimicrob. Chemother.* **22**:857–861.

106. **Colwell, R. R., R. J. Seidler, J. Kaper, S. W. Joseph, S. Garges, H. Lockman, D. Maneval, H. Bradford, N. Roberts, E. Emmers, I. Huq, and A. Huq.** 1981. Occurrence of *Vibrio cholerae* serogroup O1 in Maryland and Louisiana estuaries. *Appl. Environ. Microbiol.* **41**:555–558.

107. **Colwell, R. R., P. A. West, D. Maneval, E. F. Remmers, E. L. Elliott, and N. E. Carlson.** 1984. Ecology of pathogenic vibrios in Cheapeake Bay, p. 367–387. *In* R. R. Colwell (ed.), *Vibrios in the Environment.* John Wiley & Sons, Inc., New York, NY.

108. **Connolly, J.** 1997. Foodborne illness from seafood appears to be increasing. *Infect. Dis. News* **10**:6,10.

109. **Cook, J.** 1777. *A Voyage Towards the South Pole and Round the World,* vol. 2. Strahan and Cadell, London, United Kingdom.

110. **Cover, T. L., B. E. Dunn, R. T. Ellison, and M. J. Blaser.** 1989. Vibrio cholerae wound infection acquired in Colorado. *J. Infect. Dis.* **160**:1083.

111. **Craun, G. F.** 1986. Introduction, p. 3–11. *In* G. F. Craun (ed.), *Waterborne Diseases in the United States.* CRC Press, Boca Raton, FL.

112. **Craun, G. F.** 1986. Recent statistics of waterborne outbreaks (1981–1983), p. 161–168. *In* G. F. Craun (ed.), *Waterborne Diseases in the United States.* CRC Press, Boca Raton, FL.

113. **Cunningham, L. W., R. A. Promisloff, and A. V. Cichelli.** 1991. Pulmonary infiltrates associated with Vibrio vulnificus septicemia. *J. Am. Osteopath. Assoc.* **91**:84–86.

114. **Dakin, W. P. H., D. J. Howell, R. G. A. Sutton, M. F. O'Keefe, and P. Thomas.** 1974. Gastroenteritis due to non-agglutinable (non-cholera) vibrios. *Med. J. Aust.* **2**:487–490.

115. **D'Alessio, D. J., T. E. Minor, and C. I. Allen.** 1981. A study of the proportions of swimmers among well controls and children with enterovirus-like illness shedding or not shedding an enterovirus. *Am. J. Epidemiol.* **113**:533–541.

116. **Daniels, N., L. MacKinnon, and R. Bishop.** 2000. Vibrio parahaemolyticus infections in the United States, 1973–1998. *J. Infect. Dis.* **181**:1661–1666.

117. **Datta-Roy, K., K. Banerjee, S. P. De, and A. C. Ghose.** 1986. Comparative study of expression of hemagglutinins, hemolysins, and enterotoxins by clinical and environmental isolates of non-O1 *Vibrio cholerae* in relation to their enteropathogenicity. *Appl. Environ. Microbiol.* **52**:875–879.

118. **Davis, B. R., G. R. Fanning, and J. M. Madden.** 1981. Characterization of biochemically atypical *Vibrio cholerae* strains, and designation of a new pathogenic species, *Vibrio mimicus. J. Clin. Microbiol.* **14**:631–639.

119. **Davis, J. W., and R. K. Sizemore.** 1982. Incidence of *Vibrio* species associated with blue crabs *(Callinectes sapidus)* collected from Galveston Bay, Texas. *Appl. Environ. Microbiol.* **43**:1092–1097.

120. **DeGerome, J. H., and M. T. Smith.** 1974. Noncholera vibrio enteritis contracted in the United States by an American. *J. Infect. Dis.* **129**:587–589.

121. **De Paola, A.** 1981. Vibrio cholerae in marine foods and environmental waters: a literature review. *J. Food Sci.* **46**:66–70.

122. **Desenclos, J.-C. A., K. C. Klontz, and M. H. Wilder.** 1991. A multistate outbreak of hepatitis A caused by the consumption of raw oysters. *Am. J. Public Health* **81**:1268–1272.

123. **Desenclos, J. A., K. C. Klontz, L. E. Wolfe, and S. Hoecherl.** 1991. The risk of vibrio illness in the Florida raw oyster eating population, 1981–1988. *Am. J. Epidemiol.* **134**:290–297.

124. **Dhar, R., M. A. Ghafoor, and A. Y. Nasralah.** 1989. Unusual non-serogroup O1 *Vibrio cholerae* bacteremia associated with liver disease. *J. Clin. Microbiol.* **27**:2853–2855.

125. **Dickey, R. W., G. A. Fryxell, H. R. Granade, and D. Roelke.** 1992. Detection of the marine toxins okadaic acid and domoic acid in shellfish and phytoplankton in the Gulf of Mexico. *Toxicon* **30**:355–359.

126. **DiGaetano, M., S. F. Ball, and J. G. Straus.** 1989. Vibrio vulnificus corneal ulcer. *Arch. Ophthalmol.* **107**:323–324.

127. **Dilmore, L. A., and M. A. Hood.** 1986. Vibrios of some deep-water invertebrates. *FEMS Microbiol. Lett.* **35:**221–224.

128. **Dolin, R., J. J. Treanor, and H. P. Madore.** 1987. Novel agents of viral enteritis in humans. *J. Infect. Dis.* **155:**365–375.

129. **Donta, S. T., P. W. Smith, R. E. Levitz, and R. Quintiliani.** 1986. Therapy of Mycobacterium marinum infections: use of tetracyclines vs rifampin. *Arch. Intern. Med.* **146:**902–904.

130. **Doyle, M. P.** 1985. Food-borne pathogens of recent concern. *Annu. Rev. Nutr.* **5:**25–41.

131. **Dryden, M., M. Legarde, T. Gottlieb, L. Brady, and H. K. Ghosh.** 1989. Vibrio damsela wound infections in Australia. *Med. J. Aust.* **151:**540–541.

132. **DuPont, H. L.** 1986. Consumption of raw shellfish—is the risk now unacceptable? *N. Engl. J. Med.* **314:**707–708.

133. **Eason, R. J., and E. Harding.** 1987. Neurotoxic fish poisoning in the Solomon Islands. *P. N. G. Med. J.* **30:**49–52.

134. **Eastaugh, J., and S. Shepherd.** 1989. Infectious and toxic syndromes from fish and shellfish consumption. A review. *Arch. Intern. Med.* **149:**1735–1740.

135. **Eng, R. H. K., H. Chmel, S. M. Smith, D. Haacker, and A. Grigoriu.** 1988. Early diagnosis of overwhelming Vibrio vulnificus infections. *South. Med. J.* **81:**410–411.

136. **English, V. L., and R. B. Lindberg.** 1977. Isolation of Vibrio alginolyticus from wounds and blood of a burn patient. *Am. J. Med. Technol.* **43:**989–993.

137. **Enzenauer, R. J., J. McKoy, and D. Vincent.** 1990. Disseminated cutaneous and synovial Mycobacterium marinum infection in a patient with systemic lupus erythematosus. *South. Med. J.* **83:**471–474.

138. **Etkind, P., M. E. Wilson, K. Gallagher, and J. Cournoyer.** 1987. Bluefish-associated scombroid poisoning. *JAMA* **258:**3409–3410.

139. **Eyles, M. J., G. R. Davey, and G. Arnold.** 1985. Behavior and incidence of Vibrio parahaemolyticus in Sydney Rock oysters (Crassostrea commercialis). *Int. J. Food Microbiol.* **1:**327–334.

140. **Fang, G., V. Araujo, and R. L. Guerrant.** 1991. Enteric infections associated with exposure to animals or animal products. *Infect. Dis. Clin. N. Am.* **5:**681–701.

141. **Farmer, J. J., F. W. Hickman-Brenner, and M. T. Kelly.** 1985. Vibrio, p. 282–301. *In* G. H. Lennette, A. Balows, W. J. Hausler, and H. J. Shadomy (ed.), *Manual of Clinical Microbiology,* 4th ed. American Society for Microbiology, Washington, DC.

142. **Farmer, J. J., III.** 1979. Vibrio ("Beneckea") vulnificus, the bacterium associated with sepsis, septicemia and the sea. *Lancet* **ii:**903.

143. **Fearrington, E. L., C. H. Rand, A. Mewborn, and J. Wilkerson.** 1974. Non-cholera vibrio septicemia and meningoencephalitis. *Ann. Intern. Med.* **81:**401.

144. **Feldman, R. A., M. W. Long, and H. L. David.** 1974. Mycobacterium marinum: a leisure time pathogen. *J. Infect. Dis.* **129:**618–621.

145. **Fenner, P. J., J. A. Williamson, J. W. Burnett, et al.** 1988. The "Irukandji syndrome" and acute pulmonary oedema. *Med. J. Aust.* **149:**150–156.

146. **Field, M.** 1979. Modes of action of enterotoxins of vibrio cholerae and Escherichia coli. *Rev. Infect. Dis.* **1:**918–921.

147. **Florescu, D. P., N. Nacescu, and C. Ciufecu.** 1981. Vibrio cholerae non group O:1 associated with middle ear infection. *Arch. Roum. Pathol. Exp. Microbiol.* **40:**369–372.

148. **Fonde, E. C., J. Britton, and H. Pollock.** 1984. Marine Vibrio sepsis manifesting as necrotizing fasciitis. *South. Med. J.* **77:**933–934.

149. **Franca, S. M. C., D. L. Gibbs, P. Samuels, and W. D. Johnson, Jr.** 1980. Vibrio parahaemolyticus in Brazilian coastal waters. *JAMA* **244:**587–588.

150. **Fuhrman, F. A.** 1986. Tetrodotoxin, tarichatoxin, and chiriquitoxins. Historical perspectives. *Ann. N. Y. Acad. Sci.* **479:**1–14.

151. **Furniss, A. L., J. V. Lee, and T. J. Donovan.** 1977. Group F, a new vibrio? *Lancet* **ii:**565–566.

152. **Gerba, C. P., C. M. Goyal, and R. I. LaBelle.** 1979. Failure of indicator bacteria to reflect the occurrence of enteroviruses in marine waters. *Am. J. Public Health* **69:**1116–1119.

153. **Gerba, C. P., and S. M. Goyal.** 1986. *Development of a Qualitative Pathogen Risk Assessment Methodology for Ocean Disposal of Municipal Sludge. ALAO-CIN-493.* U.S. Environmental Protection Agency, Cincinnati, OH.

154. **Gessner, B., and M. Schloss.** 1996. A population-based study of paralytic shellfish poisoning in Alaska. *Alsk. Med.* **38:**54–58.

155. **Giannoni, C.** 2000. Swimming with tympanostomy tubes. *Arch. Otolaryngol. Head Neck Surg.* **126:**1507–1509.

156. **Gilbert, D., R. Moellering, and M. Sande.** 2002. *Sanford Guide to Antimicrobial Therapy,* 32nd ed. Antimicrobial Therapy, Inc., Hyde Park, VT.

157. **Gill, O. N., W. D. Cubitt, and D. A. McSwiggan.** 1983. Epidemic of gastroenteritis caused by oysters contaminated with small round structured viruses. *Br. Med. J.* **287:**1532–1534.

158. **Gillespie, N. C., R. J. Lewis, and J. H. Pearn.** 1986. Ciguatera in Australia: occurrence, clinical features, pathophysiology, and management. *Med. J. Aust.* **145:**584–590.

159. **Gilman, R. H., and W. M. Spira.** 1980. Invasive E. coli and V. parahaemolyticus a rare cause of dysentery in Dacca. *Trans. R. Soc. Trop. Med. Hyg.* **74:**688–689.

160. **Glasgow, H. J., J. Burkholder, D. Schmechel, P. Tester, and P. Rublee.** 1995. Insidious effects of a toxic estuarine dinoflagellate on fish survival and human health. *Toxicol. Environ. Health* **46:**501–522.

161. **Glavin, G. B., R. Bose, and C. Pinsky.** 1990. Letter. *Arch. Intern. Med.* **150:**2425.

162. **Goldsmith, R., P. O. Yarbough, and G. R. Reyes.** 1992. Enzyme-linked immunosorbent assay for diagnosis of acute sporadic hepatitis E in Egyptian children. *Lancet* **339:**328–331.

163. **Gombert, M. E., E. L. C. Goldstein, and M. L. Corrado.** 1981. Disseminated Mycobacterium marinum infection after renal transplantation. *Ann. Intern. Med.* **94:**486–487.

164. **Gorbach, S. L., J. G. Banwell, N. F. Pierce, B. D. Chatterjee, and R. C. Mitra.** 1970. Intestinal microflora in a chronic carrier of Vibrio cholerae. *J. Infect. Dis.* **121:**383–390.

165. **Goyal, S. M.** 1984. Viral pollution of the marine environment. *CRC Crit. Rev. Environ. Cont.* **14:**32.

166. **Gratton, L. M., D. Oldach, T. M. Perl, M. Lowitt, D. Matuszak, C. Dickson, C. Parrott, R. Shoemaker, C. Kauffman, M. Wasserman, J. Hebel, P. Charache, and J. Morris, Jr.** 1998. Learning and memory difficulties after environmental exposure to waterways containing toxin-producing Pfiesteria or Pfiesteria-like dinoflagellates. *Lancet* **352:**532–539.

167. **Gray, L. D., and A. S. Kreger.** 1986. Detection of anti-*Vibrio vulnificus* cytolysin antibodies in sera from mice and a human surviving *V. vulnificus* disease. *Infect. Immun.* **51:**964–965.

168. **Gray, L. D., and A. S. Kreger.** 1985. Purification and characterization of an extracellular cytolysin produced by *Vibrio vulnificus. Infect. Immun.* **48:**62–72.

169. **Greenough, W. B. I.** 1990. Vibrio cholerae, p. 1636–1646. *In* G. L. Mandell, R. G. Douglas, Jr., and J. E. Bennett (ed.), *Principles and Practice of Infectious Diseases,* 3rd ed. Churchill Livingstone, New York, NY.

170. **Grimes, D. J., J. Stemmler, and H. Hada.** 1984. Vibrio species associated with mortality of sharks held in captivity. *Microbiol. Ecol.* **10:**271–282.

171. **Gunn, R. A., H. T. Janowski, and S. Lieb.** 1982. Norwalk virus gastroenteritis following raw oyster consumption. *Am. J. Epidemiol.* **115:**348–351.

172. **Hackney, C. R., E. G. Kleeman, B. Ray, and M. L. Speck.** 1980. Adherence as a method for differentiating virulent and avirulent strains of *Vibrio parahaemolyticus. Appl. Environ. Microbiol.* **40:**652–658.

173. **Haddad, L. M., R. F. Lee, and O. McConnell.** 1983. Toxic marine life, p. 303–317. *In* L. M. Haddad and J. F. Winchester (ed.), *Clinical Management of Poisoning and Drug Overdose.* W. B. Saunders, Philadelphia, PA.

174. **Halliday, M. L., L. Kang, and T. Zhou.** 1991. An epidemic of hepatitis A attributable to the ingestion of raw clams in Shanghai, China. *J. Infect. Dis.* **164:**852–859.

175. **Halstead, B. W.** 1965. *Poisonous and Venomous Marine Animals of the World,* vol. 1, p. 59–61. U.S. Government Printing Office, Washington, DC.

176. **Halstead, B. W.** 1987. Coelenterate (Cnidarian) stings and wounds. *Clin. Dermatol.* **5:**8–13.

177. **Halstead, B. W., and E. J. Schantz.** 1984. Paralytic shellfish poisoning. *W. H. O. Offset Publ.* **1984:**1–59.

178. **Hare, P., T. Scott-Burden, and D. R. Woods.** 1983. Characterization of extracellular alkaline proteases and collagenase induction in Vibrio alginolyticus. *J. Gen. Microbiol.* **129:**1141–1147.

179. **Harris, J. R., M. L. Cohen, and E. C. Lippy.** 1981. Water-related disease outbreaks in the United States, 1981. *J. Infect. Dis.* **148:**759–762.

180. **Harrison, L. J.** 1991. Poisonous marine morsels. *J. Fla. Med. Assoc.* **78:**219–221.

181. **Heineman, H. S., S. Spitzer, and T. Pianphongsant.** 1972. Fish tank granuloma. A hobby hazard. *Arch. Intern. Med.* **130:**121–123.

182. **Heller, D., O. N. Gill, and D. Raynham.** 1986. Epidemiology: an outbreak of gastrointestinal illness associated with consumption of raw depurated oysters. *Br. Med. J.* **292:**1726–1727.

183. **Hemmert, W. H.** 1975. The public health implications of Gymnodinium breve red tides. A review of the literature and recent events, p. 489–497. *In* V. R. Locicero (ed.), *Proceedings of the First International Conference on Toxic Dinoflagellate Blooms.* Massachusetts Science and Technology Foundation, Boston, MA.

184. **Herrington, D. A., R. H. Hall, G. Losonsky, J. J. Mekalanos, R. K. Taylor, and M. M. Levine.** 1988. Toxin, toxin-coregulated pili, and the toxR regulon are essential for Vibrio cholerae pathogenesis in humans. *J. Exp. Med.* **168:**1487–1492.

185. **Hessel, D. W., B. W. Halstead, and N. H. Peckham.** 1960. Marine biotoxins. 1. Ciguatera poison: some biological and chemical aspects. *Ann. N. Y. Acad. Sci.* **90:**788–797.

186. **Hickman, F. W., J. J. Farmer, D. G. Hollis, G. R. Fanning, A. G. Steigerwalt, R. E. Weaver, and D. J. Brenner.** 1982. Identification of *Vibrio hollisae* sp. nov. from patients with diarrhoea. *J. Clin. Microbiol.* **15:**395–401.

187. **Hickman-Brenner, F. W., D. J. Brenner, and A. G. Steigerwalt.** 1984. *Vibrio fluvialis* and *Vibrio furnissii* isolated from a stool sample of one patient. *J. Clin. Microbiol.* **20:**125–127.

188. **Hill, M. K., and C. V. Sanders.** 1987. Localized and systemic infection due to Vibrio species. *Infect. Dis. Clin. N. Am.* **1:**687–707.

189. **Hirschhorn, N., J. L. Kinzie, and D. B. Sachar.** 1968. Decrease in net stool output during intestinal perfusion with glucose-containing solutions. *N. Engl. J. Med.* **279:**176.

190. **Hoashi, K., K. Ogata, H. Taniguchi, H. Yamashita, K. Tsuji, Y. Mizuguchi, and N. Ohtomo.** 1990. Pathogenesis of Vibrio parahaemolyticus: intraperitoneal and orogastric challenge experiments in mice. *Microbiol. Immunol.* **34:**355–366.

191. **Hoffman, T. J., B. Nelson, R. Darouiche, and T. Rosen.** 1988. Vibrio vulnificus septicemia. *Arch. Intern. Med.* **148:**1825–1827.

192. **Hoge, C. W., D. Watsky, R. N. Peeler, J. P. Libonati, I. E., and J. G. Morris, Jr.** 1989. Epidemiology and spectrum of vibrio infections in a Chesapeake Bay community. *J. Infect. Dis.* **160:**985–993.

193. **Hollis, D. G., R. E. Weaver, C. N. Baker, and C. Thornberry.** 1976. Halophilic *Vibrio* species isolated from blood cultures. *J. Clin. Microbiol.* **3:**425–431.

194. **Holmberg, S.** 1988. Vibrios and Aeromonas. *Infect. Dis. Clin. N. Am.* **2:**655–676.

195. **Holmgren, J., and A. Svennerholm.** 1977. Mechanisms of disease and immunity in cholerae. A review. *J. Infect. Dis.* **136**(Suppl.):105–112.

196. **Honda, T., M. Arita, T. Takeda, M. Yoh, and T. Miwatani.** 1985. Non-O1 Vibrio cholerae produces two newly identified toxins related to Vibrio parahaemolyticus haemolysin and Escherichia coli heat-stable enterotoxin. *Lancet* **ii:**163–164.

197. **Honda, T., and R. A. Finkelstein.** 1979. Purification and characterization of a hemolysin produced by *Vibrio cholerae* biotype El Tor: another toxic substance produced by cholera vibrios. *Infect. Immun.* **26:**1020–1027.

198. **Honda, T., S. Taga, T. Takeda, M. A. Hasibuan, Y. Takeda, and T. Miwatani.** 1975. Identification of lethal toxin with the thermostable direct hemolysin produced by *Vibrio parahaemolyticus* and some physicochemical properties of purified toxin. *Infect. Immun.* **13:**133–139.

199. **Hood, M. A., G. E. Ness, and G. E. Rodrick.** 1981. Isolation of *Vibrio cholerae* serotype O1 from the Eastern oyster, *Crassotrea virginica. Appl. Environ. Microbiol.* **41:**559–560.

200. **Howard, R. J., and S. Lieb.** 1988. Soft-tissue infections caused by halophilic marine vibrios. *Arch. Surg.* **123:**245.

201. **Hoyt, R. E., J. E. Bryant, and S. F. Glessner.** 1989. M marinum infections in a Chesapeake Bay community. *Va. Med.* **16:**467–470.

202. **Hu, M., T. Li, and X. Hu.** 1986. Isolation of HAV from experimentally infected shellfish, p. 688. *In Abstracts of the IXth International Congress of Infectious and Parasitic Diseases (Munich).* Infectious Disease Association, Munich, Germany.

203. **Hughes, J. M.** 1979. Epidemiology of shellfish poisoning in the United States, 1971–1977, p. 23–28. *In* D. L. Taylor and H. H. Seliger (ed.), *Toxic Dinoflagellate Blooms.* Elsevier/North Holland, New York, NY.

204. **Hughes, J. M., D. G. Hollis, E. J. Gangarosa, and R. E. Weaver.** 1978. Non-cholera vibrio infections in the United States: clinical, epidemiologic, and laboratory features. *Ann. Intern. Med.* **88:**602–606.

205. **Hughes, J. M., and M. H. Merson.** 1976. Fish and shellfish poisoning. *N. Engl. J. Med.* **295:**1117–1120.

206. **Hughes, J. M., and M. E. Potter.** 1991. Scombroid-fish poisoning. From pathogenesis to prevention. *N. Engl. J. Med.* **324:**766–768.

207. **Hughes, J. M., and R. V. Tauxe.** 1990. Food-borne disease, p. 898. *In* G. L. Mandell, R. G. Douglas, and J. E. Bennett (ed.), *Principles and Practice of Infectious Diseases,* 3rd ed. Churchill Livingstone, New York, NY.

208. **Huminer, D., S. D. Pitlik, C. Block, L. Kaufman, S. Amit, and J. B. Rosenfeld.** 1986. Aquarium-borne Mycobacterium marinum skin infection: report of a case and review of the literature. *Arch. Dermatol.* **122:**698–703.

209. **Huq, A., S. A. Huq, D. J. Grimes, M. O'Brien, K. H. Chu, J. M. Capuzzo, and R. R. Colwell.** 1986. Colonization of the gut of the blue crab *(Callinectes sapidus)* by *Vibrio cholerae. Appl. Environ. Microbiol.* **52:**586–588.

210. **Huq, A., P. A. West, E. B. Small, M. I. Huq, and R. R. Colwell.** 1984. Influence of water temperature, salinity, and pH on survival and growth of toxigenic *Vibrio cholerae* serovar O1 associated with live copepods in laboratory microcosms. *Appl. Environ. Microbiol.* **48:**420–424.

211. **Huq, M. I., A. K. M. J. Alam, and D. J. Brenner.** 1980. Isolation of *Vibrio*-like group, EF-6, from patients with diarrhea. *J. Clin. Microbiol.* **11:**621–624.

212. **Hurst, L. C., P. C. Amadio, M. A. Badalamente, J. L. Ellstein, and R. J. Dattwyler.** 1987. Mycobacterium marinum infections of the hand. *J. Hand Surg.* **12A:**428–435.

213. Reference deleted.

214. **Izumi, A. K., C. W. Hanke, and M. Higaki.** 1977. Mycobacterium marinum infections treated with tetracycline. *Arch. Dermatol.* **113:** 1067–1068.

215. **Jaffe, B. F.** 1981. Are water and tympanostomy tubes compatible? *Laryngoscope* **91:**563–564.

216. **Janda, J. M., R. Brenden, J. A. De-Benedetti, M. O. Constantino, and T. Robin.** 1986. Vibrio alginolyticus bacteremia in an immunocompromised patient. *Diagn. Microbiol. Infect. Dis.* **5:**337–340.

217. **Janda, J. M., C. Powers, R. G. Bryant, and S. L. Abbott.** 1988. Current perspectives on the epidemiology and pathogenesis of clinically significant vibrio spp. *Clin. Microbiol. Rev.* **1:** 245–267.

218. **Jean-Jacques, W., K. R. Rajashekaraiah, J. J. Farmer III, F. W. Hickman, J. G. Morris, and C. A. Kallick.** 1981. *Vibrio metschnikovii* bacteremia in a patient with cholecystitis. *J. Clin. Microbiol.* **14:**711–712.

219. **Johnston, J. M., W. A. Andes, and G. Glasser.** 1983. Vibrio vulnificus: a gastronomic hazard. *JAMA* **249:**1756–1757.

220. **Johnston, J. M., S. F. Becker, and L. M. McFarland.** 1986. Gastroenteritis in patients with stool isolates of Vibrio vulnificus. *Am. J. Med.* **80:**336–338.

221. **Johnston, J. M., S. F. Becker, and L. M. McFarland.** 1985. Vibrio vulnificus: man and the sea. *JAMA* **253:**2850–2853.

222. **Johnston, J. M., D. L. Martin, J. Perdue, L. M. McFarland, C. T. Caraway, E. C. Lippy, and P. A. Blake.** 1983. Cholera on a Gulf Coast oil rig. *N. Engl. J. Med.* **309:**523–526.

223. **Johnston, J. M., L. M. McFarland, H. C. Bradford, and C. T. Caraway.** 1983. Isolation of nontoxigenic *Vibrio cholerae* O1 from a human wound infection. *J. Clin. Microbiol.* **17:** 918–920.

224. **Jolly, H. W., and J. H. Seabury.** 1972. Infections with Mycobacterium marinum. *Arch. Dermatol.* **106:**32–36.

225. **Jones, M. W., I. A. Wahid, and J. P. Matthews.** 1988. Septic arthritis of the hand due to Mycobacterium marinum. *J. Hand Surg.* **13B:**333–334.

226. **Joseph, S. W., R. R. Colwell, and J. B. Kaper.** 1983. Vibrio parahaemolyticus and related halophilic vibrios. *CRC Crit. Rev. Microbiol.* **10:** 77–124.

227. **Kan, S. K. P., N. Singh, and M. K. C. Chan.** 1986. Oliva vidua fulminans, a marine mollusc, responsible for five fatal cases of neurotoxic food poisoning in Sabah, Malaysia. *Trans. R. Soc. Trop. Med. Hyg.* **80:**64–65.

228. **Kaneko, T., and R. R. Colwell.** 1978. The annual cycle of Vibrio parahemolyticus in Chesapeake Bay. *Microb. Ecol.* **4:**135–155.

229. **Kaneko, T., and R. R. Colwell.** 1973. Ecology of *Vibrio parahemolyticus* in Chesapeake Bay. *J. Bacteriol.* **113:**24–32.

230. **Kaper, J. B., H. Lockman, and R. R. Colwell.** 1979. Ecology, serology and enterotoxin production of *Vibrio cholerae* in Chesapeake Bay. *Appl. Environ. Microbiol.* **37:**91–103.

231. **Kaplan, J. E., R. A. Goodman, and R. C. Baron.** 1982. Epidemiology of Norwalk gastroenteritis and the role of Norwalk virus in outbreaks of acute nonbacterial gastroenteritis. *Ann. Intern. Med.* **96:**756–761.

232. **Karunasagar, I., I. Karunasagar, Y. Oshima, and T. Yasumoto.** 1990. A toxin profile for shellfish involved in an outbreak of paralytic shellfish poisoning in India. *Toxicon* **28:** 868–870.

233. **Karunasagar, I., I. Karunasagar, M. N. Venugopal, and C. N. Nagesha.** 1987. Survival of Vibrio parahaemolyticus in estuarine and seawater and in association with clams. *Syst. Appl. Microbiol.* **9:**316–319.

234. **Karunasagar, I., M. N. Venugopal, I. Karunasagar, and K. Segar.** 1987. Role of chitin in the survival of Vibrio parahaemolyticus at different temperatures. *Can. J. Microbiol.* **32:** 889–891.

235. **Kat, M.** 1983. Diarrhetic mussel poisoning in the Netherlands related to the dinoflagellate Dinophysis acuminata. *Antonie van Leeuwenhoek* **49:**417–427.

236. **Kaye, J. J.** 1990. Vibrio vulnificus infections in the hand. *J. Bone Joint Surg.* **72-A:**283–285.

237. **Kaysner, C. A., M. M. Wekell, and C. Abeyta, Jr.** 1990. Enhancement of virulence of two environmental strains of Vibrio vulnificus after passage through mice. *Diagn. Microbiol. Infect. Dis.* **13:**285–288.

238. **Kelly, M. T., and D. M. Avery.** 1980. Lactose-positive *Vibrio* in seawater: a cause of pneumonia and septicemia in a drowning victim. *J. Clin. Microbiol.* **11:**278–280.

239. **Kelly, M. T., and E. M. D. Stroh.** 1989. Urease-positive, Kanagawa-negative *Vibrio parahaemolyticus* from patients and the environment

in the Pacific Northwest. *J. Clin. Microbiol.* **27:** 2820–2822.

240. **Kerketta, J., A. Paul, V. Kirubakaran, M. Jesudason, and P. Moses.** 2002. Non-01 Vibrio cholerae septicemia and meningitis in a neonate. *Indian J. Pediatr.* **69:**909–910.

241. **Khan, M. V., and M. Shahidullah.** 1982. Epidemiologic pattern of diarrhoea caused by non-agglutinating Vibrio (NAG) and EF-6 organisms in Dacca. *Trop. Geogr. Med.* **34:**19–27.

242. **King, A. J., J. A. Fairley, and J. E. Rasmussen.** 1983. Disseminated cutaneous Mycobacterium marinum infection. *Arch. Dermatol.* **119:**268–270.

243. **Klontz, K. C.** 1990. Fatalities associated with Vibrio parahaemolyticus and Vibrio cholerae non-O1 infections in Florida (1981 to 1988). *South. Med. J.* **83:**500–502.

244. **Klontz, K. C., and J.-C. A. Desenclos.** 1990. Clinical and epidemiological features of sporadic infections with Vibrio fluvialis in Florida, USA. *J. Diarrhoeal Dis. Res.* **8:**24–26.

245. **Klontz, K. C., S. Lieb, M. Schreiber, H. T. Janowski, L. M. Baldy, and R. A. Gunn.** 1988. Syndromes of Vibrio vulnificus infections. Clinical and epidemiologic features in Florida cases, 1981–1987. *Ann. Intern. Med.* **109:**318–323.

246. **Kobayashi, M., S. Kondo, T. Yasumoto, and Y. Ohizumi.** 1986. Cardiotoxic effects of maitotoxin, a principal toxin of seafood poisoning, on guinea pig and rat cardiac muscle. *J. Pharmacol. Exp. Ther.* **238:**1077–1083.

247. **Kodama, A. M., Y. Hokama, T. Yasumoto, M. Fukui, S. J. Manea, and N. Sutherland.** 1989. Clinical and laboratory findings implicating palytoxin as cause of ciguatera poisoning due to Decapterus macrosoma (mackerel). *Toxicon* **27:**1051–1053.

248. **Kodama, H., Y. Gyobu, N. Tokuman, I. Okada, H. Uetake, T. Shimada, and R. Sakazaki.** 1984. Ecology of non-O1 Vibrio cholerae in Toyama prefecture. *Microbiol. Immunol.* **28:**311–325.

249. **Kodama, M., T. Ogata, Y. Fukuyo, T. Ishimaru, S. Wisessang, K. Saitanu, V. Panichyakarn, and T. Piyakarnchana.** 1988. Protogonyaulax cohorticula, a toxic dinoflagellate found in the Gulf of Thailand. *Toxicon* **26:** 707–712.

250. **Koff, R. S., and H. S. Sear.** 1967. Internal temperature of steamed clams. *N. Engl. J. Med.* **276:**737–739.

251. **Kothary, M. H., and S. H. Richardson.** 1987. Fluid accumulation in infant mice caused by *Vibrio hollisae* and its extracellular enterotoxin. *Infect. Immun.* **55:**626–630.

252. **Kreger, A., L. DeChatelet, and P. Shirley.** 1981. Interaction of Vibrio vulnificus with human polymorphonuclear leukocytes: association of virulence with resistance to phagocytosis. *J. Infect. Dis.* **144:**244–248.

253. **Kreger, A. S.** 1984. Cytolytic activity and virulence of *Vibrio damsela*. *Infect. Immun.* **44:**326–331.

254. **Krzanowski, J., Y. Sakamoto, and R. Duncan.** 1984. The mechanism of Ptychodiscus brevis toxin induced rat vas deferens contraction. *Pharmacologist* **26:**175.

255. **Kwo, P.** 1997. Acute hepatitis E by a new isolate acquired in the United States. *Mayo Clin Proc.* **72:**1133–1136.

256. **Lacy, J. N., S. F. Viegas, J. Calhoun, and J. T. Mader.** 1989. Mycobacterium marinum flexor tenosynovitis. *Clin. Orthop. Rel. Res.* **238:** 288–293.

257. **Lam, S., and E. Monteiro.** 1984. Isolation of mucoid *Vibrio parahaemolyticus* strains. *J. Clin. Microbiol.* **19:**87–88.

258. **Lam, S., and E. Monteiro.** 1981. Unusual Vibrio species found in diarrhoeal stools. *Singapore Med. J.* **22:**259–261.

259. **Lam, S., and M. Yeo.** 1980. Urease-positive *Vibrio parahaemolyticus* strain. *J. Clin. Microbiol.* **12:**57–59.

260. **Lam, S. Y. S., and L. T. Goi.** 1985. Isolations of "group F vibrios" from human stools. *Singapore Med. J.* **26:**300–302.

261. **Larsen, J. L., and J. F. Farid.** 1980. In vitro antibiotic sensitivity testing of Vibrio alginolyticus. *Acta Pathol. Microbiol. Scand.* **88:**307–310.

262. **Lawrence, D. N., M. B. Enriquez, R. M. Lumish, and A. Maceo.** 1980. Ciguatera fish poisoning in Miami. *JAMA* **244:**254–258.

263. **Lee, D., A. Youk, and N. Goldstein.** 1999. A meta-analysis of swimming and water precautions. *Laryngoscope* **109:**536–540.

264. **Lee, J. V., T. J. Donovan, and A. L. Furniss.** 1978. Characterization, taxonomy, and emended description of Vibrio metschnikovii. *Int. J. Syst. Bacteriol.* **28:**99–111.

265. **Lee, J. V., P. Shread, and A. L. Furniss.** 1981. Taxonomy and description of Vibrio fluvialis sp. nov. (synonym group F vibrios, group EF-6). *J. Appl. Bacteriol.* **50:**73–94.

266. **Lerke, P. A., S. B. Werner, S. L. Taylor, and L. S. Guthertz.** 1978. Scombroid poisoning: report of an outbreak. *West. J. Med.* **12:** 381–386.

267. **Lessner, A. M., R. M. Webb, and B. Rabin.** 1985. Vibrio alginolyticus conjunctivitis. *Arch. Ophthalmol.* **103:**229–230.

268. **Levesque, B., P. Giovenazzo, P. Guerrier, D. Laverdiere, and H. Prud'Homme.** 2002. Investigation of an outbreak of cercarial dermatitis. *Epidemiol. Infect.* **129:**379–386.

269. **Levine, M. M., R. E. Black, M. L. Clements, D. R. Nalin, L. Cisneros, and R. A.**

Finkelstein. 1981. Volunteer studies in development of vaccines against cholera and enterotoxigenic E. coli: a review, p. 443–459. *In* T. Holme, J. Holmgren, M. H. Merson, and R. Mollby (ed.), *Acute Enteric Infections in Children: New Prospects for Treatment and Prevention.* Elsevier/North Holland, Amsterdam, The Netherlands.

270. **Lewis, N.** 1986. Disease and development: ciguatera fish poisoning. *Soc. Sci. Med.* **23:**983–993.

271. **Limpert, G. H., and J. E. Peacock.** 1988. Soft tissue infections due to noncholera vibrios. *Am. Fam. Physician* **37:**193–198.

272. **Lin, F. Y., J. G. Morris, Jr., J. B. Kaper, T. Gross, J. Michalski, C. Morrison, J. B. Libonati, and E. Israel.** 1986. Persistence of cholera in the United States: isolation of *Vibrio cholerae* O1 from a patient with diarrhea in Maryland. *J. Clin. Microbiol.* **23:**624–626.

273. **Linell, F., and A. Norden.** 1954. Mycobacterium balnei: a new acid-fast bacillus occurring in swimming pools and capable of producing skin lesions in humans. *Acta Tuberc. Scand.* **33**(Suppl.):1–84.

274. **Link, K., F. Counselman, J. Steele, and M. Caughey.** 1999. A new hazard for windsurfers: needlefish impalement. *J. Emerg. Med.* **17:**255–259.

275. **Ljungberg, B., B. Christensson, and R. Grubb.** 1987. Failure of doxycycline treatment in aquarium-associated Mycobacterium marinum infections. *Scand. J. Infect. Dis.* **19:**539–543.

276. **Lockwood, D. E., A. S. Kreger, and S. H. Richardson.** 1982. Detection of toxins produced by *Vibrio fluvialis. Infect. Immun.* **35:**702–708.

277. **Long, R. R., J. C. Sargent, and K. Hammer.** 1990. Paralytic shellfish poisoning: a case report and serial electrophysiologic observations. *Neurology* **40:**1310–1312.

278. **Lopez-Sabater, E., J. Rodriguez-Jerez, M. Hernandez-Herrero, and M. Mora-Ventura.** 1996. Incidence of histamine-forming bacteria and histamine content in scombroid fish species from retail markets in the Barcelona area. *Int. J. Food Microbiol.* **28:**411–418.

279. **Loria, P. R.** 1976. Minocycline hydrochloride treatment for atypical acid-fast infection. *Arch. Dermatol.* **112:**517–519.

280. **Lounsbury, B. F.** 1985. Swimming unprotected with long-shafted middle ear ventilation tubes. *Laryngoscope* **95:**340–343.

281. **Love, M., D. Teebken-Fisher, J. E. Hose, J. J. Farmer III, F. W. Hickman, and G. R. Fanning.** 1981. Vibrio damsela, a marine bacterium, causes skin ulcers on the damselfish Chromis punctipinnis. *Science* **214:**1139.

282. **Lowry, P. W., L. M. McFarland, B. H. Peltier, N. C. Roberts, H. B. Bradford, J. L. Herndon, D. F. Stroup, J. B. Mathison, P. A. Blake, and R. A. Gunn.** 1989. Vibrio gastroenteritis in Louisiana: a prospective study among attendees of a scientific congress in New Orleans. *J. Infect. Dis.* **160:**978–984.

283. **Lowry, P. W., L. M. McFarland, and H. K. Threefoot.** 1986. Vibrio hollisae septicemia after consumption of catfish. *J. Infect. Dis.* **154:**730–731.

284. **Lumley, J., J. A. Williamson, and P. J. Fenner.** 1988. Fatal envenomation by Chironex fleckeri, the north Australian box jellyfish: the continuing search for lethal mechanisms. *Med. J. Aust.* **148:**527–534.

285. **Magnusson, B., and J. Gulasekharam.** 1965. A lecithin-hydrolyzing enzyme which correlates with hemolytic activity in El Tor vibrio isolates. *Nature* **206:**728.

286. **Mahoney, F. J., T. A. Farley, and K. Y. Kelso.** 1992. An outbreak of hepatitis A associated with swimming in a public pool. *J. Infect. Dis.* **165:**613–618.

287. **Mazumder, D. N. G., A. K. Ghosh, S. P. De, and B. K. Sirkar.** 1977. Vibrio parahaemolyticus infection in man. *Indian J. Med. Res.* **66:**180–188.

288. **McCabe, M. J., W. M. Hammon, and B. W. Halstead.** 1978. A fatal brain injury caused by a needlefish. *Neuroradiology* **15:**137–139.

289. **McCollum, J. P. K., R. C. M. Pearson, and H. R. Ingham.** 1968. An epidemic of mussel poisoning in north-east England. *Lancet* **ii:**767–770.

290. **McCollum, R. W., and A. J. Zuckerman.** 1981. Viral hepatitis: report on a WHO informal consultation. *J. Med. Virol.* **8:**1–29.

291. **McGuigan, M.** 1981. Shellfish poisoning. *Clin. Toxicol. Rev.* **3:**12.

292. **Mead, P., L. Slutsker, and V. Dietz.** 1999. Food-related illness and disease in the United States. *Emerg. Infect. Dis.* **5:**1–20.

293. **Meadors, M. C., and G. A. Pankey.** 1990. Vibrio vulnificus wound infection treated successfully with oral ciprofloxacin. *J. Infect.* **20:**88–89.

294. **Melnick, J. L., and C. P. Gerba.** 1980. The ecology of enteroviruses in natural waters. *CRC Crit. Rev. Environ. Contam.* **10:**65–93.

295. **Meurman, O. H., and M. J. Laine.** 1977. Rotavirus epidemics in adults. *N. Engl. J. Med.* **296:**1298–1299.

296. **Meyerhoff, W. L., T. Morizono, and C. G. Wright.** 1983. Tympanostomy tubes and otic drops. *Laryngoscope* **93:**1022–1027.

297. **Mhalu, F. S., A. M. Yusufali, J. Mbwana, and R. Nyambo.** 1982. Cholera-like diseases

due to Vibrio parahaemolyticus. *J. Trop. Med. Hyg.* **85**:169–171.

298. **Miller, C. J., B. S. Drasar, and R. G. Feacham.** 1984. Response of toxigenic Vibrio cholera O1 to physico-chemical stresses in aquatic environments. *J. Hyg.* **93**:474–496.

299. **Mills, A. R., and R. Passmore.** 1988. Pelagic paralysis. *Lancet* **331**:161–164.

300. **Mishu, B., S. C. Hadler, and V. A. Boaz.** 1990. Foodborne hepatitis A: evidence that microwaving reduces risk. *J. Infect. Dis.* **162**:655–658.

301. **Miyake, M., T. Honda, and T. Miwatani.** 1989. Effects of divalent cations and saccharides on *Vibrio metschnikovii* cytolysin-induced hemolysis of rabbit erythrocytes. *Infect. Immun.* **57**:158–163.

302. **Miyake, M., T. Honda, and T. Miwatani.** 1988. Purification and characterisation of *Vibrio metschnikovii* cytolysin. *Infect. Immun.* **56**:954–960.

303. **Miyamoto, Y., Y. Obara, T. Nikkawa, S. Yamai, T. Kato, Y. Yamada, and M. Ohashi.** 1980. Simplified purification and biophysicochemical characteristics of Kanagawa phenomenon-associated hemolysin of *Vibrio parahaemolyticus*. *Infect. Immun.* **28**:567–576.

304. **Molenda, J. R., W. G. Johnson, M. Fishbein, B. Wentz, I. J. Mehlman, and T. A. Dadisman, Jr.** 1972. Vibrio parahaemolyticus gastroenteritis in Maryland: laboratory aspects. *Appl. Microbiol.* **24**:444–448.

305. **Mollohan, C. S., and M. S. Romer.** 1961. Public health significance of swimming pool granuloma. *Am. J. Public Health* **51**:883–891.

306. **Morgan, D. R., B. D. Ball, and D. G. Moore.** 1985. Severe Vibrio cholerae sepsis and meningitis in a young infant. *Texas Med.* **81**:37–38.

307. **Morris, J. G.** 1990. Ciguatera fish poisoning: barracuda's revenge. *South. Med. J.* **83**:371–372.

308. **Morris, J. G., Jr.** 1988. Vibrio vulnificus—a new monster of the deep? *Ann. Intern. Med.* **109**:261–263.

309. **Morris, J. G., Jr., and R. E. Black.** 1985. Cholera and other vibrioses in the United States. *N. Engl. J. Med.* **312**:343–350.

310. **Morris, J. G., Jr., H. G. Miller, R. Wilson, C. O. Tacket, D. G. Hollis, F. W. Hickman, R. E. Weaver, and P. A. Blake.** 1982. Illness caused by Vibrio damsela and Vibrio hollisae. *Lancet* **i**:1294–1297.

311. **Morris, J. G., Jr., J. H. Tenney, and G. L. Drusano.** 1985. In vitro susceptibility of pathogenic *Vibrio* species to norfloxacin and six other antimicrobial agents. *Antimicrob. Agents Chemother.* **28**:442–445.

312. **Morris, J. G., Jr., R. Wilson, B. R. Davis, I. K. Wachsmuth, C. F. Riddle, H. G. Wathen, R. A. Pollard, and P. A. Blake.** 1981. Non-O group 1 Vibrio cholerae gastroenteritis in the United States: clinical, epidemiologic, and laboratory characteristics of sporadic cases. *Ann. Intern. Med.* **94**:656–658.

313. **Morris, J. G., P. Lewin, and N. T. Hargrett.** 1982. Clinical features of ciguatera fish poisoning: a study of the disease in the US Virgin Islands. *Arch. Intern. Med.* **142**:1090–1092.

314. **Morris, J. G., J. L. Picardi, S. Lieb, J. V. Lee, A. Roberts, M. Hood, R. A. Gunn, and P. A. Blake.** 1984. Isolation of nontoxigenic *Vibrio* O group 1 from a patient with severe gastrointestinal disease. *J. Clin. Microbiol.* **19**:296–297.

315. **Morris, P. D., D. S. Campbell, and J. I. Freeman.** 1990. Ciguatera fish poisoning: an outbreak associated with fish caught from North Carolina coastal waters. *South. Med. J.* **83**:379–382.

316. **Morris, P. D., D. S. Campbell, T. J. Taylor, and J. I. Freeman.** 1991. Clinical and epidemiological features of neurotoxic shellfish poisoning in North Carolina. *Am. J. Public Health* **81**:471–474.

317. **Morrow, J. D., G. R. Margolies, J. Rowland, and L. J. Roberts II.** 1991. Evidence that histamine is the causative toxin of scombroid-fish poisoning. *N. Engl. J. Med.* **324**:716–720.

318. **Morse, D. L., J. J. Guzewich, and J. P. Hanrahan.** 1986. Widespread outbreaks of clam- and oyster-associated gastroenteritis: role of Norwalk virus. *N. Engl. J. Med.* **314**:678–681.

319. Reference deleted.

320. **Mulder, G. D., T. M. Ries, and T. R. Beaver.** 1989. Nontoxigenic Vibrio cholerae wound infection after exposure to contaminated lake water. *J. Infect. Dis.* **159**:809–810.

321. **Murphey, D. K., E. J. Septimus, and D. C. Waagner.** 1992. Catfish-related injury and infection: report of two cases and review of the literature. *Clin. Infect. Dis.* **14**:689–693.

322. **Murphy, E. B., K. A. Steidinger, and B. S. Roberts.** 1975. An explanation for the Florida East Coast Gymnodinium breve red tide of November 1972. *Limnol. Oceanogr.* **20**:481–486.

323. **Murphy, M., G. S. Grohmann, and P. J. Christopher.** 1979. An Australia-wide outbreak of gastroenteritis from oysters caused by Norwalk virus. *Med. J. Aust.* **2**:329–333.

324. **Murray, C. K., G. Hobbs, and R. J. Gilbert.** 1982. Scombrotoxin and scombrotoxin-like poisoning from canned fish. *J. Hyg.* **88**:215–220.

325. **Nacescu, N., C. Ciufecu, and D. Florescu.** 1980. Vibrio alginolyticus enteritis. *Ann. Sclavo* **22:**169–172.

326. **Nataloni, R.** 1998. As more people pursue water sports, number of stings increase. *Infect. Dis. Child.* **11:**13–14.

327. **National Oceanic and Atmospheric Administration (NOAA).** 2008. *Fisheries of the United States 2007,* p. v. NOAA, Silver Spring, MD.

328. **Neafie, R. C., and W. M. Meyers.** 1991. Cutaneous larva migrans, p. 773–775. *In* G. T. Strickland (ed.), *Hunter's Tropical Medicine,* 7th ed. W. B. Saunders Co., Philadelphia, PA.

329. **Nilsen, A., and O. Boe.** 1980. Fish tank granuloma. *Acta Dermato-Venereol.* (Stockholm) **60:**451–452.

330. **Nip-Sakamoto, C. J., and F. D. Pien.** 1989. Vibrio vulnificus infection in Hawaii. *Int. J. Dermatol.* **28:**311–316.

331. **Nishibuchi, M., S. Doke, S. Toizumi, T. Umeda, M. Yoh, and T. Miwatani.** 1988. Isolation from a coastal fish of *Vibrio hollisae* capable of producing a hemolysin similar to the thermostable direct hemolysin of *Vibrio parahaemolyticus. Appl. Environ. Microbiol.* **54:**2144–2146.

332. **Nishibuchi, M., M. Ishibashi, Y. Takeda, and J. B. Kaper.** 1985. Detection of the thermostable direct hemolysin gene and related DNA sequences in *Vibrio parahaemolyticus* and other *Vibrio* species by the DNA colony hybridisation test. *Infect. Immun.* **49:**481–486.

333. **Nishibuchi, M., and R. J. Seidler.** 1983. Medium-dependent production of extracellular enterotoxins by non-O1 *Vibrio cholerae, Vibrio mimicus,* and *Vibrio fluvialis. Appl. Environ. Microbiol.* **45:**228–231.

334. **Nishibuchi, M., R. J. Seidler, D. M. Rollins, and S. W. Joseph.** 1983. *Vibrio* factors cause rapid fluid accumulation in suckling mice. *Infect. Immun.* **51:**927–931.

335. **Obara, Y., S. Yamai, T. Nikkawa, Y. Miyamoto, M. Ohashi, and T. Shimada.** 1974. Histochemical changes in the small intestine of suckling mice challenged orally with purified hemolysin from Vibrio parahaemolyticus, p. 278–284. *In* T. Fujino, G. Sakaguchi, R. Sakazaki, and Y. Takeda (ed.), *International Symposium on Vibrio parahaemolyticus.* Saikon Publ. Co., Tokyo, Japan.

336. **Oberhofer, T. R., and J. K. Podgore.** 1982. Urea-hydrolyzing *Vibrio parahaemolyticus* associated with acute gastroenteritis. *J. Clin. Microbiol.* **16:**581–583.

337. **O'Brien, A. D., M. E. Chen, R. K. Holmes, J. Kaper, and M. M. Levine.** 1984. Environmental and human isolates of Vibrio cholerae and Vibrio parahaemolyticus produce a Shigella dysenteriae 1 (Shiga)-like cytotoxin. *Lancet* **i:**77–78.

338. **Ohashi, M., T. Shimada, and H. Fukumi.** 1972. In vitro production of enterotoxin and hemorrhagic principle by Vibrio cholerae, NAG. *Jpn. J. Med. Sci. Biol.* **25:**179–194.

339. **Oliver, J. D.** 1981. Lethal cold stress of *Vibrio vulnificus* in oysters. *Appl. Environ. Microbiol.* **41:**710–717.

340. **Oliver, J. D., R. A. Warner, and D. R. Cleland.** 1983. Distribution of *Vibrio vulnificus* and other lactose-fermenting vibrios in the marine environment. *Appl. Environ. Microbiol.* **45:**985–998.

341. **Oliver, J. D., J. E. Wear, and M. B. Thomas.** 1981. Production of extracellular enzymes and cytotoxicity by V. vulnificus. *Diagn. Microbiol. Infect. Dis.* **5:**99–111.

342. **Opal, S. M., and J. R. Saxon.** 1986. Intracranial infection by *Vibrio alginolyticus* following injury in saltwater. *J. Clin. Microbiol.* **23:**373–374.

343. **O'Reilly, G., G. Isbister, P. Lawrie, G. Treston, and B. Currie.** 2001. Prospective study of jellyfish stings from tropical Australia, including the major box jellyfish Chironex fleckeri. *Med. J. Aust.* **175:**652–655.

344. **Palafox, N., L. Jain, A. Pinano, T. Gulick, R. Williams, and I. Schatz.** 1988. Successful treatment of ciguatera fish poisoning with intravenous mannitol. *JAMA* **259:**2740–2742.

345. **Palasuntheram, C., and S. Selvarajah.** 1981. Vibrio parahaemolyticus in Colombo environment. *Indian J. Med. Res.* **73:**13–17.

346. **Park, S. D., H. S. Shon, and N. J. Joh.** 1991. Vibrio vulnificus septicemia in Korea: clinical and epidemiologic findings in seventy patients. *J. Am. Acad. Dermatol.* **24:**397–403.

347. **Park, S. D., H. S. Sohn, and J. W. Koh.** 1986. Effect of hydrogen ions on the growth of Vibrio vulnificus. *Kor. J. Dermatol.* **24:**354–357.

348. **Pavia, A. T., J. A. Bryan, K. L. Maher, T. R. Hester, Jr., and J. J. Farmer III.** 1989. Vibrio carchariae infection after a shark bite. *Ann. Intern. Med.* **111:**85–86.

349. **Perl, T. M., L. Bedard, T. Kosatsky, J. C. Hockin, E. C. D. Todd, and R. S. Remis.** 1990. An outbreak of toxic encephalopathy caused by eating mussels contaminated with domoic acid. *N. Engl. J. Med.* **322:**1775–1780.

350. **Peterson, E. M., P. Jemison-Smith, L. M. de la Maza, and D. Miller.** 1982. Cholecystitis: its occurrence with cholelithiasis associated with a non-O1 Vibrio cholerae. *Arch. Pathol. Lab. Med.* **106:**300–301.

351. **Peterson, J. W., and L. G. Ochoa.** 1989. Role of prostaglandins and cAMP in the secretory effects of cholera toxin. *Science* **245:**857–859.

352. **Pien, F. D., K. S. Ang, and N. T. Nakashima.** 1983. Bacterial flora of marine penetrating injuries. *Diagn. Microbiol. Infect. Dis.* **1:**229–232.

353. **Plotkin, B. J., S. G. Kilgore, and L. McFarland.** 1990. Polyvibrio infections: Vibrio vulnificus and Vibrio parahaemolyticus dual wound and multiple site infections. *J. Infect. Dis.* **161:**364–365.

354. **Poli, M. A., R. J. Lewis, R. W. Dickey, S. M. Musser, C. A. Buckner, and L. G. Carpenter.** 1997. Identification of Caribbean ciguatoxins as the cause of an outbreak of fish poisoning among U.S. soldiers in Haiti. *Toxicon* **35:**733–741.

355. **Pool, M. D., and J. D. Oliver.** 1978. Experimental pathogenicity and mortality in ligated ileal loop studies of the newly reported halophilic lactose-positive *Vibrio* sp. *Infect. Immun.* **20:**126–129.

356. **Portnoy, B. L., P. A. Mackowiak, and C. T. Caraway.** 1975. Oyster-associated hepatitis: failure of shellfish certification programs to prevent outbreaks. *JAMA* **233:**1065–1068.

357. Reference deleted.

358. **Prevost, E., E. M. Walker, Jr., A. J. Kreutner, and J. Manos.** 1982. Mycobacterium marinum infections: diagnosis and treatment. *South. Med. J.* **75:**1349–1352.

359. **Prociv, P.** 1978. Vibrio alginolyticus in Western Australia. *Med. J. Aust.* **2:**296.

360. **Quilliam, M. A., and J. L. C. Wright.** 1989. The amnesic shellfish poisoning mystery. *Anal. Chem.* **61:**1053–1059.

361. **Rainer, M. D.** 1972. Mode of action of ciguatoxin. *Fed. Proc.* **31:**1139–1145.

362. **RaLonde, R.** 1996. Paralytic shellfish poisoning: the Alaska problem. *Alsk. Mar. Resour.* **8(2):**1–20.

363. **Ramamurthy, T., S. Garg, and R. Sharma.** 1993. Emergence of novel strain of Vibrio cholerae with epidemic potential in southern and eastern India. *Lancet* **341:**703–704.

364. **Ramia, S.** 1985. Transmission of viral infections by the water route: implications for developing countries. *Rev. Infect. Dis.* **7:**180–188.

365. **Rank, E. L., I. B. Smith, and M. Langer.** 1988. Bacteremia caused by *Vibrio hollisae*. *J. Clin. Microbiol.* **26:**375–376.

366. **Reichelt, J. L., P. Baumann, and L. Baumann.** 1976. Study of genetic relationships among marine species of the genus Beneckea and Photobacterium by means of in vitro DNA/DNA hybridization. *Arch. Microbiol.* **110:**101–120.

367. **Reid, T. M. S., and H. G. Robinson.** 1987. Frozen raspberries and hepatitis A. *Epidemiol. Infect.* **98:**109–112.

368. **Rhodes, J. B., D. Schweitzer, and J. E. Ogg.** 1985. Isolation of non-O1 *Vibrio cholerae* associated with enteric disease of herbivores in Western Colorado. *J. Clin. Microbiol.* **22:**572–575.

369. **Rhodes, J. B., H. L. Smith, and J. E. Ogg.** 1986. Isolation of non-O1 *Vibrio cholerae* serovars from surface waters in Western Colorado. *Appl. Environ. Microbiol.* **51:**1216–1219.

370. **Richards, C. A.** 1998. Pfiesteria piscicida studies underway in six states. *Infect. Dis. News* **11:**14–15.

371. **Ries, K. M., G. L. White, Jr., and R. T. Murdock.** 1990. Atypical mycobacterial infection caused by Mycobacterium marinum. *N. Engl. J. Med.* **322:**633.

372. **Risk, M., K. Werrbach-Perez, and J. R. Perez-Polo.** 1979. Mechanism of action of the major toxin from Gymnodinium breve davis, p. 367–372. *In* D. L. Taylor and H. H. Seliger (ed.), *Toxic Dinoflagellate Blooms.* Elsevier/Holland, New York, NY.

373. **Robinson, A. C.** 1989. Evaluation for waterproof ear protectors in swimmers. *J. Laryngol. Otol.* **103:**1154–1157.

374. **Rodrick, G. E., M. A. Hood, and N. J. Blake.** 1982. Human vibrio gastroenteritis. *Med. Clin. N. Am.* **66:**665–673.

375. **Rodrigue, D. C., R. A. Etzel, S. Hall, E. De Porras, O. H. Velasquez, R. V. Tauxe, E. M. Kilbourne, and P. A. Blake.** 1990. Lethal paralytic shellfish poisoning in Guatemala. *Am. J. Trop. Med.* **42:**267–281.

376. **Roland, F., R. Bertini, and J. Jhang.** 1985. Vibrio parahaemolyticus osteomyelitis of 12 years duration. *Rhode Island Med. J.* **68:**553–555.

377. **Roos, B.** 1956. Hepatitis epidemic transmitted by oysters. *Sven. Lakartidn.* **53:**989–1003.

378. **Rosenberg, C. E.** 1962. *The Cholera Years: The United States in 1832, 1849, and 1866.* University of Chicago Press, Chicago, IL.

379. **Rosenblum, L. S., I. R. Mirkin, and D. T. Allen.** 1990. A multifocal outbreak of hepatitis A traced to commercially distributed lettuce. *AJPH* **80:**1075–1079.

380. **Rubin, L. G., J. Altman, L. K. Epple, and R. H. Yolken.** 1981. Vibrio cholerae meningitis in a neonate. *J. Pediatr.* **98:**940–942.

381. **Russell, F. E.** 1961. Injuries by venomous animals in the US. *JAMA* **177:**85.

382. **Ryan, A. J.** 1989. Nontraumatic medical problems, p. 391–414. *In* A. J. Ryan and F. L. Allman (ed.), *Sports Medicine,* 2nd ed. Academic Press, Inc., San Diego, CA.

383. **Sacks-Berg, A., M. J. Strampfer, and B. A. Cunha.** 1987. Vibrio vulnificus bacteremia: report of a case and review of the literature. *Heart Lung* **16:**706–709.

384. **Safrin, S., J. G. Morris, Jr., M. Adams, V. Pons, R. Jacobs, and J. E. Conte, Jr.** 1988. Non-O:1 Vibrio cholerae bacteremia: case report and review. *Rev. Infect. Dis.* **10:**1012–1017.

385. **Sakamoto, Y., R. F. Lockey, and J. J. Krzanowski, Jr.** 1987. Shellfish and fish poisoning related to the toxic dinoflagellates. *South. Med. J.* **80:**866–872.

386. **Sakamoto, Y., J. Krzanowski, R. Lockey, et al.** 1985. The mechanism of Ptychodiscus brevis toxin-induced contraction of rat vas deferens. *J. Allergy Clin. Immunol.* **76:**117–122.

387. **Sakazaki, R.** 1968. Proposal of Vibrio alginolyticus for the biotype 2 of Vibrio parahaemolyticus. *Jpn. J. Med. Sci. Biol.* **21:**359–362.

388. **Saliba, L. J., and R. Helmer.** 1990. Health risks associated with pollution of coastal bathing waters. *World Health Stat. Q.* **43:**177–187.

389. **Salmaso, S., D. Greco, B. Bonfiglio, M. Castellani-Pastoris, G. De Filip, A. Bracciotti, G. Sitzia, A. Congiu, G. Piu, G. Angioni, L. Barra, A. Zampieri, and W. B. Baine.** 1980. Recurrence of pelecypod-associated cholera in Sardinia. *Lancet* **ii:**1124–1127.

390. **Samadi, A. R., M. I. Huq, and N. S. Shahid.** 1983. Classical Vibrio cholerae biotype displaces El Tor in Bangladesh. *Lancet* **i:**805–807.

391. **Sanders, W. E., Jr.** 1987. Intoxications from the seas: ciguatera, scombroid, and paralytic shellfish poisoning. *Infect. Dis. Clin. N. Am.* **1:** 665–676.

392. **Sarkar, B. L., G. B. Nair, A. K. Banerjee, and S. C. Pal.** 1985. Seasonal distribution of *Vibrio parahaemolyticus* in freshwater environs and in association with freshwater fishes in Calcutta. *Appl. Environ. Microbiol.* **49:**132–136.

393. **Sarnaik, A. P., M. P. Vohra, S. W. Sturman, and W. M. Belenky.** 1986. Medical problems of the swimmer. *Clin. Sports Med.* **5:** 47–64.

394. **Schandevyl, P., E. Van Dyck, and P. Piot.** 1984. Halophilic *Vibrio* species from seafish in Senegal. *Appl. Environ. Microbiol.* **48:**236–238.

395. **Scheid, R., F. Deinhardt, and G. Frosner.** 1982. Inactivation of hepatitis A and B virus and risk of iatrogenic transmission, p. 627–628. *In* W. Szmuness, H. J. Alter, and H. E. Maynard (ed.), *Viral Hepatitis*. Franklin Institute Press, Philadelphia, PA.

396. **Schiraldi, O., V. Benvestito, C. DiBari, R. Moschetta, and G. Pastore.** 1974. Gastric abnormalities in cholera: epidemiologic and clinical considerations. *Bull. W. H. O.* **51:**349–352.

397. **Schmidt, V., H. Chmel, and C. Cobbs.** 1979. *Vibrio alginolyticus* infections in humans. *J. Clin. Microbiol.* **10:**666–668.

398. **Schonherr, U., G. O. H. Naumann, G. K. Lang, and A. A. Bialasiewicz.** 1989. Sclerokeratitis caused by Mycobacterium marinum. *Am. J. Ophthalmol.* **108:**607–608.

399. **Schuller, D. E., and R. A. Bruce.** 1991. Ear, nose, throat, and eye, p. 189–203. *In* R. Strauss (ed.), *Sports Medicine*, 2nd ed. W. B. Saunders Co., Philadelphia, PA.

400. **Seidler, R. J., D. A. Allen, and R. R. Colwell.** 1980. Biochemical characteristics and virulence of environmental group F bacteria isolated in the United States. *Appl. Environ. Microbiol.* **40:**715–720.

401. **Seidler, R. J., and T. M. Evans.** 1984. Computer-assisted analysis of Vibrio field data: four coastal areas, p. 411–426. *In* R. R. Colwell (ed.), *Vibrios in the Environment*. John Wiley & Sons, Inc., New York, NY.

402. **Shandera, W. X., J. M. Johnston, B. R. Davis, and P. A. Blake.** 1983. Disease from infection with Vibrio mimicus, a newly recognized Vibrio species: clinical characteristics and epidemiology. *Ann. Intern. Med.* **99:**169–171.

403. **Shirai, H., H. Ito, T. Hirayama, Y. Nakamoto, N. Nakabayashi, K. Kumagai, T. T., and M. Nishibuchi.** 1990. Molecular epidemiologic evidence for association of thermostable direct hemolysin (TDH) and TDH-related hemolysin of *Vibrio parahaemolyticus* with gastroenteritis. *Infect. Immun.* **58:**3568–3573.

404. **Simpson, L. M., and J. D. Oliver.** 1983. Siderophore production by *Vibrio vulnificus. Infect. Immun.* **41:**644–649.

405. **Sims, J. K.** 1986. Pufferfish poisoning: emergency diagnosis and management of mild human tetrodotoxin. *Ann. Emerg. Med.* **15:**1094–1098.

406. **Sims, J. K.** 1987. A theoretical discourse on the pharmacology of toxic marine ingestions. *Ann. Emerg. Med.* **16:**1006–1015.

407. **Singleton, F. L., R. Attwell, S. Jangi, and R. R. Colwell.** 1982. Effects of temperature and salinity on *Vibrio cholerae* growth. *Appl. Environ. Microbiol.* **44:**1047–1058.

408. **Singleton, F. L., R. W. Attwell, S. Jangi, and R. R. Colwell.** 1982. Influence of salinity and organic nutrient concentration on survival and growth of *Vibrio cholerae* in aquatic microcosms. *Appl. Environ. Microbiol.* **43:**1080–1085.

409. **Sircar, B. K., P. Dutta, S. P. De, S. N. Sikdar, B. C. Deb, and S. C. Pal.** 1981. ABO blood group distributions in diarrhoea

cases including cholera in Calcutta. *Ann. Human Biol.* **8:**289–291.

410. **Smith, G. C., and J. R. Merkel.** 1982. Collagenolytic activity of *Vibrio vulnificus*: potential contribution to its invasiveness. *Infect. Immun.* **35:**1155–1156.

411. **Sodeman, W. A., Jr.** 1991. Venomous marine animals, p. 869–875. *In* G. T. Strickland (ed.), *Hunter's Tropical Medicine,* 7th ed. W. B. Saunders Co., Philadelphia, PA.

412. **Soppe, G. G.** 1989. Marine envenomation and aquatic dermatology. *Am. Fam. Physician* **40:**97–106.

413. **Sreenivasan, M. A., K. Banerjee, and P. G. Pandya.** 1978. Epidemiologic investigations of an outbreak of infectious hepatitis in Ahmedabad City during 1975–76. *Indian J. Med. Res.* **67:**197–206.

413a.**Stafford-Deitsch, J.** 1991. *Reef: a Safari through the Coral World.* Sierra Club Books, San Francisco, CA.

414. **Stahr, B., S. T. Threadgill, T. L. Overman, and R. C. Noble.** 1989. Vibrio vulnificus sepsis after eating raw oysters. *J. Ky. Med. Assoc.* **87:**219–222.

415. **Steidinger, K. A.** 1979. Collection, enumeration, and identification of free-living marine dinoflagellates, p. 435–442. *In* D. L. Taylor and H. H. Seliger (ed.), *Toxic Dinoflagellate Blooms.* Elsevier/North Holland, New York, NY.

416. **Steinkuller, P. G., M. T. Kelly, S. J. Sands, and J. C. Barber.** 1980. Vibrio parahaemolyticus endophthalmitis. *J. Pediatr. Ophthalmol. Strabismus* **17:**150–153.

417. **Stewart, J. P.** 1951. Chronic exudative otitis externa. *J. Laryngol. Otol.* **65:**24.

418. **Subba Rao, D. V., M. A. Quilliam, and R. Pocklington.** 1988. Domoic acid—a neurotoxic amino acid produced by the marine diatom Nitzschia pungens in culture. *Can. J. Fish. Aquat. Sci.* **45:**2076–2079.

419. **Sullivan, J. J., and W. T. Iwaoka.** 1983. High pressure liquid chromatographic determination of toxins associated with paralytic shellfish poisoning. *J. Assoc. Off. Anal. Chem.* **66:**297–303.

420. **Swerdlow, D. L., and A. A. Ries.** 1992. Cholera in the Americas. Guidelines for the clinician. *JAMA* **267:**1495–1499.

421. **Swift, S., and H. Cohen.** 1962. Granulomas of the skin due to Mycobacterium balnei after abrasions from a fish tank. *N. Engl. J. Med.* **267:**1244–1246.

422. **Tacket, C. O., T. J. Barrett, G. E. Sanders, and P. A. Blake.** 1982. Panophthalmitis caused by *Vibrio parahaemolyticus. J. Clin. Microbiol.* **16:**195–196.

423. **Tacket, C. O., F. Brenner, and P. A. Blake.** 1984. Clinical features and an epidemiological study of Vibrio vulnificus infections. *J. Infect. Dis.* **149:**558–561.

424. **Tacket, C. O., F. Hickman, and G. V. Pierce.** 1982. Diarrhea associated with *Vibrio fluvialis* in the United States. *J. Clin. Microbiol.* **16:**991–992.

425. **Tamplin, M., G. E. Rodrick, N. J. Blake, and T. Cuba.** 1982. Isolation and characterization of *Vibrio vulnificus* from two Florida estuaries. *Appl. Environ. Microbiol.* **44:**1466–1470.

426. **Tan, C. T. T., and E. J. D. Lee.** 1986. Paralytic shellfish poisoning in Singapore. *Ann. Acad. Med. Singapore* **15:**77–79.

427. **Tang, Y. W., J. X. Wang, and Z. Y. Xu.** 1991. A serologically confirmed, case-control study, of a large outbreak of hepatitis A in China, associated with consumption of clams. *Epidemiol. Infect.* **107:**651–657.

428. **Taylor, R., M. McDonald, G. Russ, M. Carson, and E. Lukaczynski.** 1981. Vibrio alginolyticus peritonitis associated with ambulatory peritoneal dialysis. *Br. Med. J.* **283:**275.

429. **Taylor, S. L., J. E. Stratton, and J. A. Nordlee.** 1989. Histamine poisoning (scombroid fish poisoning): an allergy-like intoxication. *J. Toxicol. Clin. Toxicol.* **27:**225–240.

430. **Tefany, F. J., S. Lee, and S. Shumack.** 1990. Oysters, iron overload and vibrio vulnificus septicaemia. *Australas. J. Dermatol.* **31:**27–31.

431. **Teitelbaum, J. S., R. J. Zatorre, S. Carpenter, D. Gendron, E. C. Evans, A. Gjedde, and N. R. Cashman.** 1990. Neurologic sequelae of domoic acid intoxication due to the ingestion of contaminated mussels. *N. Engl. J. Med.* **322:**1781–1787.

432. **Tester, P. A., P. K. Fowler, and J. T. Turner.** 1990. Gulf stream transport of the toxic red tide dinoflagellate Ptychodiscus brevis from Florida to North Carolina, p. 349–358. *In* E. M. Cosper, E. J. Carpenter, and V. M. Bricelj (ed.), *Novel Phytoplankton Blooms: Causes and Impact of Recurrent Brown Tides and Other Unusual Blooms.* Springer-Verlag, Berlin, Germany.

433. **Thekdi, R. J., A. G. Lakhani, V. B. Rale, and M. V. Panse.** 1990. An outbreak of food poisoning suspected to be caused by Vibrio fluvialis. *J. Diarrhoeal Dis. Res.* **8:**163–165.

434. **Thibaut, K., P. Van de Heying, and S. R. Pattyn.** 1986. Isolation of non-O1 Vibrio cholerae from ear tracts. *Eur. J. Epidemiol.* **2:**316–317.

435. **Tibballs, J., D. Williams, and S. Sutherland.** 1998. The effects of antivenom and verapamil on the haemodynamic actions of Chironex fleckeri (box jellyfish) venom. *Anaesth. Intensive Care* **26:**40–45.

436. **Ticehurst, J., L. L. J. Rhodes, and K. Krawczynski.** 1992. Infection of owl monkeys (Aotus trivirgatus) and cynomolgus monkeys (Macaca fascicularis) with hepatitis E virus from Mexico. *J. Infect. Dis.* **165:**835–845.

437. **Tison, D. L., and M. T. Kelly.** 1984. Vibrio species of medical importance. *Diagn. Microbiol. Infect. Dis.* **2:**263–276.

438. **Tison, D. L., and M. T. Kelly.** 1984. *Vibrio vulnificus* endometritis. *J. Clin. Microbiol.* **20:**185–186.

439. **Tison, D. L., M. Nishibuchi, R. J. Seidler, and R. J. Sieberling.** 1986. Isolation of non-O1 *Vibrio cholerae* serovars from Oregon coastal waters. *Appl. Environ. Microbiol.* **51:**444–445.

440. **Togias, A. G., J. W. Burnett, A. Kagey-Sobotka, and L. M. Lichtenstein.** 1985. Anaphylaxis after contact with a jellyfish. *J. Allergy Clin. Immunol.* **75:**672–675.

441. **Trestrail, J. H., III, and Q. M. al-Mahasneh.** 1989. Lionfish sting experiences of an inland poison center: a retrospective study of 23 cases. *Vet. Hum. Toxicol.* **31:**173–175.

442. **Tripuraneni, J., A. Koutsoris, L. Pestic, P. De Lanerolle, and G. Hecht.** 1997. The toxin of diarrheic shellfish poisoning, okadaic acid, increases intestinal epithelial paracellular permeability. *Gastroenterology* **112:**100–108.

443. **Truwit, J. D., D. B. Badesch, A. M. Savage, and M. Shelton.** 1987. Vibrio vulnificus bacteremia with endocarditis. *South. Med. J.* **80:**1457–1459.

444. **Tsega, E., K. Krawczynski, and B. G. Hansson.** 1991. Outbreak of hepatitis E virus infection among military personnel in Northern Ethiopia. *J. Med. Virol.* **34:**232–236.

445. **Tu, A. T.** 1987. Biotoxicology of sea snake venoms. *Ann. Emerg. Med.* **16:**1023–1028.

446. **Tu, A. T.** 1990. Neurotoxins from sea snake and other vertebrate venoms, p. 336–346. *In* S. Hall and G. Strichartz (ed.), *Marine Toxins. Origin, Structure, and Molecular Pharmacology.* American Chemical Society, Washington, DC.

447. **Twedt, R. M.** 1989. Vibrio parahaemolyticus, p. 543–568. *In* M. P. Doyle (ed.), *Foodborne Bacterial Pathogens.* Marcel Dekker, New York, NY.

448. **Twedt, R. M., J. M. Madden, J. M. Hunt, D. W. Francis, J. T. Peeler, A. P. Duran, W. O. Herbert, S. G. McCay, C. N. Roderick, G. T. Spite, and T. J. Wazenski.** 1981. Characterization of *Vibrio cholerae* isolated from oysters. *Appl. Environ. Microbiol.* **41:**1475–1478.

449. **Vancouver, G.** 1798. *A Voyage of Discovery to the North Pacific Ocean and Round the World,* vol. 2, p. 284–286. Robinson, London, England.

450. **van der Sar, A.** 1982. Ciguatera poisoning and T-wave changes. *JAMA* **247:**1345.

451. **Van Dyke, J. J., and K. B. Lake.** 1975. Chemotherapy for aquarium granuloma. *JAMA* **233:**1380–1381.

452. **Vartian, C. V., and E. J. Septimus.** 1990. Osteomyelitis caused by Vibrio vulnificus. *J. Infect. Dis.* **161:**363.

453. **Vincenzi, C., F. Bardazzi, and A. Tosti.** 1992. Fish tank granuloma: report of a case. *Cutis* **49:**275–276.

454. **Viswanathan, R.** 1957. Infectious hepatitis in Delhi (1955–56): a critical study; epidemiology. *Indian J. Med. Res.* **45**(Suppl.):1–30.

455. **Wagner, R. W., Jr., A. B. Tawil, A. J. Colletta, L. C. Hurst, and L. D. Yecies.** 1981. Mycobacterium marinum tenosynovitis in a Long Island fisherman. *N. Y. State J. Med.* **81:**1091–1094.

456. **Walker, S. T.** 1884. Fish mortality in the Gulf of Mexico. *Proc. U. S. Natl. Museum* **6:**105–109.

457. **Wallace, C. K., N. F. Pierce, P. N. Anderson, T. C. Brown, G. W. Lewis, S. N. Sanyal, G. V. Segre, and R. H. Waldman.** 1967. Probable gallbladder infection in convalescent cholera patients. *Lancet* **i:**865–868.

458. **Wanke, C. A., and R. L. Guerrant.** 1987. Viral hepatitis and gastroenteritis transmitted by shellfish and water. *Infect. Dis. Clin. N. Am.* **1:**649–664.

459. **Watsky, D.** 1983. Vibrio fluvialis and Vibrio mimicus associated with terminal ileitis. *Clin. Microbiol. Newsl.* **5:**111.

459a.**Weinberg, S., N. Prose, and L. Kristal.** 1998. *Color Atlas of Pediatric Dermatology,* 3rd ed. McGraw-Hill, New York, NY.

460. **Weissman, J. B., W. E. DeWitt, J. Thompson, C. N. Muchnick, B. L. Portnoy, J. C. Feeley, and E. J. Gangarosa.** 1975. A case of cholera in Texas, 1973. *Am. J. Epidemiol.* **100:**487–498.

461. **West, B., R. Silberman, and W. Otterson.** 1998. Acalculous cholecystitis and septicemia caused by non-O1 Vibrio cholerae: first reported case and review of biliary infections with Vibrio cholerae. *Diagn. Microbiol. Infect. Dis.* **30:**187–191.

462. **West, P. A.** 1986. Hazard analysis critical control point (HACCP) concept: application to bivalve shellfish purification systems. *J. R. Soc. Health* **106:**133–140.

463. **West, P. A.** 1989. The human pathogenic vibrios—a public health update with environmental perspectives. *Epidemiol. Infect.* **103:**1–34.

464. **West, P. A., and J. V. Lee.** 1982. Ecology of Vibrio species, including Vibrio cholerae, in natural waters in Kent, England. *J. Appl. Bacteriol.* **52:**435–448.

465. **West, P. A., P. C. Wood, and M. Jacob.** 1985. Control of food poisoning risks associated with shellfish. *J. R. Soc. Health* **105:**15–21.

466. **Wickboldt, I. G., and C. V. Sanders.** 1983. Vibrio vulnificus infection: case report and update since 1970. *J. Am. Acad. Dermatol.* **9:**243–251.

467. **Williams, C. S., and D. C. Riordan.** 1973. Mycobacterium marinum (atypical acid-fast bacillus) infections of the hand: a report of six cases. *J. Bone Joint Surg.* **55A:**1042–1050.

468. **Williams, L. A., and P. A. La Rock.** 1985. Temporal occurrence of *Vibrio* species and *Aeromonas hydrophila* in estuarine sediments. *Appl. Environ. Microbiol.* **50:**1490–1495.

469. **Wilson, R., S. Lieb, A. Roberts, S. Stryker, H. Janowski, R. Gunn, B. Davis, C. F. Riddle, T. Barrett, J. G. Morris, Jr., and P. A. Blake.** 1981. Non-O group 1 Vibrio cholerae gastroenteritis associated with eating raw oysters. *Am. J. Epidemiol.* **114:**293–298.

470. **Withers, N. W.** 1982. Ciguatera fish poisoning. *Annu. Rev. Med.* **33:**97–111.

471. **Wong, D. C., R. H. Purcell, and M. A. Sreenivasan.** 1980. Epidemic and endemic hepatitis in India: evidence for a non-A, non-B hepatitis etiology. *Lancet* **ii:**876–879.

472. **World Health Organization.** 1986. Aquatic (marine and freshwater) biotoxins, p. 73–75. *In Environmental Health Criteria.* World Health Organization, Geneva, Switzerland.

473. **World Health Organization.** 1980. Cholera and other vibrio-associated diarrhoeas. *Bull. W. H. O.* **58:**353–374.

474. **World Health Organization.** 1969. Outbreak of gastroenteritis by non-agglutinable (NAG) vibrios. *W. H. O. Wkly. Epidemiol. Rec.* **44:**10.

475. **World Health Organization.** 1970. *Principles and Practice of Cholera Control 40.* World Health Organization, Geneva, Switzerland.

476. **World Health Organization.** 1980. Rotavirus and other viral diarrhoeas. *Bull. W. H. O.* **58:**183–198.

477. **Wozniak, D. F., G. R. Stewart, J. P. Miller, and J. W. Olney.** 1991. Age-related sensitivity to kainate neurotoxicity. *Exp. Neurol.* **114:**250–253.

478. **Wright, A. C., L. M. Simpson, and J. D. Oliver.** 1981. Role of iron in the pathogenesis of *Vibrio vulnificus* infections. *Infect. Immun.* **34:**503–507.

479. **Wright, A. C., L. M. Simpson, J. D. Oliver, and J. G. Morris, Jr.** 1990. Phenotypic evaluation of acapsular transposon mutants of *Vibrio vulnificus. Infect. Immun.* **58:**1769–1773.

480. **Wright, D. N., and J. M. Alexander.** 1974. Effect of water on the bacterial flora of swimmer's ears. *Arch. Otolaryngol.* **99:**15–18.

481. **Yamamoto, K., Y. Ichinose, N. Nakasone, M. Tanabe, M. Nagahama, J. Sakurai, and M. Iwanaga.** 1986. Identity of hemolysins produced by *Vibrio cholerae* non-O-1 and *V. cholerae* O1, biotype El Tor. *Infect. Immun.* **51:**927–931.

482. **Yamamoto, K., Y. Takeda, T. Miwatani, and J. P. Craig.** 1983. Evidence that a non-O1 *Vibrio cholerae* produces enterotoxin that is similar but not identical to cholera enterotoxin. *Infect. Immun.* **41:**896–901.

483. **Yamashita, T., K. Sakae, Y. Ishihara, and S. Isomura.** 1992. A 2-year survey of the prevalence of enteric viral infections in children compared with contamination in locally-harvested oysters. *Epidemiol. Infect.* **108:**155–163.

484. **Yasumoto, J.** 1985. Recent progress in the chemistry of dinoflagellate toxins, p. 259–270. *In* D. M. Anderson, A. W. White, and D. G. Baden (ed.), *Toxic Dinoflagellates.* Elsevier, New York, NY.

485. **Yasumoto, T., A. Inoue, and R. Bagnis.** 1979. Ecological survey of a toxic dinoflagellate associated with ciguatera, p. 221–224. *In* D. L. Taylor and H. H. Seliger (ed.), *Toxic Dinoflagellate Blooms.* Elsevier/North Holland, New York, NY.

486. **Yoh, M., T. Honda, and T. Miwatani.** 1986. Purification and partial characterization of a Vibrio hollisae hemolysin that relates to the thermostable direct hemolysin of Vibrio parahaemolyticus. *Can. J. Microbiol.* **32:**632–636.

487. **Yokoo, A.** 1950. Chemical studies on tetrodotoxin. III. Isolation of spheroidine. *J. Chem. Soc. Jpn.* **71:**591–592.

488. **Yoshida, S., M. Ogawa, and Y. Mizuguchi.** 1985. Relation of capsular materials and colony opacity to virulence of *Vibrio vulnificus. Infect. Immun.* **47:**446–451.

489. **Yoshii, Y., H. Nishino, K. Satake, and K. Umeyama.** 1987. Isolation of Vibrio fluvialis, an unusual pathogen in acute suppurative cholangitis. *Am. J. Gastroenterol.* **82:**903–905.

490. **Yu, S. L., and O. Uy-Yu.** 1984. Vibrio parahaemolyticus pneumonia. *Ann. Intern. Med.* **100:**320.

491. **Zen-Yoji, H., Y. Kudoh, H. Igarashi, K. Ohta, and K. Fukai.** 1974. Purification and identification of enteropathogenic toxins "a" and "a'" produced by Vibrio parahaemolyticus and their biological and pathological activities, p. 237–243. *In* T. Fujino, G. Sakaguchi, R. Sakazaki, and Y. Takeda (ed.), *International Symposium on Vibrio parahaemolyticus.* Saikon Publishing Co., Tokyo, Japan.

FRESHWATER: FROM LAKES TO HOT TUBS

Bertha S. Ayi and David Dworzack

2

This chapter focuses on infections acquired in nonmarine environments, including natural freshwater environments (lakes, ponds, rivers, and streams) and man-made aquatic environments (swimming pools, hot tubs, whirlpools, and spas). The discussion is limited to infections associated with immersion or other exposure to aquatic macro- or microenvironments. An appreciation of the wide variety of potential pathogens that occasionally cause problems for patients exposed to freshwater can be gained from Table 1.

Swimming is a popular activity in most places. In most countries, people enjoy rivers, lakes, and untreated water bodies. In several industrialized countries, most hotels and community centers have swimming pools (9, 21). In the United States, swimming is the second-most-common recreational activity. There are an estimated 7.4 million swimming pools in public places or in people's homes, and more than 360 million visits are recorded for rec-

reational water avenues (69, 70). These recreational activities, however, place users at an increased risk of illness acquired from these venues. Recreational water illnesses (RWIs) are illnesses acquired from using bodies of water for recreation. Of these illnesses, infections are particularly common, because waterborne pathogens may enter the body through inhalation, aspiration, direct application to intact or injured skin, or invasion of respiratory or gastrointestinal mucosae. Over the last 2 decades, RWIs have been on the increase, partly due to chlorine-resistant organisms like *Cryptosporidium* spp. and partly due to inadequate pool maintenance (12, 70). The pathogens may be native to the environments where infections are acquired, or they may proliferate there because of the influence of humans or their waste products. Infections produced by these pathogens range from skin infections to brain infections; however, gastrointestinal infections are the most common (70, 100). These infections are often merely nuisances; however, on occasion, they can be life-threatening or cause severe long-term sequelae.

A bacterium or protozoan was responsible for most of these outbreaks. In one study that reviewed outbreaks over 3 decades from 1971 to 2000 in the United States, the most com-

Bertha S. Ayi, Mercy Infectious Disease and Epidemiology Center, 801 5th St., Sioux City, IA 51103. *David Dworzack,* Department of Medical Microbiology and Immunology and Section of Infectious Diseases, Department of Internal Medicine, Creighton University Medical Center, Omaha, NE 68131.

Infections of Leisure, Fourth Edition, Edited by David Schlossberg,
© 2009 ASM Press, Washington, DC

TABLE 1 Infections associated with exposure to freshwater

Skin and soft tissue infections
P. aeruginosa dermatitis/folliculitis
P. aeruginosa hot-foot syndrome
Acute diffuse otitis externa (swimmer's ear)
Schistosome dermatitis (swimmer's itch, clam digger's itch)
Nontuberculous mycobacterial infections (*M. marinum, M. ulcerans,* rapidly growing mycobacteria)
Gram-negative bacilli *(Aeromonas, Edwardsiella)*
Prototheca infection
Cyanobacterium infection
Methicillin-resistant *Staphylococcus aureus* (MRSA) infections

Ocular infections
Pharyngoconjunctival fever (swimming pool conjunctivitis)
Amoebic keratitis (*Acanthamoeba* spp.)
P. aeruginosa keratitis

Urinary tract infections
P. aeruginosa infection

Pulmonary infections
Legionella infection (pneumonia, Pontiac fever)
P. aeruginosa pneumonia
M. avium infection
Pneumonia following near drowning
  Aerobic gram-negative bacteria (*P. aeruginosa, Aeromonas* spp., *B. pseudomallei, Legionella* spp.)
  S. pneumoniae
  Aspergillus spp.
  P. boydii

Gastrointestinal infections
Cryptosporidium parvum
Giardia
Shigella
Escherichia coli O157
Norovirus

Disseminated infections
Leptospirosis
C. violaceum

Central nervous system infections
PAM *(N. fowleri)*
P. boydii brain abscess and meningitis
Coxsackieviruses

mon agents were *Cryptosporidium* (15%), *Pseudomonas* (14%), *Shigella* (13%), *Naegleria* (11%), *Giardia* (6%), and toxigenic *Escherichia coli* (6%) (23). While *Shigella, Naegleria,* and *E. coli* were more likely to cause outbreaks in freshwater, such as in lakes, ponds, and rivers, *Cryptosporidium* and *Giardia* were more likely to cause infections and outbreaks in treated waters, like in swimming pools.

SKIN AND SOFT TISSUE INFECTIONS
Skin, soft tissue, and wound infections acquired in aquatic, nonmarine environments run the gamut from relatively benign conditions which resolve without specific therapy to life-threatening processes requiring intensive medical and surgical care. Infections caused by pyogenic bacteria, mycobacteria, parasites, and algae have all been reported previously (8).

Pseudomonas Dermatitis/Folliculitis
Pseudomonas dermatitis/folliculitis, a superficial infection which is usually recognized in cluster or localized outbreaks, was first reported in 1975 by McCausland and Cox (65). That original outbreak, like most others reported since, was associated with exposure to heated water in a hotel whirlpool (51). Similar outbreaks have occurred from the use of home spas as well as swimming pools (16). The largest (265 cases from 650 people exposed) and first outbreak involving exposure at a water slide was in Salt Lake City, UT, in 1983 (15). Since then, more outbreaks involving water slides have been reported (30). More unusual are reports associated with the use of neoprene diving suits and contaminated synthetic sponges used in bathing. These outbreaks may be more common in the summer, when outdoor activities are common.

In most outbreaks, faulty maintenance of water in man-made pools has been associated with overgrowth of *Pseudomonas aeruginosa.* Recommendations for the treatment of pool water include maintaining the pH between 7.2 and 7.5 and free-chlorine levels above 2 mg/liter (17, 101). In one outbreak, however, the pH and the chlorine content of contaminated water were found to be within these guidelines, suggesting that some strains of *P. aeruginosa* may be resistant to recommended chlorine concentrations (51). In another, more recent outbreak involving swimming pool water in which adequate chlorination had been maintained, the source of the infection was traced to inflatables used by children (92). These inflatables serve as obstacle courses and are kept inflated by an air pump during use and deflated after use. Microorganisms can grow on these devices when they are kept outside the pool and not allowed to dry, or they can be contaminated from residual water inside the inflatable. Folliculitis occurs after skin contact with a contaminated inflatable.

There have been more outbreaks associated with whirlpools or spas than with swimming pools, indicating that the environment of the former is more conducive to the growth of organisms that cause folliculitis. In part, this appears to be related to the difficulty in maintaining a stable free-chlorine level in whirlpools compared to that in swimming pools because of the higher temperature of the water, mechanical agitation and aeration by pressurized jets, and a higher concentration of organic material due to the larger number of bathers per volume of water (78). For this reason, some have recommended higher concentrations of free chlorine (1 to 3 mg/liter) in whirlpool or spa water (84). The use of cyanuric acid to stabilize chlorine levels in indoor pools and hot tubs may also decrease the antimicrobial capacity of free chlorine (16). In addition, due to the predisposing environmental factors mentioned above, dilatation of skin pores because of the higher water temperature may facilitate entry of the *P. aeruginosa* organisms contained in the water (99).

Some outbreaks have been due to faulty chlorination systems in swimming pools. Occasionally, a source of the organism is found. In one recent water slide outbreak (30), *P. aeruginosa* was isolated from the water butt used to draw water for games as well as the tank of the fire engine that supplied the water. Guidelines for swimming pools have been proposed (17).

The source of *P. aeruginosa* infection in patients with diving suit-associated lesions was less clear. Although the suits were worn in salt water, which poorly supports the growth of *P. aeruginosa,* the microenvironment next to the skin was not salty, and the source might have been skin colonization (both patients were health care workers). Alternatively, freshwater used to rinse the suits after use may have contained *P. aeruginosa*. The use of synthetic sponges to bathe has given rise to family outbreaks as well as sporadic cases of folliculitis (53). It is hypothesized that the minor trauma of rubbing the skin with a contaminated sponge might favor the entrance of the organism into the skin. Some outbreaks may occur at home, related to bath toys, infected bathroom faucets, wells, loofah sponges, or beauty aids. Sporadic cases after depilation of the legs have been traced to contaminated sponges or cosmetics (26). Loofah sponges must be allowed to dry after use or be decontaminated intermittently.

Most outbreaks have been associated with serogroup O-11 *P. aeruginosa,* although other serogroups have been implicated occasionally, including O-1, O-3, O-4, O-6, O-7, O-8, O-9, O-10, and O-16 (15, 55, 56). An outbreak due to O-4 seemed to be associated with systemic symptoms. The systemic involvement may have been due to the higher pathogenicity of serogroup O-4.

Clinically, *P. aeruginosa* dermatitis/folliculitis presents after an incubation period which averages 48 h, with a range of 8 to 120 h. Younger patients (<20 years old) appear to be predisposed to infection, as do those who are exposed to contaminated water for a long period or frequently (34). Showering after exposure to *P. aeruginosa*-laden water does not appear to prevent the development of infection, suggesting that the organism rapidly gains access to the deeper regions of the skin pores during water exposure. This was confirmed in a recent outbreak (92). *P. aeruginosa* is not a component of normal skin flora; certain factors may predispose people to colonization and multiplication. Initially, the infection is manifest as pruritic follicular papules 2 to 10 mm in diameter, generally located on the buttocks, thighs, arms, and axillae, with the palms, soles, and mucous membranes spared. These are areas in which apocrine sweat glands, which open into hair follicles, are located. Other skin areas can be involved as well. Women not infrequently develop a low-grade mastitis through infection of the glands of Montgomery. A greater intensity of rash in areas covered by tight bathing suits has been reported. Application to the skin of felt pads wetted with water containing pseudomonads and covered with an occlusive dressing has been shown to induce a maculopustular rash on superhydrated skin, similar to the eruptions described for patients. The face and scalp are generally not affected, as these parts of the body are typically not immersed when the patient is using a whirlpool or spa. With time, pinpoint pustules develop in the middle of the papules, and the rash generally heals within 2 to 5 days without scarring. Some rashes may last for a week (7). Deeper infections with nodules have been noted (55). Hyperpigmentation may persist at the site of the papules for some time. In most patients, this eventually resolves; however, a rare case of persistent hyperpigmentation and residual scarring has been noted despite the use of therapeutic UV light and tetracycline. Fever, if present at all, is usually low grade. Malaise and headache are uncommon; however, in some outbreaks, headache, fatigue, muscle aches, and burning eyes have occurred in more than 30% of patients. Secondary infections involving friends or family members have not been documented, except for cases involving contaminated bath sponges.

Systemic or topical antibiotic therapy is not required, and topical corticosteroid therapy may delay resolution of folliculitis.

P. aeruginosa "Hot-Foot" Syndrome

The *Pseudomonas* "hot-foot" syndrome has been described previously (31). In one such outbreak, 33 children at a pool party were affected, and 2 of them required hospital admission (104). This is a condition characterized pathologically by perivascular and perieccrine neutrophilic infiltrates or microab-

scesses and clinically by painful erythematous plantar nodules and pustular lesions. Unlike lesions in *Pseudomonas* folliculitis, these lesions are nodular and involve the soles of the feet, which may have been predisposed to invasion by the abrasive nature of the pool floor. Similar hot, tender, plantar nodules of this nature have been noted in past hot tub outbreaks (75). The syndrome resolves without specific therapy.

Acute Diffuse Otitis Externa (Swimmer's Ear)

Acute diffuse otitis externa is also usually caused by *P. aeruginosa* and may be similar to *Pseudomonas* folliculitis in its pathogenesis. Both conditions may occur in the same patient (36). Swimmer's ear has been seen more frequently in swimming pool users than in whirlpool and spa users, who usually keep their heads out of the water. However, an outbreak has been reported related to the use of redwood hot tubs (14). Clinical manifestations of swimmer's ear include discharge from a pruritic and painful external auditory canal that, on examination, is erythematous, edematous, and filled with debris. Usually, systemic antibiotic therapy is unnecessary, as most cases resolve spontaneously without serious complications. However, one patient was reported to have developed purulent otitis externa with a temperature of 104°F, severe dermatitis, and axillary lymphadenopathy and required hospitalization and the use of an intravenous antibiotic (15). Most mild infections respond to 2% acetic acid otic solution, which impairs the growth of *P. aeruginosa*. Eardrops containing topical steroids and antibiotics are also employed. Infection is often recurrent in swimmers.

Schistosome Dermatitis (Swimmer's Itch or Clam Digger's Itch)

Schistosome dermatitis is caused when the cercariae of schistosome parasites present in environmental water penetrate human skin, are unable to proceed any further, and are destroyed, causing a pruritic skin rash. Schistosomes are trematodes whose life cycle involves a definitive host (humans, other mammals, or birds) and an intermediate host, usually snails, from which cercariae are released into a body of water. Dermatitis can occasionally be seen in patients with human schistosomiasis *(Schistosoma mansoni* and *Schistosoma haematobium);* however, this dermatitis is usually more severe and occurs more often when cercariae of nonhuman (usually waterfowl or nonprimate-mammal) schistosomes penetrate human skin. The disease was first noted in the United States by Cort in 1928 among patients who had waded in Douglas Lake in Michigan (22). Since then, more than 20 species of cercariae from freshwater snails and at least four species from marine snails have been found to produce the illness. It has been described in North, Central, and South America, as well as Oceania, India, Europe, and Africa. More recently, an outbreak in Iceland was reported (54). In the United States, the illness following swimming or wading in lakes in the north-central states has been most frequent. Marine outbreaks in Florida, southern California, and Hawaii have also been reported.

The association of 317 cases of schistosome dermatitis with the limnological characteristics of a northern Michigan lake has been investigated (60). Patients were more likely to have had exposure to lake water in the morning and to have been exposed in shallower water and in water with a high algal content. Dermatitis was most frequent during June and early July. These characteristics are related to the emergence and peak population of cercariae in water.

Clinical manifestations include an initial "prickling" sensation, typically felt when the film of water evaporates on the skin. This is followed by urticaria, which spontaneously subsides, usually within an hour, with persistence of pruritic macules. With time, these macules may evolve into papules or pustules, which reach their peak intensity in 48 to 72 h. The severity of the reaction varies markedly from person to person and appears to increase with repeated exposures, as the patient be-

comes sensitized. In most patients, symptoms subside in 4 to 7 days, but severely allergic individuals may be symptomatic for more than a week.

Histopathologically, the cercariae are unable to penetrate human skin, become walled off, and evoke an acute inflammatory response, with infiltration of lymphocytes, neutrophils, and eosinophils.

There is no specific antihelminthic therapy. The illness is treated with topical and systemic medications to control the pruritus. Prevention is largely keyed to control of the intermediate host by application of molluscicides, such as copper sulfate and copper carbonate, to the water. Newer methods under development to assist in identifying infested water bodies and to minimize parasitic exposure include traps impregnated with linoleic acid to stimulate the attachment of cercariae as well as PCR amplification techniques to detect cercariae. The rash must be differentiated from sea bather's eruption (caused by *Linuche unguiculata* [thimble jellyfish]), which occurs under swimsuits after swimming in marine environments.

Skin and Soft Tissue Infections Caused by Nontuberculous Mycobacteria

Several nontuberculous mycobacteria cause skin infections (5). *Mycobacterium marinum* is the most frequently identified mycobacterial species causing skin and subcutaneous infections associated with immersion. The organism is a photochromogen that grows best at 30 to 32°C and poorly at 37°C or more. It inhabits both fresh- and saltwater environments (including aquariums and swimming pools) as a free-living organism. Aronson first recognized it as a pathogen in aquarium fish in 1926 (2). Human infection was described definitely in 1954, when an outbreak of 80 cases of infection acquired in a swimming pool was reported. The responsible organism was initially identified as *"Mycobacterium balnei,"* later shown to be synonymous with *M. marinum* (61). Further swimming pool-related outbreaks were reported prior to the institution of guidelines for swimming pool disinfection (67). *M. marinum* does not survive chlorine concentrations of 0.6 mg/liter. In one study, it was repeatedly isolated from pool water when chlorine levels dropped to 0.2 mg/liter but could not be isolated at concentrations above 0.5 to 0.6 mg/liter. Better adherence to current guidelines for swimming pool disinfection may explain why skin infections acquired in pools are now unusual. Currently, fish tank exposure has proven to be the most consistent risk factor for acquiring this infection, with 84% of the largest series of patients (a total of 63) reporting fish tank exposure. Other recreational activities associated with this infection include skin diving, dolphin training, and boating activities (3, 11, 33, 58).

Human infection is usually associated with trauma, such as abrasions, injuries from fish spines, or pricks from crustaceans or shellfish (3). The skin injury itself may be trivial, may have healed, or may be an open cutaneous lesion. Usually the infection is confined to cooler areas of the body, such as the extremities. The incubation period appears to be several weeks, although the mean time to diagnosis is 3 to 4 months, with initial lesions appearing as groups of small papules, a nodule, or a plaque with a verrucous surface. Often there is progression to shallow ulcerations. However, there is considerable pleomorphism in the appearance of infections, with "sporotrichoid" variants, in which nodules appear in the afferent lymphatics, simulating sporotrichosis. Sporotrichosis has been found to be the more common presentation in certain studies (3). Fewer than half of the patients experience pain, and systemic symptoms are uncommon. Adults are more commonly infected due to direct exposure to contaminated environmental water. Children who develop infections usually have fish tanks in their homes (86).

Involvement of deeper structures in the hand, such as the synovium, tendons, and bones, has been demonstrated. Dissemination in both immunosuppressed and immunocompetent patients has been reported. Human immunodeficiency virus–associated *M. marinum* infections, usually acquired from home aquariums, have also been reported. The use of rubber or plastic gloves to handle fish and to clean aquariums has been recommended for these patients and may be useful for the general public as well, especially if preexisting skin lesions are present.

Diagnosis is made most readily from tissue biopsy. The specimen should be submitted for mycobacterial culture as well as histology, since the organism frequently cannot be identified microscopically in the biopsy sample. Growth of the organism in the laboratory is facilitated by incubation at 30 to 32°C. Pulsed-field gel electrophoresis and pattern restriction site analysis after PCR have enhanced the accuracy and speed of identification from culture. A range of histopathological findings is possible, with some lesions showing suppuration and others showing granulomas with various degrees of organization. The tuberculin skin test may be positive.

Skin lesions caused by *M. marinum* can spontaneously resolve. This quality makes it difficult to judge the broad clinical applicability of anecdotal reports describing successful interventional drug or surgical therapy. Many smaller lesions are adequately resected at the time of biopsy and require no further therapy. Surgical debridement is sometimes required for infections of the hand, where closed spaces may be involved.

Of the antimicrobial agents commonly used to treat other mycobacteria, *M. marinum* is usually susceptible to rifampin, rifabutin, ethambutol, trimethoprim-sulfamethoxazole, tetracyclines, and amikacin (59). It is usually resistant to isoniazid and streptomycin. Because antimicrobial therapy is felt to shorten the duration of this frequently painful illness, patients are usually given such therapy, especially if the lesion is on the hand.

Successes as well as failures have been reported with tetracyclines and trimethoprim-sulfamethoxazole. Rifampin, with or without ethambutol, has generally been reported to produce favorable results, even in cases where tetracycline has failed (28). Rifampin and rifabutin seem to be the most active agents in vitro, with MICs at which 90% of isolates are inhibited being 0.5 and 0.06 mg/ml, respectively. Clarithromycin with or without additional agents such as ethambutol has also shown clinical benefit in studies involving limited numbers of patients. This has been confirmed in a more recent study involving a larger series of patients. In addition to surgical therapy, the use of clarithromycin was endorsed by the American Thoracic Society in 2007 (35). Increasing experience with this antibiotic has led some authors to recommend it as a first-line agent in any combination therapy. Azithromycin, a newer macrolide, has recently been reported to produce clinical cure when used with ethambutol, even though in vitro MICs have been shown to be in the range of 8 to 128 mg/ml, higher than typical peak concentrations in serum. Quinolones have also been used successfully in the treatment of *M. marinum* infections. Moxifloxacin and sparfloxacin appear to be active in vitro, with MICs of 1 and 2 mg/ml, respectively. Clinical use of the quinolones for these infections has been limited. Attainable peak concentrations in serum are close to measured MICs. Levofloxacin has been reported to be effective in a patient infected with a multidrug-resistant isolate, while a combination of rifabutin and ciprofloxacin was curative in a patient for whom six previous regimens had failed (57). Linezolid, an oxazolidinone, has been shown to have excellent in vitro antimicrobial activity, with a MIC of 0.5 to 4 mg/ml. These concentrations are below those usually achieved in serum and tissue at conventional dosages. Clinical experience with this agent is limited. In general, susceptibility testing with the agar dilution method or the Etest may be used to guide therapy, although more-recent reports have validated the better accuracy of the agar dilution method. Combination therapy with two or three agents is associated with better

cure rates. Monotherapy should probably be avoided, especially for deep infections, due to a high failure rate. The proper duration of therapy is uncertain, with most authors recommending 6 to 24 weeks. However, the duration of therapy also depends on clinical response; some deep infections may require as much as 25 months of treatment (5).

Mycobacterium ulcerans is a nontuberculous mycobacterium responsible for Buruli or Bairnsdale ulcer, a chronic cutaneous ulceration seen in parts of Africa, Australia, Papua New Guinea, Malaysia, Suriname, Mexico, Peru, Japan, and China (1). Worldwide, this ulceration is the third-most-common mycobacterial disease after tuberculosis and leprosy. This infection has been associated with rivers and bodies of water used for recreation. Transmission is thought to be through minor trauma or skin abrasions. The lesions initially appear as painless plaques, papules, or nodules on the extremities and gradually develop into undermined ulcers. These lesions often heal with resultant severe contracture deformities as well as loss of organs such as the eye, breast, or genitalia. In earlier studies, isolation of the organism from water was difficult; however, recently, the use of PCR has considerably improved our ability to detect *M. ulcerans* from bodies of water suspected of containing the organism. PCR techniques have also suggested a very close genetic relationship between *M. marinum* and *M. ulcerans*. *M. ulcerans* has not been isolated from skin lesions in the United States, although with frequent international travel, infections acquired abroad may be diagnosed in this country. Such infections are found more commonly in children in poor communities who frequent contaminated water. No gender predilection has been noted, and there does not appear to be an increased risk in patients with human immunodeficiency virus infection. Most patients have a positive tuberculin skin test. Drugs with in vitro activity include clarithromycin, rifampin, rifabutin, streptomycin, and amikacin; however, antimicrobial treatment has been unsuccessful. Thus far, surgery is the only consistently effective management. Application of heat to affected areas has resulted in cure in a few cases (66).

It is unusual to encounter community-acquired skin and soft tissue infections caused by mycobacteria other than *M. marinum* and *M. ulcerans* for which immersion in freshwater is an epidemiological factor. A new species of mycobacterium with significant DNA sequence homology with *M. ulcerans, M. marinum,* and *Mycobacterium tuberculosis* has recently been isolated from the Chesapeake Bay in Maryland from fish with skin lesions (77). This may become a potential source of infection. Occasional infections by rapidly growing mycobacteria *(Mycobacterium fortuitum, Mycobacterium chelonae,* or *Mycobacterium abscessus)* have occurred following injuries in water, but far more common are a history of injury caused by objects contaminated with soil. An outbreak of *M. fortuitum* furunculosis involving 110 patients occurred among customers of a nail salon who had used 10 different whirlpool footbaths. These infections were severe and protracted and resulted in scarring. The same strain of *M. fortuitum* was recovered from the footbaths and the tap water in the salon. The patients were more likely than controls to have shaved their legs with a razor before the pedicure (102). Sporotrichoid lesions due to *M. abscessus* occurred in two women who worked at a public bath (57). The rapidly growing mycobacteria are resistant to most antituberculous agents but are often susceptible to amikacin, ciprofloxacin, cefoxitin, doxycycline, and rifampin. Extensive debridement, coupled with combination antimicrobial agent therapy, appears to offer the best chance of cure.

Soft Tissue Infections Caused by Gram-Negative Bacilli

Aeromonas species are ubiquitous gram-negative straight or curved bacilli found in freshwater (including fish tanks, swimming pools, and tap water) as well as brackish water worldwide. They have been known to cause infection in cold-blooded animals (fish, rep-tiles, and amphibians). Their pathogenicity for humans was noted in 1968 (98). They have been implicated as a cause of gastroenteritis, traumatic and surgical wound infections, myonecrosis, gangrene, osteomyelitis, and, rarely, lower respiratory tract and ocular infections. *Aeromonas hydrophila* is the species most commonly associated with soft tissue infections.

Traumatic wound infections in which *A. hydrophila* appears to have been acquired from contaminated freshwater or salt water have been reported frequently. These infections tend to occur on the lower extremities or hand and are often sustained while wading or swimming (52). The spectrum of severity is broad ranging, from mild cellulitis to rapidly progressive, life-threatening myonecrosis with gangrene. Presumably, the virulence of the infecting strain, the severity of the injury, and the immune status of the patient are all factors determining this severity. Janda has provided an excellent review of *Aeromonas* virulence factors and pathogenicity (43).

Cases of cellulitis related not only to injuries that occur during immersion in environmental water but also to an abrasion associated with a fish tank, to a boating accident, to an unusual football injury, to blunt trauma while diving, and to swimming in river water in which no injuries were sustained have been described previously. The incubation period may be as short as 8 h. The cellulitis is characterized by fever, pain, warmth, erythema, edema, and a foul "fishy" odor. Characteristic subcutaneous abscesses may form and were noted in 91% of patients in one series. The cellulitis is clinically indistinguishable from that due to beta-hemolytic streptococci. The infections have also been noted to occur in warm weather, emphasizing the role of water exposure. Burn wound infections have also been known to occur in patients following immersion in untreated water. These may be complicated by rapidly evolving deep infection. Cellulitis "one step removed" from freshwater has been reported as a complication of the use of the medicinal freshwater leech *Hirudo medicinalis* for the treatment of vascular congestion after surgical procedures. *A. hydrophila* is part of the normal gut flora of this annelid, and *Aeromonas* infections have occurred in up to 20% of patients treated with leeches, leading to the use of prophylactic antibiotics at the time of leech application. No definite aeromonad infections have been reported in cases of naturally acquired leech bites.

More-severe aeromonad tissue infections, including myonecrosis with or without gas gangrene, have been reported. In a number of these cases, the original injury occurred in association with freshwater. Some patients had underlying conditions associated with immune defects, such as diabetes or corticosteroid use, while others appeared to be immunocompetent. The latter group included a 19-year-old man whose leg was lacerated by a motorboat propeller and an 88-year-old woman who cut her hand on a fish bone (85). Bacteremia may complicate these severe soft tissue infections, and it appears to significantly worsen the prognosis. Heckerling et al., in their case report and literature review, found no survivors among patients with *Aeromonas* myonecrosis complicated by bacteremia (39). In their article on human infections caused by *Aeromonas* species, Janda and Duffrey reviewed studies of patients with bacteremia previously reported in the literature; mortality ranged from 29 to 73% (44). Most of these bacteremic patients did not have associated severe soft tissue infections. In fact, the precipitating event was not apparent for many patients, although some had a history of contact with water. *Aeromonas* bacteremia may give rise to ecthyma gangrenosum, which has a clinical appearance identical to that seen in *P. aeruginosa* septicemia. In addition to traumatic injuries, hematologic malignancies, solid tumors, and hepatobiliary disorders all appear to predispose to *Aeromonas* bacteremia.

Aeromonas soft tissue infections, which complicate trauma in freshwater, can lead to contiguous osteomyelitis. Karam et al. reported two such cases occurring in immunologically healthy patients (48).

In vitro, *A. hydrophila* is generally susceptible to broad-spectrum cephalosporins, chloramphenicol, trimethoprim-sulfamethoxazole, fluoroquinolones, aztreonam, and aminoglycosides. *Aeromonas sobria* tends to be more susceptible to cephalothin but is more varied in susceptibility to chloramphenicol and amikacin. Broad-based beta-lactam resistance may develop in *Aeromonas* species through stable depression of inducible beta-lactamases. Clinical reports have generally described therapy with combinations of antibiotics, often broad-spectrum cephalosporins combined with aminoglycosides. Surgical debridement is usually required and may lead to favorable outcomes even in situations where the initial antibiotic choice was not appropriate.

Edwardsiella tarda is a gram-negative bacterium that has been isolated from reptiles, fish, mammals, birds, and environmental water sources. It is a rare cause of human infections and is associated with gastroenteritis in 0.80% of cases. Soft tissue infections, the second-most-common infections caused by *E. tarda,* have been associated with injuries sustained in freshwater. They are more common in the warm-weather months. Clinically, these infections appear to be similar to *Aeromonas* cellulitis. Coinfection with these organisms can occur, which emphasizes their common source. The cellulitis may be complicated by abscess formation and necrotizing fasciitis. The first reported case of cellulitis complicated by myonecrosis due to *E. tarda* occurred in a man who sustained an injury while crab fishing (83). In one case of neonatal sepsis, a mother who was immersed in lake water during the sixth month of gestation also had vaginal and gastrointestinal colonization with the same strain of *E. tarda.* The organism is susceptible in vitro to ampicillin, chloramphenicol, aminoglycoside, cephalosporins, tetracyclines, fluoroquinolones, and trimethoprim-sulfamethoxazole.

Bacteria of the genus *Vibrio* can also cause extensive skin and soft tissue infection, usually after exposure to brackish water. This is discussed elsewhere in this book (chapter 1).

Prototheca Skin and Soft Tissue Infections

Prototheca species are unicellular achlorophyllous algae. They are found in aquariums, freshwater or stagnant water, and other moist environments. Of the four identified species (*Prototheca wickerhamii, Prototheca zopfii, Prototheca filamenta,* and *Prototheca stagnora*), *P. wickerhamii* and *P. zopfii* are known to infect humans, with the former being a more common cause of infections. Since Davies et al. described the first human infection in 1964 (25), about 108 cases have been described. Several types of human infections have been described. The most frequent have been papulonodular or ulcerative skin lesions, which have generally followed minor trauma or surgical incisions, particularly on the extremities or face. Often, patients with these wound infections report exposure to environments known to harbor this organism. Another type of infection is olecranon bursitis, usually following minor (even nonpenetrating) trauma. In the United States, most *Prototheca* infections have been reported from southern or central states. Immunosuppression appears to be a risk factor for both localized and disseminated infections and has been reported for over half the affected patients, although healthy patients may also be infected. In a recent report of infection in an AIDS patient, there was a history of bathing in an urban pond (73). Nasopharyngeal ulceration complicating prolonged endotracheal intubation, as well as meningitis in a patient with AIDS, has also been reported, but this was apparently not related to water exposure. Four other cases in association with AIDS were also cutaneous.

Diagnosis is best established by biopsy and culture. Sporangia with symmetrically arranged endospores (spoked-wheel appearance) are characteristic. Microabscesses and granulomas are seen histologically. Fungal stains, such as Gomori's methenamine-silver, usually identify the organism in the biopsied tissue. Histologically, *Prototheca* species must be differentiated from *Coccidioides immitis, Cryptococcus neoformans, Rhinosporidium seeberi, Blastomyces dermatitidis,* and *Acanthamoeba* species,

which may have similar clinical presentations. *Prototheca* grows on Sabouraud agar, producing whitish colonies.

Antimicrobial and/or surgical therapy is usually necessary; few lesions have resolved spontaneously. Amphotericin B and ketoconazole have been used in larger lesions; smaller ones can often be resected successfully. In more-recent studies, itraconazole has appeared to be the most effective antimicrobial agent for these infections, although surgical intervention has been utilized as first-line management for olecranon bursitis. Fluconazole has also been used successfully (47).

Cyanobacterium (Blue-Green Alga) Infection

Both dermatologic (rash, pruritus, and blistering) and gastrointestinal (abdominal pain, nausea and vomiting, and diarrhea) symptoms have been statistically linked to domestic (showering or bathing) and recreational water use during periods of high concentrations of blue-green algae (89–91). These ill effects are thought to be caused by exposure to various toxins produced by these organisms. The organisms themselves are killed by chlorination, although the toxins appear to be unaffected.

MRSA Infections

Staphylococcus aureus is a common cause of skin and soft tissue infections such as abscesses and cellulitis. The methicillin-resistant strains have notably caused widespread disease in recent years. Although no waterborne outbreaks have been reported, methicillin-resistant *Staphylococcus aureus* (MRSA) seems to be more viable in nonmarine environments like swimming pools than in marine environments and may be spread in recreational settings (93).

OCULAR INFECTIONS

Pharyngoconjunctival Fever (Swimming Pool Conjunctivitis)

Pharyngoconjunctival fever, a pediatric and occasionally adult syndrome, has been associated with a number of adenoviruses, most commonly of serotypes 3 and 7 in the United

States and of serotype 4 in Asia and Latin America. Pharyngoconjunctival fever often occurs in outbreaks or small epidemics and has been reported as a hazard at children's summer camps.

The illness is characterized by fever as high as 38°C, bulbar and palpebral conjunctivitis, pharyngitis, and enlargement of the adenoids. Abdominal pain may occur. Usually, symptoms begin in one eye but ultimately involve both. Occasionally, symptoms other than conjunctivitis are lacking. The illness usually lasts 3 to 5 days, is not complicated by bacterial superinfections, and can be treated symptomatically. Outbreaks can usually be terminated or prevented by adequate chlorination of pool water (>0.2 mg/liter).

Amoebic Keratitis

Free-living amoebae of the genus *Acanthamoeba* have been responsible for several hundred reported cases of keratitis since the original description of a case in a Texas rancher in 1975 (97). This infection has proven difficult to treat, often resulting in severe impairment or loss of vision.

Acanthamoeba species are found in a variety of environmental settings, including soil, water, and air. They have even been isolated from the respiratory tracts of healthy people. The species reported to cause keratitis in humans include *Acanthamoeba hatchetti, Acanthamoeba castellanii, Acanthamoeba polyphaga, Acanthamoeba culbertsoni,* and *Acanthamoeba rhysodes. Acanthamoeba* species exist in nature only in the trophozoite or cyst stage. Identifying markers of trophozoites include a diameter of 14 to 40 mm; a single nucleus containing a centrally placed, prominent nucleolus; and spinelike plasma membrane projections (acanthopodia). Motility is sluggish. Cysts are 12 to 16 mm in diameter and have a wrinkled, double-layered wall with pores.

Acanthamoeba species are capable of producing a granulomatous encephalitis in debilitated or immunosuppressed patients. In contrast, the keratitis that they produce can occur in healthy people, as well as those with underlying diseases. Most, if not all, of these pa-

tients have been soft contact lens wearers. The illness has been associated with minor corneal trauma and exposure to contaminated water. A case control study of soft contact lens wearers found that patients with *Acanthamoeba* keratitis were more likely than controls to use homemade saline for rinsing and as a wetting agent and to wear their lenses while swimming. They also appear to disinfect their lenses less frequently than recommended by the manufacturers. Other authors remarked on the use of chemical rather than thermal disinfection of contact lenses as a risk factor. There is no gender predilection, and most cases have been reported in the United States (88).

Histologically, both trophozoites and cysts are found within the cornea in association with an acute inflammatory infiltrate. Giant cells may be present. Corneal neovascularization is variably present. Involvement of the posterior chamber of the eye in amoebic keratitis occurs only rarely.

Symptoms of amoebic keratitis generally begin with a sensation of a foreign body in the eye, followed by pain, photophobia, tearing, blepharospasm, and altered visual acuity. In isolated cases, the infection may be painless. The progression of symptoms is variable and may take place over several days to several months. Periods of remission are not unusual, and when these coincide with a change in therapy, an erroneous impression of the etiology may occur. Findings on examination in one-half or more of patients include iritis, a ring-shaped corneal infiltrate, and recurrent epithelial breakdown or cataracts. Less commonly found are hypopyon, increased intraocular pressure, or anterior nodular scleritis. The ring-shaped corneal infiltrate has been described as a characteristic finding in amoebic keratitis and is probably caused by the presence of antigen-antibody complexes in the cornea and the resultant chemoattraction of neutrophils. Although this ring-shaped infiltration has occasionally been reported to occur under other conditions, such as herpes simplex, fungal, or bacterial keratitis, its presence should signal the need for microbiological studies to determine if amoebae are present.

Elevated corneal epithelial lines also appear to be a clinical indication of *Acanthamoeba* infection. Histopathological examination of scrapings of these lines has revealed both trophozoites and cysts. Dendriform epithelial involvement has also been reported as an early finding for *Acanthamoeba* keratitis. The infection may be complicated by chorioretinitis as well as painful sclerokeratitis.

The definitive diagnosis of amoebic keratitis requires a demonstration of *Acanthamoeba* in corneal scrapings, biopsy specimens, or culture. Motile trophozoites can sometimes be identified in wet mounts of scrapings. Cysts and trophozoites can be identified in fixed material with several different stains, including hematoxylin-eosin, Wright stain, Giemsa stain, and periodic acid-Schiff stain. Calcofluor white, a chemofluorescent dye, has been reported to facilitate the identification of trophozoites in cysts in tissue. Routine culture methods are frequently misleading in the diagnosis of *Acanthamoeba* keratitis. Because of colonization of the corneal scrapings or contamination, culture may reveal potential bacterial pathogens. A nonnutrient agar with an *Escherichia coli* or *Aerobacter aerogenes* overlay has been shown to successfully grow *Acanthamoeba* from the majority of positive biopsy specimens. Cultures of contact lenses or lens solutions may also be helpful diagnostically. A variety of nonmorphological identification criteria, including restriction fragment length polymorphism analysis of mitochondrial or genomic DNA, PCR, and immunofluorescence, have also been described (71).

Effective treatment of *Acanthamoeba* keratitis requires both surgical and medical components. Diagnosis early in the course can sometimes lead to successful management by employing debridement of abnormal epithelium in combination with topical medication for 3 to 4 weeks. In many cases, however, penetrating keratoplasty is necessary for pain relief and to improve vision. Deep lamellar keratectomy with a corneal flap is a recent surgical approach that has been used with success in refractory cases. Topical medications that have been reported to be beneficial include the following:

1. A combination of 1% miconazole nitrate, 0.1% propamidine isethionate, and Neosporin

2. A combination of 1% clotrimazole, 0.1% propamidine isethionate, and Neosporin

3. 0.1% propamidine isethionate and 0.15% dibromopropamidine

4. 0.02% polyhexamethylene biguanide

5. 0.02% chlorhexidine

Unfortunately, propamidine and dibromopropamidine, both analogs of stilbamidine, are not available commercially in the United States. Topical steroids are also frequently, but not universally, employed to inhibit neovascularization in the cornea. However, some experimental evidence suggests that when used for *Acanthamoeba* keratitis, steroids may not be effective for this purpose. The use of systemic steroids has appeared to be useful for *Acanthamoeba* sclerokeratitis, a painfully disabling complication of amoebic keratitis that may require enucleation. In vitro, *A. culbertsoni* and *A. polyphaga* are killed at relatively low concentrations of azithromycin, but there are no reports regarding the efficacy of macrolide therapy of amoebic keratitis.

Prevention of *Acanthamoeba* keratitis in contact lens wearers is possible. Microwave irradiation has been shown to effectively kill trophozoites and cysts in as little as 3 min without affecting the integrity of the lens. Heat disinfection of contact lenses is preferable to chemical disinfection. Homemade saline solutions should be avoided for lens cleaning and storage, and contact lenses should not be worn while swimming in freshwater (87).

P. aeruginosa Keratitis

P. aeruginosa keratitis usually occurs in contact lens wearers with no history of freshwater immersion. However, it has been reported in conjunction with *P. aeruginosa* folliculitis. A patient who had *P. aeruginosa* folliculitis during a whirlpool exposure outbreak developed a corneal ulcer that resolved with antibiotics.

URINARY TRACT INFECTIONS

P. aeruginosa Urinary Tract Infections

In addition to causing dermatitis/folliculitis, keratitis, and pneumonia, *P. aeruginosa* has been known to cause urinary tract infection in whirlpool users (80). Three previously healthy outpatients developed *Pseudomonas* urinary tract infection within 48 h after exposure to whirlpools. *P. aeruginosa* was later isolated from the whirlpool associated with each case.

PULMONARY INFECTIONS

Legionella spp.

Members of the genus *Legionella* are fastidious, non-spore-forming, gram-negative bacilli. *Legionella pneumophila* is the major pathogen for humans and causes infections in healthy hosts as well as those with underlying disease. Nineteen other *Legionella* species have been isolated from humans, usually immunosuppressed patients. Most legionellae have been found growing naturally in a variety of freshwater habitats. *L. pneumophila* and other species have been isolated from flowing streams and rivers as well as lakes, thermal ponds, and groundwater. They can gain access to man-made water supplies, such as air-conditioning cooling towers, potable-water systems, and whirlpools or spas. They tolerate water temperatures in excess of 60°C. Aerosols from both natural and man-made water sources appear to be the usual source for human respiratory tract infections investigated since the first identified outbreak in 1976. It has been thought that legionellae may be non-free-living microorganisms. There is some evidence that they live on the products of blue-green and thermophilic algae as well as bacteria such as *Pseudomonas* and *Flavobacterium* spp., which commonly share the same environment. In addition, legionellae are capable of intracellular survival and multiplication in free-living amoebae.

L. pneumophila causes pneumonia, Pontiac fever (an influenza-like illness with less severe respiratory symptoms), and occasional soft tissue infections. Although most outbreaks of *Legionella* pneumonia or Pontiac fever have resulted from exposure to airborne bacteria from air-conditioning systems, hospital potable-water systems, or machine tool grinding coolants, infections related to immersion have also been reported. A 1982 outbreak of Pontiac fever related to the use of a whirlpool spa was reported (62). Fourteen female members of a church group who used a health club whirlpool developed chills, fever, chest pain, cough, and nausea within 2 days. Most of these patients seroconverted to antigen from *L. pneumophila* serogroup 6. This organism was recovered from the whirlpool water. It was hypothesized that legionellae seeded the whirlpool from an air conditioner condensation pan with a blocked drain. The organism can reach high numbers in heated, agitated, and underchlorinated water. Whirlpool aerators produce droplets of 2 to 8 mm, which are capable of reaching the alveolar air spaces when inhaled. Two similar outbreaks, one involving 34 cases of Pontiac fever and the other involving 7 cases of pneumonia, were reported in 1982, associated with a whirlpool at a Vermont inn. Six college students on a ski trip to Vermont developed Pontiac fever (five cases) or Legionnaires' disease (one case) after using a whirlpool. Pontiac fever was confirmed in a mother and possibly occurred in her two children after similar exposures. In 1996, an outbreak consisting of 50 confirmed or probable cases of Legionnaires' disease associated with exposure to whirlpool spas during a total of nine cruises on a single ship was reported. Infection was associated not only with immersion but also with spending time in the area around the spas. Bacterium-laden aerosols generated from the spas presumably infected the patients of that outbreak. *L. pneumophila* of serogroup 1 was isolated from the sand filter in the spa water treatment system. An isolate matching the spa strain by monoclonal antibody subtyping and arbitrarily primed PCR was recovered from one patient. It was felt that the brominator in the system

36

did not adequately disinfect the spa water after it passed through the sand filter (45).

A hospital-associated wound infection caused by *L. pneumophila* of serogroup 4 was related to immersion in a Hubbard tank. The pathogenic isolate and *L. pneumophila* strains of other serogroups were grown from the Hubbard tank as well as a small whirlpool tank near it. Povidone-iodine, which was used to disinfect the tank and was added to the water used to immerse the patients, was ineffective in killing *L. pneumophila* at concentrations under 1,000 ppm. An outbreak of three cases of sternal wound infection caused by *L. pneumophila* and *Legionella dumoffii* has also been reported. The authors presented evidence that the infections were acquired from tap water baths in the intensive care unit. Both *Legionella* species were recovered from water taps in the intensive care unit.

Most patients with Pontiac fever have recovered from their illness without specific therapy. This holds true for those involved in the above-mentioned whirlpool-associated outbreaks. Before the advent of the newer macrolides, erythromycin, with frequent addition of rifampin in severe cases, was the therapy of choice for *L. pneumophila* pneumonia as well as infections caused by other species of *Legionella*. Azithromycin, a newer macrolide with more-potent intracellular activity, better lung penetration, fewer side effects, and once-daily dosing, is currently the preferred agent. Tetracycline, trimethoprim-sulfamethoxazole, and ciprofloxacin have been used with success in smaller numbers of patients. The newer quinolones, including levofloxacin and moxifloxacin, have also shown efficacy in vitro and have been used as monotherapy for patients with community-acquired pneumonia when *L. pneumophila* was considered to be a possible pathogen. Rifampin may be added to any of the macrolides or quinolones.

Disinfection of hospital water systems colonized by *Legionella* has been accomplished thermally, through hyperchlorination, and by use of silver-copper ion generators. *Legionella*

is relatively chlorine tolerant and even more resistant to bromine, which is used occasionally for whirlpool disinfection. Levels of residual chlorine of 2 to 6 ppm are effective but, as discussed earlier, difficult to maintain in whirlpools, spas, and hot tubs.

P. aeruginosa

Pneumonia caused by *P. aeruginosa* has been reported for a patient with a 50-year-long history of smoking but no other underlying medical problems who sat in a whirlpool spa for 90 min 1 day prior to the onset of respiratory symptoms (79). The sputum culture and the cultures of the spa water grew identical serogroups of *P. aeruginosa*. It was hypothesized that prolonged inhalation of the *P. aeruginosa*-laden aerosol from the spa was responsible for the development of pneumonia in this patient, whose pulmonary clearance mechanisms were probably impaired from heavy smoking. In this regard, the pathogenesis is similar to the development of nosocomial *P. aeruginosa* pneumonia after inhalation of contaminated humidified air during mechanical ventilation. *P. aeruginosa* has also been implicated in pneumonia associated with near drowning in hot tubs.

Mycobacterium avium Complex

A previously healthy young woman apparently developed widespread pulmonary infection with *M. avium* complex acquired from a hot tub. Isolates from the patient and the hot tub water had identical enzymatic profiles by multilocus enzyme electrophoresis. In addition, a high degree of relatedness of their insertion sequence, IS*1245,* was demonstrated by restriction fragment length polymorphism analysis.

Pneumonia following Near Drowning

The risk of pneumonia in submersion victims has been related to the severity of the pulmonary insult. Patients with abnormal lung examination results after submersion and those requiring ventilation have developed pneumonia more frequently than patients with milder lung injuries. A wide variety of respiratory pathogens have been recovered from these patients. However, in many cases, it has been difficult to differentiate pathogens acquired from the aquatic environment from those that colonized or infected the patients prior to the near drowning or later in the hospital setting.

Aerobic Gram-Negative Bacteria

Aeromonas species are found in both freshwater and brackish water. In addition to causing soft tissue infections associated with immersion, discussed earlier in this chapter, *Aeromonas* species can also cause pneumonia, usually complicated by septicemia, in individuals who have nearly drowned. Several such cases have been reported, but it is difficult to discern whether there was actual pulmonary parenchyma infection in all cases (76). Sometimes the patients' pulmonary findings have been more compatible with noncardiogenic pulmonary edema when the *Aeromonas* organisms have been recovered only from blood cultures. Although *A. hydrophila* was identified as the species causing infection in most of the cases noted above, more recently differentiated *Aeromonas* species, such as *A. sobria*, *Aeromonas caviae*, and *Aeromonas veronii*, may have been responsible. The mortality of patients with *Aeromonas* pneumonia associated with near drowning has been reported to exceed 50%.

The antimicrobial susceptibility of *Aeromonas* species and the therapy of infections are discussed in "Skin and Soft Tissue Infections" above.

Burkholderia pseudomallei, the cause of melioidosis, has been associated with pneumonia related to near drowning in tropical Asian countries where the organism is endemic, including the Philippines, Thailand, Vietnam, and Taiwan. This agent is also associated with dissemination from the lungs and a high risk of mortality. The organism is usually susceptible to antipseudomonal penicillins, cefoperazone, ceftazidime, ampicillin-sulbactam, amoxicillin-clavulanate, chloramphenicol, and tetracyclines. Fluoroquinolone susceptibility is varied, and most isolates demonstrate resistance to trimethoprim-sulfamethoxazole and aminoglycosides.

Pneumonia definitely or probably associated with *Legionella* species has been associated with near drowning in a hot spring spa, in dirty swamp water, and in swimming pool water (82). Only one of the pathogens in these cases was identified as *L. pneumophila*.

Streptococcus pneumoniae

S. pneumoniae has been linked to pneumonia associated with near drowning in three fatal pediatric cases, two of which occurred in freshwater (95).

Aspergillus spp.

Invasive pulmonary aspergillosis has been reported following the near drowning of a 27-year-old man in a ditch after a motor vehicle accident (96). Preexisting bronchiectasis was present in this patient. He was successfully treated with amphotericin B and flucytosine. Of the newer antifungal therapies, voriconazole and caspofungin have been approved in the United States for the treatment of invasive aspergillosis that is refractory to other therapies and have been used successfully.

Pseudallescheria boydii

P. boydii has been isolated from polluted water, sewage sludge, soil, and animal manure. This fungus has caused pulmonary infections in severely immunocompromised patients and, occasionally, in previously healthy individuals who have aspirated contaminated water. The organism appears to have a propensity for spreading from the initial site of infection in the lungs, often producing widespread metastasis, including brain abscesses (6). On one occasion, infected kidneys from a patient with a fatal disseminated case were transplanted into two recipients, both of whom developed *P. boydii* infections (94). Therapy with antifungal drugs has been disappointing overall. In vitro susceptibility tests usually indicate resistance to amphotericin B and flucytosine, with susceptibility to miconazole and, to a lesser extent, ketoconazole. The last two agents have been used successfully to treat human pulmonary and bone infections. Itraconazole has been used successfully to treat a patient with *P. boydii* and *Aspergillus terreus* coinfection in the lungs. Voriconazole, a newer triazole antifungal agent, is approved for pulmonary infection due to *P. boydii,* having achieved some clinical success.

GASTROINTESTINAL INFECTIONS

Cryptosporidium parvum

C. parvum is a protozoan parasite associated with recreational diarrhea. It was first described in 1907 but was not associated with human disease until 1976. 1n 1993, it was responsible for a large outbreak of diarrhea that affected over 400,000 in Milwaukee, WI, as a result of fecal contamination of municipal water (19). It is a common affliction of individuals infected with human immunodeficiency virus. It continues to be an important cause of diarrhea in the summer months and is related to the use of swimming pools (29, 40, 81, 103). In some of these outbreaks, significant risk factors included swallowing the water and heavy usage by children still in diapers (13, 63). Over the last few years, it has come to assume an unpleasantly important role in RWIs. Between 1994 and 2004 it was responsible for an annual average of five outbreaks; however, in 2006 and 2007 it caused 22 and 29 outbreaks, respectively (70).

Symptoms include nonbloody diarrhea, abdominal cramps, nausea, and fever. The major problems with attempts to control this infection include the facts that it is resistant to the usual levels of chlorine in most recreational water bodies, it is very small (only 5 μm wide), infected individuals continue to shed cysts for about a week after their symptoms resolve, and average daily shedding of infective cysts runs in the millions, while only about 50 cysts are required for infection. Due to its incubation period of 1 to 14 days, infected children and individuals may shed the cysts for days before they develop symptoms, during which time many users of a swimming pool will be exposed (101). An example is the outbreak in the "spray park" at the Seneca Lake State Park in upstate New York, which infected over 4,000 individuals and lasted for months, partly because the park lacked modern ultrafiltration systems and also because people who were infected visited the park multiple times during the outbreak (19).

Giardia

Giardia is similar to *Cryptosporidium* in its tendency to require a very low dose for infection. Only 10 cysts are needed to cause infection (12). It is also relatively chlorine resistant and is excreted in large quantities per stool, making it highly infectious. Symptoms include abdominal pain and cramps, diarrhea, and gaseous abdominal distension. Prevalence studies of swimming pools in the absence of outbreaks have shown that about 1% of swimming pools harbor *Giardia* alone, while up to 8% may harbor both *Giardia* and *Cryptosporidium* (81).

Shigella

Shigella is a highly infectious bacterium that is transmitted through direct or indirect contact with feces of infected individuals, mostly through contaminated food or water or by person-to-person transmission. However, outbreaks related to the use of recreational water have been reported (42). It causes a more severe illness than the two above-named organisms. Symptoms include fever, vomiting, headaches, and bloody diarrhea.

Escherichia coli O157:H7

E. coli O157 is a bacterium that is usually transmitted through contaminated food and water and infected animals. However, an outbreak involving seven children who had used a contaminated stream as a source of recreation was reported in England (41). Other outbreaks have involved 9 and 14 children, respectively (10, 72). Its presence has been documented in lakes and other freshwater bodies (4). Its relation to petting animals is discussed elsewhere in this book.

Noroviruses

Noroviruses are an important cause of foodborne diarrhea. However, occasionally, recreational water use has been noted to be a risk factor (18, 64, 74).

DISSEMINATED INFECTIONS

Leptospirosis

Leptospires are aerobic, motile, spiral, flexible microorganisms with hooked ends. They can be cultured in artificial media containing rabbit serum or bovine serum albumin and long-chain fatty acids, although the incubation time for optimal growth can range from a few days to a few weeks.

Two species are recognized as causes of disseminated infections. *Leptospira biflexa* is considered saprophytic and is found in surface and potable water. *Leptospira interrogans* is pathogenic and may be carried for prolonged periods in proximal renal tubular cells of many different mammalian species. Members of these two *Leptospira* species can be distinguished biochemically, but within each species, members can be divided into serovars only on the basis of their agglutinogenic characteristics in rabbit antiserum. More than 210 serovars of *L. interrogans* are known. Mammals are affected year-round in the tropical regions and during warm and rainy seasons in temperate regions. From the site of infection in the kidney, leptospires are shed into the urine in variable numbers. With some serovars in some hosts, this excretion may be lifelong. With other host-serovar combinations, however, urine shedding may persist for only a few months.

Human leptospirosis is a zoonosis that has been found to be an occupational risk for cattle, dairy, or swine farmers; rice farmers; farmers in marshy areas; cray fishers; veterinarians; and abattoir workers. Humans can also be infected by exposure, such as when swimming or wading in water contaminated with animal urine. The first reported waterborne outbreak of leptospirosis occurred in 1939 (37). Since then, similar outbreaks and small epidemics have occurred regularly. Crawford et al. have reviewed 12 such outbreaks in the United States associated with swimming in natural freshwater pools, streams, and rivers (24). In several outbreaks, contamination of water with animal urine or offal was proven. They pointed out that sporadic cases of leptospirosis may occur as a result of various kinds of contact but that epidemics are usually associated with swimming or other types of water immersion. Tropical river rafting (Costa Rica and Thailand) was the apparent mode of transmission in two reported cases. Infections related to water sports have also been reported. Human infections appear to be more common in tropical regions. Within the United States, Hawaii has been the state with the highest incidence. In 2005 and 2006, two outbreaks occurred in the United States (103).

Many human cases of leptospirosis are asymptomatic. Human illness varies in severity from a mild influenza-like syndrome to severe renal and hepatic failure accompanied by hemorrhage, shock, and confusion. The severe form of leptospirosis is called Weil's disease or Weil syndrome, after the initial describer of the illness.

Leptospires may enter the body through intact mucosal membranes, the conjunctiva, or abraded skin. They are rapidly disseminated hematogenously. The incubation period is usually 7 to 12 days. During the influenza-like septicemic phase of anicteric leptospirosis, the organism can be cultured from blood, cerebrospinal fluid, and other tissues. Despite its presence in spinal fluid, patients usually have no meningeal signs in this phase of the illness, although headache is usually present, as are fever, nausea, vomiting, anorexia, myalgia, and fatigue. The most common physical finding is conjunctival suffusion in the absence of purulent discharge. After 4 to 7 days, the illness resolves for a day or two, followed in many patients by an "immune" stage of the illness, which can last up to a month.

#39

Circulating immunoglobulin M antibody can be detected, and patients may have meningismus, uveitis, and rash. Blood and cerebrospinal fluid cultures are usually negative during this phase, but the organism can be found in the urine and the aqueous humor of the eye. Cerebrospinal fluid pleocytosis, a variably elevated protein level, and a normal glucose level, although sterile, characterize the meningitis in the immune stage. Eye findings of photophobia, ocular pain, and conjunctival hemorrhage are common.

In icteric leptospirosis, there is less distinction between the septicemic and immune phases, although the renal and hepatic complications generally are not present before 3 to 7 days. The jaundice usually does not reflect hepatocellular necrosis, and no residual hepatic dysfunction has been found in survivors. Elevation of liver enzymes is relatively modest. Creatine kinase levels are quite high, however. Renal failure usually does not progress to the point where the patient requires dialysis, and this dysfunction resolves completely. Thrombocytopenia occurs in about one-half of patients and is correlated with renal failure. Death is usually related to vascular collapse, thought to be caused by vasculitis and hemorrhagic myocarditis, which occurs in about 50% of fatal cases.

Diagnosis may be established by serologic means or by culturing the organism from clinical specimens (usually blood, cerebrospinal fluid, or urine). Tween 80-albumin agar is usually commercially available and is used in clinical laboratories. Cultures are incubated for 5 to 6 weeks in the dark; growth is usually apparent by 2 weeks, however. Leptospires can also be identified in clinical specimens by dark-field examination and by immunostaining and can be faintly stained by Giemsa or Wright's stain. In tissue specimens, the organism can be detected by silver staining.

Most diagnoses are made serologically. The microscopic agglutination test is used most frequently but is highly serovar specific and requires the use of a battery of antigens. Titers of 1:100 are considered significant. Macroscopic agglutination tests with single or pooled Formalin-fixed antigens are also available, as are enzyme-linked immunosorbent assays and an indirect hemagglutination test. PCR assays for leptospiral DNA detection in clinical specimens afford rapid diagnosis, while the use of DNA primers may allow for rapid serovar identification.

Traditional antibiotic therapy for leptospirosis has been penicillin G or tetracycline. Evidence from humans indicates that therapy is effective even in severe disease treated after the initial septicemic period. Animal studies indicate that penicillins, tetracyclines, and some cephalosporins are effective, while other cephalosporins are not. Intravenous penicillin or ampicillin should be used for severe disease; oral ampicillin or doxycycline should be used for mild symptoms. Therapy should be given for 5 to 7 days. A recent prospective randomized control trial showed that the times to defervescence were the same for ceftriaxone and penicillin G (3 days), and the former can be used once daily; it suggested that it should be the preferred agent in regions of the world where it is affordable. Because of the year-round occurrence of leptospirosis and its relation to water immersion recreational activities, a proposal to give weekly prophylactic doxycycline to those travelers intending to participate in water sports has been made.

Chromobacterium violaceum

C. violaceum is a gram-negative, facultatively anaerobic, fermentative bacillus that is a normal inhabitant of soil and water and has caused human infections, primarily in tropical and subtropical areas. Most reports have not linked infection to freshwater exposure, but cases in which immersion appears to play a role have been reported. One case occurred in a 44-year-old woman who sustained a wasp sting while bathing in a Paraguayan lagoon. One month later, she developed septicemia in association with inflammation of the sting site and purplish ulcerating nodular lesions on her thigh, abdomen, and back. Blood and skin lesion cultures grew *C. violaceum*. She responded to mezlocillin and gentamicin therapy despite shock and renal failure. However, the infection recurred 2 weeks after the antibiotic course was completed, leading to her demise (49).

A second patient (a 53-year-old man), who nearly drowned in a Florida river, developed multiple liver abscesses, lung infiltrates, and a pustular skin rash 2 months after the accident. Blood and pustule cultures grew *C. violaceum,* and the patient responded to chloramphenicol, ampicillin, and carbenicillin.

Other fatal cases have been linked to exposure to stagnant water. The features of the disseminated infections in these patients were a long incubation period and skin lesions as well as hepatic and pulmonary abscesses.

This organism is usually susceptible to fluoroquinolones, trimethoprim-sulfamethoxazole, tetracyclines, aminoglycosides, extended-spectrum penicillins, and chloramphenicol.

CENTRAL NERVOUS SYSTEM INFECTIONS

Primary Amoebic Meningoencephalitis
Amoebic meningoencephalitis was first described in 1965 in Australia (Fig. 1) (20, 32). *Naegleria fowleri,* a thermophilic free-living

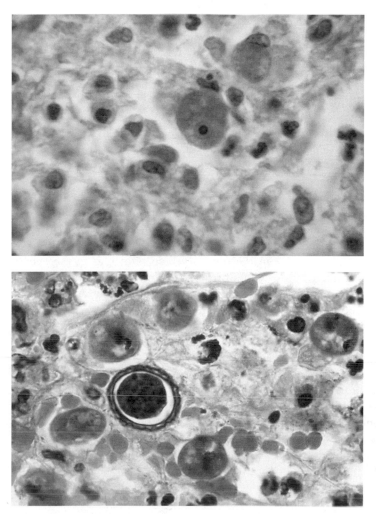

FIGURE 1 (Top) Trophozoite of an *Acanthamoeba* sp. or *Naegleria fowleri;* (bottom) cysts of an *Acanthamoeba* sp. from brain tissue. Source: CDC Public Health Image Library (http://phil.cdc.gov).

amoeba that inhabits freshwater ponds, lakes, and rivers; minimally chlorinated pools; and hot springs causes amoebic meningoencephalitis throughout the world. Other free-living amoebae include *Acanthamoeba* and *Balamuthia* spp. These amphizoic amoebae, so called because they can exist as parasites or free-living organisms, may cause fulminant rapidly progressive central nervous system infection called primary amoebic meningoencephalitis (PAM) (due to *Naegleria fowleri*) or chronic slowly progressive disease called granulomatous amoebic encephalitis (GAE), primarily caused by several species of *Acanthamoeba* and by *Balamuthia mandrillaris*. PAM was so named to distinguish it from metastatic amoebic abscesses involving the brain caused by *Entamoeba histolytica*. PAM was originally thought to be caused by an *Acanthamoeba* species. Some *B. mandrillaris* meningitis cases were originally diagnosed as caused by *Acanthamoeba,* and the true cause of the disease was recognized only after death. GAE caused by *Acanthamoeba* species occurs in debilitated or immunosuppressed patients, while that due to *B. mandrillaris* occurs in healthy hosts. The pathogenesis of GAE does not appear to be related to immersion. Rather, the *Acanthamoeba* species reach the brain via the hematogenous route from a primary focus, usually thought to be the lungs or skin. It is hypothesized that dusts, aerosols, or air containing the *Acanthamoeba* cysts infects these primary foci.

N. fowleri is a small amoeba, measuring 10 to 35 mm. In unfavorable environments, it transforms into a pear-shaped biflagellate stage. The amoebae may also encyst. The cysts are spherical and smooth walled, have mucus-plugged pores, and measure 7 to 15 mm. *N. fowleri* is a thermophilic organism and tolerates water as warm as 45°C. It has worldwide distribution in naturally warm as well as thermally polluted waters. The concentration of amoebae in warm water frequently exceeds one organism per 25 ml. With its wide distribution in water frequently used for recreation, it is apparent that millions of people have been exposed. Human cases, however, number in

the range of 150 to 200. Eighty-one cases had been reported in the United States as of 1 October 1996. In 1998, four more cases were identified, and during the period from 1999 to 2000, four additional fatal cases were reported in the United States. These last patients were all less than 19 years old; three had exposure to recreational water, and the fourth fell into stagnant water during a Jet Ski accident. In 2002, six more U.S. cases were reported—two each in Texas, Arizona, and Florida. Between 2005 and 2006, three fatal cases were reported in the United States (103). Only eight survivors of PAM have been documented in the literature to date. What factors provide immunity to *N. fowleri* in the majority of exposed individuals is uncertain. Most patients have been healthy prior to infection, although one case in a patient with AIDS has been reported. The majority of cases occur in children in the summer months. Antibody to the amoeba can be demonstrated in the human population, but its protective role is unclear.

The organism is thought to enter the central nervous system via the nasal route. Amoebae from contaminated water are deposited on the olfactory mucosal epithelium and penetrate the submucosal nervous plexus and cribriform plate. Olfactory neuroepithelium is capable of active phagocytosis, and the amoebae travel to the terminus of the olfactory nerve in the olfactory bulb, which is in the subarachnoid space and surrounded by cerebrospinal fluid. Multiplication of the amoebae occurs in the meninges and in neural tissue, and eventually a diffuse hemorrhagic necrotic meningoencephalitis develops. Cortical gray matter is severely affected, with hemorrhage and edema, often leading to uncal or cerebellar herniation. Trophozoites can be identified in the necrotic olfactory bulbs as well as the adventitia and perivascular spaces of small- to medium-sized arteries and cerebrospinal fluid. No cysts are found. Tissue necrosis in response to *Naegleria* infections, seen in the nasal mucosa as well as in the neural tissue, has been ascribed to the release of lysosomal enzymes

#42

or cytopathic toxins by the amoebae or to enzymes on the surface of the organism.

Unfortunately, there is little in the clinical picture of PAM to distinguish it from acute bacterial meningitis. As a result, clinicians often do not consider PAM in their initial differential diagnosis when a patient presents with purulent meningitis. The period between exposure and the onset of symptoms may vary from 2 to 14 days, although most cases have occurred within 5 days. The majority of cases have involved children and young adults. Initially, the patient may notice some alteration of taste or smell. This is rapidly followed by fever, headache, anorexia, nausea, vomiting, and meningismus. The majority of patients also exhibit confusion at the time of presentation (50). This progresses to coma, and the infection is usually fatal within a week. Outside the central nervous system, focal myocarditis has been described to occur in fatal cases of PAM. The pathogenesis is unclear, however, since the amoebae have not been demonstrated in myocardial tissue.

PAM should be considered in any case of acute pyogenic meningitis, which occurs in a patient with a history of swimming in water potentially contaminated with amoebae. Cerebrospinal fluid pressure is often elevated, and the fluid generally has an increased number of erythrocytes, sometimes sufficient to appear grossly hemorrhagic. Leukocyte counts in the cerebrospinal fluid can vary widely, but there is a predominance of neutrophils. Glucose levels may be normal or slightly reduced, with an elevated protein level. It is of paramount diagnostic importance to do a wet-mount microscopic examination of the spinal fluid to detect motile trophozoites. Phase-contrast or dark-field microscopy may aid in this detection. Trophozoites are not usually recognized by Gram staining because of disruption of the amoebae by the fixation process. Cerebrospinal fluid can be examined by Giemsa or other stains after preparation of the sample by cytospinning and fixation. Confirmation of the diagnosis requires cultures of clinical specimens (as mentioned earlier in the discussion

43

of *Acanthamoeba* keratitis) or an indirect immunofluorescent-antibody test. A PCR assay has been described. Serologic tests may be positive for asymptomatic individuals and are not helpful in the diagnosis of acute infections. Computed tomographic scanning studies have been reported for a few patients. Cerebral edema and diffuse-contrast enhancement of the gray matter have been reported. Magnetic resonance imaging may show meningeal enhancement or ring-enhancing lesions with a predilection for diencephalon, thalamus, brain stem, and posterior fossa structures.

A successful clinical outcome is related to early diagnosis and appropriate aggressive therapy. Amphotericin B is the drug that has shown the greatest clinical activity, and it has been employed in the therapy of all survivors. The drug is given in high doses both intravenously and intrathecally. Even when given within 24 h of admission, its use has not been universally successful. Rifampin has also been given in combination with amphotericin B to several survivors. Azithromycin has shown better activity than amphotericin B in vitro and in a mouse model. It may be a useful adjunct to therapy in human infections.

P. boydii

As noted earlier in this chapter, *P. boydii* can be found in polluted waters as well as other sources. Most central nervous system infections have been preceded by aspiration of potentially contaminated material in individuals who nearly drowned, often associated with loss of consciousness from closed-head trauma and asphyxiation. Usually, but not always, pneumonia in which *P. boydii* is cultured from the sputum precedes the development of central nervous system infection. Both meningitis and brain abscesses have been reported, although most cases of meningitis have been associated with abscess formation. Rarely, meningitis has occurred alone in association with trauma and contiguous infection or spinal anesthesia. Both solitary and multiple brain abscesses may occur, although patients who develop central nervous system infection after

#37

aspiration and pneumonia usually have multiple abscesses. That these abscesses are caused by fungemia is evidenced by the frequency of documented abscesses elsewhere in these patients (thyroid, kidney, heart, lungs, and skin).

Surgical therapy appears to be effective in solitary or contiguous brain abscesses where the abscesses were adequately drained. Indeed, one patient with a solitary abscess survived after drainage even though amphotericin B (to which the isolate was resistant in vitro) was used therapeutically (8). In addition to surgical drainage, factors that may improve survival include prolonged high-dose antifungal drug administration and avoidance of corticosteroid therapy. Most isolates have been resistant to amphotericin B and flucytosine and somewhat more susceptible to miconazole than to ketoconazole. The survival of two patients who developed multiple brain abscesses (as well as other foci of infection) was reported following prolonged, high-dose intravenous miconazole therapy (up to 90 mg/kg of body weight/day). One of these patients also had probable meningitis and was treated intrathecally with miconazole as well. It was noted for both patients that frequent dosage increases were necessary in order to keep blood drug levels above the MICs for the isolates. Miconazole is extensively metabolized by hepatic enzymes, and it is possible that with prolonged dosing, this metabolism is facilitated. Unfortunately, miconazole is no longer available in the United States and cannot be obtained even for compassionate use. As mentioned earlier in this chapter, itraconazole has been used successfully for pulmonary P. boydii infections. However, there is no information regarding its efficacy in central nervous system infections. Fluconazole has good central nervous system penetration but does not appear to be active in vitro. The newer azoles have shown promise in the treatment of disseminated infections due to P. boydii. In a mouse model of disseminated infection with P. boydii, posaconazole at high doses was found to be more effective than itraconazole in preventing death and

clearing the organisms from tissues. Voriconazole, a triazole antifungal, has proven effective in the therapy of disseminated infections in immunosuppressed and immunocompetent patients. The Food and Drug Administration has approved it for patients with P. boydii infections that are intolerant or refractory to other agents. Of all tested antifungal agents, it appears to have the lowest MIC for P. boydii. It is available in both intravenous and oral forms, has 90% bioavailability, and achieves concentrations in cerebrospinal fluid and the brain that are 50 and 200% of that in serum. In vitro data also suggest good activity by the echinocandins. There are reports of successful treatment of this infection with voriconazole and intraventricular caspofungin (46, 68).

Coxsackieviruses

Coxsackieviruses are members of the genus Enterovirus, along with polioviruses, echovirus, and enteroviruses 68 to 71. Coxsackieviruses are divided into groups A and B based on their infection patterns in mice and growth in primate cells. Twenty-three serotypes of group A and six serotypes of group B have been recognized.

Most infections caused by coxsackieviruses either are asymptomatic or take the form of undifferentiated febrile illness. Aseptic meningitis, encephalitis, paralysis, myopericarditis, pleurodynia, conjunctivitis, exanthema, enanthema, pharyngitis, and lower respiratory tract infections are additional infection patterns that can be caused by various coxsackievirus serotypes.

Apparent waterborne infections caused by coxsackieviruses B_5 and A_{16} have been described. Hawley et al. reported a summer outbreak of illness caused by coxsackievirus B_5 at a boys' camp on Lake Champlain in Vermont. The illness included conjunctivitis, meningitis, and/or gastroenteritis. The virus was also recovered from a roped-off swimming area in the lake adjacent to the camp (38).

Denis et al. reported an illness that consisted of fever, vomiting, anorexia, diarrhea, and myalgia in five children who had swum in a lake in France (27). Coxsackievirus A$_{16}$ was cultured from a patient and from the lake water. Both of the boys tested had increased titers of antibody to this virus.

Transmission of enteroviruses between humans is mostly by the fecal-oral route. Coxsackieviruses are often shed simultaneously from both the upper respiratory and the gastrointestinal tracts. Coxsackievirus A$_{21}$, which causes upper respiratory tract infections, is thought to be spread additionally by the respiratory-oral route. Urban sewage sampling, especially in summer months, commonly shows enteroviruses, and it may be that outbreaks of freshwater coxsackievirus infection are caused by contamination with sewage or the presence of infected swimmers who spread the virus.

CONCLUSIONS

In conclusion, infections related to recreational water use are many and varied. Mostly, the source of the infections is from bathers themselves. Increasing trends noticed over the last few years indicate that treatments and maintenance strategies for pools must be improved. In the United States, the Centers for Disease Control and Prevention (CDC) have improved reporting systems for these illnesses by making them available online (70). Owners of swimming facilities need to pay more attention to maintenance, operation, disinfection, and filtration. While these issues are being resolved, some practical measures will come in handy to prevent further infections and associated outbreaks.

PRACTICAL TIPS

- Shower thoroughly before using a public pool.
- Avoid sharing swimming pools if you have an open wound.
- Check toddlers frequently for soiling and change their diapers in the bathroom.
- Do not swim if you have diarrhea.
- Avoid swallowing pool water.
- Clean yourself properly after using the bathroom.

REFERENCES

1. **Amofah, G., F. Bonsu, C. Tetteh, J. Okrah, K. Asamoa, K. Asiedu, and J. Addy.** 2002. Buruli ulcer in Ghana: results of a national case search. *Emerg. Infect. Dis.* **8:**167–170.
2. **Aronson, J. D.** 1926. Spontaneous tuberculosis in saltwater fish. *J. Infect. Dis.* **39:**315–319.
3. **Aubry, A., O. Chosidow, E. Caumes, J. Robert, and E. Cambau.** 2002. Sixty-three cases of *Mycobacterium marinum* infection: clinical features, treatment, and antibiotic susceptibility of causative isolates. *Arch. Intern. Med.* **162:**1746–1752.
4. **Avery, L. M., A. P. Williams, K. Killham, and D. L. Jones.** 2008. Survival of Escherichia coli O157:H7 in waters from lakes, rivers, puddles and animal-drinking troughs. *Sci. Total Environ.* **389:**378–385.
5. **Bartralot, R., V. Garcia-Patos, D. Sitjas, L. Rodriguez-Cano, J. Mollet, N. Martin-Casabona, P. Coll, A. Castells, and R. M. Pujol.** 2005. Clinical patterns of cutaneous nontuberculous mycobacterial infections. *Br. J. Dermatol.* **152:**727–734.
6. **Bell, W. E., and M. G. Myers.** 1978. *Allescheria (Petriellidium) boydii* brain abscess in a child with leukemia. *Arch. Neurol.* **35:**386–388.
7. **Bhatia, A., and R. T. Brodell.** 1999. 'Hot tub folliculitis.' Test the waters—and the patient—for *Pseudomonas. Postgrad. Med.* **106:**43–46.
8. **Bisno, A. L.** 1984. Cutaneous infections: microbiologic and epidemiologic considerations. *Am. J. Med.* **76:**172–179.
9. **Bowen, A. B., J. C. Kile, C. Otto, N. Kazerouni, C. Austin, B. C. Blount, H. N. Wong, M. J. Beach, and A. M. Fry.** 2007. Outbreaks of short-incubation ocular and respiratory illness following exposure to indoor swimming pools. *Environ Health Perspect.* **115:**267–271.
10. **Bruce, M. G., M. B. Curtis, M. M. Payne, R. K. Gautom, E. C. Thompson, A. L. Bennett, and J. M. Kobayashi.** 2003. Lake-associated outbreak of Escherichia coli O157:H7 in Clark County, Washington, August 1999. *Arch. Pediatr. Adolesc. Med.* **157:**1016–1021.
11. **Casal, M., and M. M. Casal.** 2001. Multicenter study of incidence of *Mycobacterium marinum* in humans in Spain. *Int. J. Tuberc. Lung Dis.* **5:**197–199.
12. **Castor, M. L., and M. J. Beach.** 2004. Reducing illness transmission from disinfected rec-

reational water venues: swimming, diarrhea and the emergence of a new public health concern. *Pediatr. Infect. Dis. J.* **23**:866–870.

13. **Causer, L. M., T. Handzel, P. Welch, M. Carr, D. Culp, R. Lucht, K. Mudahar, D. Robinson, E. Neavear, S. Fenton, C. Rose, L. Craig, M. Arrowood, S. Wahlquist, L. Xiao, Y. M. Lee, L. Mirel, D. Levy, M. J. Beach, G. Poquette, and M. S. Dworkin.** 2006. An outbreak of Cryptosporidium hominis infection at an Illinois recreational waterpark. *Epidemiol. Infect.* **134**:147–156.

14. **Centers for Disease Control and Prevention.** 1982. Otitis due to *Pseudomonas aeruginosa* serotype O-10 associated with mobile redwood hot tub system—North Carolina. *MMWR Morb. Mortal. Wkly. Rep.* **31**:541–542.

15. **Centers for Disease Control and Prevention.** 1983. An outbreak of *Pseudomonas* folliculitis associated with a waterslide—Utah. *MMWR Morb. Mortal. Wkly. Rep.* **32**:425–427.

16. **Centers for Disease Control and Prevention.** 2000. *Pseudomonas* dermatitis/folliculitis associated with pools and hot tubs—Colorado and Maine, 1999–2000. *MMWR Morb. Mortal. Wkly. Rep.* **49**:1087–1091.

17. **Centers for Disease Control and Prevention.** 2001. Responding to fecal accidents in disinfected swimming venues. *MMWR Morb. Mortal. Wkly. Rep.* **50**:416–417.

18. **Centers for Disease Control and Prevention.** 2004. An outbreak of norovirus gastroenteritis at a swimming club—Vermont, 2004. **53**:793–795.

19. **Clark, B. T.** 2007. Cryptosporidiosis: a recreational water threat that hasn't gone away. *J. Environ. Health* **69**:65–66.

20. **Cooter, R.** 2002. The history of the discovery of primary amoebic meningoencephalitis. *Aust. Fam. Physician* **31**:399–400.

21. **Cornall, P., S. Howie, A. Mughal, V. Sumner, F. Dunstan, A. Kemp, and J. Sibert.** 2005. Drowning of British children abroad. *Child Care Health Dev.* **31**:611–613.

22. **Cort, W. W.** 1928. Schistosome dermatitis in the United States (Michigan). *JAMA* **90**:1027–1029.

23. **Craun, G. F., R. L. Calderon, and M. F. Craun.** 2005. Outbreaks associated with recreational water in the United States. *Int. J. Environ. Health Res.* **15**:243–262.

24. **Crawford, R. P., J. M. Heinemann, W. F. McCulloch, and S. L. Diesch.** 1971. Human infections associated with waterborne Leptospires, and survival studies on serotype pomona. *J. Am. Vet. Med. Assoc.* **159**:1477–1484.

25. **Davies, R. R., H. Spencer, and P. O. Wakelin.** 1964. A case of human protothecosis. *Trans. R. Soc. Trop. Med. Hyg.* **58**:448–451.

26. **De La Cuadra, J., P. Gil-Mateo, and R. Llucian.** 1996. *Pseudomonas aeruginosa* folliculitis after depilation. *Ann. Dermatol. Venereol.* **123**:268–270. (In French.)

27. **Denis, F. A., E. Blanchouin, A. de Lignieres, and P. Flamen.** 1974. Coxsackie A16 infection from lake water. *JAMA* **228**:1370–1371.

28. **Donta, S. T., P. W. Smith, R. E. Levitz, and R. Quintiliani.** 1986. Therapy of *Mycobacterium marinum* infections. Use of tetracyclines vs rifampin. *Arch. Intern. Med.* **146**:902–904.

29. **Eisenstein, L., D. Bodager, and D. Ginzl.** 2008. Outbreak of giardiasis and cryptosporidiosis associated with a neighborhood interactive water fountain—Florida, 2006. *J. Environ. Health* **71**:18–22, 49–50.

30. **Evans, M. R., E. J. Wilkinson, R. Jones, K. Mathias, and P. Lenartowicz.** 2003. Presumed *Pseudomonas* folliculitis outbreak in children following an outdoor games event. *Commun. Dis. Public Health* **6**:18–21.

31. **Fiorillo, L., M. Zucker, D. Sawyer, and A. N. Lin.** 2001. The *Pseudomonas* hot-foot syndrome. *N. Engl. J. Med.* **345**:335–338.

32. **Fowler, M., and R. F. Carter.** 1965. Acute pyogenic meningitis probably due to *Acanthamoeba* spp.: a preliminary report. *Br. Med. J.* **5464**:740–742.

33. **Gluckman, S. J.** 1995. *Mycobacterium marinum.* *Clin. Dermatol.* **13**:273–276.

34. **Gregory, D. W., and W. Schaffner.** 1987. *Pseudomonas* infections associated with hot tubs and other environments. *Infect. Dis. Clin. N. Am.* **1**:635–648.

35. **Griffith, D. E., T. Aksamit, B. A. Brown-Elliott, A. Catanzaro, C. Daley, F. Gordin, S. M. Holland, R. Horsburgh, G. Huitt, M. F. Iademarco, M. Iseman, K. Olivier, S. Ruoss, C. F. von Reyn, R. J. Wallace, Jr., and K. Winthrop.** 2007. An official ATS/IDSA statement: diagnosis, treatment, and prevention of nontuberculous mycobacterial diseases. *Am. J. Respir. Crit. Care Med.* **175**:367–416.

36. **Gustafson, T. L., J. D. Band, R. H. Hutcheson, Jr., and W. Schaffner.** 1983. *Pseudomonas* folliculitis: an outbreak and review. *Rev. Infect. Dis.* **5**:1–8.

37. **Havens, W. P., C. J. Buchner, and H. A. Reinmann.** 1941. Leptospirosis: a public health hazard. Report of a small outbreak of Weil's disease in bathers. *JAMA* **116**:289–291.

38. **Hawley, H. B., D. P. Morin, M. E. Geraghty, J. Tomkow, and C. A. Phillips.** 1973. Coxsackievirus B epidemic at a boy's summer camp. Isolation of virus from swimming water. *JAMA* **226**:33–36.

39. **Heckerling, P. S., T. M. Stine, J. C. Pottage, Jr., S. Levin, and A. A. Harris.** 1983.

Aeromonas hydrophila myonecrosis and gas gangrene in a nonimmunocompromised host. *Arch. Intern. Med.* **143:**2005–2007.

40. **Ichinohe, S., T. Fukushima, K. Kishida, K. Sanbe, S. Saika, and M. Ogura.** 2005. Secondary transmission of cryptosporidiosis associated with swimming pool use. *Jpn. J. Infect. Dis.* **58:**400–401.

41. **Ihekweazu, C., M. Barlow, S. Roberts, H. Christensen, B. Guttridge, D. Lewis, and S. Paynter.** 2006. Outbreak of E. coli O157 infection in the southwest of the UK: risks from streams crossing seaside beaches. *Euro Surveill.* **11:**128–130.

42. **Iwamoto, M., G. Hlady, M. Jeter, C. Burnett, C. Drenzek, S. Lance, J. Benson, D. Page, and P. Blake.** 2005. Shigellosis among swimmers in a freshwater lake. *South. Med. J.* **98:**774–778.

43. **Janda, J. M.** 1991. Recent advances in the study of the taxonomy, pathogenicity, and infectious syndromes associated with the genus *Aeromonas*. *Clin. Microbiol. Rev.* **4:**397–410.

44. **Janda, J. M., and P. S. Duffrey.** 1988. Mesophilic aeromonads in human disease: current taxonomy, laboratory identification, and infectious disease spectrum. *Rev. Infect. Dis.* **10:**980–997.

45. **Jernigan, D. B., J. Hofmann, M. S. Cetron, C. A. Genese, J. P. Nuorti, B. S. Fields, R. F. Benson, R. J. Carter, P. H. Edelstein, I. C. Guerrero, S. M. Paul, H. B. Lipman, and R. Breiman.** 1996. Outbreak of Legionnaires' disease among cruise ship passengers exposed to a contaminated whirlpool spa. *Lancet* **347:**494–499.

46. **Kanafani, Z. A., Y. Comair, and S. S. Kanj.** 2004. Pseudallescheria boydii cranial osteomyelitis and subdural empyema successfully treated with voriconazole: a case report and literature review. *Eur. J. Clin. Microbiol. Infect. Dis.* **23:**836–840.

47. **Kantrow, S. M., and A. S. Boyd.** 2003. Protothecosis. *Dermatol. Clin.* **21:**249–255.

48. **Karam, G. H., A. M. Ackley, and W. E. Dismukes.** 1983. Posttraumatic *Aeromonas hydrophila* osteomyelitis. *Arch. Intern. Med.* **143:**2073–2074.

49. **Kaufman, S. C., D. Ceraso, and A. Schugurensky.** 1986. First case report from Argentina of fatal septicemia caused by *Chromobacterium violaceum*. *J. Clin. Microbiol.* **23:**956–958.

50. **Kaushal, V., D. K. Chhina, S. Ram, G. Singh, R. K. Kaushal, and R. Kumar.** 2008. Primary amoebic meningoencephalitis due to *Naegleria fowleri*. *J. Assoc. Physicians India* **56:**459–462.

51. **Khabbaz, R. F., T. W. McKinley, R. A. Goodman, A. W. Hightower, A. K. Highsmith, K. A. Tait, and J. D. Bandin.** 1983. *Pseudomonas aeroginosa* O:9. New cause of whirlpool–associated dermatitis. *Am. J. Med.* **74:**73–77.

52. **Khardori, N., and V. Fainstein.** 1988. *Aeromonas* and *Plesiomonas* as etiologic agents. *Annu. Rev. Microbiol.* **42:**395–419.

53. **Kitamura, M., S. Kawai, and T. Horio.** 1998. *Pseudomonas aeruginosa* folliculitis: a sporadic case from use of a contaminated sponge. *Br. J. Dermatol.* **139:**359–360.

54. **Kolarova, L., K. Skirnisson, and P. Horak.** 1999. Schistosome cercariae as the causative agent of swimmer's itch in Iceland. *J. Helminthol.* **73:**215–220.

55. **Kosatsky, T., and J. Kleeman.** 1985. Superficial and systemic illness related to a hot tub. *Am. J. Med.* **79:**10–12.

56. **Lacour, J. P., P. el Baze, J. Castanet, D. Dubois, M. Poudenx, and J. P. Ortonne.** 1994. Diving suit dermatitis caused by *Pseudomonas aeruginosa*: two cases. *J. Am. Acad. Dermatol.* **31:**1055–1056.

57. **Lee, W. J., T. W. Kim, K. B. Shur, B. J. Kim, Y. H. Kook, J. H. Lee, and J. K. Park.** 2000. Sporotrichoid dermatosis caused by *Mycobacterium abscessus* from a public bath. *J. Dermatol.* **27:**264–268.

58. **Lewis, F. M., B. J. Marsh, and C. F. von Reyn.** 2003. Fish tank exposure and cutaneous infections due to *Mycobacterium marinum*: tuberculin skin testing, treatment, and prevention. *Clin. Infect. Dis.* **37:**390–397.

59. **Liang, R. B., P. J. Flegg, B. Watt, and C. L. Leen.** 1997. Antimicrobial treatment of fishtank granuloma. *J. Hand Surg. (Br.)* **22:**135–137.

60. **Lindblade, K. A.** 1998. The epidemiology of cercarial dermatitis and its association with limnological characteristics of a northern Michigan lake. *J. Parasitol.* **84:**19–23.

61. **Linell, F., and A. Nordin.** 1954. *Mycobacterium blanei*: a new acid-fast bacillus occurring in swimming pools and capable of producing skin lesions in humans. *Acta Tuberc. Pneumol. Scand.* **33**(Suppl.):1–5.

62. **Mangione, E. J., R. S. Remis, K. A. Tait, H. B. McGee, G. W. Gorman, B. B. Wentworth, P. A. Baron, A. W. Hightower, J. M. Barbaree, and C. V. Broome.** 1985. An outbreak of Pontiac fever related to whirlpool use, Michigan 1982. *JAMA* **253:**535–539.

63. **Mathieu, E., D. A. Levy, F. Veverka, M. K. Parrish, J. Sarisky, N. Shapiro, S. Johnston, T. Handzel, A. Hightower, L. Xiao, Y. M. Lee, S. York, M. Arrowood, R. Lee, and**

J. L. Jones. 2004. Epidemiologic and environmental investigation of a recreational water outbreak caused by two genotypes of Cryptosporidium parvum in Ohio in 2000. *Am. J. Trop. Med. Hyg.* **71:**582–589.

64. Maunula, L., S. Kalso, C. H. Von Bonsdorff, and A. Ponka. 2004. Wading pool water contaminated with both noroviruses and astroviruses as the source of a gastroenteritis outbreak. *Epidemiol. Infect.* **132:**737–743.

65. McCausland, W. J., and P. J. Cox. 1975. *Pseudomonas* infection traced to motel whirlpool. *J. Environ. Health* **37:**455–459.

66. Meyers, W. M., W. M. Shelly, and D. H. Connor. 1974. Heat treatment of *Mycobacterium ulcerans* infections without surgical excision. *Am. J. Trop. Med. Hyg.* **23:**924–929.

67. Mollohan, C. S., and M. S. Romer. 1961. Public health significance of swimming pool granuloma. *Am. J. Public Health* **51:**883–891.

68. Mursch, K., S. Trnovec, H. Ratz, D. Hammer, R. Horre, A. Klinghammer, S. de Hoog, and J. Behnke-Mursch. 2006. Successful treatment of multiple Pseudallescheria boydii brain abscesses and ventriculitis/ependymitis in a 2-year-old child after a near-drowning episode. *Childs Nerv. Syst.* **22:**189–192.

69. Otto, C., III. 2006. Recreational water-illness-prevention = healthy swimming. *J. Environ. Health* **68:**54–55.

70. Otto, C., and P. S. Joe. 2008. Recreational water illness prevention, 2008. *J. Environ. Health* **70:**57–58.

71. Pasricha, G., S. Sharma, P. Garg, and R. K. Aggarwal. 2003. Use of 18S rRNA gene-based PCR assay for diagnosis of *Acanthamoeba* keratitis in non-contact lens wearers in India. *J. Clin. Microbiol.* **41:**3206–3211.

72. Paunio, M., R. Pebody, M. Keskimaki, M. Kokki, P. Ruutu, S. Oinonen, V. Vuotari, A. Siitonen, E. Lahti, and P. Leinikki. 1999. Swimming-associated outbreak of Escherichia coli O157:H7. *Epidemiol. Infect.* **122:**1–5.

73. Piyophirapong, S., R. Linpiyawan, P. Mahaisavariya, C. Muanprasat, A. Chaiprasert, and P. Suthipinittharm. 2002. Cutaneous protothecosis in an AIDS patient. *Br. J. Dermatol.* **146:**713–715.

74. Podewils, L. J., L. Zanardi Blevins, M. Hagenbuch, D. Itani, A. Burns, C. Otto, L. Blanton, S. Adams, S. S. Monroe, M. J. Beach, and M. Widdowson. 2007. Outbreak of norovirus illness associated with a swimming pool. *Epidemiol. Infect.* **135:**827–833.

75. Rasmussen, J. E., and W. H. Graves III. 1982. *Pseudomonas aeruginosa,* hot tubs, and skin infections. *Am. J. Dis. Child.* **136:**553–554.

76. Reines, H. D., and F. V. Cook. 1981. Pneumonia and bacteremia due to *Aeromonas hydrophila.* *Chest* **80:**264–267.

77. Rhodes, M. W., H. Kator, S. Kotob, P. van Berkum, I. Kaattari, W. Vogelbein, F. Quinn, M. M. Floyd, W. R. Butler, and C. A. Ottinger. 2003. *Mycobacterium shottsii* sp. nov., a slowly growing species isolated from Chesapeake Bay striped bass *(Morone saxatilis). Int. J. Syst. Evol. Microbiol.* **53:**421–424.

78. Rinke, C. M. 1983. Hot tub hygiene. *JAMA* **250:**2031.

79. Rose, H. D., T. R. Franson, N. K. Sheth, M. J. Chusid, A. M. Macher, and C. H. Zeirdt. 1983. *Pseudomonas* pneumonia associated with use of a home whirlpool spa. *JAMA* **250:**2027–2029.

80. Salmen, P., D. M. Dwyer, H. Vorse, and W. Kruse. 1983. Whirlpool-associated *Pseudomonas aeruginosa* urinary tract infections. *JAMA* **250:**2025–2026.

81. Shields, J. M., E. R. Gleim, and M. J. Beach. 2008. Prevalence of Cryptosporidium spp. and Giardia intestinalis in swimming pools, Atlanta, Georgia. *Emerg. Infect. Dis.* **14:**948–950.

82. Shiota, R., K. Takeshita, K. Yamamoto, K. Imada, E. Yabuuchi, and L. Wang. 1995. *Legionella pneumophila* serogroup 3 isolated from a patient of pneumonia developed after drowning in bathtub of a hot spring spa. *Kansenshogaku Zasshi* **69:**1356–1364. (In Japanese.)

83. Slaven, E. M., F. A. Lopez, S. M. Hart, and C. V. Sanders. 2001. Myonecrosis caused by *Edwardsiella tarda:* a case report and case series of extraintestinal *E. tarda* infections. *Clin. Infect. Dis.* **32:**1430–1433.

84. Smith, G. L. 1982. Methods for preventing *Pseudomonas* folliculitis. *Cutis* **29:**378, 381.

85. Smith, J. A. 1980. *Aeromonas hydrophila:* analysis of 11 cases. *Can. Med. Assoc. J.* **122:**1270–1272.

86. Speight, E. L., and H. C. Williams. 1997. Fish tank granuloma in a 14-month-old girl. *Pediatr. Dermatol.* **14:**209–212.

87. Stehr-Green, J. K., T. M. Bailey, F. H. Brandt, J. H. Carr, W. W. Bond, and G. S. Visvesvara. 1987. *Acanthamoeba* keratitis in soft contact lens wearers. A case-control study. *JAMA* **258:**57–60.

88. Stehr-Green, J. K., T. M. Bailey, and G. S. Visvesvara. 1989. The epidemiology of *Acanthamoeba* keratitis in the United States. *Am. J. Ophthalmol.* **107:**331–336.

89. Stewart, I., I. M. Robertson, P. M. Webb, P. J. Schluter, and G. R. Shaw. 2006. Cutaneous hypersensitivity reactions to freshwater cyanobacteria—human volunteer studies. *BMC Dermatol.* **6:**6.

90. **Stewart, I., P. M. Webb, P. J. Schluter, L. E. Fleming, J. W. Burns, Jr., M. Gantar, L. C. Backer, and G. R. Shaw.** 2006. Epidemiology of recreational exposure to freshwater cyanobacteria—an international prospective cohort study. *BMC Public Health* **6:**93.

91. **Stewart, I., P. M. Webb, P. J. Schluter, and G. R. Shaw.** 2006. Recreational and occupational field exposure to freshwater cyanobacteria—a review of anecdotal and case reports, epidemiological studies and the challenges for epidemiologic assessment. *Environ. Health* **5:**6.

92. **Tate, D., S. Mawer, and A. Newton.** 2003. Outbreak of *Pseudomonas aeruginosa* folliculitis associated with a swimming pool inflatable. *Epidemiol. Infect.* **130:**187–192.

93. **Tolba, O., A. Loughrey, C. E. Goldsmith, B. C. Millar, P. J. Rooney, and J. E. Moore.** 2008. Survival of epidemic strains of healthcare (HA-MRSA) and community-associated (CA-MRSA) methicillin-resistant Staphylococcus aureus (MRSA) in river-, sea- and swimming pool water. *Int. J. Hyg. Environ. Health* **211:**398–402.

94. **van der Vliet, J. A., G. Tidow, G. Kootstra, H. F. van Saene, R. A. Krom, M. J. Sloof, J. J. Weening, A. M. Tegzess, S. Meijer, and W. P. van Boven.** 1980. Transplantation of contaminated organs. *Br. J. Surg.* **67:**596–598.

95. **Vernon, D. D., W. Banner, Jr., G. P. Cantwell, B. H. Holzman, R. G. Bolte, and J. M. Dean.** 1990. *Streptococcus pneumoniae* bacteremia associated with near-drowning. *Crit. Care Med.* **18:**1175–1176.

96. **Vieira, D. F., H. K. Van Saene, and D. R. Miranda.** 1984. Invasive pulmonary aspergillosis after near-drowning. *Intensive Care Med.* **10:**203–204.

97. **Visvesvara, G. S.** 1995. Pathogenic and opportunistic free living amoeba, p. 1196–1203. *In*

P. R. Murray, E. J. Baron, M. A. Pfaller, F. C. Tenover, and R. H. Yolken (ed.), *Manual of Clinical Microbiology,* 6th ed. American Society for Microbiology, Washington, DC.

98. **Von Graevenitz, A., and A. H. Mensch.** 1968. The genus *Aeromonas* in human bacteriology report of 30 cases and review of the literature. *N. Engl. J. Med.* **278:**245–249.

99. **Washburn, J., J. A. Jacobson, E. Marston, and B. Thorsen.** 1976. *Pseudomonas aeruginosa* rash associated with a whirlpool. *JAMA* **235:** 2205–2207.

100. **Weber, C. J.** 2005. Update on recreational water illnesses. *Urol. Nurs.* **25:**289–290.

101. **Wheeler, C., D. J. Vugia, G. Thomas, M. J. Beach, S. Carnes, T. Maier, J. Gorman, L. Xiao, M. J. Arrowood, D. Gilliss, and S. B. Werner.** 2007. Outbreak of cryptosporidiosis at a California waterpark: employee and patron roles and the long road towards prevention. *Epidemiol. Infect.* **135:**302–310.

102. **Winthrop, K. L., M. Abrams, M. Yakrus, I. Schwartz, J. Ely, D. Gillies, and D. J. Vugia.** 2002. An outbreak of mycobacterial furunculosis associated with footbaths at a nail salon. *N. Engl. J. Med.* **346:**1366–1371.

103. **Yoder, J. S., M. C. Hlavsa, G. F. Craun, V. Hill, V. Roberts, P. A. Yu, L. A. Hicks, N. T. Alexander, R. L. Calderon, S. L. Roy, and M. J. Beach.** 2008. Surveillance for waterborne disease and outbreaks associated with recreational water use and other aquatic facility-associated health events—United States, 2005–2006. *MMWR Surveill. Summ.* **57:**1–29.

104. **Yu, Y., A. S. Cheng, L. Wang, W. M. Dunne, and S. J. Bayliss.** 2007. Hot tub folliculitis or hot hand-foot syndrome caused by Pseudomonas aeruginosa. *J. Am. Acad. Dermatol.* **57:**596–600.

THE CAMPER'S UNINVITED GUESTS

Gordon E. Schutze and Richard F. Jacobs

3

Venturing into wilderness environments can be exhilarating, and each year millions of people take time off to enjoy this pastime. During this relaxing endeavor, the majority of adventurers come into contact with different species of biting arthropods. Ticks, mosquitoes, lice, fleas, mites, bees, wasps, scorpions, and spiders can make time spent outdoors unpleasant, and they are potential carriers of disease. These biting arthropods may identify humans not only as enemies but also as potential sources of food. Biting, therefore, can be an act of feeding, probing, or defending. Contact with the host can be transient (mosquito) or prolonged (tick) and may result in the inoculation of salivary fluids or the regurgitation of digestive tract contents. Organisms present in these fluids are able to cause many different diseases in their human hosts.

In the United States, the majority of illnesses attributed to biting arthropods are due to ticks and mosquitoes. Although potentially serious, the majority of bites from bees, wasps, scorpions, and spiders are simply painful. Physicians should consider arthropod-transmitted diseases during all seasons, but suspicions should be heightened during the summer, when arthropods are most abundant. Children are especially prone to encounter ticks due to their frequent contact with animals and tick habitats. The spectrum of disease caused by these arthropods is broad and can be confusing for the clinician. A history of rural travel, travel to areas where arthropod-borne diseases are endemic, tick bites, or wilderness exposure may aid in obtaining a diagnosis.

TICKS

The major diseases in the United States which are transmitted to humans by ticks include Lyme disease, human monocytic ehrlichiosis (HME), human granulocytic anaplasmosis (HGA), Rocky Mountain spotted fever (RMSF), and tularemia. Each of these disorders has a causative agent that is passed from a specific tick to the host. The two types of ticks usually encountered are the soft (argasid) tick and the hard (ixodid) tick. The hard ticks are of greater concern, since they are more frequently encountered, are difficult to re-

Gordon E. Schutze, Section of Retrovirology and Baylor International Pediatric AIDS Initiative, Baylor College of Medicine, Texas Children's Hospital, Houston, TX 77030. *Richard F. Jacobs,* Department of Pediatrics, University of Arkansas for Medical Sciences, Arkansas Children's Hospital Research Institute, and Pediatric Infectious Diseases, Arkansas Children's Hospital, 800 Marshall St., Little Rock, AR 72202-3591.

Infections of Leisure, Fourth Edition, Edited by David Schlossberg,
© 2009 ASM Press, Washington, DC

move, and are more likely to transmit disease to humans.

Nonspecific Fever

Data from areas in northwest Wisconsin, where tick-borne disease is endemic, demonstrated that 27% of patients evaluated for a nonspecific fever without a rash ($n = 62$) had laboratory evidence of a tick-borne infection (3). In a reevaluation of the military experience in Fort Chaffee, AR, 162 of 1,067 persons (15.2%) had antibodies to one or more tick-borne pathogens following training exercises and contact with wooded areas (36). Finally, two recent seroprevalence surveys of children (aged 1 to 17 years) in the southeastern United States found seropositivity rates of 2% to 22% for antibodies to RMSF or HME antigens in randomly selected blood specimens (32, 33). These data suggest that tick-borne infections may be more common than has previously been recognized and that these organisms are responsible for a significant amount of subclinical or self-limited disease.

Lyme Disease

Lyme disease is the most common tick-borne disease in the United States, with approximately 20,000 cases reported per year to the Centers for Disease Control and Prevention. Lyme disease has been reported in most states, but cases remain concentrated in well-established areas of prevalence in the northeastern, north-central, and Pacific Coast states (7, 8). In these regions of endemicity, the incidence of disease over a 3-year period was recently reported to be 29.2/100,000 people (6, 57). This multisystem inflammatory disease is caused by the spirochetal organism *Borrelia burgdorferi*. Ticks from the *Ixodes ricinus-Ixodes persulcatus* complex (e.g., *Ixodes scapularis* and *Ixodes pacificus*) are responsible for transmitting *B. burgdorferi* to humans. Even when engorged, these *Ixodes* ticks are quite small, and therefore, histories of tick bites are infrequently obtained.

The clinical presentation of Lyme disease is divided into three stages. These stages are de-fined by the chronological relationship to the original tick bite (Table 1). The major manifestation of the first stage of the disease (early, localized infection) is the localized skin rash termed erythema migrans, which is present in up to 80% of patients (Fig. 1). This rash usually begins anywhere from 4 to 21 days after the tick bite and consists of an erythematous papule which gradually enlarges to form a large plaque-like annular lesion (5 cm or more in diameter, with a median of 15 cm, sometimes with partial central clearing). The average duration of the untreated lesion is approximately 3 weeks. If appropriate antibiotics are given, the rash may resolve in several days. Patients in this stage of disease may also have fever, regional adenopathy, or other minor constitutional symptoms (46, 50–52).

The second stage of Lyme disease (early disseminated infection) is the result of dissemination by the spirochete into the circulation. Although the potential clinical manifestations

TABLE 1 Major clinical manifestations of Lyme disease[a]

Stage 1 (early localized infection)
Erythema migrans
Headache
Arthralgias
Regional lymphadenopathy

Stage 2 (early disseminated infection)
Recurrent erythema migrans
Migratory bone and joint pain
Meningitis
Bell's palsy
Peripheral radiculoneuropathy
Atrioventricular block
Myocarditis
Pancarditis
Conjunctivitis
Mild hepatitis
Hematuria and proteinuria
Malaise and fatigue

Stage 3 (late infection)
Acrodermatitis chronica atrophicans
Prolonged arthritis
Chronic neurological syndromes
Keratitis

[a] Adapted from references 52 and 57.

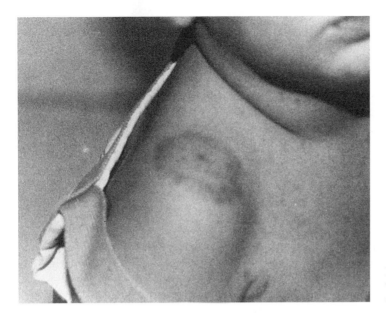

FIGURE 1 Annular lesion of erythema migrans on the shoulder of a child.

of this dissemination are extensive, the major characteristics are seen in the skin and the nervous and musculoskeletal systems. Patients in this stage may appear quite ill, with debilitating malaise and fatigue as the major symptoms. A secondary annular skin lesion may occur in approximately one-half of the patients. The musculoskeletal discomfort is generally migratory in joints, bursae, tendons, muscle, and bone, lasting only a few hours or days in one location (52). Disease of the nervous system is found in approximately 15% of the reported cases and usually begins approximately 4 weeks after the tick bite. The characteristic triad of findings includes meningitis, cranial nerve palsies, and a peripheral radiculoneuropathy (49). The most common manifestation of meningitis is usually a headache and a stiff neck, which is not generally associated with a Kernig or Brudzinski sign. Unilateral or bilateral facial nerve involvement (Bell's palsy) is the most common nerve palsy and may represent the only neurological abnormality (10). Other cranial nerves may also be involved. Cardiac involvement is limited to less than 10% of patients, with problems ranging from atrioventricular block to myopericarditis and

left ventricular dysfunction (41). The length of cardiac involvement can be as brief as 3 days.

The third stage (late infection) is highlighted by chronic complaints of arthritis. Although present very early in children, episodes of arthritis in adults become longer during the second and third years of illness, lasting months instead of weeks or days. Large joints, often those that were very close to the initial rash, are most commonly involved. The knee is the principal joint that is involved in the majority of patients (17). The involved joints tend to become swollen, warm, and painful but rarely red. Other clinical manifestations of the third stage of the disease include acrodermatitis chronica atrophicans, which is a progressive dermatologic condition that develops with increasing erythema and pigmentation changes of the skin surfaces. Chronic neurological complications, keratitis, and fatigue may also be seen. Late disease is uncommon in children who are treated with antibiotics in the early stages of disease (46).

Physicians remained concerned that pregnant women could be at risk for transplacental passage of *B. burgdorferi* to their fetuses. No causal relationship between Lyme disease in

#45

pregnancy and abnormalities or congenital disease has been confirmed. No evidence that Lyme disease can be transmitted via breast milk exists. The risk of an adverse outcome is quite low (56).

Lyme disease can easily be diagnosed if erythema migrans is present. Without this characteristic rash, a broad range of diseases should be considered. The primary rash is sometimes confused with staphylococcal or streptococcal cellulitis, erythema multiforme, or erythema marginatum. Other forms of arthritis that can be confused with Lyme disease include pauciarticular juvenile rheumatoid arthritis; Reiter syndrome; psoriatic arthritis; gonococcal arthritis; reactive arthritis due to *Salmonella, Shigella,* or *Yersinia* species; parvovirus B19 arthritis; postinfectious (streptococcal) arthritis; and septic arthritis.

The specific diagnosis is made with clinical and epidemiological data and can be established early if erythema migrans is present. Otherwise, serologic studies will be needed to establish the diagnosis. Antibodies may not rise until 2 or 3 weeks after the infection and may be aborted with antimicrobial therapy. Antibodies are not detected in most patients with erythema migrans. Routine serologic tests are not recommended for children with typical signs and symptoms. A two-step approach is recommended for the diagnosis of Lyme disease. Serum specimens that give positive or equivocal results to screening tests by enzyme immunoassay or immunofluorescent antibody assay should undergo confirmatory Western blot testing (11).

For patients with stage 1 disease (early infection), isolated Bell's palsy, arthritis, or mild carditis, oral antimicrobial therapy is recommended (11, 57). For those patients over 9 years of age, doxycycline, cefuroxime axetil, or amoxicillin is recommended. Children less than 9 years of age should receive amoxicillin or cefuroxime axetil. Macrolides (e.g., erythromycin, clarithromycin, and azithromycin) are not recommended as first-line therapy and should be used only for patients who cannot tolerate the recommended regimens (57). The

oral regimens are given until the patients demonstrate a clinical response, which is usually after a total of between 10 and 30 days of therapy. For those patients with persistent arthritis, severe carditis, meningitis, or encephalitis, parenteral medications should be used. Penicillin G, ceftriaxone, or cefotaxime for 14 to 21 days is recommended as the medication of choice.

The risk of Lyme disease following a tick bite is low. Animal studies indicate that prolonged attachment (36 h) by infected ticks is required to transmit *B. burgdorferi*. Current recommendations support the use of a single dose of doxycycline (4 mg/kg of body weight or 200 mg maximum) for adults and children ≥8 years of age if the following apply: (i) if an *I. scapularis* tick has been attached for ≥36 h, (ii) if prophylaxis can be started within 72 h of tick removal, (iii) if ecologic information indicates that the local rate of infection of the *Ixodes* ticks is ≥20%, and (iv) if doxycycline is not contraindicated (57). There are no current recommendations for chemoprophylaxis for patients who are unable to take doxycycline (e.g., pregnant women and children <8 years of age). Prophylaxis after *I. pacificus* bites is generally not needed because of low rates of infection with *B. burgdorferi* in most instances. However, if the ecologic data demonstrate a ≥20% infection rate of the *I. pacificus* ticks in a specific geographic location, there chemoprophylaxis should be considered as outlined above. There is currently no vaccine available for prevention.

Ehrlichioses

Ehrlichiosis is a tick-borne disease that is caused most commonly by *Ehrlichia chaffeensis* (HME) or *Anaplasma phagocytophilum* (HGE). These organisms are intraleukocytic rickettsiae spread from a tick bite to the human host. Ehrlichiosis has been recognized as a disease in dogs since 1935, but human disease caused by this organism in the United States has been recognized only since 1986 (30). Circulating white blood cells are the target of these organisms, and the diseases that they cause are often named after the specific white blood cells that they infect (e.g., *E. chaffeensis* infects human monocytes, and the infection is called HME). HME in humans is caused by *E. chaffeensis*. The exact incidence of HME is unknown but has been described to be as high as 330 to 414/100,000 people in regions of the United States where ticks are endemic (40, 47). The geographic distribution of illness closely overlaps that of RMSF, as the tick vectors are identical *(Amblyomma americanum* and *Dermacentor variabilis)*. From the first year that it became a reportable disease in 1999 until 2006, a mean of 300 cases per year (range, 99 to 578) was reported to the Centers for Disease Control and Prevention in the United States (7, 8). The majority of reported cases, however, are from the southeastern part of the United States, with approximately 80% of reported cases occurring during the months of May and June.

HGA is caused by *Anaplasma phagocytophilum* and is transmitted from the same *Ixodes* ticks that transmit Lyme disease. The prevalence of HGA is not well documented, but rates as high as 52 to 58 cases/100,000 people have been described to occur in regions of high endemicity, Connecticut and Wisconsin, in the United States (1, 37). From 1999 to 2006, there was a mean of 457 cases/year (range, 203 to 786) of HGA reported to the Centers for Disease Control and Prevention (7, 8). Most HGA infections are diagnosed between April and September, and more than two-thirds occur in rural residents. Tick and human studies suggest a potential coinfection with comorbidity for HGA and Lyme borreliosis or babesiosis (38). HGA has also been demonstrated to be transmitted perinatally as well as by blood transfusion (16, 27). The interval from tick exposure to the development of the illness from either form of ehrlichia is 2 days to 3 weeks.

Fever, rash, headache, myalgia, and hepatosplenomegaly are common abnormalities encountered on physical examination in patients with HME (19, 45). The rash associated with HME is more commonly encountered in children than in adults, is generally distributed over the trunk or extremities, and may be macular, maculopapular, petechial, or a combination of all three types.

The most important feature of HGA is a lack of abnormal findings on physical examination (2). Symptoms similar to those of HME are found, but the rash is usually absent (Table 2). Peripheral neuropathies (e.g., brachial plexus, demyelinating polyneuropathy, and isolated facial palsy) can occur in HGA patients and may persist for weeks or months (19).

The recognition of ehrlichiosis can be difficult. Patients who are evaluated during the summer with a history of tick attachment should be considered to be at risk. Elevated liver function test results, thrombocytopenia, and leukopenia (with lymphopenia [HME] or neutropenia [HGA]) are the most common laboratory abnormalities noted (1, 19, 27). Patients may also have hyponatremia, anemia, and cerebrospinal fluid abnormalities (i.e., pleocytosis with a predominance of lymphocytes and an elevated total protein concentration), but none of these laboratory tests are specific for the diagnosis. Although examination of the peripheral smear with a Wright

TABLE 2 Comparison of symptoms of HME and HGA[a]

Sign, symptom, or finding	% of patients with:	
	HME	HGA
Fever	97	93
Myalgia	57	77
Headache	80	76
Malaise	82	94
Nausea	64	38
Arthralgia	41	46
Vomiting	33	26
Diarrhea	23	16
Rash	31	6
Stiff neck	3	21
Confusion	19	17
Leukopenia	62	49
Thrombocytopenia	71	71
Elevated liver function test	83	71

[a]Adapted from reference 19.

stain looking for intracytoplasmic inclusions (morulae) in the monocytes (HME) or neutrophils (HGA) has been described previously, it is a very insensitive method for establishing the diagnosis (1, 19). In addition, doxycycline treatment will adversely affect the ability to detect these inclusions. Likewise, in vitro cultivation of the organism, immunohistology or immunocytology, or PCR is not widely available. The use of serologic testing is therefore required for confirmation in patients with compatible histories and clinical findings (5). HME can be diagnosed with a minimum titer of antibody to *E. chaffeensis* of ≥1:64 or a fourfold or greater change in antibody titers from acute- and convalescent-phase sera by indirect fluorescent antibody testing. Currently, testing for HGA requires identification of indirect fluorescent antibodies to preparations of *Anaplasma phagocytophila* and a fourfold increase in titer between acute- and convalescent-phase sera. If a rash is present, ehrlichiosis may be clinically indistinguishable from RMSF. The inability to distinguish the two clinically is not important since the antimicrobial and supportive therapy for these two diseases is the same. Treatment of ehrlichioses is discussed below, at the end of the section on RMSF.

Rocky Mountain Spotted Fever

RMSF is the most important and severe disease in the spotted-fever group, and it is caused by *Rickettsia rickettsii*. From 1999 to 2006, there was a mean of 1,237 cases/year (range, 495 to 2,236 cases) of RMSF reported in the United States (7, 8). Of these cases, approximately 90% occurred between April and September. Approximately two-thirds of the cases occurred in children <15 years of age, with the highest age-specific incidence occurring between 5 and 9 years of age (46). Although the disease is rare in infants, RMSF has been described to occur in more than one family member at the same time. In the United States, RMSF is most common in the South and southeastern states. Ticks that transmit the disease vary by region. In the western

United States, wood ticks *(Dermacentor andersoni)* are the primary carriers and vectors of infection, whereas the dog tick *(Dermacentor variabilis)* and the Lone Star tick *(Amblyomma americanum)* represent the most common arthropod hosts in the eastern United States and the south-central region, respectively. Even in areas where most human cases are reported, only approximately 1 to 3% of the tick population carries the causative agent, *Rickettsia rickettsii,* and very few humans actually become infected despite suffering a tick bite (46).

The incubation period for RMSF is usually 7 days but ranges from 1 to 14 days, depending on the size of the rickettsial inoculum (35, 46). The illness is usually characterized by a short prodromal period with headache, malaise, and myalgia (4, 22, 44). The classic triad of fever, headache, and a centrifugal petechial rash, plus a history of exposure to ticks, is present in only 3 to 18% of patients at their initial evaluation (4, 22). The onset of fever is usually abrupt and high grade (40 to 40.5°C [104 to 104.9°F]). The skin rash, however, begins to appear, on average, 2 to 3 days after the onset of illness as blanching, 1- to 4-mm macules that later become petechial (Fig. 2) (4, 15, 35). The skin rash begins peripherally (e.g., on the wrists and ankles) and spreads centrally; it is common to have involvement of the palms and soles. It is important to note, however, that only 50% of patients have a rash during the first 3 days of illness and that as many as 20% of adults and 5% of children may never develop a rash (4, 15, 22). Care should also be taken when dealing with patients with darkly pigmented skin, because the rash may not be appreciated. The absence of a rash should never delay the institution of appropriate antimicrobial therapy if the historical, clinical, and laboratory findings are compatible with the diagnosis of RMSF. Although physicians rely greatly on a history of tick exposure, in a reported series of cases, such information was confirmed in only one-half to two-thirds of documented infections.

Other clinical manifestations include headache, mental confusion, and myalgia. The

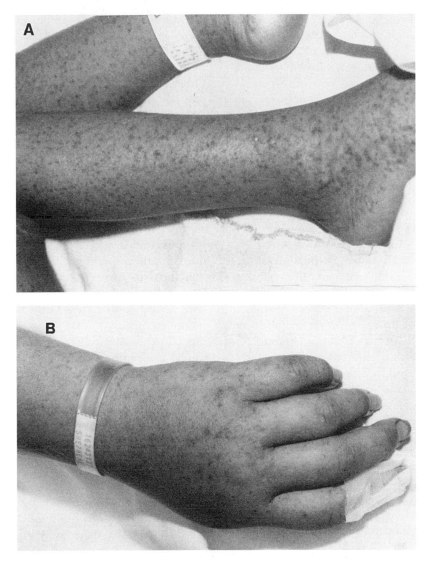

FIGURE 2   Maculopapular rash of RMSF on the legs (A) and hand (B).

headache is described by adults and older children as being the most severe headache they have ever experienced, persisting throughout the day and being unresponsive to any pain medications. Most of the major complications of this illness occur as a result of a vasculitic mechanism of injury. Complications of severe illness include encephalitis, meningitis, pulmonary edema, respiratory distress syndrome, cardiac arrhythmias, coagulopathy, gastrointestinal bleeding, hepatitis, and skin necrosis

(4, 15, 35). Long-term sequelae that have been described include paraparesis; hearing loss; peripheral neuropathy; cerebellar, vestibular, and motor dysfunction; language disorders; behavioral disturbances; learning disabilities; bladder and bowel incontinence; and limb amputation (25, 26, 34, 55). The mortality rate associated with RMSF is 20 to 25% if untreated and 5% with appropriate antimicrobial therapy. Risk factors for an adverse outcome include nonwhite race, male gender, absence of headache,

_#50_

#49

no history of tick attachment, delay in initiating therapy, gastrointestinal symptoms, and no treatment by the fifth day of illness.

The diagnosis of RMSF must be based only on the history and physical examination findings, because specific laboratory tests may not become positive until the second week of infection. Although laboratory abnormalities, such as thrombocytopenia, hyponatremia, leukopenia, and elevated liver function test results, may be present in patients with RMSF, none are specific for this illness and therefore cannot be used to confirm a diagnosis (4, 22, 35). Specific serologic testing should be performed to confirm a diagnosis of RMSF (5). This can be accomplished by demonstrating a fourfold increase in antibody titer between acute- and convalescent-phase sera as determined by one or more of the specific serologic tests or by a number of other methods, including complement fixation, immunofluorescent assays, latex agglutination, indirect hemagglutination, or microagglutination tests. Testing is available in most state and local laboratories in regions of high endemicity, as well as at the Centers for Disease Control and Prevention in Atlanta, GA. A single titer of >1: 128 can also be used to confirm the diagnosis. _Rickettsia rickettsii_ has been identified by immunofluorescent staining of skin biopsy specimens obtained at the site of the rash, with 70% sensitivity and 100% specificity (15). A PCR assay has been developed to detect _R. rickettsii_ in blood and biopsy specimens during the acute phase of illness, but it is not currently widely available and its use has been limited due to its inferior sensitivity in detecting _R. rickettsii_ in the blood.

Doxycycline and tetracycline are the antimicrobial agents of choice for most rickettsial infections (RMSF and ehrlichioses), and its use should not be delayed in suspected cases. Despite years of intensive education, clinicians in regions of tick endemicity still delay in starting empirical antirickettsial therapy (4, 42). In the past, chloramphenicol was used for children younger than 9 years of age because of the side effects (e.g., tooth staining) attrib-

uted to the use of tetracycline agents. In children with RMSF, however, the mortality is higher for those treated with chloramphenicol than for those treated with doxycycline (14). Other important issues include the lack of oral preparations of chloramphenicol in the United States, the knowledge that the staining of teeth by the tetracyclines is dose related, and the lack of teeth staining with doxycycline (28). Because of this, doxycycline is the drug of choice for use at any age. The optimal duration of antimicrobial therapy has not been well established for any of the rickettsial diseases because very few comparative clinical trials have examined short-course versus conventional antibiotic management. Patients should, therefore, be managed individually, and a briefer course should be reserved for those with mild illness or for those with a rapid response to therapy. However, as a general approach for more-difficult patients, therapy should be continued until patients have been afebrile for 48 to 72 h and have clinically improved.

Tularemia

Tularemia is a bacterial infection caused by _Francisella tularensis_. This acute febrile illness is a zoonotic disease for which humans are susceptible hosts. There are more than 100 species in the animal kingdom that carry this bacterium (23). The organism is usually associated with lagomorphs (hares and rabbits) but is quite commonly found among rodents, raccoons, opossums, and cats. The infection is transmitted to humans by ingestion of infected animal tissue; by direct contact with infected animals or through the bite of infected animals, ticks, or other arthropods; by inhalation of infected vapors; or by consumption of water that is contaminated.

There are currently three subspecies of _F. tularensis_ that are recognized based upon biochemical characteristics and virulence for domestic rabbits (24). _F. tularensis_ subsp. _tularensis_ (type A) is highly virulent to rabbits and found most commonly in North America, _F. tularensis_ subsp. _holarctica_ (type B) is less virulent and found mostly in the Northern Hemisphere, and *F. tularensis* subsp. *mediasiatica* is similar to organisms of the subspecies *holarctica* but has been found only in Kazakhstan and Turkmenistan in Central Asia. A fourth subspecies, *F. tularensis* subsp. *novicida,* is found in North America. Life-threatening disease is most commonly found with subsp. *tularensis* (type A), which does not appear to be commonly found outside North America.

F. tularensis is a highly infectious bacterium, with as few as 10 organisms required to produce systemic disease in humans. The organism will gain access to the body through the skin, oropharynx, conjunctiva, respiratory tract, or gastrointestinal tract. After the organism gains entry into the body, further dissemination may occur via the blood or lymphatic system.

Ticks are the major vectors in the southern part of the United States for the transmission of this disease. *A. americanum* (the Lone Star tick), *D. andersoni* (the wood tick), and *D. variabilis* (the dog tick) are the principal tick vectors known not only to transmit but also to serve as reservoirs for this disease. Other vectors, such as fleas, mites, deer flies, and mosquitoes, are also known to transmit the disease.

The incubation period for this disorder is usually 3 to 4 days (range, 1 to 21 days). The onset of symptoms is usually quite abrupt; the symptoms consist of fever, chills, headache, myalgia, vomiting, and photophobia. Children are more likely to suffer from adenopathy and fever than adults. Six forms of the disease have been described. The most common is the ulceroglandular form; the others are the glandular, oculoglandular, oropharyngeal, typhoidal, and pneumonic forms (Table 3) (20).

In the ulceroglandular form of the disease, the organisms gain entry through the skin via an embedded tick. After approximately 2 days, patients will complain of tender, swollen lymph nodes, most commonly in the axillary or inguinal regions in adults and the cervical nodes in children. At the site of entry, there is often a painful, swollen papule. This papule

TABLE 3 Common forms of tularemia

Form	% of patients with form
Ulceroglandular	50
Glandular	9
Oculoglandular	1
Oropharyngeal	2
Typhoidal	8
Pneumonic	15
Unclassified	15

will rupture, leaving a punched-out ulcer with raised borders. This ulcer may persist for months. The swollen lymph node may become inflamed and, in many cases, will suppurate and drain. The glandular form of the disease is very similar, except that the skin lesion is lacking.

The conjunctival space is thought to be the portal of entry in the oculoglandular form of tularemia. The eye becomes involved, due to contact with infected secretions, most often from rubbing the eyes. The eyelids become edematous, inflamed, and extremely painful. Occasionally, multiple small, yellowish nodules or ulcers will appear on the palpebral conjunctiva or sclera (Fig. 3). Preauricular, submaxillary, and cervical adenopathy may also be evident.

In oropharyngeal tularemia, the organisms are introduced to the oropharyngeal mucosa through contaminated food and water. Complaints of a sore throat are usually out of proportion to the pharyngitis seen on examination. Cervical adenopathy may also be present.

The typhoidal form of tularemia often presents as an acute septicemia. The onset is usually quite abrupt, with fever, myalgia, and vomiting. Patients often have meningitis, delirium, and pulmonary involvement. In children, in whom typhoidal tularemia can be the result of the ingestion of the organism, necrotic lesions may be present throughout the bowel.

The pneumonic form of tularemia is uncommon, but when it presents, it is quite severe. This disorder has been limited to laboratory workers in the past. Pneumonia,

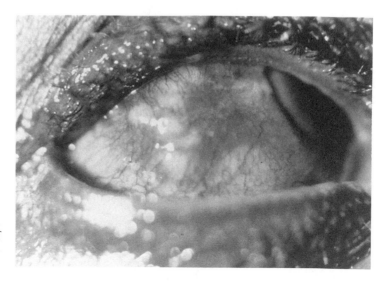

FIGURE 3 Small nodules on palpebral conjunctiva and sclera of a patient with oculoglandular tularemia.

however, may occur in up to 15% of cases of ulceroglandular disease and 80% of typhoidal tularemia cases.

The overall mortality rate for tularemia is approximately 2% (54). Patients with a poor outcome are more likely to have electrolyte or renal abnormalities, pneumonia, pleural effusion, rhabdomyolysis with elevated serum creatine phosphokinase, and *F. tularensis* bacteremia (43).

The diagnosis of tularemia is established based upon history, physical examination, and serology. The agglutination test is the usual method employed for diagnosing tularemia. Antibody usually develops in the second week of illness. A titer of ≥1:160 is a presumptive diagnostic test, which suggests a current or past infection, while a fourfold rise in titer in convalescent-phase serum, in the range of 1:1,280 to 1:2,560, is an easy way to document a current infection (53). Culture of *F. tularensis* should not be attempted in routine clinical laboratories due to the risk of infection of the workers.

Streptomycin was previously the drug of choice for tularemia. Gentamicin, however, has become the principal medication due to side effects and manufacturing problems with streptomycin (53). Although tetracycline and chloramphenicol have been demonstrated to cause a prompt response in patients with tu-

laremia, a relatively high rate of relapse makes these medications less desirable. Recent data support the use of ciprofloxacin for the treatment of tularemia after institution of appropriate medication (gentamicin, 5.0 mg/kg twice daily); patients demonstrate improvement within 24 to 48 h. The duration of treatment is usually 7 to 10 days, with the patient having at least 4 afebrile days prior to discontinuation of the medication. Recent uncontrolled studies have demonstrated the quinolone ciprofloxacin to be an effective treatment. Some experts recommend ciprofloxacin treatment of tularemia in adults, but most treatment data are restricted to its use against type B tularemia; there are currently few data supporting its use for type A disease. Ciprofloxacin should not be used in patients less than 18 years of age.

Prevention of Tick-Transmitted Diseases

A proper wardrobe is essential in preventing tick-transmitted diseases. Protective clothing that covers the arms, legs, and other usually exposed areas; ankle-high footwear; and pant legs that cinch at the ankles or are worn tucked into the socks can help protect the wilderness adventurer from unwanted travel companions. Permethrin can be sprayed on clothing to prevent tick attachment, and insect repellents that employ *N,N*-diethyl-3-methylbenzamide (DEET) can be applied to the skin for further protection (12). Concentrations of more than 35% DEET should also be avoided, since they are not proven to be more effective than the lower concentrations and have a greater risk for complications due to overdose (12, 21). DEET repels a variety of mosquitoes, chiggers, ticks, fleas, and biting flies. In the United States, DEET is available in formulations of 5 to 40% and 100% (48). DEET at 20% provides complete protection for 1 to 3 h.

Close and regular inspections of all body parts are essential for the adventurer. Adult ticks are usually on the body for 1 to 2 h prior to attachment. The duration of tick feeding may be directly related to disease transmission (13). If ticks are discovered, they should be removed. The recommended method for tick removal is to grasp the tick as close to the skin as possible with tweezers or protected fingers and then pull the tick straight out with steady, even pressure. Care should be taken to avoid twisting or jerking the tick, as this might cause mouthparts to break off and be left in the skin. Crushing or puncturing the body of the tick is also not suggested, since the body fluids may contain infective agents. After the tick is removed, the bite site should be disinfected (39). Traditional methods of tick removal, such as the application of fingernail polish or isopropyl alcohol to the tick or the use of a hot match, may induce the tick to salivate or regurgitate into the wound, thus spreading its infected secretions. The empirical use of antimicrobial agents after a tick bite to prevent the acquisition of tick-borne disease has been demonstrated not to be useful except as outlined for Lyme disease.

MOSQUITOES, LICE, FLEAS, AND MITES

There are many diseases transmitted by mosquitoes around the world, but very few are encountered in the United States (Table 4). The use of proper clothing can help prevent these diseases. Items that should be considered include long-sleeve shirts, protective facial

TABLE 4 Mosquito-borne infections

Disease	Agent
Western equine encephalitis	Alphavirus
Eastern equine encephalitis	Alphavirus
St. Louis encephalitis	Flavivirus
California virus encephalitis	Bunyavirus
Dengue	Flavivirus
Venezuelan encephalitis	Alphavirus
Tularemia	*F. tularensis*
West Nile fever	Flavivirus

netting, and mosquito netting for sleeping. These garments and nets should be used in areas with large mosquito populations. Insect repellents that employ DEET will also aid in the battle against these biting arthropods. Lice are the main vectors for epidemic typhus. This disease, which is rarely reported in North America, is caused by *Rickettsia prowazekii*. Louse-borne disease is especially prominent in areas of poverty, overcrowding, and poor sanitation. The disease in the United States has been attributed to contact with flying squirrels in Virginia, West Virginia, and North Carolina (18). The disease is characterized by an influenza-like illness with headache, fever, and malaise. A rash begins approximately 4 to 7 days into the illness. This rash usually begins on the trunk and then spreads to involve the extremities. Illness usually varies from moderate to fatal and, if left untreated, will last approximately 2 weeks. Epidemic typhus is treated with tetracycline or chloramphenicol.

A second zoonotic infection transmitted by the flea is murine (endemic) typhus. This disorder is caused by the organism *Rickettsia typhi* or *Rickettsia felis* and is transmitted from rats or cats to humans by the rat or cat flea. Fever, headache, malaise, and rash are the common clinical symptoms of this disease. Typhus is endemic in the southwestern regions of the United States and is treated with tetracycline (9).

Infections due to mites have been recognized for many years. The larval form of the mite is commonly referred to as the chigger and is responsible for many of these diseases. Scabies, rickettsialpox, and scrub typhus are all transmitted by mites. In the wilderness, most humans have trouble only with the bite of the chigger. Within 24 to 48 h, these bites become intensely pruritic and may develop small hemorrhagic papules or nodules. The inflammation is proportional to the host's hypersensitivity to the oral secretions of the mite. These bites may persist for 5 to 6 days and occur mostly on the lower legs or other exposed regions.

OTHER ARTHROPODS

Some other arthropod envenomations may be particularly severe. Stings of hymenopteran insects (bees, wasps, hornets, and ants) are the most common cause of envenomation, especially in children. They usually produce local pain, swelling, and erythema. If a stinger remains after the envenomation, it should be removed by carefully brushing it away. Grasping the stinger to remove it may squeeze the remaining venom into the wound (31). The application of ice or cool compresses often helps to reduce the pain and swelling. In older children, the use of oral antihistamines may provide relief. Early signs of generalized pruritus, urticaria, angioedema, or bronchospasm necessitate a medical evaluation emergently. If the patient cannot be evaluated, epinephrine is the drug of choice for systemic reactions and should be given in the field (21).

Although lethal scorpion bites are a serious problem throughout the world, in the United States, the only dangerous species encountered is *Centruroides sculpturatus* (also known as *Centruroides exilicauda* or the bark scorpion). This scorpion is found mostly in the desert climate of the Southwest. Symptoms are usually limited to local pain, but children younger than 2 years of age may experience multisystem organ failure (29). The brown recluse *(Loxosceles reclusa)* and black widow *(Latrodectus mactans)* spiders may also cause painful bites. If signs of systemic envenomation develop, the victim requires medical evaluation. Antivenin is available for black widow and bark scorpion bites.

PRACTICAL TIPS

- Only a very few individuals who are bitten by a tick in regions of Lyme endemicity are candidates for chemoprophylaxis.
- RMSF and HME are clinically indistinguishable from each other.
- Concentrations of DEET above 35% in repellants are not more effective than lower concentrations and have a greater risk for side effects.
- The recommended method for tick removal is to grasp the tick as close to the skin as possible with tweezers or protected fingers and then pull the tick straight out with steady even pressure.
- If a stinger remains after envenomation from a bee, wasp, or hornet, it should be removed by carefully brushing it away.

REFERENCES

1. **Bakken, J. S., P. Goellner, M. Van Etten, D. Z. Boyle, O. L. Swonger, S. Mattson, J. Krueth, R. L. Tilden, K. Asanovich, J. Walls, and J. S. Dumler.** 1998. Seroprevalence of human granulocytic ehrlichiosis among permanent residents of northwestern Wisconsin. *Clin. Infect. Dis.* **27:**1491–1496.
2. **Bakken, J. S., and J. S. Dumler.** 2006. Clinical diagnosis and treatment of human granulocytotropic anaplasmosis. *Ann. N. Y. Acad. Sci.* **1078:**236–247.
3. **Belongia, E. A., K. D. Reed, P. D. Mitchell, N. Mueller-Rizner, M. Vandermause, M. F. Finkel, and J. Kazmierczak.** 2001. Tickborne infections as a cause of nonspecific febrile illness in Wisconsin. *Clin. Infect. Dis.* **32:**1434–1439.
4. **Buckingham, S. C., G. S. Marshall, G. E. Schutze, C. R. Woods, M. A. Jackson, L. E. Patterson, and R. F. Jacobs.** 2007. Clinical and laboratory features, hospital course, and outcome of Rocky Mountain spotted fever in children. *J. Pediatr.* **150:**180–184.
5. **Centers for Disease Control and Prevention.** 2006. Diagnosis and management of tickborne rickettsial diseases: Rocky Mountain spotted fever, ehrlichioses, anaplasmosis—United States. A practical guide for physicians and other healthcare and public health professionals. *MMWR Recommend. Rep.* **55**(RR04)**:**1–27.
6. **Centers for Disease Control and Prevention.** 2007. Lyme disease—United States, 2003–2005. *MMWR Morb. Mortal. Wkly. Rep.* **56:**573–576.

7. **Centers for Disease Control and Prevention.** 2007. Summary of notifiable diseases—United States, 2005. *MMWR Morb. Mortal. Wkly. Rep.* **54:**2–92.

8. **Centers for Disease Control and Prevention.** 2008. Summary of notifiable diseases—United States, 2006. *MMWR Morb. Mortal. Wkly. Rep.* **55:**1–94.

9. **Civen, R., and V. Ngo.** 2008. Murine typhus: an unrecognized suburban vectorborne disease. *Clin. Infect. Dis.* **46:**913–918.

10. **Clark, J. R., R. D. Carlson, C. T. Sasaki, A. R. Pachner, and A. C. Steere.** 1985. Facial paralysis in Lyme disease. *Laryngoscope* **95:**1341–1345.

11. **Committee on Infectious Diseases.** 2006. Lyme disease, p. 428–433. *In* L. K. Pickering, C. J. Baker, S. S. Long, and J. A. McMillan (ed.), *Red Book: 2006 Report of the Committee on Infectious Diseases,* 27th ed. American Academy of Pediatrics, Elk Grove Village, IL.

12. **Committee to Advise on Tropical Medicine and Travel (CATMAT).** 2005. Statement on personal protective measures to prevent arthropod bites. *Can. Commun. Dis. Rep.* **31:**1–20.

13. **Costello, C. M., A. C. Steere, R. E. Pinkerton, and H. M. Feder, Jr.** 1989. A prospective study of tick bites in an endemic area for Lyme disease. *J. Infect. Dis.* **159:**136–139.

14. **Dalton, M. J., M. J. Clarke, R. C. Holman, J. W. Krebs, D. B. Fishbein, J. G. Olson, and J. E. Childs.** 1995. National surveillance for Rocky Mountain spotted fever, 1981–1992: epidemiologic summary and evaluation of risk factors for fatal outcome. *Am. J. Trop. Med. Hyg.* **52:**405–413.

15. **Dantas-Torres, F.** 2007. Rocky Mountain spotted fever. *Lancet Infect. Dis.* **7:**724–732.

16. **Dhand, A., R. B. Nadelman, M. Aguero-Rosenfeld, F. A. Haddad, D. P. Stokes, and H. W. Horowitz.** 2007. Human granulocytic anaplasmosis during pregnancy: case series and literature review. *Clin. Infect. Dis.* **45:**589–593.

17. **Doughty, R. A.** 1984. Lyme disease. *Pediatr. Rev.* **6:**20–25.

18. **Duma, R. J., D. E. Sonenshine, F. M. Bozeman, J. M. Veazey, Jr., B. L. Elisberg, D. P. Chadwick, N. I. Stocks, T. M. McGill, G. B. Miller, Jr., and J. N. MacCormack.** 1981. Epidemic typhus in the United States associated with flying squirrels. *JAMA* **245:**2318–2323.

19. **Dumler, J. S., J. E. Madigan, N. Pusteria, and J. S. Bakken.** 2007. Ehrlichioses in humans: epidemiology, clinical presentation, diagnosis, and treatment. *Clin. Infect. Dis.* **45:**S45–S51.

20. **Eliasson, H., T. Broman, M. Forsman, and E. Bäck.** 2006. Tularemia: current epidemiology and disease management. *Infect. Dis. Clin. N. Am.* **20:**289–311.

21. **Gentile, D. A., and B. C. Kennedy.** 1991. Wilderness medicine for children. *Pediatrics* **88:**967–981.

22. **Helmick, C. G., K. W. Bernard, and L. J. D'Angelo.** 1984. Rocky Mountain spotted fever: clinical, laboratory, and epidemiological features of 262 cases. *J. Infect. Dis.* **150:**480–488.

23. **Hopla, C. E.** 1974. The ecology of tularemia. *Adv. Vet. Sci. Comp. Med.* **18:**25–53.

24. **Keim, P., A. Johansson, and D. M. Wagner.** 2007. Molecular epidemiology, evolution, and ecology of *Francisella. Ann. N. Y. Acad. Sci.* **1105:**30–66.

25. **Kirk, J. L., I. X. Fine, D. J. Sexton, and H. G. Muchmore.** 1990. Rocky Mountain spotted fever: a clinical review based upon 48 cases, 1943–1986. *Medicine* **69:**35–45.

26. **Kirkland, K. B., P. K. Marcorn, D. J. Secton, J. S. Dumler, and D. H. Walker.** 1993. Rocky Mountain spotted fever complicated by gangrene: report of six cases and review. *Clin. Infect. Dis.* **16:**629–634.

27. **Leiby, D. A., A. P. Chung, R. G. Cable, J. Trouern-Trend, J. McCollough, M. J. Homer, L. D. Reynolds, R. L. Houghton, M. J. Lodes, and D. H. Persing.** 2002. Relationship between tick bites and the seroprevalence of *Babesia microti* and *Anaplasma phagocytophila* (previously *Ehrlichia* sp.) in blood donors. *Transfusion* **42:**1585–1591.

28. **Lochary, M. E., P. B. Lockhart, and W. T. Williams, Jr.** 1998. Doxycycline and staining of permanent teeth. *Pediatr. Infect. Dis. J.* **17:**429–431.

29. **LoVecchio, F., and C. McBride.** 2003. Scorpion envenomations in young children in central Arizona. *J. Toxicol. Clin. Toxicol.* **41:**937–940.

30. **Maeda, K., N. Markowitz, R. C. Hawley, M. Ristic, D. Cox, and J. E. McDade.** 1987. Human infection with *Ehrlichia canis*, a leukocytic rickettsia. *N. Engl. J. Med.* **316:**853–856.

31. **Maguire, J. F., and R. S. Geha.** 1986. Bee, wasp, and hornet stings. *Pediatr. Rev.* **8:**5–11.

32. **Marshall, G. S., R. F. Jacobs, G. E. Schutze, H. Paxton, S. C. Buckingham, J. P. DeVincenzo, M. A. Jackson, V. H. San Joaquin, S. M. Standaert, and C. R. Woods for the Tick-Borne Infections in Children Study Group.** 2002. *Ehrlichia chaffeensis* seroprevalence among children in the southeast and south-central regions of the United States. *Arch. Pediatr. Adolesc. Med.* **156:**166–170.

33. **Marshall, G. S., G. G. Stout, R. F. Jacobs, G. E. Schutze, H. Paxton, S. C. Buckingham, J. P. DeVincenzo, M. A. Jackson,**

V. H. San Joaquin, S. M. Standaert, C. R. Woods, and the Tick-Borne Infections in Children Study (TICS) Group. 2003. Antibodies reactive to Rickettsia rickettsii among children living in the southeast and south central regions of the United States. *Arch. Pediatr. Adolesc. Med.* **157:**443–448.

34. Massey, E. W., T. Thames, C. E. Coffey, and H. A. Gallis. 1985. Neurologic complications of Rocky Mountain spotted fever. *South. Med. J.* **78:**1288–1290.

35. Masters, E. J., G. S. Olson, S. J. Weiner, and C. D. Paddock. 2003. Rocky Mountain spotted fever. *Arch. Intern. Med.* **163:**769–774.

36. McCall, C. L., A. T. Curns, L. D. Roz, J. A. Singleton, T. A. Treadwell, J. A. Comer, W. L. Nicholson, J. G. Olson, and J. E. Childs. 2001. Fort Chaffee revisited: the epidemiology of tick-borne rickettsial and ehrlichial diseases at a natural focus. *Vector Borne Zoonotic Dis.* **1:**119–127.

37. McQuiston, J. H., C. D. Paddock, R. C. Holman, and J. E. Childs. 1999. The human ehrlichiosis in the United States. *Emerg Infect. Dis.* **5:**635–642.

38. Mitchell P. D., K. D. Reed, and J. M. Hofkes. 1996. Immunoserologic evidence of coinfection with *Borrelia burgdorferi, Babesia microti,* and human granulocytic *Ehrlichia* species in residents of Wisconsin and Minnesota. *J. Clin. Microbiol.* **3:**724–727.

39. Needham, G. R. 1985. Evaluation of five popular methods for tick removal. *Pediatrics* **75:**997–1002.

40. Olano, J. P., E. Masters, W. Hogrefe, and D. H. Walker. 2003. Human monocytic ehrlichiosis, Missouri. *Emerg. Infect. Dis.* **9:**1579–1586.

41. Olson, L. J., E. C. Okafor, and I. P. Clements. 1986. Cardiac involvement in Lyme disease: manifestations and management. *Mayo Clin. Proc.* **61:**745–749.

42. O'Reilly, M., C. Paddock, B. Elchos, J. Goddard, J. Childs, and M. Currie. 2003. Physician knowledge of the diagnosis and management of Rocky Mountain spotted fever, Mississippi, 2002. *Ann. N. Y. Acad. Sci.* **990:**295–301.

43. Penn, R. L., and G. T. Kinasewitz. 1987. Factors associated with a poor outcome in tularemia. *Arch. Intern. Med.* **147:**265–268.

44. Razzaq, S., and G. E. Schutze. 2005. Rocky Mountain spotted fever: a physician's challenge. *Pediatr. Rev.* **26:**125–129.

45. Schutze, G. E., S. C. Buckingham, G. S. Marshall, C. R. Woods, M. A. Jackson, L. E. Patterson, and R. F. Jacobs. 2007. Human monocytic ehrlichiosis in children. *Pediatr. Infect. Dis. J.* **26:**475–479.

46. Shapiro, E. D., and M. A. Gerber. 2002. Lyme disease: fact versus fiction. *Pediatr. Ann.* **31:**170–177.

47. Standaert, S. M., T. Yu, M. A. Scott, J. E. Childs, C. D. Paddock, W. L. Nicholson, J. Singelton, Jr., and M. J. Blaser. 2000. Primary isolation of *Ehrlichia chaffeensis* from patients with febrile illnesses: clinical and molecular characteristics. *J. Infect. Dis.* **181:**1082–1088.

48. Staub, D., M. Debrunner, L. Amsler, and R. Steffen. 2002. Effectiveness of a repellent containing DEET and EBAAP for preventing tick bites. *Wilderness Environ. Med.* **13:**12–20.

49. Stechenberg, B. W. 1988. Lyme disease: the latest great imitator. *Pediatr. Infect. Dis. J.* **7:**402–409.

50. Steere, A. C., N. H. Bartenhagen, J. E. Craft, G. J. Hutchinson, J. H. Newman, D. W. Rahn, L. H. Sigal, P. N. Spieler, K. S. Stenn, and S. E. Malawista. 1983. The early clinical manifestations of Lyme disease. *Ann. Intern. Med.* **99:**76–82.

51. Steere, A. C., E. Taylor, M. L. Wilson, J. F. Levine, and A. Spielman. 1986. Longitudinal assessment of the clinical and epidemiological features of Lyme disease in a defined population. *J. Infect. Dis.* **154:**295–300.

52. Steere, A. C. 2001. Lyme disease. *N. Engl. J. Med.* **345:**115–125.

53. Tärnvik, A., and M. C. Chu. 2007. New approaches to diagnosis and therapy of tularemia. *Ann. N. Y. Acad. Sci.* **1105:**378–404.

54. Taylor, J. P., G. R. Istre, T. C. McChesney, F. T. Satalowich, R. L. Parker, and L. M. McFarland. 1987. Epidemiologic characteristics of human tularemia in the Southwest-Central States, 1981–1987. *Am. J. Epidemiol.* **133:**1032–1038.

55. Thorner, A. R., D. H. Walker, and W. A. Petri, Jr. 1998. Rocky Mountain spotted fever. *Clin. Infect. Dis.* **27:**1353–1359.

56. Walsh, C. A., E. W. Mayer, and L. V. Baxi. 2008. Lyme disease in pregnancy: case report and review of the literature. *Obstet. Gynecol. Surv.* **62:**41–50.

57. Wormser, G. P., R. J. Dattwyler, E. D. Shapiro, J. J. Halperin, A. C. Steere, M. S. Klempner, P. J. Krause, J. S. Bakken, F. Strle, G. Stanek, L. Bockenstedt, D. Fish, J. S. Dumler, and R. B. Nadelman. 2006. The clinical assessment, treatment, and prevention of Lyme disease, human granulocytic anaplasmosis, and babesiosis: clinical practice guidelines by the Infectious Diseases Society of America. *Clin. Infect. Dis.* **43:**1089–1134.

INFECTIONS IN THE GARDEN

Burke A. Cunha and Diane H. Johnson

4

Although there are many infections that one may acquire in the garden, people have gardened for years without becoming infected, yet others may become ill after a rather limited time in the garden. Being in the garden presents a series of complex possibilities from an infectious disease standpoint, and the likelihood of one acquiring an infectious disease while gardening depends upon many factors. Gardens are usually near the home and may be the closest that many people get to being in the great outdoors, especially in urban or suburban environments. The time spent in the garden is not nearly as important as the age and nature of the gardener, his friends, or his family (2, 6, 7, 12, 20).

Gardening may be a salutary experience for the well, but it is conceivably more dangerous to a patient with impaired immunity than to healthy individuals. For example, if a compromised host contracts coccidioidomycosis, histoplasmosis, or the organism responsible for cat scratch fever, he or she would be at increased risk for dissemination. Elderly patients are fortunately relatively well-off in terms of acquiring diseases in the garden. While elderly individuals can still acquire a variety of infections from the soil, animals, or animal-related insect bites, as a group they are not at increased risk for acquiring disorders solely on account of their age. Of course, if excavations are taking place or there is construction nearby, if the aquatic areas have *Legionella* species, and if the wind is right, then an elderly person would be more likely to acquire or have a more severe case of Legionnaires' disease than his or her younger gardening counterparts.

Since many gardens are an extension of the home, children of various ages may frequent the garden or the land close to the house alone or with gardening adults. Many infectious diseases acquired in the garden are age specific; e.g., small children are more likely than adults to get *Strongyloides stercoralis* or hookworm infections in the appropriate locale. The garden not only is inhabited by plants and visited by humans but also may be a stopping point or refuge for birds and animals. Because of its proximity to the house, household pets frequently wander freely throughout the backyard and the garden. Even if you do not have pets, it is not uncommon that pets from the neighborhood will spend various lengths of time and perform various bodily functions

Burke A. Cunha and Diane H. Johnson, Infectious Disease Division, Winthrop-University Hospital, Mineola, NY 11501, and State University of New York School of Medicine, Stony Brook, NY.

Infections of Leisure, Fourth Edition, Edited by David Schlossberg,
© 2009 ASM Press, Washington, DC

while passing through your garden. Therefore, if dogs, cats, or rodents are in the area, it is wise to consider that your garden and yard present the potential for contact with these animals or their excreta. *Toxocara* species organisms may be picked up by your dog or cat by ingestion and later transmitted via petting to children, for example. A stray neighborhood cat giving birth in or near your garden immediately sets the stage for the possibility of Q fever. The possibilities are almost endless. Birds may fly over, nest above, or be found sick or dead in the garden. Due to bird droppings in wood stacked for winter or in nests near the soil, the potential for histoplasmosis or blastomycosis exists. Lastly, we come to the soil and plants themselves, which are, after all, the purpose of having a garden. What potential pathogens soil contains is largely a function of the animal life in the area as well as the particular location of the garden. For example, if the garden is located near moist, humid environments along riverbanks in the South, then blastomycosis becomes a diagnostic consideration. In contrast, if the garden is in the Southwest, then coccidioidomycosis and even plague, if an appropriately infected rodent is in the area, also become diagnostic possibilities. Rosebush thorn or sphagnum moss contact should immediately suggest the possibility of sporotrichosis. In the southeastern United States, where soil in moist areas may be contaminated with hookworm or *Strongyloides* larvae, these worms add to the potential diseases that can be acquired by contact of unprotected skin with the soil alone. The *Ixodes* species

ticks that transmit Lyme disease, babesiosis, and ehrlichiosis in areas of endemicity may be found in the lawn grass adjacent to the garden, so Lyme disease, babesiosis, and/or ehrlichiosis may literally be acquired in your own backyard or garden. Therefore, the soil, by the nature of the organisms that normally reside in specific locations, e.g., spores of *Coccidioides immitis* or larvae of hookworm, presents infectious disease hazards that need to be reckoned with, as do the contributions made by various animals to the soil either by their presence or by contamination with their body fluids. One can easily appreciate the large array of infectious diseases that confront a person simply slipping out of the house and walking across the yard to do a little gardening!

THE DIAGNOSTIC APPROACH

In trying to analyze diagnostic possibilities for someone who has become ill and has spent time in the garden, it is necessary to consider the diagnosis from three different perspectives. First, one should consider the potential nature of contact, either passive or active, that the individual has had with sources of infection. If there has been extensive soil contact, then sporotrichosis is a diagnostic possibility. If piles of stacked or old moldy wood have been moved in association with wood gardening, then blastomycosis and histoplasmosis become additional possibilities. Nearby excavations with aerosolization of soil and water may suggest the possibility of Legionnaires' disease. If the particular location of the patient is one where Lyme disease (Table 1), babesiosis, or

TABLE 1 Clinical features of Lyme disease

Stage	Clinical feature(s)			
	Dermatologic	Neurologic	Rheumatologic	Cardiac
1	Erythema migrans	Possible headache, myalgias	Arthralgias	
2	Multiple and/or recurrent erythema migrans	Meningoencephalitis, peripheral neuritis	Arthralgias	Carditis
3	Acrodermatitis chronica atrophicans		Chronic arthritis	

ehrlichiosis is endemic, then these diagnoses should be considered with the appropriate clinical presentation. Similarly, as mentioned in the introduction, specific locations suggest specific soil organisms, e.g., hookworms, *Coccidioides immitis, Histoplasma capsulatum,* etc. Additionally, potential animal contact needs to be considered from a variety of standpoints. The person's own pets and their interaction with insect vectors and other animals in the area should be carefully ascertained and considered. In addition to considering the gardener's own pets, one needs to consider the pets in the neighborhood as well as any wild animals interacting with the gardener or the gardener's pet(s). One should inquire specifically about dead birds or other animals that the gardener may have found and buried in the garden. Specific inquiry should be made as to the potential for contact with rodents or rabbits in the wild or runaway pets in the area. Only rarely is a disease actively transmitted from an animal to a human, and the situations are usually found to be straightforward if the proper question is asked. As has been mentioned previously, some infectious diseases may be acquired actively or passively; for example, sporotrichosis may be acquired by simple handling of sphagnum moss or may be actively acquired as the result of a puncture wound from the thorn of a rose. The epidemiological associations with infectious diseases acquired from plants, soil, or animal vectors are presented in Table 2.

The next step in the diagnostic process is to determine end organ involvement by the infectious disease process to limit diagnostic possibilities and suggest specific disease entities. For example, if the patient presents with lymphadenopathy and a history of garden contact, then diagnostic possibilities are narrowed to toxoplasmosis, cat scratch fever, sporotrichosis, and occasionally Lyme disease. Cat contact increases the likelihood that these lesions are due to cat scratch fever or toxoplasmosis, whereas nodular lymphangitis immediately suggests sporotrichosis. Obviously, there are many causes of adenopathy that have

nothing to do with gardening or being in the garden, and the clinician must always be careful not to fail to consider the usual causes of lymph node involvement. However, if the adenopathy is most likely associated with gardening, then diagnostic possibilities are greatly reduced. If there are other associated findings, this also helps to limit diagnostic possibilities. It is a good diagnostic principle for infectious diseases as well as in internal medicine to combine two diagnostic findings, even if they are nonspecific, to increase diagnostic specificity. For example, if the patient with a history of gardening and axillary adenopathy has in addition a mild, nonexudative pharyngitis and a few atypical lymphocytes, then the likelihood of acquired toxoplasmosis is enhanced. Similarly, the likelihood of Lyme disease being present in a patient with lymph node enlargement is enhanced if the patient has a facial nerve palsy. The more variables that one can combine, the easier it is to arrive at a definitive diagnosis. For example, if a patient presents with an ill-defined infiltrate on chest X ray, abdominal pain, and a cough, accompanied by mental confusion and some diarrhea, then the chances of that individual having Legionnaires' disease are very great. These would not be the findings for a patient with another atypical pneumonia, i.e., Q fever, psittacosis, or *Mycoplasma pneumoniae* pneumonia. The diagnosis of worms producing cough or pneumonitis during their pulmonary-migration phase may be a much more challenging diagnostic problem. Once again, by looking for associated features, one can increase diagnostic specificity and limit the differential diagnosis. For example, if a nonspecific pulmonary infiltrate is associated with eosinophilia, then strongyloidiasis becomes a very likely explanation for the patient's problem. Mental confusion, especially in a young child, with persistent eosinophilia, may suggest visceral larva migrans, especially if there has been a history of cat or dog contact. The differential diagnosis of infectious diseases by organ involvement is presented in Fig. 1. The clinician should remember that other diseases may pro-

TABLE 2 Epidemiological considerations for infections from the garden

Focus or vectors	Infectious disease or organism(s)[a]	
	Passively acquired	Actively acquired
Soil and plants	Sporotrichosis	Sporotrichosis
	Blastomycosis	Legionnaires' disease
	Histoplasmosis	Nocardiosis
	Strongyloidosis	
	Hookworm	
	Nocardiosis	
Animals		
Cats	Toxoplasmosis	Cat scratch disease
	Q fever	*Pasteurella multocida*
	Tularemia	Rabies
	CLM (*Ancylostoma* spp.)	
	VLM *(Toxocara cati)*	
	Strongyloides	
	Campylobacter spp.	
	Giardiasis	
	Yersinia pestis	
	Salmonella enterica	
	Dermatophytes	
Dogs	Group A streptococci	*P. multocida*
	VLM *(Toxocara canis)*	*Capnocytophaga* spp.
	CLM (*Ancylostoma* spp.)	Rabies
	Leptospirosis	
	Brucellosis	
	Cryptosporidium spp.	
	Dirofilaria immitis	
	S. enterica	
	Giardiasis	
	Campylobacter spp.	
	RMSF (via tick bite)	
	Listeria spp.	
	Dermatophytes	
Birds	Blastomycosis	
	Histoplasmosis	
	Cryptococcosis	
	Q fever	
Rabbits	Tularemia	Tularemia
	Brucellosis	
Rats	Leptospirosis	Rat bite fever
Other rodents	Plague (via flea bite)	
	Relapsing fever (via tick bite)	
	Lyme disease (white-footed mouse)	
	Leptospirosis	
	S. enterica	
	LCM (hamsters)	

[a]CLM, cutaneous larva migrans; VLM, visceral larva migrans; LCM, lymphocytic choriomeningitis.

Skin (rash)
CLM
Lyme disease
RMSF
Dermatophytes
Histoplasmosis (erythema nodosum)
Tularemia
Pasteurella multocida
Group A streptococci
Strongyloides stercoralis

Lungs (infiltrates)
Legionnaires' disease
Q fever
Psittacosis
Dirofilaria immitis
Helminths (migratory lung phase)

Lymph Nodes (adenopathy)
Toxoplasmosis
Cat scratch disease
Sporotrichosis (nodular)
Lyme disease

Eyes
Chorioretinitis
Ocular larva migrans
Toxoplasmosis
Cranial Nerve Abnormalities
Lyme disease
Conjunctival Suffusion
RMSF
Leptospirosis
Relapsing fever

Central Nervous System (encephalopathy)
Lyme disease
VLM
Toxoplasmosis
Cat scratch disease
Legionnaires' disease

Pharynx (sore throat)
Toxoplasmosis
Cat scratch disease
Lyme disease

Gastrointestinal Tract (diarrhea)
Dirofilaria immitis
Strongyloides stercoralis
Cryptosporidium spp.
Campylobacter spp.
Yersinia enterocolitica
Giardia lamblia

Liver (increased serum transaminases)
Legionnaires' disease
RMSF
Q fever
Psittacosis
Lyme disease
Leptospirosis
Histoplasmosis
Cat scratch disease

Spleen (splenomegaly)
Q fever
Lyme disease
Psittacosis
Histoplasmosis

FIGURE 1 Infectious disease diagnostic considerations by organ involvement. CLM, cutaneous larva migrans; RMSF, Rocky Mountain spotted fever; VLM, visceral larva migrans.

duce similar end organ dysfunction and clinical manifestations, but Fig. 1 is particularly helpful if gardening is an important epidemiological factor to consider in assessing the patient's problem.

Laboratory tests represent the last approach to making the diagnosis. With all of the diseases potentially acquired by working in the garden, the clinician needs to establish a working diagnosis as described above and then arrive at a definitive diagnosis by ordering the appropriate specific tests. Aside from the specific laboratory tests needed to make a diagnosis, the clinician needs to have some clues that suggest the proper tests to be ordered for the individual patient. Therefore, nonspecific tests are most helpful when applied in the appropriate clinical context and combined with epidemiological and/or characteristic end organ manifestations. For example, anemia in a small child from a rural area of the southeastern United States should immediately prompt a search for hookworm or *Strongyloides*. The liver is involved in many infectious disease processes, and therefore the finding of abnormal liver function is an important clue to a whole range of infectious diseases. With respect to the gardening population, an increased bilirubin count in a patient with pneumonitis may suggest Legionnaires' disease, and in a patient with conjunctival suffusion, it should suggest leptospirosis. Mild increases in the alkaline phosphatase or the serum transaminases may occur with dissimilar diseases, such as toxoplasmosis and Rocky Mountain spotted fever (Table 3). If the patient has an atypical pneumonia, i.e., an ill-defined infiltrate and mild to moderately abnormal liver function tests, then diagnostic possibilities are quickly narrowed to Legionnaires' disease, psittacosis, and Q fever. Once again, it is important not to interpret diagnostic tests in a vacuum but rather to combine them with some other factor in the history of physical diagnosis that quickly limits the diagnostic possibilities and provides the rationale for the working diagnosis (Fig. 2).

SPECIFIC INFECTIOUS DISEASES

Sporotrichosis

The classic fungus associated with the soil is *Sporothrix schenckii. S. schenckii* is a dimorphic fungus which on culture produces conidia arranged in a "daisy" cluster on top of a conidiophore. In tissue, the organism assumes an oval or cigar-shaped yeast form. The organism may be introduced into the skin via a minor abrasion, such as a thorn or splinter, resulting in the development of a suppurative lymphangitis of the skin and subcutaneous tissues, although, rarely, hematogenous dissemination to the lungs, bones, and joints does occur. Alcoholics seem particularly prone to developing disseminated sporotrichosis, so this diagnostic point should be kept in mind when assessing patients who work in gardens and consume alcohol. The skin lesions of sporotrichosis usually begin as a small, gradually enlarging papular nodule which may become pustular and eventually ulcerates. Spread is distal to proximal along the lymphatics, and the lesions are characteristically not painful. While other diseases, such as tularemia, may resemble sporotrichosis, the indolent course of the illness along the lymphatics, with bridges of normal skin between painless lesions, is highly suggestive of sporotrichosis. Diagnosis of sporotrichosis is made by culturing the mycelial form of the organism from the affected tissue;

however, repeat cultures may need to be performed. Direct examination of tissue for the presence of the yeast form may be helpful, but the organisms are generally rare. Serologic testing is generally not useful in the diagnosis of sporotrichosis (3, 14, 17).

Histoplasmosis

Histoplasmosis is caused by the dimorphic fungus *Histoplasma capsulatum,* which has a wide geographic distribution but is most heavily concentrated in North America along the Ohio and Mississippi river valleys. The organism has been associated with the presence of birds or bats and survives well in warm, moist soil contaminated by their droppings. Excavation, cleaning, or demolition of fecally contaminated organic material usually results in inhalation followed by acute pneumonitis in a nonimmune individual. Obviously, the use of bird droppings as fertilizer enhances the likelihood of acquiring acute pulmonary histoplasmosis in nonimmune individuals. Although many infections are asymptomatic, acute pulmonary histoplasmosis manifests as a flu-like illness with cough and headache. Rarely, patients may have arthralgias or erythema nodosum. Infants, the elderly, or immunosuppressed persons may be predisposed to disseminated disease. Manifestations include fever, hepatosplenomegaly, and pancytopenia. Patients with chronic lung disease may develop chronic histoplasmosis, the symptoms of which resemble tuberculosis. In persons infected with human immunodeficiency virus (HIV), preexisting histoplasmosis can reactivate and present with a septicemia-like picture, with hepatic and renal involvement that may progress to a shock-like state. Persons with HIV should take particular care to avoid gardening situations in which exposure to *H. capsulatum* is likely. Definitive diagnosis is made by culturing the organism or identifying the yeast phase of the organism in tissue or through serologic techniques or urinary antigen testing, which is both rapid and sensitive (4, 9, 16, 21, 30–32) (Fig. 3 and Table 4).

Other fungi are very uncommon or only distantly associated with gardening per se. Blastomycosis and cryptococcosis are unusual

TABLE 3 Differential diagnosis of Rocky Mountain spotted fever[a]

Sign(s) and/or symptom(s)	Rocky Mountain spotted fever	Meningococcal meningitis	Dengue fever	Leptospirosis	Atypical measles
Mental confusion	±	±	−	±	−
Headache	+++	+++	+++	+++	−
Photophobia	−	+	−	−	±
Myalgias, arthralgias	+++	++	+++	+++	−
Nausea, vomiting	±	±	−	±	−
Abdominal pain	±	−	−	±	−
Rash	Petechial on ankles, wrists	"Palpable" petechiae diffusely	Petechial, truncal	Maculopapular, truncal	Urticarial, maculopapular, truncal
Jaundice	±	−	−	±	−
Splenomegaly	+[b]	−	±	±	−
Periorbital edema	++	−	−	+	−
Conjunctival suffusion	−	−	−	+	−
Abnormal LFTs	−	−	±	+++	−
Eosinophilia	−	−	−	−	+++
Infiltrates on chest film	−	−	−	−	+

[a]LFTs, liver function tests; +, present; −, absent; ++, severe manifestation; +++, extremely severe manifestation; ±, present or absent.
[b]The size of the spleen increases by 50%.

Thrombocytopenia
RMSF

Atypical Lymphocytes
Toxoplasmosis

Eosinophilia
Strongyloides stercoralis
VLM
Group A streptococci
Ascariasis
Hookworm

Anemia
Hookworm
Strongyloides stercoralis
Histoplasmosis

Elevated Alkaline Phosphatases/Transaminases
Legionnaires' disease
RMSF
Q fever
Leptospirosis
Toxoplasmosis

Elevated Bilirubin
Legionnaires' disease
Leptospirosis

Chest X-Ray Findings
Infiltrates
Q fever
Legionnaires' disease
Histoplasmosis
Blastomycosis
Ascariasis
Tularemia
Coin Lesion
Dirofilaria immitis

Abnormal Brain CT Scan
VLM (mass lesions)

Abnormal Urinalysis
Legionnaires' disease
Leptospirosis (microscopic hematuria)
Brucellosis (sterile pyuria)

CSF Pleocytosis
Toxoplasmosis
Lyme disease
LCM
Cat scratch disease
VLM
Leptospirosis
RMSF

**Stools + for Enteric Pathogens
or Ova/Parasites**
Giardia lamblia
Campylobacter spp.
Yersinia enterocolitica
Ascariasis
Hookworm
Strongyloides stercoralis
Salmonella spp.
Cryptosporidium spp.

FIGURE 2 Infectious disease differential diagnostic considerations by laboratory and roentgen findings. CT, computed tomography; RMSF, Rocky Mountain spotted fever; VLM, visceral larva migrans; LCM, lymphocytic choriomeningitis.

and are associated with typical clinical findings which should lead one to the diagnosis (Table 4).

Blastomycosis

Blastomyces dermatitidis is the dimorphic fungus responsible for the development of blastomycosis. This organism has proven difficult to isolate from environmental sources; however, exposure to organically rich, warm, moist soil appears to be a risk factor for the development of infection. Blastomycosis is endemic in the southeastern and midwestern United States

and has been classically associated with the Ohio and Mississippi river valley regions. The fungus enters via the lungs and can result in asymptomatic disease, acute infection that mimics a bacterial pneumonia, or chronic pulmonary infection which may be confused clinically with tuberculosis. *B. dermatitidis* often disseminates hematogenously, with the skin being the most frequent site of extrapulmonary infection. The skin lesions are characteristically verrucous or ulcerative in nature.

Osteomyelitis due to *B. dermatitidis* occurs as well. Genitourinary tract involvement man-

Hematologic
Thrombocytopenia
Anemia
Leukopenia
Pancytopenia
Splenomegaly
Generalized adenopathy
Eosinophilia

Pulmonary
Apical infiltrates
Hilar adenopathy
"Buckshot" calcifications
Miliary calcifications
"Thick-walled" cavities
"Marching cavities"
Superior vena cava obstruction*

Ear, Nose, and Throat
Nose ulcers
Lip ulcers
Gum ulcers
Mouth ulcers
Tongue ulcers
Laryngeal ulcers

Dermatologic
Erythema nodosum
Erythema multiforme
Skin ulcers

Cardiac
Endocarditis
Pericarditis

Neurologic
Chronic meningitis
Focal cerebritis
Spinal cord compression*

Gastrointestinal
Esophageal obstruction*
Granulomatous hepatitis
Diarrhea
Intestinal ulceration

Other
Addison's disease

FIGURE 3 Clinical spectrum of histoplasmosis. ★, secondary to lymph node compression or mediastinal fibrosis.

ifests as prostatitis and/or epididymo-orchitis in males, but involvement of the female genitourinary tract is rare. Central nervous system infection resulting in meningitis or a brain abscess is seen most commonly in immunocompromised individuals, especially in persons with AIDS (1, 5, 28).

The diagnosis of blastomycosis is confirmed by isolating the organism in culture or from a biopsy specimen, where the fungus appears in its yeast phase. The organism may also be observed on KOH preps of clinical specimens such as sputum, pus, or prostatic secretions. Serologic testing remains unreliable and should be used only in conjunction with isolation of the organism.

Legionnaires' Disease

Legionnaires' disease can be acquired in the garden only if the organism is in soil that is being excavated nearby and there is airborne spread of the organism in the garden area. Legionnaires' disease is varied in its distribution; some areas have a relatively high incidence of Legionnaires' disease, while the disease is unheard of in other locations. Legionnaires' disease is most common in the late spring and

early fall, and infection may begin with a flu-like illness. The course may be subacute or fulminant, and the illness most typically presents as a pneumonia. However, a nonpulmonary form, i.e., Pontiac fever, is a manifestation of *Legionella* infection without associated pneumonitis. Legionnaires' disease should be considered in the diagnosis of all community-acquired pneumonias, and specific diagnostic features should be looked for to arrive at a working diagnosis. The clue to all of the atypical pneumonias lies in their extrapulmonary manifestations, since they are all systemic infections. With Legionnaires' disease, the patient's extrapulmonary manifestations commonly include changes in mental status, nonspecific abdominal pain, or diarrhea. In contrast to *Mycoplasma* pneumonia, Legionnaires' disease is not associated with otitis or pharyngitis. If the patient has a temperature in excess of 102°F on presentation to the physician and the patient does not have an arrhythmia, does not have a pacemaker, and is not on beta-blockers, then a pulse-temperature deficit provides the single most important clue to the diagnosis. Relative bradycardia is present in virtually all patients with

TABLE 4 Differential diagnosis of histoplasmosis[a]

Factor	Histoplasmosis	Tuberculosis	Blastomycosis
Fever			
Double-quotidian fever	−	±	−
Morning temperature spikes	−	+	−
Laboratory tests			
Pancytopenia	+[b]	+	−
Hypergammaglobulinemia	−	−	−
Leukemoid reaction	−	+	−
Chest X ray			
Miliary calcifications	+	±	−
Hilar adenopathy	+	±	−
Pleural effusion	−	+	−
Abdominal X ray			
Liver/splenic calcifications	+	±	−
Organ involvement			
Meningitis	+[b]	+	−
Oropharyngeal ulcers	+[b]	−	−
Pulmonary infiltrates	+	+	±
Endocarditis	+	−	−
Addison's disease	+[b]	+	−
Granulomatous hepatitis	+	+	−
Splenomegaly	+[b]	±	−
Generalized adenopathy	+	±	−
Intestinal ulcers	+[b]	−	−
Bone/joint lesions	+	+	−
Glomerulonephritis	−	−	−
Epididymo-orchitis	−	+	+
Granulomatous prostatitis	+	−	+
Skin ulcers	+[b]	±	+
Erythema nodosum	+	+	±

[a]Symbols: +, present; −, absent; ±, variously present or absent.
[b]Only in disseminated histoplasmosis.

Legionnaires' disease presenting with a temperature of 102°F, and if the pulse is charted with a temperature, a pulse-temperature deficit is readily seen by simple inspection. However, if one desires to calculate if there is relative bradycardia present, then one takes the temperature in degrees Fahrenheit, takes the last digit, decreases it by 1, multiplies that number by 10, and adds that number to 100. For example, if the temperature is 105°F, the 5 is reduced to 4 and multiplied by 10 to get 40, and this is added to 100 to get 140.

Therefore, any pulse of <140 in a patient with a 105°F temperature indicates a pulse-temperature deficit even if the patient is "tachying along" at 120 beats/min.

Chest X rays do not have specificic characteristics, but they usually "behave" in a typical way. Legionnaires' disease on chest X ray is characterized by a rapidly progressive asymmetrical infiltrate(s). While not all *Legionella* species infections behave in this fashion, this is nevertheless the most typical roentgen manifestation. In terms of laboratory tests, a decreased serum phosphate level, when present, is a most helpful finding. A decreased serum sodium level appears to be more commonly associated with Legionnaires' disease than with other pneumonias, but it is not specific for *Legionella* infections. A decrease in sodium on the basis of the syndrome of inappropriate secretion of antidiuretic hormone may occur with any pulmonary process, whether it is infectious, inflammatory, or neoplastic. In contrast, a depressed serum phosphate level is uniquely associated with Legionnaires' disease. An elevated bilirubin count in association with an atypical pneumonia is more helpful and limits diagnostic possibilities to pneumococcal pneumonia and Legionnaires' disease. The serum transaminases are almost always modestly elevated in patients with Legionnaires' disease, and this is also true for other *Legionella* species. This is another important laboratory clue to the presence of an atypical pneumonia, since only Legionnaires' disease, Q fever, and psittacosis are frequently associated with abnormal liver function tests, in contrast to *Mycoplasma* pneumonia. Therefore, a working diagnosis can readily be obtained by combining the aforementioned features, while a definitive diagnosis depends upon demonstrating the organism with direct fluorescent-antibody assay of sputum or pleural fluid, urinary antigen testing, or indirect fluorescent-antibody assay serologic methods. The organism may also be cultured directly from sputum or appropriate samples of lung or pleural fluid. The differential diagnostic features of Legionnaires' disease are presented in Table 5 (8, 10, 15, 22, 23, 25).

Hookworm

Hookworm disease is caused by two intestinal nematodes, *Ancylostoma duodenale* and *Necator americanus*. The environmental conditions of the southeastern United States, with its warmth, high humidity, and heavy rainfall, are ideal for the life cycles of these nematodes. In contaminated soil, the eggs hatch in approximately 24 h and become rhabditiform larvae. The rhabditiform larvae incubate in the warm,

moist soil for 5 to 10 days, developing into the infectious filariform larvae. This form can survive for up to 1 month in the soil. Human infection occurs when the filariform larvae penetrate exposed skin, usually through bare feet. When *N. americanus* is involved, there is often a local skin reaction consisting of erythema and a pruritic papular or vesicular eruption near the entry site. This is less commonly seen with *A. duodenale*. These larvae enter the venous circulation, where they are carried to the lungs. Pulmonary complaints such as cough, wheezing, or pulmonary infiltrates can be seen at this time. The filariform larvae then migrate into the pharynx, where they are swallowed. They mature into adult worms in the small intestine, where they attach and feed on the blood of the host and liberate more eggs. Symptoms at this time generally consist of nonspecific abdominal complaints such as pain, bloating, nausea, or symptoms attributable to anemia. Laboratory findings may consist of a hypochromic, microcytic anemia, the degree of which is a function of the worm burden and consequent blood loss, eosinophilia, and hypoproteinuria. Diagnosis of hookworm disease is made by finding the characteristic oval eggs in a direct stool smear. Stool studies may be negative during early infections, and infections with light worm burdens require stool concentration techniques. Fresh stools should be examined immediately since eggs may hatch into rhabditiform larvae resembling the rhabditiform larvae of *Strongyloides* (13).

Strongyloides stercoralis

Strongyloidiasis, or threadworm infection, results from infection with the nematode *Strongyloides stercoralis*. It is less commonly encountered than hookworm infection, and the threadworm is unique among the nematodes in its ability to cause autoinfection due to its peculiar triphasic life cycle. The filariform larvae of *Strongyloides* penetrate the skin in a manner analogous to that of the hookworm. A pruritic maculopapular eruption or larva currens, which is a migrating serpiginous lin-

TABLE 5 Diagnostic features of atypical pneumonias[a]

Manifestation	Mycoplasma pneumonia	Legionnaires' disease	Psittacosis	Q fever	Tularemia
Symptoms					
Mental confusion	−	+	−	−	−
Headache	±	+	+	+	−
Meningismus	±	−	−	−	−
Myalgias	+	+	+	+	−
Ear pain	±	−	−	±	−
Pleuritic pain	−	±	±	−	±
Abdominal pain	−	+	−	−	+
Diarrhea	±	±	−	−	−
Hoarseness	−	−	−	−	±
Signs					
Rash	± (erythema multiforme)	−	± (Horder's spots)	−	−
Raynaud's phenomenon	+	−	−	−	−
Nonexudative pharyngitis	+	−	−	−	−
Hemoptysis	−	+	−	−	+
Lobar consolidation	−	±	±	±	±
Cardiac involvement	±	±	±	±	+
Splenomegaly	−	−	+	+	+
Relative bradycardia	−	+	+	+	−
Chest film findings					
Infiltrates	Patchy	Patchy/consolidation	Patchy/consolidation	Ovoid infiltrates	Patchy/consolidation
Bilateral hilar adenopathy	−	−	−	−	+
Pleural effusion	± (small)	±	±	−	+ (bloody)
Laboratory findings					
Leukocytosis	+	+	−	−	−
Hypophosphatemia	−	+	−	−	−
Elevated SGOT/SGPT	−	+	+	+	−
Cold agglutinins	+	−	−	±	−
Microscopic hematuria	−	+	−	−	−

[a] Adapted from reference 10. SGOT/SGPT, serum glutamic oxaloacetic transaminase/serum glutamic pyruvic transaminase; +, present; −, absent; ±, variously present or absent.

#58

ear rash, may be seen at that time. The filariform larvae are carried by the venous circulation to the lungs. In a healthy host, this pulmonary migration is usually asymptomatic, but in an immunocompromised host, cough, wheezing, dyspnea, and fleeting pulmonary infiltrates accompanied by peripheral eosinophilia may provide a clue to the diagnosis. The filariform larvae ascend and are swallowed to complete their life cycle within the small intestine of the host, where the presence of the nematode may cause abdominal pain, diarrhea, and weight loss. Autoinfection occurs when, while still in the intestine, the rhabditiform larvae develop into infectious filariform larvae, which in turn penetrate the colonic mucosa or perirectal skin, reinfecting the host. In immunocompromised individuals, a hyperinfection syndrome may be seen, which occurs when there is widespread dissemination of the filariform larvae via the bloodstream. Secondary bacterial infections are common in this condition due to large numbers of filariform larvae migrating from the intestine. Mortality associated with hyperinfection syndrome is quite high.

The diagnosis of strongyloidiasis is made by demonstrating the rhabditiform larvae in concentrated stool specimens or duodenal fluid. Stool concentration techniques may increase yield. Peripheral eosinophilia is generally present in immunocompetent (but not immunocompromised) individuals, and total immunoglobulin E may be evaluated. The filariform larvae may be present in the stool, urine, sputum, or bronchoalveolar lavage fluid of immunocompromised persons (19, 24, 29).

Nocardiosis

Nocardia species are soil-borne aerobic actinomycetes that can cause localized or disseminated infection in humans. *Nocardia asteroides* is most frequently implicated in human illness, followed by *Nocardia brasiliensis* or *Nocardia otitidiscaviarum,* although infections with other species have been reported. These organisms are recovered throughout the world from warm, moist soil as well as from other environmental sources. Clinical infection with *Nocardia* occurs most commonly in immunocompromised individuals, such as transplant recipients or persons with collagen vascular disease, lymphoreticular malignancies, or chronic steroid use. Persons infected with HIV are also at risk for nocardiosis. The organism enters the body via inhalation into the lungs, although the portal is occasionally the gastrointestinal tract or the skin through traumatic implantation.

#59

Pulmonary infection is characterized by the formation of multiple suppurative abscesses. The clinical symptoms of pulmonary nocardiosis are similar to those of tuberculosis, with fever, malaise, cough, weight loss, and night sweats. Sinus tract formation from the lungs can occur. Radiographically, the infiltrates of patients with nocardiosis may present as consolidated, alveolar, or reticular infiltrates. Cavitation and pleural involvement are common, and empyema occurs in about one-quarter of patients. Pulmonary *Nocardia* infection can have a protracted course, but it may also remit spontaneously or have an acute self-limited course. Hematogenous spread of *Nocardia* from the lungs to distant sites can occur. Concurrent pulmonary symptoms may be absent at the time of discovery. The central nervous system is a common site of dissemination. The clinical picture is generally that of a brain abscess or tumor, with fever, headache, nausea, vomiting, and focal neurological deficits. There is frequent dissemination of the pathogen to the eyes, kidneys, heart, bones, and subcutaneous tissues. Dissemination can occur in the absence of pulmonary involvement. Cutaneous or subcutaneous manifestations are seen after traumatic inoculation through the skin. When subcutaneous abscesses form, they are generally discrete, firm, nonindurated nodules, which, in contrast to those of actinomycosis, do not form draining fistulas. One exception to this is when *Nocardia* species are the causative agents in maduromycosis; in these cases, draining of sinus tracts occurs.

The diagnosis of nocardiosis is made by isolation of the organism from a clinical speci-

#60

men. Gram staining should be performed on pus or sputum. When *Nocardia* organisms are present, they appear as weakly gram-positive, branching, filamentous rods, often looking "beaded." Many species of *Nocardia* are acid fast. *Nocardia* species grow well on standard laboratory media; however, growth may take longer than 48 h when the organisms are present in mixed culture. They grow poorly on routinely used fungal media. No useful serologic tests are available at present (11, 18, 26, 27).

CONCLUSIONS

Gardening is a wonderful pastime, and the garden is a very peaceful place to enjoy one's vocation. However, the garden may be a treacherous place for very young or compromised hosts when one takes into account the infectious potential residing in the soil, as well as the insect vectors on plants and animals. The location of the garden and the characteristics of the soil play a part in determining its infectious potential. The most important factor making the garden an infectious and dangerous place is the number and interaction of animals, whether they are pets or in the wild, that temporarily use the garden for part of their daily activities. The clinician should always ask about garden exposure, which will help in eliminating the diagnostic possibilities for the patient. The diagnostic approach is to utilize epidemiological principles in concert with clinical clues, which together should suggest a reasonable list of diagnostic possibilities. Organ involvement and specific laboratory tests will help further narrow the differential diagnosis and will determine the specific tests necessary to make a definitive diagnosis.

PRACTICAL TIPS

- Alcoholics are particularly prone to developing disseminated sporotrichosis. Sporotrichosis should be considered in persons who regularly consume alcohol and work in the garden.
- In backyard gardens near chicken coops or caves, patients developing a flu-like illness

should be suspected of having histoplasmosis.

- Patients whose gardens are near water or outdoor construction sites and who develop rapidly progressive asymmetrical infiltrates on chest X rays should be suspected of having Legionnaires' disease.
- Strongyloidiasis with peripheral eosinophilia occurs in immunocompetent patients but may be absent in immunocompromised hosts.
- Pneumonia accompanied by headache after mowing the lawn around garden beds should suggest the possibility of tularemia.

REFERENCES

1. **Bradsher, R. W., S. W. Chapman, and P. G. Pappas.** 2003. Blastomycosis. *Infect. Dis. Clin. N. Am.* **17:**21–40.
2. **Braude, A. I. (ed.).** *Infectious Diseases and Medical Microbiology,* 2nd ed. W. B. Saunders Company, Philadelphia, PA.
3. **Centers for Disease Control.** 1988. Multistate outbreak of sporotrichosis in seedling handlers, 1988. *MMWR Morb. Mortal. Wkly. Rep.* **37:**652.
4. **Centers for Disease Control and Prevention.** 2001. Update: outbreak of acute febrile respiratory illness among college students—Acapulco, Mexico, March 2001. *MMWR Morb. Mortal. Wkly. Rep.* **50:**359–360.
5. **Chapman, S. W., R. W. Bradsher, Jr., G. D. Campbell, Jr., P. G. Pappas, and C. A. Kauffman.** 2000. Practice guidelines for the management of patients with blastomycosis. *Clin. Infect. Dis.* **30:**679–683.
6. **Cohen, J., and W. G. Powderly.** 2004. *Infectious Diseases,* 2nd ed. Mosby, New York, NY.
7. **Cook, G. C., and A. I. Zumia (ed.).** 2003. *Manson's Tropical Diseases,* 21st ed. Elsevier Science, Ltd., Edinburgh, Scotland.
8. **Cunha, B. A.** 2008. The clinical diagnosis of Legionnaire's disease: diagnostic value of combining non-specific laboratory tests. *Infection* **6:**395–397.
9. **Cunha, B. A.** 2006. The atypical pneumonias: clinical diagnosis and importance. *Clin. Microbiol. Infect.* **12:**12–24.
10. **Cunha, B. A.** 2008. Atypical pneumonias: current clinical concepts focusing on Legionnaire's disease. *Curr. Opin. Pulm. Med.* **14:**183–194.
11. **Dorman, S. E., S. V. Guide, P. S. Conville, E. S. DeCarlo, H. L. Malech, J. I. Gallin, F. G. Witebsky, and S. M. Holland.** 2002.

Nocardia infection in chronic granulomatous disease. *Clin. Infect. Dis.* **35:**390–394.

12. **Gorbach, S. L., J. G. Bartlett, and N. R. Blacklow (ed.).** 2003. *Infectious Diseases,* 3rd ed. W. B. Saunders Company, Philadelphia, PA.

13. **Grencis, R. K., and E. S. Cooper.** 1996. Enterobius, Trichuris, Capillaria, and hookworm including Ancylostoma caninum. *Gastroenterol. Clin. N. Am.* **25:**579–597.

14. **Hajjeh, R., S. McDonnell, S. Reef, C. Licitra, M. Hankins, B. Toth, A. Padhye, L. Kaufman, L. Pasarell, C. Cooper, L. Hutwagner, R. Hopkins, and M. McNeil.** 1997. Outbreak of sporotrichosis among tree nursery workers. *J. Infect. Dis.* **176:**499–504.

15. **Johnson, R. D., M. Raff, and J. van Arsdall.** 1984. Neurologic manifestations of legionnaires' disease. *Medicine* (Baltimore) **63:**303.

16. **Karimi, K., L. J. Wheat, P. Connolly, G. Cloud, R. Hajjeh, E. Wheat, K. Alves, C. da Silva Lacaz, and E. Keath.** 2002. Differences in histoplasmosis in patients with acquired immunodeficiency syndrome in the United States and Brazil. *J. Infect. Dis.* **186:**1655–1660.

17. **Kauffman, C. A.** 2007. Histoplasmosis: a clinical and laboratory update. *Clin. Microbiol. Rev.* **20:**115–132.

18. **Lerner, P. I.** 1996. Nocardiosis. *Clin. Infect. Dis.* **22:**891–903.

19. **Mahmoud, A. A.** 1996. Strongyloides. *Clin. Infect. Dis.* **23:**949–952.

20. **Mandell, G. L., J. E. Bennett, and R. Dolin (ed.).** 2000. *Principles and Practice of Infectious Diseases,* 5th ed. Churchill Livingstone, Philadelphia, PA.

21. **Medeiros, A. A., S. D. Marty, F. E. Tosh, and T. D. Y. Chin.** 1966. Erythema nodosum and erythema multiforme as clinical manifesta-

tions of histoplasmosis in a community outbreak. *N. Engl. J. Med.* **274:**415.

22. **Murdoch, D. R.** 2003. Diagnosis of Legionella infection. *Clin. Infect. Dis.* **36:**64–69.

23. **Murray, H. W., and C. Tuazon.** 1980. Atypical pneumonias. *Med. Clin. N. Am.* **64:**507.

24. **Siddiqui, A. A., and S. L. Berk.** 2001. Diagnosis of Strongyloides stercoralis infection. *Clin. Infect. Dis.* **33:**1040–1047.

25. **Speil, C., and N. Khardori.** 2008. Histoplasmosis—an endemic mycosis. *Infect. Dis. Pract.* **32:**735–739.

26. **Threlkeld, S. C., and D. C. Hooper.** 1997. Update on management of patients with Nocardia infections. *Curr. Clin. Top. Infect. Dis.* **17:**1–23.

27. **Van Burik, J. A., R. C. Hackman, S. Q. Nadeem, J. W. Hiemenz, M. H. White, M. E. Flowers, and R. A. Bowden.** 1997. Nocardiosis after bone marrow transplantation: a retrospective study. *Clin. Infect. Dis.* **24:**1154–1160.

28. **Wallace, J.** 2002. Pulmonary blastomycosis: a great masquerader. *Chest* **121:**677–679.

29. **Wehner, J. H., and C. M. Kirsch.** 1997. Pulmonary manifestations of strongyloidiasis. *Semin. Respir. Infect.* **12:**122–129.

30. **Wheat, J.** 1997. Histoplasmosis. Experience during outbreaks in Indianapolis and review of the literature. *Medicine* (Baltimore) **76:**339–354.

31. **Wheat, L. J., A. G. Freifeld, M. B. Kleiman, J. W. Baddley, D. S. McKinsey, J. E. Loyd, and C. A. Kauffman.** 2007. Clinical practice guidelines for the management of patients with histoplasmosis: 2007 update by the Infectious Diseases Society of America. *Clin. Infect. Dis.* **45:**807–825.

32. **Wheat, L. J., and C. A. Kauffman.** 2003. Histoplasmosis. *Infect. Dis. Clin. N. Am.* **17:**1–19.

WITH MAN'S BEST FRIEND

Julie M. Collins and Bennett Lorber

5

The relationship between humans and dogs is an ancient one. The dog has been our workmate, protector, guide, and companion. No one would question the merit of the long history of valuable service that dogs have provided to humans; it is the stuff of legend and literature. We even have evidence that a dog companion may be good for our physical health given that contact with dogs has been shown to lower blood pressure, ameliorate depression, and produce a survival benefit after myocardial infarction (7, 63, 163). Occasionally, however, pathogens may be transmitted from dogs to human beings, resulting in problems ranging from a trivial rash to life-threatening bacteremia. These infections are reviewed in this chapter.

Considering that there are an estimated 72 million pet dogs in the United States, physicians need to be familiar with the potential illnesses that can result from canine exposure (30, 51). An inquiry into animal contact is an important part of a medical history. Some clinical conditions, along with etiologies to be considered in persons with a canine exposure, are listed in Table 1.

LOCAL INFECTIONS FOLLOWING DOG BITES

Epidemiology

Animal bites are a major public health problem and account for about 0.5 to 1% of emergency room visits; dogs are responsible for 75 to 90% of reported bites (51, 75, 184). Almost 5 million persons in the United States suffer a dog bite each year, and approximately 15% of these require medical attention. In most instances, the dog belongs to the bite victim, a friend, or a neighbor (30, 108). Most bites occur in warm-weather months, and bites are located most frequently on the hand and upper extremity. One-half to two-thirds of bites occur in children, with a peak incidence in those 5 to 9 years of age; in adult life, letter carriers, veterinarians, and animal control officers have a high incidence (30, 185).

The risk of infection following a dog bite is considerably lower than with cat bites, and infection rates are generally reported in the range of 3 to 18%, with a mean of about 5% (169, 184).

Julie M. Collins, Department of Medicine, Temple University Hospital, Philadelphia, PA 19140. *Bennett Lorber,* Section of Infectious Diseases, Department of Medicine, Temple University School of Medicine and Hospital, Philadelphia, PA 19140.

Infections of Leisure, Fourth Edition, Edited by David Schlossberg,
© 2009 ASM Press, Washington, DC

TABLE 1 Etiologies to consider in patients with canine exposure

Clinical picture	Pathogen(s)
Skin and soft tissue	
Local infection after a bite	
Less than 24 h	*Pasteurella multocida*
More than 24 h	*Streptococcus* and *Pasteurella* species
	Staphylococcus spp., anaerobes
Chronic	*Blastomyces dermatitidis*
Tinea (ringworm)	*Microsporum canis*
Pruritic papules	*Sarcoptes scabiei* var. *canis*, *Cheyletiella*, *Ctenocephalides*
Creeping eruption	*Ancylostoma* species
Erythema migrans	*Borrelia burgdorferi*
Lymph nodes (regional lymphadenopathy)	*Bartonella henselae* (cat scratch)
	Francisella tularensis
	Yersinia pestis
Respiratory	
Pharyngitis	*Streptococcus pyogenes*[a]
Pneumonitis	*Toxocara canis*
	Coxiella burnetii
Pulmonary embolism	*Dirofilaria immitis*
Solitary pulmonary nodule	*Dirofilaria immitis*
Gastrointestinal	
Diarrhea	*Campylobacter jejuni*
	Salmonella enterica serovar Enteritidis
	Cryptosporidium species
	Isospora belli[a]
	Giardia lamblia
	Trichuris vulpis
	Dipylidium caninum
Pruritus ani	*Dipylidium caninum*
Hepatitis	*Leptospira interrogans*
Hepatomegaly	*Toxocara canis*
Articular (arthritis)	*Borrelia burgdorferi*[a]
Neurological	
Aseptic meningitis	*Leptospira interrogans*
	Borrelia burgdorferi[a]
Pyogenic meningitis	*Capnocytophaga canimorsus*
	Pasteurella multocida
	Bergeyella zoohelcum
Visual disturbances	*Toxocara canis*
Encephalitis	Rabies virus
Systemic	
Septicemia (shock, DIC)	*Capnocytophaga canimorsus*
	Pasteurella multocida
Endocarditis	*Coxiella burnetii*
	Brucella canis
	Capnocytophaga canimorsus
	Pasteurella multocida
	Staphylococcus aureus
Fever and rash	*Rickettsia rickettsii*
Fever without localizing symptoms	*Salmonella enterica* serovar Enteritidis
	Brucella canis
	Ehrlichia and *Anaplasma* species
	Leptospira interrogans
Other	
Visceral mass	*Echinococcus granulosus*
Eosinophilia	*Toxocara canis*

[a]Transmission from dogs is controversial or unproved.

Microbiology #61

The oral flora of the dog is complex, plentiful, and made up of many aerobic and anaerobic species (169). Uninfected bite wounds should not be cultured, since they typically grow multiple species, and initial cultures do not predict infection and show little correlation with later cultures from infected bites (51, 60, 184).

Most infections following a dog bite are polymicrobial, typically yielding five or more species on wound culture (169). Common organisms are *Pasteurella* species, including *Pasteurella canis* and *Pasteurella multocida,* along with various anaerobes, streptococcal species, and staphylococcal species (76, 169). *P. multocida* is less common in dog bite infections than in cat bites or scratches. Rarely, chronic cutaneous infection with the fungus *Blastomyces dermatitidis* has been reported after a dog bite injury from an infected dog (73).

Initial Bite Management

Wounds should be irrigated under high pressure with large amounts of sterile saline (158, 184). Studies suggest that, following such irrigation, it is safe to close most bite wounds up to 12 h after injury (158). Puncture wounds should be covered with a topical antimicrobial agent and an absorbent dressing and allowed to heal by secondary intention. Standard recommendations for rabies and tetanus prophylaxis should be followed.

Antibiotic Prophylaxis

Controlled studies have not shown a beneficial effect of antibiotics in preventing infection (50), but these studies were small and may be subject to statistical error since infection rates following canine bites are low. A systematic review of antimicrobial prophylaxis for mammalian bites showed a beneficial infection rate reduction only for bites to the hand (119). Many authorities recommend prophylactic antibiotics for wounds of the hands and face, for deep puncture wounds that cannot be irrigated adequately, and for immunocompromised persons, particularly postsplenectomy

(2). There is no consensus regarding drug choice. Amoxicillin-clavulanate at 500 mg by mouth three times a day is a reasonable choice, with tetracycline at 500 mg four times a day as an alternative for penicillin-allergic individuals.

Treatment of Infection

There are no good large-scale trials evaluating antibiotic treatment of infected dog bite wounds. Most infections are polymicrobial, and treatment should be adequate for *P. canis, P. multocida,* anaerobes, and streptococcal and staphylococcal species. Those persons whose infection began more than 24 h after the bite should have therapy guided by Gram staining and culture, when possible (51). Reasonable initial therapeutic choices include amoxicillin-clavulanate alone, ciprofloxacin or levofloxacin plus clindamycin, or trimethoprim-sulfamethoxazole (TMP-SMX) plus clindamycin. Infections that manifest (pain, erythema) within a few hours to within 24 h of the bite are usually due to *P. multocida;* penicillin is the drug of choice, with tetracycline, TMP-SMX, or a quinolone as an alternative in penicillin-allergic persons.

Prevention of Dog Bites

Large breeds of dogs (shepherds) and guard dogs account for a disproportionate percentage of bites. Children should not be left unattended with large dogs; should be educated never to disturb dogs of any size who are eating, sleeping, or caring for puppies; and should be encouraged to avoid unfamiliar animals entirely.

LIFE-THREATENING SYSTEMIC INFECTIONS

Capnocytophaga canimorsus (Dog Bite Septicemia)

C. canimorsus, formerly DF-2 (dysgonic fermenter 2), is a fastidious gram-negative rod which can cause serious systemic illness following a dog bite. Since it was first reported about 30 years ago, more than 125 human cases have been described (136). The bacterium has been isolated from the normal gingival flora of 16% of dogs (184).

Sixty to 80% of patients have a predisposing condition (87, 109, 136, 175), most commonly splenectomy (35%), alcohol abuse (35%), or evidence of immune dysfunction due to steroid therapy, hematologic malignancy, or autoimmune disease (17%). More than 75% of cases involved previous exposure to a dog, through either ownership or a direct bite (109, 127).

The clinical illness is typically one of severe septicemia; shock and disseminated intravascular coagulation are common. Manifestations of *C. canimorsus* septicemia include cellulitis, gangrene, arthritis, endocarditis (146), meningitis (109), brain abscess, rash, hemolytic-uremic syndrome (125), thrombotic thrombocytopenic purpura, purpura fulminans, adrenal hemorrhage (Waterhouse-Friderichsen syndrome), myocardial infarction with normal coronary arteries and without evidence of endocarditis (49, 121), mycotic aortic aneurysm (175), and mononeuropathy by occlusion of vasa nervorum and infarction of the nerve (11). The mortality rate is about 30% (87, 109, 125, 127, 136, 175).

C. canimorsus infection must be considered in a febrile, severely ill patient with a history of a dog bite or dog exposure (cats may also transmit this infection). Diagnosis depends on isolation of the organism from blood, other fluids, or tissues. Organisms may be seen in buffy coat smears, particularly for splenectomized patients. However, *C. canimorsus* is often misidentified or not isolated by routine culture. Recently, 16S rRNA gene sequencing and PCR amplification techniques have improved the ability to correctly diagnose *C. canimorsus* infection (92).

Penicillin is thought to be the drug of choice. The bacterium is also susceptible to piperacillin, imipenem, erythromycin, vancomycin, clindamycin, expanded-spectrum cephalosporins, chloramphenicol, rifampin, TMP-SMX, ciprofloxacin, and tetracyclines. Resistance to aminoglycosides has been demonstrated (127).

Any person who has had a splenectomy should be warned about this rare but devastating infection and advised to take prophylactic antibiotics following a dog bite or contamination of an open wound with dog saliva.

Endocarditis

Coxiella burnetii, the cause of Q fever, is a well-described cause of culture-negative endocarditis; humans have acquired the infection from dog exposure. On occasion, endocarditis, in addition to rare instances of endocarditis due to *C. canimorsus,* has been reported as a complication of infection with *Brucella canis* and *P. multocida.* One instance of *Staphylococcus aureus* endocarditis was reported to occur in a dog breeder after minor bite trauma without evidence of infection at the bite site (19).

Rabies

The important problem of rabies and its ancient association with dog bites is considered in chapter 10.

BACTERIAL ZOONOTIC INFECTIONS

Bacterial zoonoses transmissible from dogs to human beings include campylobacteriosis, salmonellosis, leptospirosis, and brucellosis.

Campylobacteriosis

Campylobacteriosis is found throughout the world and is an important cause of human bacterial diarrhea, being as common as or more common than salmonellosis and shigellosis. The vast reservoir of *Campylobacter* in animals is probably the ultimate source for most human enteric infections. *Campylobacter* infections occur most often as sporadic cases after contact with contaminated raw or undercooked poultry or with contaminated feces from dogs or other animals. Outbreaks are less common and have been reported following ingestion of unpasteurized milk or contaminated water.

Approximately 50% of all pet dogs are carriers of *Campylobacter,* with colonization rates being higher in puppies than in mature dogs and higher in kennel populations than among household dogs (16, 52). Investigations of healthy pet dogs below 1 year of age have revealed carrier rates of up to 75%. The most common species isolated was *Campylobacter upsaliensis,* followed by *Campylobacter jejuni* (52 79, 103). *C. jejuni* is a cause of canine diarrhea but is also found in dogs without gastrointestinal symptoms (103, 186).

People who live with pet dogs are at increased risk of acquiring *Campylobacter* infection (172). Several case studies have shown an association between human *Campylobacter* enteritis and a history of close contact with sick puppies (17, 145). Epidemiological investigation of these cases revealed that the only common factor was exposure to sick puppies. Subsequently, the transmission of *Campylobacter* from a puppy to an infant, resulting in neonatal sepsis, has been confirmed by genetic analysis of the infecting bacteria from both hosts (188). Young children have particularly close exposure to puppies and are, therefore, more susceptible to fecal-oral transmission.

The clinical picture of *Campylobacter* enteritis is usually one of abrupt onset, with fever, abdominal pain, and diarrhea, and sometimes includes malaise, headache, myalgia, arthralgia, nausea, and vomiting. A history of grossly bloody stools is common, and many patients have at least 1 day of illness, with eight or more bowel movements (18). Severe abdominal pain before the onset of diarrhea can mimic appendicitis (139). Most patients recover within a week. Nonsuppurative complications of *C. jejuni* enteritis include reactive arthritis, Guillain-Barré syndrome, and, rarely, myocarditis (81, 98, 105).

Confirmation of the diagnosis of *C. jejuni* infection is based upon positive stool cultures, which must be placed on special selective media. Serologic testing can be done, but a low titer may reflect previous infection (16). Recently, *C. upsaliensis* has been identified by use of longer incubation periods and specific culture media as the second-most-common *Campylobacter* species to cause enteritis in humans (106).

Fluid and electrolyte replacement is an important therapy in any diarrheal illness. *Campylobacter* enteritis is largely self-limiting, and only in cases with severe prolonged symptoms are antibiotics warranted. *C. jejuni* is sensitive to a wide variety of antibiotics, including erythromycin, tetracyclines, and quinolones. Erythromycin remains the treatment of choice for *C. jejuni* infections. The newer macrolides (azithromycin, clarithromycin) are also effective, but they are more expensive and have no proven advantage over erythromycin. Unlike with *Salmonella* infection, treatment with antimicrobial agents does not prolong carriage of *C. jejuni;* on the contrary, erythromycin eliminates carriage within 72 h in most patients. #64 Even though erythromycin does not alter the clinical course of infection, therapy has been suggested, in some instances, to prevent person-to-person transmission (6). The emerging resistance of organisms to fluoroquinolones has diminished their usefulness (24, 27). Fluoroquinolones may be the best choice when bacterial gastroenteritis is suspected, but no organisms have yet been isolated (3).

Salmonellosis

Nontyphoidal *Salmonella* species may be relatively common inhabitants of the canine intestinal tract (186). The reported prevalence rate of *Salmonella* colonization in healthy dogs ranges from 1 to 36% (23, 59). Since dogs can shed the bacteria for 6 weeks or more after exposure, it is difficult to determine the true prevalence rate. Dogs may act as a reservoir for human infection with transmission through the fecal-oral route (39). However, only about 1% of human salmonellosis cases are secondary to contact with household pets (59). Recently, contaminated dry dog food and dog treats (made from pig ears, salmon, and beef) have been linked to multiple *Salmonella* outbreaks in humans. Humans may acquire the infection through direct contact with the contaminated food products or through contact with their pet dogs (26, 29, 59).

The clinical features of canine infection vary with the virulence of the strain, inoculum size, and host factors. Most dogs shedding *Sal-*

monella organisms in their stools are asymptomatic. The common clinical presentation of canine salmonellosis consists of fever, vomiting, and diarrhea (varying from watery to mucoid to bloody). Abortion and stillbirth may occur and have epidemiological importance, as the meconium, membranes, and discharge contain the organism.

Humans who have acquired salmonellosis have similar clinical findings, with fever, nausea, vomiting, colicky abdominal pain, and diarrhea (with or without mucus and blood).

Diagnosis is confirmed by isolation of the organism from stool or blood.

Clinical management should be based upon severity of disease. Human *Salmonella* gastroenteritis is self-limiting and requires antimicrobial treatment only in special cases (the very young, the very old, the immunocompromised, and those with prostheses) (78). TMP-SMX, fluoroquinolones, and expanded-spectrum cephalosporins can be used as the initial therapy in high-risk patients or those suspected of being bacteremic. The rate of TMP-SMX resistance is significant (13%) but decreasing, while resistance to fluoroquinolones is low (<3%) but increasing (27, 129). The intracellular nature of salmonellae may occasionally create discrepancies between in vitro sensitivity and clinical response.

With regard to public health risk, infected dogs typically shed *Salmonella* organisms for 20 to 40 days but sometimes up to 100 days. If one or more family members have confirmed salmonellosis without a known focus of exposure, the family pet should be tested regardless of symptoms. A thorough investigation should attempt to identify a common source for both human and pet.

Leptospirosis

Leptospires are finely coiled, motile spirochetes that are unique among pathogenic spirochetes in that they can be cultivated readily on artificial media. Historically, leptospires have been classified by antigenic determinants, with pathogenic serovars making up the species *Leptospira interrogans*. Recently, molecular analysis of *Leptospira* isolates has led to the reorganization of these bacteria into over 15 species. In clinical practice, however, leptospires continue to be identified by serotype, which can provide important epidemiological information (serotype Canicola, dogs; serotype Grippotyphosa, raccoons; serotype Icterohaemorrhagiae, rats; serotype Pomona, pigs and cattle) (13, 111).

Leptospirosis is a common zoonosis of livestock, pet animals, and wildlife in the United States and other parts of the world. Dogs are important vectors of human illness. Canine seroprevalence ranges from 5% to 60%, with higher rates in stray dogs, males, and animals over 1 year old (94, 143, 148). Leptospirosis has a wide range of presentations in dogs; it varies from being asymptomatic to fatal. When canine infection is clinically apparent, the most-common presenting symptoms and signs are anorexia, lethargy, vomiting, weakness, polyuria, polydipsia, and abdominal tenderness. Fever and icterus may also be present. Laboratory testing frequently reveals azotemia and elevated alkaline phosphatase, transaminases, and bilirubin (15, 67).

Canine shedder or carrier states develop after infection; leptospires can survive in the distal convoluted tubules of the host kidney after they have disappeared from the host tissues. In the carrier state, the host may have leptospiruria for months or for the remainder of its life, potentially contaminating the surrounding environment. Optimal factors that determine the length of survival of leptospires outside the host are acid urine, neutral or slightly alkaline environment, temperature of 22°C or higher, and aqueous or wet soil. Given these conditions, leptospires may survive for several weeks.

Humans are accidental hosts, becoming infected (i) directly from the urine or tissue of affected animals or (ii) indirectly through contact with water or soil that has been contaminated. Most human infections occur through exposed mucous membranes or abrasions of the skin (111). Leptospirosis can occur at all ages and in all seasons, but it presents primarily in young adults, in tropical climates, and in men (99).

Most humans develop a subclinical infection. Patients who do have clinically apparent disease typically experience a self-limited febrile illness, with only 10% of patients developing severe, life-threatening systemic disease. Leptospirosis is classically described as a biphasic illness; however, the phases may not be distinct in severe disease, and patients may present in the second phase. After an incubation period of 7 to 12 days, the initial septicemic phase, lasting 4 to 7 days, is characterized by fever, headache, myalgia, conjunctival suffusion, jaundice, proteinuria, and, less often, abdominal pain, diarrhea, and rash. The second phase is immunologically mediated and is manifested by aseptic meningitis, recurrent fever, uveitis, myositis, pulmonary symptoms, acute renal failure, and leptospiruria (99, 111). The most severe form of leptospirosis, known as Weil's disease, is characterized by hepatic and renal dysfunction, hemorrhage, and circulatory collapse (13). Reviews by Bharti et al. (13) and Levett (111) provide a detailed description of individual organ manifestations.

Definitive diagnosis requires isolation of leptospires from a clinical specimen or demonstration of seroconversion. Leptospires can be isolated from the blood, cerebrospinal fluid, or tissue in the acute phase of infection and identified by dark-phase microscopy or culture. In the immune phase, the organism is found in tissues and the urine (111). Growth may be very slow, and cultures should be incubated in the dark for 6 weeks at 30°C (74). Laboratory diagnosis is usually made on the basis of serologic tests. Agglutinins appear between the 6th and 12th days of illness, and a specific diagnosis is usually based on the demonstration of a fourfold rise in antibody titer. The microscopic agglutination test (MAT) is the current standard for diagnosis, but it is a complex test performed only in reference laboratories. Other methods have been developed for rapid screening prior to performance of the MAT. The enzyme-linked immuno-sorbent assay (ELISA) and dot ELISA have the highest sensitivities and specificities of these rapid tests and may be able to detect antibodies earlier than the MAT (9).

Treatment of leptospirosis remains controversial, as it is usually a nonfatal, self-limiting disease. Despite early studies with conflicting data regarding the benefit of treatment with penicillin, most authorities recommend treating moderate-to-severe leptospirosis with antimicrobial agents (182). Comparisons of penicillin to ceftriaxone, cefotaxime, and doxycycline in severe leptospirosis have demonstrated that all drugs are equally effective in shortening the duration of fever and reducing complications. Mortality rates in the different treatment groups were similar as well (132, 166). Treatment with ceftriaxone, cefotaxime, or doxycycline also provides broader antimicrobial coverage when the diagnosis is not clear in patients with undifferentiated febrile illness. The Jarisch-Herxheimer reaction is frequently observed during treatment (152).

There are several vaccines available to prevent leptospirosis in dogs, and they appear to be effective in preventing clinical illness. However, immunity wanes rapidly and vaccination is required annually (101). There have also been case reports of dogs that have had leptospires isolated from their urine despite vaccination within the previous year (57). Human vaccines have been used for some overseas populations, but no licensed preparation is available for use in the United States. Prophylaxis with doxycycline (200 mg weekly) for Americans traveling to a high-risk environment has been demonstrated to decrease the rate of leptospirosis (167).

Brucellosis

Dogs are the primary host for *Brucella canis*, an intracellular, gram-negative coccobacillus whose cell membrane contains rough lipopolysaccharides, unlike the other pathogenic species of *Brucella*. Transmission between dogs occurs during mating or, less often, through oronasal contact. Dogs infected with *B. canis* are asymptomatic or have disease manifested

#65

by spontaneous abortion, orchitis, epididymitis, fever, lymphadenopathy, or uveitis. Infected dogs characteristically have prolonged bacteremia (183). It may be difficult to eradicate canine infection, and some authorities have recommended euthanasia for infected dogs.

Human infection due to *B. canis* is rare, but like with other forms of brucellosis, it may be protean in its manifestations (138). Patients may have a nonspecific febrile illness with headache, myalgia, arthralgia, and malodorous perspiration or may demonstrate findings consistent with focal infection. Osteoarticular disease, such as peripheral arthritis, sacroiliitis, and spondylitis, is the most common localized manifestation. Endocarditis, epididymoorchitis, hepatitis, epidural abscess, uveitis, and involvement of the central nervous system have been described previously (133, 140).

The combination of potential exposure, consistent clinical features, and positive serology or culture confirms the diagnosis of brucellosis (147). Since antibodies to *B. canis* do not react with the standard antigens used when testing for *Brucella abortus, Brucella suis,* and *Brucella melitensis,* specific serology for *B. canis* must be performed when infection with this organism is suspected (133, 138). The serum agglutination test is the most commonly employed method for laboratory diagnosis, although indirect ELISA and PCR have recently become available (133). Cultures of blood and bone marrow are positive in 50 to 70% of cases. It may be necessary to hold culture bottles for up to 6 weeks.

Single-agent therapy and relatively short courses (less than 8 weeks) of combination treatments are associated with a high incidence of failure and relapse. Two regimens are the mainstay of treatment: (i) doxycycline plus an aminoglycoside (with streptomycin or gentamicin being equally effective [83]) and (ii) doxycycline plus rifampin. A meta-analysis found that the streptomycin regimen was slightly more effective at preventing relapse (161). A fluoroquinolone combined with either doxycycline or rifampin is an alternative option for second-line use (53).

Ehrlichiosis and Anaplasmosis

Ehrlichiosis is a zoonotic infection caused by small, obligately intracellular, gram-negative bacteria that reside and proliferate within cytoplasmic phagosomes called morulae (45). The causative bacteria have recently been reorganized taxonomically as members of the family *Anaplasmataceae. Anaplasma phagocytophila* and *Ehrlichia canis* cause human and canine monocytic ehrlichiosis, respectively, and *Ehrlichia chaffeensis* and *Ehrlichia ewingii* cause the granulocytic form of disease in humans and canines, respectively (44). However, all species have been reported to cause infection in both humans and dogs (22, 28, 44, 135). Ticks transmit these bacteria between hosts, and deer are the likely reservoirs.

Canine ehrlichiosis is manifested by uveitis, depression, anorexia, lymphadenopathy, splenomegaly, petechiae, and fever (104).

In the United States, most cases of human ehrlichiosis occur from April to September. Clinical features include acute onset of fever, malaise, and headache; rash is absent in granulocytic ehrlichiosis but may be present in the monocytic form. Laboratory features include leukopenia, thrombocytopenia, and liver function abnormalities (28). Most patients have a history of tick bite, and the diagnosis is established serologically or by PCR (45). Doxycycline has been reported to be effective and is the recommended treatment (191).

Q Fever

Q fever is a worldwide zoonosis caused by *Coxiella burnetii,* a strictly intracellular bacterium (116). Farm animals, such as cattle, sheep, and goats, are the most common reservoirs for human infection, which begins with inhalation of contaminated aerosols from parturient fluids of infected animals. Human infection may be asymptomatic or can result in pneumonia, a nonspecific febrile illness, hepatitis, or endocarditis. A dog-related outbreak of Q fever in which *C. burnetii* pneumonia developed in all three members of one family 8 to 12 days following exposure to an infected parturient dog was reported (20). Diagnosis is made serologically, and the preferred treatment is with doxycycline or a fluoroquin-olone.

Cat Scratch Disease

Cat scratch disease, reviewed in chapter 6, rarely has been reported following dog bites or scratches.

Streptococcosis

Streptococcus pyogenes, the group A beta-hemolytic bacterium, is a common cause of pharyngitis in children and adults. There are reports of dogs acting as reservoirs for this organism. In one study, a family of four had recurrent group A streptococcal pharyngitis which was not eradicated until the family dog was treated (117). Canine reservoirs for human streptococcal pharyngitis are probably exceedingly rare; that they occur at all is controversial (187). Nevertheless, it is probably prudent to consider a canine source in families with recurrent hemolytic streptococcal infection and a pet dog.

Streptococcus canis, a group G beta-hemolytic organism, is a commensal flora of the skin and oropharynx in healthy dogs and rarely is involved in human infection. In one large series, *S. canis* accounted for only 1% of all streptococcal isolates from human infections (65). Several case reports do identify infection with *S. canis* secondary to dog exposure. In one case, the patient was inoculated through a bite wound on the thigh and was treated twice for recurrent bacteremia (168); in another, bacteremia occurred following presumed entrance through venostasis ulcerations of the legs (12); and, in three instances, dog owners developed infections complicating chronic ulcers (107).

Urinary Tract Infection

Escherichia coli is the most common cause of urinary tract infections (UTI) in humans. The fecal flora from the patient is often the immediate source of these uropathogenic bacteria. Two studies (95, 96) have demonstrated household sharing of *E. coli* strains between humans and dogs. Thus, the family dog may serve as a reservoir of uropathogenic *E. coli*

that can colonize the human gastrointestinal tract and potentially cause UTI. In one family, an *E. coli* strain causing an acute UTI in the mother was found at the same time in fecal samples from the mother, father, and dog and at later time points in fecal samples from the three children, father, and dog (95). While sharing of *E. coli* strains between household members has been documented at similar rates in the presence and absence of dogs, dogs may be more likely to carry strains that are pathogenic to humans (96).

PARASITIC INFECTIONS

Many dogs harbor intestinal parasites; autopsy data have shown that more than 50% are infested with one or more such parasites (84). Some of these canine parasites may be transmitted to human beings, in whom they may produce symptomatic illness.

Cryptosporidiosis and Isosporiasis

Cryptosporidium spp. are ubiquitous coccidian protozoan parasites of the gastrointestinal tract, related to *Isospora* and *Toxoplasma* spp., that have been identified in a large variety of animals. *Cryptosporidium* has six major developmental stages, all of which occur within a single host. Morphologically, the oocysts of all cryptosporidia are extremely similar, but an increasing number of distinct species and genotypes are now being identified by molecular and genetic studies. For example, *Cryptosporidium hominis,* which affects humans, and *Cryptosporidium canis,* whose primary host is dogs, are now recognized as unique species separate from *Cryptosporidium parvum,* which infects humans, dogs, and farm animals (192). In a review of over 2,400 cases of human cryptosporidiosis, the majority of cases were caused by *C. parvum* (56%) and *C. hominis* (42%), while only 0.04% of cases were due to *C. canis* (110).

The parasite is acquired by the ingestion of fecally contaminated material, such as from the water supply, swimming pool water, food, fomites, and sexual activities that favor fecal-oral inoculation (34). An increasing number of cases of cryptosporidiosis are now being re-

#66

ported, which may reflect a true increase in the incidence of the disease or increased testing for and reporting of the disease by physicians (195).

Dogs can act as reservoirs for *C. parvum* and are the primary host for *C. canis* (34, 40, 55, 85, 193). The disease seems to be limited to puppies, but one study showed antibodies to cryptosporidia in 80% of all dogs tested (181). Worldwide, the reported rates of fecal shedding of *Cryptosporidium* oocysts in dogs ranges from 0% to 45%. These reports did not distinguish between species or genotype (56, 80).

To date, direct transmission of *Cryptosporidium* from dogs to humans has not been definitively proven. However, outbreaks involving veterinary students suggest that human cryptosporidiosis may be acquired from dogs and/or cats (54). Additionally, in 2007, a case of possible transmission of *C. canis* between two children and a dog living in the same household was reported (194).

Human cryptosporidiosis is characterized by watery diarrhea and cramping abdominal pain; fever is not prominent. It is an important source of illness in AIDS patients, in whom it causes a protracted, wasting diarrheal illness that may be complicated by extraintestinal infection such as biliary tract disease. In immunocompetent hosts, it produces a self-limiting diarrheal illness of 1 to 2 weeks (34); fecal leukocytes and blood are absent.

Diagnosis is made by microscopic identification of the organism in a fresh stool sample by microscopy, immunofluorescence, or enzyme immunoassays (165). After diagnosis, treatment of immunocompetent individuals may not be necessary. However, nitazoxanide has been shown to reduce the duration of diarrhea compared to placebo in these patients (142) and is now approved for cryptosporidiosis in both children and adults. For immunocompromised patients who are unable to clear the infection on their own, treatment has been frustrating and unsuccessful in most cases (40), although paromomycin sulfate has had limited success. In human immunodeficiency virus (HIV)/AIDS patients, initiation of antiretroviral therapy is the treatment of choice

because the resulting immune reconstitution allows patients to clear the infection. Protease inhibitors may also act directly against *Cryptosporidium* by reducing host cell invasion and parasite development (160). One large clinical study indicates that nitazoxanide is also effective for cryptosporidiosis in patients with AIDS; however, this study was not randomized or controlled (141).

The Centers for Disease Control and Prevention and the U.S. Public Health Service have issued guidelines for the prevention of opportunistic infections, including cryptosporidiosis, in persons with HIV infection (31). To prevent cryptosporidial infection, contact with human and animal feces should be avoided, and it is prudent to use disposable gloves for or immediately wash hands after contact with human feces (for example, changing diapers). Pet handling, gardening, or other contact with soil warrants similar precautions. Newly acquired puppies should be more than 6 months old, should not have diarrhea, and should not be stray. HIV-infected persons who wish to acquire a puppy younger than 6 months of age should have the puppy's stool examined for *Cryptosporidium* before contact.

The related protozoan *Isospora belli* causes clinical illness similar to that caused by *Cryptosporidium* and is diagnosed by identification of oocysts in fecal specimens. The size and shape (large and ovoid) of *Isospora* distinguish it from *Cryptosporidium* (smaller and round); both are acid fast.

Isospora canis is the predominant form of the parasite found in dogs, although *I. belli* has been isolated from canine feces as well (112, 176). Transmission to humans has not been proven. Treatment of humans with a week of oral TMP-SMX is curative; AIDS patients have a high frequency of recurrence but respond to retreatment.

Giardiasis

The flagellated enteric protozoan *Giardia lamblia* (also known as *Giardia intestinalis* or *Giardia duodenalis*) is an important worldwide cause of waterborne diarrhea in humans. Fecal-oral spread may also occur, particularly in day care settings, in custodial institutions, and among those who have oral-anal sexual contact.

Giardia colonization is relatively common in dogs. Studies have shown carriage prevalence rates of 4 to 25% in dogs (70). Rates are higher in puppies (35 to 50%) and kenneled dogs (100%) (164, 173). Canine infection is usually asymptomatic but may cause diarrhea (173).

There is growing evidence for the role of dogs in human giardiasis (51). One study found that humans living with dogs were more likely to be infected with *Giardia* than humans living in canine-free households (177). Humans living with infected dogs were more likely to have giardiasis than humans living with *Giardia*-free dogs. In addition, genetically similar isolates of *Giardia* have been identified in humans and dogs sharing the same household (177). While this evidence confirms the zoonotic potential for *Giardia* transmission to humans, information about the frequency of zoonotic transmission is lacking. Case-control studies have failed to demonstrate an association between contact with dogs and human giardiasis (196). Compared to the risk of transmission from other sources, the risk of direct zoonotic transmission is thought to be small (70, 90).

Human infection is manifested initially by watery diarrhea without fever. Cramps, bloating, flatulence, and sulfuric belching are common. Later in the illness, stools may become greasy and foul smelling and may float.

Giardiasis should be considered in all patients with prolonged diarrhea (more than 2 weeks' duration) or malabsorption symptoms. Diagnosis is achieved by identifying cysts or trophozoites in stool specimens by microscopy or ELISA or by sampling duodenal contents. Collection of multiple stool samples on different days may be needed to establish the diagnosis, because giardial cysts are excreted intermittently (196). Giardiasis can be treated with tinidazole, metronidazole, or nitazoxanide (64, 66). Efficacy rates for a single dose of tinidazole and for a 5 day course of metronidazole are similar (66). A recent study indicated that a 3-day course of nitazoxanide is equivalent to a 5-day course of metronidazole in the treatment of giardiasis in children (130).

Dirofilariasis

The dog heartworm, *Dirofilaria immitis* (L. *dirus,* evil; *filum,* thread), and the related parasite *Dirofilaria repens* are found worldwide in warm climates. The majority of human infections occur in Mediterranean countries, where the disease is endemic in animals (156). In the United States, canine and human dirofilariasis are most prevalent along the East Coast and Gulf Coast and in the Great Lakes region and the Mississippi River Valley (36). Dirofilariasis should be considered in patients with appropriate symptoms or signs (described below) who reside in or have visited any of these areas (126).

Classically, *D. immitis* causes pulmonary dirofilariasis, while *D. repens* causes the subcutaneous form. However, both species have been reported to cause both types of disease (156).

In the canine host, the adult worm lives in the right ventricle and pulmonary artery and releases microfilaria into circulation (157). Mosquito vectors transmit the microfilarial form of the parasite from dog to dog and from dog to human being. Infected dogs are often asymptomatic but may have dermatitis, subcutaneous nodules, hemoptysis, pulmonary embolism, or evidence of heart failure secondary to right ventricular outflow obstruction (10, 137).

In humans, larvae cannot develop into adults; most die before reaching the heart. Occasionally, a larva may reach the right ventricle, die, and embolize to the lung. Symptoms are rare but, when present, may mimic pulmonary thromboembolism (pleuritic pain, fever, hemoptysis) (41, 179). The granulomatous lung reaction to the embolized larva produces the roentgenographic finding of a solitary pulmonary nodule, described as a coin lesion (82, 120). The intracellular bacterium *Wolbachia* sp. resides symbiotically in *Dirofilaria* and plays an integral role in activating the immune response in the human host (156).

Subcutaneous nodules are hard and erythematous. They occur most frequently on the upper extremities and head, including within the orbits and periorbital structures (8, 156). Nodules in the breast, scrotum, bladder, and abdominal cavity have also been reported (8, 102). Depending on the location, the nodule of dirofilariasis may mimic malignancy (lung, breast, or scrotum), other infections (tuberculosis or pulmonary fungal infection), or other benign masses (cyst or hamartoma) (126).

Canine infection is diagnosed by demonstrating microfilariae in smears of peripheral blood. The ELISA has excellent sensitivity and specificity (170). Treatment of dogs and prophylaxis in areas of endemicity should be under veterinary supervision. Diagnosis of human infection is established histologically following resection, and further treatment is unnecessary.

Toxocariasis

Toxocara canis is a roundworm that infects most puppies and many adult dogs in the United States, and it is the primary cause of visceral larva migrans (VLM) in humans.

Infection in dogs follows ingestion of embryonated eggs, ingestion of larvae in other infected hosts, or vertical transmission. After hatching in the stomach, the larvae penetrate the intestinal mucosa, entering lymph and blood vessels. They are transported to the liver, lungs, and heart and then by systemic circulation. The larvae can move through capillary walls and migrate into any tissue, where they may survive for years (42, 115). Hormonal changes in a pregnant bitch stimulate these larvae, resulting in transplacental migration of the larvae to the litter or passage of larvae in the bitch's milk (150). Larvae in circulation can also reenter the intestines via the lungs; some of the larvae pass through the bronchioles to the trachea and pharynx and are swallowed. These larvae or larvae that have remained in the intestine since hatching may then develop into adults in the intestine (72).

Adult worms live for an average of four months in the proximal small intestine of dogs. The female roundworm can produce 200,000 eggs per day. Eggs are then passed in the feces but are noninfectious until embryonation occurs over approximately a 2-week period (115). Depending on the temperature and moisture of the environment, eggs can remain viable for months.

Transmission from dogs to humans occurs by ingestion of eggs from the soil or from contaminated hands and fomites. Twenty to 60% of soil samples recovered from residential backyards, public parks, and children's sandboxes are contaminated with *T. canis* eggs. Children 1 to 6 years of age are most prone to infection, particularly those with a history of pica and exposure to puppies (71, 131). Despite uniformly high levels of toxocariasis in dogs throughout the United States, the diagnosis of VLM in children is made most frequently in the south-central and southeastern regions of the country.

Human infection follows a pattern similar to that of canine infection. After ingestion, eggs hatch in the small intestine. Larvae penetrate the intestinal mucosa, enter circulation, and then migrate across capillaries into tissue (115). However, the life cycle of *T. canis* is not completed in human hosts: larvae do not mature into adult worms.

The clinical manifestations of human toxocariasis are classified as VLM, ocular larva migrans, and neurological toxocariasis (115). Infections may also be asymptomatic (4).

In VLM, the most frequently involved organs are the liver and lungs. Liver involvement presents as abdominal pain and hepatomegaly, with low-density lesions seen on computed tomography (CT) (115). Pulmonary manifestations are present in 20 to 80% of cases and range from cough and wheezing to eosinophilic pneumonia (35). Chest radiograph may be normal or show bilateral infiltrates. A CT scan may reveal multiple subpleural nodules with halos or ground glass opacities. These radiographic findings may be migratory on repeat imaging (35, 144). Cases of myocarditis and nephritis secondary to VLM have been reported as well (1, 155).

Ocular larva migrans is caused by the larvae of *Toxocara* entering the eye; it is typically a unilateral disease but occasionally occurs bilaterally. Presenting complaints are varied, and there is no pathognomonic pattern. Patients may complain of failing vision, strabismus, leukocoria, eye pain, fixed pupil, or red eye. Funduscopic exam findings may vary from a solitary posterior pole lesion or peripheral granuloma in an asymptomatic eye to severe exudative endophthalmitis with retinal detachment. Ocular cases are more frequently reported for adults than for children and are usually seen in the absence of visceral symptoms (5).

Neurological toxocariasis is an uncommon occurrence, with less than 50 possible cases reported by 2003. Involvement of the central nervous system presents most frequently as encephalitis, meningitis, or myelitis. Cerebrospinal fluid analysis usually reveals eosinophilic pleocytosis, and cerebral lesions may be visualized by magnetic resonance imaging (47). In addition, *T. canis* has been implicated as a risk factor for epilepsy. Skin testing for *Toxocara* in healthy persons and those with epilepsy showed positive tests in 2.1 and 7.5% of individuals, respectively (189). Studies have also shown significantly higher *Toxocara* titers in epileptic children and adults than in nonepileptic controls (72, 128). However, children with *Toxocara* are more likely to have lead poisoning than noninfected children, and the two groups have the same risk factors: pica and lower socioeconomic status. Further studies are necessary to define the significance of *T. canis* in children with respect to neurological function and to distinguish the effects from those of lead (71).

A definitive diagnosis of toxocariasis is established by demonstration of the larvae in pathological specimens (biopsy or autopsy). However, in practice, the diagnosis of VLM is usually based on the clinical scenario and laboratory data, avoiding the need for biopsy (42). Eosinophilia is a common but nonspe-

cific laboratory finding for toxocariasis. Elevated serum immunoglobulin E levels are also associated with infection (115). Stool samples are not useful, as the larvae do not mature in human beings. Serologic tests using ELISA are the mainstay of diagnosis and have been reported to be 91% sensitive and 86% specific (91). A positive ELISA, however, may indicate prior or current infection and must be interpreted with regard to the clinical situation (115). Serologic tests are less likely to be positive in cases of ocular larva migrans, and diagnosis is made by ophthalmologic exam (42).

The disease is usually self-limiting, and only in rare instances have there been fatalities resulting from an exaggerated immune response in the heart, central nervous system, or lungs. Glucocorticoids may be employed to reduce inflammatory complications. Available antihelminthic drugs, including diethylcarbamazine, thiabendazole, mebendazole, and albendazole, reduce clinical manifestations in 50 to 70% of cases (115). Treatment of ocular disease is unsatisfactory, and the role of glucocorticoids or antihelminthic drugs in the management of ocular disease is controversial (113).

Preventive measures are essential to reduce the frequency of accidental ingestion of infective eggs. Children exposed to dogs treated for roundworm infection are less likely to have positive serologic tests for *T. canis* than children exposed to untreated dogs (37). Other preventive measures include removing children with pica from environments thought to be contaminated, prohibiting canine access to children's game areas, and frequently turning over sand in public parks (89).

Cutaneous Larva Migrans

The dog intestinal hookworm *Ancylostoma braziliense* is the nematode that causes human cutaneous larva migrans, also known as creeping eruption (69). Larvae enter human skin after direct contact in areas contaminated with canine feces, such as beaches and playgrounds. Cutaneous larva migrans is a common cause of skin problems among those returning from

70

travel in tropical areas (93). The larvae do not possess the enzymes necessary to penetrate the dermis and remain confined to the epidermis, in which they migrate. About 2 weeks after exposure, skin eruptions manifested by serpiginous, pruritic, red tunnels occur and spread a few millimeters per day. Lesions may appear on any area of the body but are typically found on the feet and legs. The skin appearance is diagnostic, and infection is self-limiting but may last for several weeks.

Although cutaneous larva migrans is a self-limiting problem, treatment is employed to relieve symptoms and prevent superinfection. Effective therapies include a single oral dose of albendazole or ivermectin (25). A rare eosinophilic enteritis syndrome due to *Ancylostoma caninum* is manifested by abdominal pain and may be treated with mebendazole (97).

Trichuriasis

Human infection with the dog whipworm, *Trichuris vulpis,* has been reported (46). In that case, a 49-year-old woman with previous surgery for duodenal ulcer disease developed diarrhea, abdominal pain, and nausea. Ova of the dog whipworm were seen on stool exam, and her symptoms responded to mebendazole treatment. She owned five dogs.

Echinococcosis

Echinococcus granulosus is a tapeworm that resides in the small intestines of its definitive hosts, dogs and wolves. Ten genotypes of *E. granulosus* have been identified, some of which may become recognized as distinct species in the future. The majority of human echinococcosis is caused by the sheep strain G1.

Gravid segments of the adult cestode release eggs which are shed in the stool and may remain viable in the environment for up to a year. Following ingestion by an intermediate host (sheep, humans, cattle, pigs, goats, horses), the eggs hatch in the upper small intestine and oncospheres are released. The oncospheres penetrate the intestinal mucosa and obtain passage to the liver via portal veins. Most of the oncospheres are trapped in the liver; however, a few may pass through the liver and arrest in the lung or continue to the heart. Those embryos that reach the systemic circulation may seed any organ, where the parasite is then destroyed by an inflammatory reaction or develops into a hydatid cyst. Cysts contain multiplying larvae and enlarge slowly over many years.

Upon the death of the intermediate host, the larval hydatid may be ingested by a dog through eating infected offal. The released scolices attach to the small intestinal mucosa. These scolices mature over a period of 6 to 8 weeks into adult tapeworms 3 to 6 mm long, completing the life cycle (77, 151). Dogs harboring the tapeworm are asymptomatic.

The prevalence of human echinococcosis is dependent upon the direct association of humans with infected canines. The frequency of infection is much higher in those regions where livestock is a major industry, especially in sheep-raising areas, where dogs feed on uncooked offal (77, 118). In the United States, affected individuals are typically immigrants from areas of endemicity (Iceland, Italy, Greece, the Middle East, and parts of Asia), inhabitants of Alaska, or sheep ranchers in Arizona and New Mexico. No new cases have been reported in Utah since 1996 (124).

The majority of human infections with *E. granulosus* are asymptomatic. The disease is indolent, as cysts enlarge slowly over many years. The growing cysts may remain unilocular or become multilocular with the formation of daughter cysts. Some of the cysts die, shrink, become heavily calcified, and remain asymptomatic (48, 149). Overall, approximately 75% of infected patients remain asymptomatic (62).

Symptomatic infections present with features of a space-occupying lesion specific to the organ(s) involved. Multiple case series have found similar anatomical distributions of cysts in the liver (63 to 75% of cases); lung (17 to 25%); muscles, bone, kidney, and spleen (all less than 5%); and brain, heart, thyroid, breast, prostate, parotid gland, and pancreas (all less than 1%) (77, 134).

The most important complications of hydatid cysts are rupture, secondary bacterial infection, and problems caused by compression. For example, hepatic cysts may cause secondary cholangitis by rupturing in the biliary tree or by obstructing the bile duct by compression of the biliary ductal system. Leaking cysts can precipitate a wide range of reactions, from urticaria to anaphylaxis. Scolices that are released may lead to the establishment of secondary or metastatic hydatid infections elsewhere in the body (77, 149).

Diagnosis is made primarily from characteristic findings upon imaging studies, such as ultrasound, X ray, CT, and magnetic resonance imaging. Eosinophil counts or liver function tests may or may not be abnormal and should not be relied upon. Ultrasound is most frequently used to assess abdominal cysts, with several findings, such as intracystic septations, being pathognomonic for hepatic hydatid lesions. Pulmonary cysts can be identified by chest X ray, which usually shows a round, uniformly dense, noncalcified lesion 1 to 20 cm in diameter.

Immunodiagnostic techniques are used to confirm cases of human echinococcosis suggested by imaging findings. The ELISA is the most commonly employed test to detect serum antibodies to *E. granulosus,* with a sensitivity of 68 to 80% and a specificity of 73 to 88% (114). Approximately 10% of patients with liver cysts and 25% of patients with lung cysts do not have detectable serum antibodies.

Historically, aspiration of the cyst for diagnosis was not recommended, since leakage of contents or rupture of the cyst can lead to secondary infection or an anaphylactic reaction. However, ultrasound-guided cyst puncture, which was introduced in 1986, has been demonstrated to be a safe technique that may be used in cases where the diagnosis remains unclear after the standard assessments (134).

Therapy for echinococcosis is based on consideration of the size, location, and manifestations of cysts and the overall health of the patient. The available options are surgery, puncture-aspiration-injection-reaspiration (PAIR), chemotherapy, or observation. Surgical treatment results in cure if the cyst is able to be completely removed. Risks during surgery from leakage of fluid include anaphylaxis and dissemination of infection. Operative mortality ranges from 0.5 to 4%. Secondary spread of infection has been minimized by the instillation of scolicidal solutions and perioperative chemotherapy (154). Albendazole or mebendazole should be given at least 4 days before surgery and for 1 month or 3 months postoperatively, respectively. A longer (1- to 3-month) preoperative course of albendazole significantly decreases the number of viable parasites present at the time of surgery, which may translate to a lower risk of recurrence (14).

PAIR with concomitant chemotherapy is a minimally invasive technique that is indicated as treatment for most hepatic cysts, infected cysts, inoperable cysts, patients at high surgical risk, and patients who refuse surgery. In a recent controlled trial, percutaneous drainage, combined with albendazole therapy, was found to be an effective and safe alternative to surgery for the treatment of uncomplicated hydatid cysts of the liver (100). A review of 756 cases in which PAIR was used to treat abdominal hydatid cysts reported minor complications (fever, rash, nausea, vomiting, infection of the cavity, and intracystic hemorrhage) in 13.7% of cases, anaphylactic shock in 0.5% of cases, and death in 0.13% of cases (58). The failure rate was 0.26%, while the rate of recurrence was 1.6%. PAIR may also be used for cysts in the spleen, kidney, and nonvertebral bones, but it should not be used for cysts in the spine, brain, or heart (190).

Chemotherapy alone is less successful than surgery or PAIR, with 20 to 40% of cysts showing no morphological changes 12 months after the initiation of treatment with benzimidazoles (albendazole or mebendazole). However, 30% of patients are cured (cyst disappearance), and 30 to 50% show improvement (degeneration of cysts and/or significant size reduction). Chemotherapy is indicated for inoperable patients with primary liver or lung echinococcosis, for patients with multiple cysts in two or more organs, for peritoneal cysts, and for perioperative use in patients undergoing surgery or PAIR (134). Response rates may be higher with albendazole, which is better absorbed after oral administration, than with mebendazole (43, 61, 88). Praziquantel has also been used for therapy. A few reports suggest that the combination of albendazole and praziquantel as medical therapy or as postspillage prophylaxis is more effective than either therapy alone (122, 171).

Control of *E. granulosus* in dogs has been shown to decrease rates of human echinococcosis. In the United Kingdom, the incidence of human infection significantly declined when dogs were treated with praziquantel every 6 weeks. When canine treatment was replaced by an education program for dog owners, the rates of human hydatid disease increased again (21).

Dipylidiasis

Dipylidium caninum, a common tapeworm of dogs, has been reported sporadically as a cause of human infection, with fewer than 100 case reports in the English-language literature. Human infection typically occurs in children, with one-third of cases occurring in infants 6 months of age or younger (33, 123, 180). Dogs are the definitive hosts, with adult, proglottid-shedding worms residing in the intestine. Egg-containing proglottids are passed in the feces and disintegrate, releasing ova which are ingested by fleas, the usual intermediate hosts. Cysticercoid larvae develop in the flea, and dogs or children may acquire infection while nipping or accidentally ingesting fleas. The larvae grow to maturity in the intestine in about 1 month.

Infected humans typically are asymptomatic, but abdominal discomfort, diarrhea, and pruritus ani may occur (51). One case report describes colic and feeding difficulties associated with dipylidiasis (180).

Clinical diagnosis usually follows observation by a parent of white, motile, cucumber-seed-shaped proglottids in the stool or diaper of an infant. Worms migrating from the anus may lead to a misdiagnosis of pinworms by history. Definitive diagnosis is made through identification of typical egg-containing proglottids.

Treatment consists of praziquantel as a single dose, with niclosamide as alternative therapy. Prevention of infection in both dogs and humans is achieved most effectively by keeping pets free from fleas or tapeworms (68, 170).

SUPERFICIAL FUNGAL INFECTIONS (DERMATOPHYTOSIS)

Dermatophytosis is a common superficial fungal infection of dogs, cats, and humans. Zoophilic dermatophytes are occasionally transmitted to humans, causing tinea (ringworm). Dermatophytes rarely invade the skin and produce disease by releasing allergens and creating an inflammatory reaction.

The most common fungi causing dermatophytosis in dogs are species of *Epidermophyton, Microsporum,* and *Trichophyton.* The cutaneous signs are variable and not characteristic for a specific dermatophyte. By far, the most common dog dermatophyte to cause human skin infection is *Microsporum canis.*

Diagnosis is established based on history, physical examination, Wood's lamp examination, KOH preparation, skin biopsy, and fungal culture. Fungal culture is necessary to confirm the etiology. In urban settings, 10 to 30% of human cases of tinea corporis (ringworm) are estimated to be of animal origin (51).

Effective eradication of the infection should include treatment of the source animal as well as the human patient with topical agents, such as clotrimazole, miconazole, and ketoconazole. In severe cases, treatment with oral fluconazole or itraconazole is effective. The living environment, which may retain animal hair or dander, should be thoroughly cleansed (170).

An intensive care nursery outbreak due to *Malassezia pachydermatis* has been well documented (32). The organism, which caused fungemia, UTI, meningitis, and asymptomatic colonization in infants, was introduced into the intensive care nursery on a health care worker's hands, which had become colonized from contact with pet dogs at home.

ECTOPARASITE-ASSOCIATED ILLNESS

Dogs that frequent the outdoors may disseminate the flea and tick vectors responsible for such serious human diseases as plague, Rocky Mountain spotted fever, tularemia, and Lyme disease. Thus, a pet owner need not leave home to be exposed to these infections; his or her dog can bring the vectors right into the living room.

Other canine ectoparasites (mites and fleas) may cause vexing dermatoses in humans. The most common ectoparasite-induced dermatoses of dogs are canine scabies, cheyletiellosis, and fleas. It has been estimated that over 5% of the cases presenting to human dermatology clinics are directly attributable to animal ectoparasites (86).

Canine Scabies

Sarcoptes scabiei var. *canis* causes canine scabies (sarcoptic mange), a nonseasonal, pruritic, contagious infestation of the skin of dogs that is transmissible to humans. The adult female mite penetrates to the level of the stratum granulosum, where she feeds. She deposits her eggs in a burrow, in which they hatch and give rise to larvae. The larvae migrate to the surface and molt through nymphal and adult forms. This maturation process occurs over 10 to 21 days.

Canine scabies has no age, sex, or breed preferences and is characterized by intense pruritus followed by an erythematous, nonfollicular papular dermatitis. These lesions, frequently found on the pinnae, face, limbs, and ventrolateral trunk, become excoriated and crusted. In the absence of early diagnosis or treatment, extension of these lesions may involve the entire animal, with accompanying alopecia (174). It is thought that prolonged skin-to-skin exposure is important for transmission to take place from a dog to a human

being; 30 to 50% of human contacts of a canine case may be affected.

Hypersensitivity appears to play a role in canine and human scabies. In both species, dermatologic manifestations are out of proportion to the number of mites present.

Diagnosis is generally established by history, clinical findings, or response to scabicides, since human skin scrapings frequently fail to demonstrate mites. Canine scrapings are more often positive, but in one study only 51% of canine scrapings were positive for ova or mites (153).

There is no correlation between the severity and duration of the canine disease and transmission to humans. The lesions in humans consist of vesicles, erythematous papules, wheals, crusts, and excoriations occurring in areas of pet contact. Therefore, it is seen especially on the arms, legs, abdomen, and chest. Unlike with human scabies, there are no burrows and no involvement of the hands, finger webs, or genitalia. Human infestation may occur in small epidemics (159).

The severity of the eruption and its extent and duration can vary considerably. Generally, the lesions are self-limiting without treatment after the infected animal has been removed. Human scabies and papular urticaria are the main conditions to be differentiated from canine scabies in humans. A history of exposure to an infested pet, a different distribution pattern, a lack of burrows, and demonstration of the causative organism on examination of the pet will aid in making the diagnosis.

Infested dogs are easily treated with weekly applications of scabicidal dips (especially lindane or lime sulfur) until 2 weeks after clinical cure is achieved (153). All dogs in a household or those exposed to an infested dog should be treated. In addition, a single washing of fomites in hot water and detergent is recommended.

For human treatment, permethrin is highly effective and relatively nontoxic. Orally administered ivermectin appears to be effective as a scabicide. Alternative scabicides, including benzyl benzoate, crotamine cream, and sulfur ointment, may be preferred for infants, pregnant women, or unsupervised mass treatments (162).

Cheyletiellosis

Cheyletiella species dermatitis ("walking dandruff") is a nonseasonal, variably pruritic, transmissible infestation of the skin of dogs and cats caused by nonburrowing mites which live in skin surface keratin. They move about rapidly but occasionally pierce the skin with their hooks and become engorged with tissue fluids (153).

As with scabies, there is no apparent predilection for breed or sex. Pruritus is variously found, but there is usually some degree of dorsal scaling, crusting, and dermatitis (153). Adult dogs can be symptomatic carriers of mites, but puppies are most often clinically affected.

Rarely, a human dermatitis produced by *Cheyletiella* mites has been reported (38, 178). The lesions begin as single or grouped erythematous macules, which rapidly evolve into papules; these lesions frequently become vesicular or pustular. Old lesions develop a very characteristic central necrosis, which is of diagnostic significance. The pruritus may be intense and involve any portion of the body but rarely the face. Other eruptions that may be produced by these mites include bullae, urticaria, erythema multiforme, and generalized pruritus without dermatitis.

Diagnosis is based on historical and physical findings, positive skin scrapings or Scotch tape preparations, and response to miticidal agents. However, skin scrapings from humans are rarely positive.

Human infestations are self-limiting; *Cheyletiella* mites are unable to complete their life cycle on humans. The source of mites must be removed or treated with topical miticides. Dogs in contact with affected animals must be treated, and their environment must be vigorously cleaned. With humans, dermatoses resolve within 3 weeks without specific treatment.

Fleas

Fleas can cause asymptomatic infestation or severe hypersensitivity skin disease in dogs and humans. In the United States, the genera of most importance are *Ctenocephalides* and *Pulex* (153). Although flea bites in humans are generally trivial and not more than a nuisance, they may play a role in the transmission of systemic disease, such as *Bartonella henselae* infection (170).

Hypersensitivity to flea salivary antigens plays a critical role in dermatoses. The typical lesion on human beings is an urticarial papule. Lesions favor exposed distal extremities and are extremely pruritic.

In diagnosing human flea bites, it is important to demonstrate fleas in the environment. This is often done by having the patient walk through infested areas wearing white knee socks to better visualize the fleas.

Treatment involves flea control measures as well as topical or systemic anti-inflammatory medication (if the reaction is severe). Effective flea control requires treatment of the affected pets, their areas, and other animal contacts. Flea bombs or sprays are needed to kill larval forms and prevent reinfection. Pets should not be allowed to forage in areas where *Yersinia pestis* is prevalent.

MEASURES TO MINIMIZE DOG-ASSOCIATED ILLNESS

- Children should not be left unattended with dogs, unfamiliar dogs should be avoided, and feeding or sleeping dogs should not be disturbed.
- Dogs should be vaccinated for rabies and possibly for leptospirosis.
- Prophylaxis for dirofilariasis should be given in areas of endemicity.
- Newly acquired puppies should be treated for intestinal parasites before being taken into the home.
- Dogs should not be permitted to defecate on beaches or playgrounds, and animal feces on lawns should be removed at least weekly. Sand in public parks should be turned over frequently.

- Feces should not be used as fertilizer.
- Dogs should not be allowed to eat offal.
- Hands should be washed after animals are handled, and diarrhea in pets should lead to increased attention to hygiene.
- Animals should be inspected regularly for fleas and ticks.

PRACTICAL TIPS

- Advise persons who have undergone splenectomy that a dog bite could result in a life-threatening infection (*Capnocytophaga* bacteremia); in the event of a bite, they should seek medical attention immediately.
- HIV-infected persons who wish to acquire a puppy younger than 6 months of age should have the puppy's stool examined for *Cryptosporidium* before contact.
- Persons with ringworm or a pruritic, papular rash may have acquired a fungus or ectoparasite from a pet dog; in patients with such skin eruptions one should inquire about canine exposure.

REFERENCES

1. **Abe, K., H. Shimokawa, T. Kubota, Y. Nawa, and A. Takeshita.** 2002. Myocarditis associated with visceral larva migrans due to *Toxocara canis. Intern. Med.* **41:**706–708.
2. **Aghababian, R. V., and J. E. Conte, Jr.** 1980. Mammalian bite wounds. *Ann. Emerg. Med.* **9:**79–83.
3. **Allos, B. M., and M. J. Blaser.** 2002. Campylobacter species, p. 157–168. *In* V. L. Yu, R. Weber, and D. Raoult (ed.), *Antimicrobial Therapy and Vaccines,* 2nd ed., vol. 1. Apple Trees Productions, LLC, New York, NY.
4. **Altcheh, J., M. Nallar, M. Conca, M. Biancardi, and H. Freilij.** 2003. Toxocariasis: clinical and laboratory features in 54 patients. *An. Pediatr.* (Barcelona) **58:**425–431. (In Spanish.)
5. **Ament, C. S., and L. H. Young.** 2006. Ocular manifestations of helminthic infections: onchocerciasis, cysticercosis, toxocariasis, and diffuse unilateral subacute neuroretinitis. *Int. Ophthalmol. Clin.* **46:**1–10.
6. **Anders, B. J., B. A. Lauer, J. W. Paisley, and L. B. Reller.** 1982. Double-blind placebo controlled trial of erythromycin for treatment of *Campylobacter* enteritis. *Lancet* **i:**131–132.
7. **Anderson, W. P., C. M. Reid, and G. L. Jennings.** 1992. Pet ownership and risk factors for cardiovascular disease. *Med. J. Aust.* **157:**298–301.
8. **Angeli, L., R. Tiberio, R. Zuccoli, G. Annali, A. Ramponi, and G. Leigheb.** 2007. Human dirofilariasis: ten new cases in Piedmont, Italy. *Int. J. Dermatol.* **46:**844–847.
9. **Bajani, M. D., D. A. Ashford, S. L. Bragg, C. W. Woods, T. Aye, R. A. Spiegel, B. D. Plikaytis, B. A. Perkins, M. Phelan, P. N. Levett, and R. S. Weyant.** 2003. Evaluation of four commercially available rapid serologic tests for diagnosis of leptospirosis. *J. Clin. Microbiol.* **41:**803–809.
10. **Baneth, G., Z. Volansky, Y. Anug, G. Favia, O. Bain, R. E. Goldstein, and S. Harrus.** 2002. *Dirofilaria repens* infection in a dog: diagnosis and treatment with melarsomine and doramectin. *Vet. Parasitol.* **105:**173–178.
11. **Benerjee, T. K., W. Grubb, C. Otero, M. McKee, B. O. Brady, and N. W. Barton.** 1993. Musculocutaneous mononeuropathy complicating *Capnocytophaga canimorsus* infection. *Neurology* **43:**2411–2412.
12. **Bert, F., and N. Lambert-Zechovsky.** 1997. Septicemia caused by *Streptococcus canis* in a human. *J. Clin. Microbiol.* **35:**777–779.
13. **Bharti, A. R., J. E. Nally, J. N. Ricaldi, M. A. Matthias, M. M. Diaz, M. A. Lovett, P. N. Levett, R. H. Gilman, M. R. Willig, E. Gotuzzo, and J. M. Vinetz.** 2003. Leptospirosis: a zoonotic disease of global importance. *Lancet Infect. Dis.* **3:**757–771.
14. **Bildik, N., A. Cevik, M. Altintas, H. Ekinci, M. Canberk, and M. Gulmen.** 2007. Efficacy of preoperative albendazole use according to months in hydatid cyst of the liver. *J. Clin. Gastroenterol.* **41:**312–316.
15. **Birnbaum, N., S. C. Barr, S. A. Center, T. Schermerhorn, J. F. Randolph, and K. W. Simpson.** 1998. Naturally acquired leptospirosis in 36 dogs: serological and clinicopathological features. *J. Small Anim. Pract.* **39:**231–236.
16. **Blaser, M. J., D. N. Taylor, and R. A. Feldman.** 1983. Epidemiology of *Campylobacter jejuni* infections. *Epidemiol. Rev.* **5:**157–176.
17. **Blaser, M. J., J. Cravens, B. W. Powers, and W. L. Wang.** 1978. *Campylobacter* enteritis associated with canine infection. *Lancet* **ii:**979–981.
18. **Blaser, M. J., and L. B. Reller.** 1981. *Campylobacter* enteritis. *N. Engl. J. Med.* **305:**1444–1452.
19. **Bradshaw, S.** 2003. Endocarditis due to *Staphylococcus aureus* after minor dog bite. *South. Med. J.* **96:**407–409.
20. **Buhariwalla, F., B. Cann, and T. J. Marrie.** 1996. A dog related outbreak of Q fever. *Clin. Infect. Dis.* **23:**753–755.

21. **Buishi, I., T. Walters, Z. Guildea, P. Craig, and S. Palmer.** 2005. Reemergence of canine *Echinococcus granulosus* infection, Wales. *Emerg. Infect. Dis.* **11:**568–571.

22. **Buller, R. S., M. Arens, S. P. Hmiel, C. D. Paddock, J. W. Sumner, Y. Rikihisa, A. Unver, M. Gaudreault-Keener, F. A. Manian, A. M. Liddell, N. Schmulewitz, and G. A. Storch.** 1999. *Ehrlichia ewingii,* a newly recognized agent of human ehrlichiosis. *N. Engl. J. Med.* **341:**148–155.

23. **Buogo, C., A. P. Burnens, J. Perrin, and J. Nicolet.** 1995. Presence of *Campylobacter* spp., *Clostridium difficile, C. perfringens,* and salmonellae in litters of puppies and adult dogs in a shelter. *Schweiz. Arch. Tierheilkd.* **137:**165–171.

24. **Butzler, J. P.** 2004. *Campylobacter,* from obscurity to celebrity. *Clin. Microbiol. Infect.* **10:**868–876.

25. **Caumes, E.** 2000. Treatment of cutaneous larva migrans. *Clin. Infect. Dis.* **30:**811–814.

26. **Centers for Disease Control and Prevention.** 2008. Multistate outbreak of human *Salmonella* infections caused by contaminated dry dog food—United States, 2006–2007. *MMWR Morb. Mortal. Wkly. Rep.* **57:**521–524.

27. **Centers for Disease Control and Prevention.** 2007. National antimicrobial resistance monitoring system for enteric bacteria (NARMS): human isolates final report, 2004, p. 41–44. CDC, U.S. Department of Health and Human Services, Atlanta, GA.

28. **Centers for Disease Control and Prevention.** 2006. Diagnosis and management of tickborne rickettsial disease: Rocky Mountain spotted fever, ehrlichiosis, and anaplasmosis—United States: a practical guide for physicians and other healthcare and public health professionals. *MMWR Morb. Mortal. Wkly. Rep.* **55:**1–36.

29. **Centers for Disease Control and Prevention.** 2006. Human salmonellosis associated with animal-derived pet treats—United States and Canada, 2005. *MMWR Morb. Mortal. Wkly. Rep.* **55:**702–705

30. **Centers for Disease Control and Prevention.** 2003. Nonfatal dog bite-related injuries treated in hospital emergency departments—United States, 2001. *MMWR Morb. Mortal. Wkly. Rep.* **52:**605–610.

31. **Centers for Disease Control and Prevention.** 2002. Guidelines for preventing opportunistic infections among HIV-infected persons—2002. *MMWR Morb. Mortal. Wkly. Rep.* **51:**1–46.

32. **Chang, H. J., H. L. Miller, N. Watkins, M. J. Arduino, D. A. Ashford, G. Midgley, S. M. Aguero, R. Pinto-Powell, F. Von Reyn, W. Edwards, M. M. McNeil, and W. R. Jarvis.** 1998. An epidemic of *Malassezia pachydermatis* in an intensive care nursery associated with colonization of health care workers' pet dogs. *N. Engl. J. Med.* **338:**706–711.

33. **Chappell, C. L., and H. M. Penn.** 1990. *Dipylidium caninum,* an underrecognized infection in infants and children. *Pediatr. Infect. Dis. J.* **9:**745–747.

34. **Chen, X. M., J. S. Keithly, C. V. Paya, and N. F. LaRusso.** 2002. Cryptosporidiosis. *N. Engl. J. Med.* **1346:**1723–1731.

35. **Chitkara, R. K., and G. Krishna.** 2006. Parasitic pulmonary eosinophilia. *Semin. Respir. Crit. Care Med.* **27:**171–184.

36. **Ciferri, F.** 1982. Human pulmonary dirofilariasis in the United States: a critical review. *Am. J. Trop. Med. Hyg.* **31:**302–303.

37. **Coelho, L. M., M. V. Silva, C. Y. Dini, A. A. Giacon Neto, N. F. Novo, and E. P. Silveira.** 2004. Human toxocariasis: a seroepidemiological survey in schoolchildren of Sorocaba, Brazil. *Mem. Inst. Oswaldo Cruz* **162:**533–557.

38. **Cohen, S. R.** 1980. *Cheyletiella* dermatitis. A mite infestation of rabbit, cat, dog, and man. *Arch. Dermatol.* **116:**435–437.

39. **Cook, G. C.** 1989. Canine-associated zoonoses: an unacceptable hazard to human health. *Q. J. Med.* **70:**5–26.

40. **Current, W. L.** 1988. The biology of *Cryptosporidium. ASM News* **54:**605–611.

41. **Dayal, Y., and R. C. Neafie.** 1975. Human pulmonary dirofilariasis: a case report and review of the literature. *Am. Rev. Respir. Dis.* **112:**437–443.

42. **Despommier, D.** 2003. Toxocariasis: clinical aspects, epidemiology, medical ecology, and molecular aspects. *Clin. Microbiol. Rev.* **16:**265–272.

43. **Dogru, D., N. Kiper, U. Ozcelik, E. Yalcin, and A. Gocmen.** 2005. Medical treatment of pulmonary hydatid disease: for which child? *Parasitol. Int.* **54:**135–138.

44. **Dumler, J. S., A. F. Barbet, C. P. J. Bekker, G. A. Dasch, G. H. Palmer, S. C. Ray, Y. Rikihisa, and F. R. Rurangirwa.** 2001. Reorganization of genera in the families *Rickettsiaceae* and *Anaplasmataceae* in the order *Rickettsiales:* unification of some species of *Ehrlichia* with *Anaplasma, Cowdria* with *Ehrlichia* and *Ehrlichia* with *Neorickettsia,* descriptions of six new species combinations and designation of *Ehrlichia equi* and 'HGE agent' as subjective synonyms of *Ehrlichia phagocytophila. Int. J. Syst. Evol. Microbiol.* **51:**2145–2165.

45. **Dumler, J. S., and J. S. Bakken.** 1995. Ehrlichial diseases of humans: emerging tick-borne infections. *Clin. Infect. Dis.* **20:**1102–1110.

46. **Dunn, J. J., S. T. Columbus, W. E. Aldeen, M. Davis, and K. C. Carroll.** 2002. *Trichuris vulpis* recovered from a patient with chronic diarrhea and five dogs. *J. Clin. Microbiol.* **40:**2703–2704.

47. **Eberhardt, O., R. Bialek, T. Nagele, and J. Dichgans.** 2005. Eosinophilic meningomyelitis in toxocariasis: case report and review of the literature. *Clin. Neurol. Neurosurg.* **107:**432–438.

48. **Eckert, J., and P. Deplazes.** 2004. Biological, epidemiological, and clinical aspects of echinococcosis, a zoonosis of increasing concern. *Clin. Microbiol. Rev.* **17:**107–135.

49. **Ehrbar, H. U., J. Gubler, S. Harbarth, and B. Hirschel.** 1996. *Capnocytophaga canimorsus* sepsis complicated by myocardial infarction in two patients with normal coronary arteries. *Clin. Infect. Dis.* **23:**335–336.

50. **Elenbaas, R. M., W. K. McNabney, and W. A. Robinson.** 1981. Prophylactic antibiotics and dog bite wounds. *JAMA* **246:**833–834.

51. **Elliot, D. L., S. W. Tolle, L. Goldberg, and J. B. Miller.** 1985. Pet-associated illness. *N. Engl. J. Med.* **313:**985–995.

52. **Engvall, E. O., B. Brandstrom, L. Andersson, V. Baverud, G. Trowald-Wigh, and L. Englund.** 2003. Isolation and identification of thermophilic *Campylobacter* species in faecal samples from Swedish dogs. *Scand. J. Infect. Dis.* **35:**713–718.

53. **Falagas, M. E., and I. A. Bliziotis.** 2006. Quinolones for treatment of human brucellosis: critical review of the evidence from microbiological and clinical studies. *Antimicrob. Agents Chemother.* **50:**22–33

54. **Fang, G., V. Araujo, and R. L. Guerrant.** 1991. Enteric infections associated with exposure to animals or animal products. *Infect. Dis. Clin. N. Am.* **5:**681–700.

55. **Fayer, R., and B. L. P. Ungar.** 1986. Cryptosporidium spp. and cryptosporidiosis. *Microbiol. Rev.* **50:**458–483.

56. **Fayer, R., J. M. Trout, L. Xiao, U. M. Morgan, A. A. Lal, and J. P. Dubey.** 2001. *Cryptosporidium canis* n. sp. from domestic dogs. *J. Parasitol.* **87:**1415–1422.

57. **Feigin, R. D., L. A. Lober, D. Anderson, and L. Pickering.** 1973. Human leptospirosis from immunized dogs. *Ann. Intern. Med.* **79:**777–785.

58. **Filice, C., E. Brunetti, R. Bruno, F. G. Crippa, et al.** 2000. Percutaneous drainage of echinococcal cysts (PAIR—puncture, aspiration, injection, reaspiration): results of a worldwide survey for assessment of its safety and efficacy. *Gut* **47:**156–157.

59. **Finley, R., R. Reid-Smith, and J. S. Weese.** 2006. Human health implications of *Salmonella*-contaminated natural pet treats and raw pet food. *Clin. Infect. Dis.* **42:**686–691.

60. **Fleisher, G. R.** 1999. The management of bite wounds. *N. Engl. J. Med.* **340:**138–140.

61. **Franchi, C., B. Di Vico, and A. Teggi.** 1999. Long-term evaluation of patients with hydatidosis treated with benzimidazole carbamates. *Clin. Infect. Dis.* **29:**304–309.

62. **Frider, B., E. Larrieu, and M. Odriozola.** 1999. Long-term outcome of asymptomatic liver hydatidosis. *J. Hepatol.* **30:**228–231.

63. **Friedmann, E., A. H. Katcher, J. J. Lynch, and S. A. Thomas.** 1980. Animal companions and one-year survival of patients after discharge from a coronary care unit. *Public Health Rep.* **95:**307–312.

64. **Fox, L. A., and L. D. Saravolatz.** 2005. Nitazoxanide: a new thiazolide antiparasitic agent. *Clin. Infect. Dis.* **40:**1173–1180.

65. **Galpérine, T., C. Cazoria, E. Blanchard, F. Boineau, J.-M. Ragnaud, and D. Neau.** 2007. *Streptococcus canis* infections in humans: a retrospective study of 54 patients. *J. Infect.* **55:**23–26.

66. **Gardner, T. B., and D. R. Hill.** 2001. Treatment of giardiasis. *Clin. Microbiol. Rev.* **14:**114–128.

67. **Geisen, V., C. Stengel, S. Brem, W. Muller, C. Greene, and K. Hartmann.** 2007. Canine leptospirosis infections—clinical signs and outcomes with different suspected *Leptospira* serogroups (42 cases). *J. Small Anim. Pract.* **48:**324–328.

68. **Georgi, J. R.** 1987. Tapeworms. *Vet. Clin. N. Am. Small Anim. Pract.* **17:**1285–1305.

69. **Gillespie, S. H.** 2004. Cutaneous larva migrans. *Curr. Infect. Dis. Rep.* **6:**50–53.

70. **Glaser, C. A., F. J. Angulo, and J. A. Rooney.** 1994. Animal-associated opportunistic infections among persons infected with the human immunodeficiency virus. *Clin. Infect. Dis.* **18:**14–24.

71. **Glickman, L. T., and F. S. Shofer.** 1987. Zoonotic visceral and ocular larva migrans. *Vet. Clin. N. Am. Small Anim. Pract.* **17:**39–53.

72. **Glickman, L. T., and P. M. Schantz.** 1981. Epidemiology and pathogenesis of zoonotic toxocariasis. *Epidemiol. Rev.* **3:**230–250.

73. **Gnann, J. W., G. S. Bressler, C. A. Bodet, and C. K. Avent.** 1983. Human blastomycosis after a dog bite. *Ann. Intern. Med.* **160:**48–49.

74. **Goldstein, E. J. C.** 1991. Household pets and human infections. *Infect. Dis. Clin. N. Am.* **5:**117–130.

75. **Goldstein, E. J. C.** 1999. Current concepts on animal bites: bacteriology and therapy. *Curr. Clin. Top. Infect. Dis.* **19:**99–111.

76. **Goldstein, E. J. C., D. M. Citron, B. Wield, V. Blachman, V. L. Sutter, T. A. Miller, and S. M. Finegold.** 1978. Bacteriology of human and animal bite wounds. *J. Clin. Microbiol.* **8:**667–672.

77. **Grove, D. I., K. S. Warren, and A. A. F. Mahmoud.** 1976. Algorithms in the diagnosis and management of exotic diseases. X. Echinococcosis. *J. Infect. Dis.* **133:**354–358.

78. **Guerrant, R. L., T. van Gilder, T. S. Steiner, N. M. Thielman, L. Slutsker, R. V. Tauxe, T. Hennessy, P. M. Griffin, H. DuPont, R. B. Sack, P. Tarr, M. Neill, I. Nachamkin, L. B. Reller, M. T. Osterholm, M. L. Bennish, and L. K. Pickering.** 2001. Practice guidelines for the management of infectious diarrhea. *Clin. Infect. Dis.* **32:**331–351.

79. **Hald, B., K. Pederson, M. Waino, J. C. Jorgensen, and M. Madsen.** 2004. Longitudinal study of excretion patterns of thermophilic *Campylobacter* spp. in young pet dogs in Denmark. *J. Clin. Microbiol.* **42:**2003–2012.

80. **Hamnes, I. S., B. K. Gjerde, and L. J. Robertson.** 2007. A longitudinal study on the occurrence of *Cryptosporidium* and *Giardia* in dogs during their first year of life. *Acta Vet. Scand.* **49:**22–31.

81. **Hannu, T., L. Mattila, H. Rautelin, A. Siitonen, and M. Leirisalo-Repo.** 2005. Three cases of cardiac complications associated with *Campylobacter jejuni* infection and review of the literature. *Eur. J. Clin. Microbiol. Infect. Dis.* **24:**619–622.

82. **Harrison, E. G., Jr., and J. H. Thompson.** 1965. Dirofilariasis of human lung. *Am. J. Clin. Pathol.* **43:**224–234.

83. **Hasanjani Roushan, M. R., M. Mohraz, M. Hajiahmadi, A. Ramzani, and A. A. Valayati.** 2006. Efficacy of gentamicin plus doxycycline versus streptomycin plus doxycycline in the treatment of brucellosis in humans. *Clin. Infect. Dis.* **42:**1075–1080.

84. **Hasi, D. K., J. A. Collins, and S. C. Flick.** 1978. Canine parasitism. *Canine Pract.* **2:**42–47.

85. **Havin, T. R., and D. D. Juranek.** 1984. Cryptosporidiosis: clinical, epidemiologic and parasitologic review. *Rev. Infect. Dis.* **6:**313–327.

86. **Hewitt, M., G. S. Walton, and M. Waterhouse.** 1971. Pet animal infestations and human skin lesions. *Br. J. Dermatol.* **85:**215–225.

87. **Hicklin, H., A. Verghese, and S. Alvarez.** 1987. Dysgonic fermenter-2 septicemia. *Rev. Infect. Dis.* **9:**884–890.

88. **Horton, R. J.** 1997. Albendazole in treatment of human cystic echinococcosis: 12 years of experience. *Acta Trop.* **64:**79–93.

89. **Humbert, P., S. Buchet, and T. Barde.** 1995. Toxocariasis: a cosmopolitan parasitic zoonosis. *Allerg. Immunol.* (Paris) **27:**284–291.

90. **Hunter, P. R., and R. C. A. Thompson.** 2005. The zoonotic transmission of *Giardia* and *Cryptosporidium*. *Int. J. Parasitol.* **35:**1181–1190.

91. **Jacquier, P., B. Gottstein, Y. Stingelin, and J. Eckert.** 1991. Immunodiagnosis of toxocariasis in humans: evolution of a new enzyme-linked immunosorbent assay kit. *J. Clin. Microbiol.* **29:**1831–1835.

92. **Janda, J. M., M. H. Graves, D. Lindquist, and W. S. Probert.** 2006. Diagnosing *Capnocytophaga canimorsus* infections. *Emerg. Infect. Dis.* **12:**340–342.

93. **Jelinek, T., H. Maiwald, H. D. Nothdurft, and T. Löscher.** 1994. Cutaneous larva migrans in travelers: synopsis of histories, symptoms, and treatment of 98 patients. *Clin. Infect. Dis.* **19:**1062–1066.

94. **Jimenez-Coello, M., I. Vado-Solis, M. F. Cardenas-Marrufo, J. C. Rodriguez-Buenfil, and A. Ortega-Pacheco.** 2008. Serological survey of canine leptospirosis in the tropics of Yucatan Mexico using two different tests. *Acta Trop.* **106:**22–26.

95. **Johnson, J. R., and C. Clabots.** 2006. Sharing of virulent *Escherichia coli* clones among household members of a woman with acute cystitis. *Clin. Infect. Dis.* **43:**e101–e108.

96. **Johnson, J. R., K. Owens, A. Gajewski, and C. Clabots.** 2008. *Escherichia coli* colonization patterns among human household members and pets, with attention to acute urinary tract infection. *J. Infect. Dis.* **197:**218–224.

97. **Juckett, G.** 1997. Pets and parasites. *Am. Fam. Physician* **56:**1763–1774.

98. **Kaldor, J., and B. R. Speed.** 1984. Guillain-Barré syndrome and *Campylobacter jejuni*: a serologic study. *Br. Med. J.* **288:**1867–1870.

99. **Katz, A. R., V. E. Ansdell, P. V. Effler, C. R. Middleton, and D. M. Sasaki.** 2001. Assessment of the clinical presentation and treatment of 353 cases of laboratory confirmed leptospirosis in Hawaii, 1974–1998. *Clin. Infect. Dis.* **33:**1834–1841.

100. **Khuroo, M. S., N. A. Wani, G. Javid, B. A. Khan, G. N. Yattoo, A. H. Shah, and S. G. Jeelani.** 1997. Percutaneous drainage compared with surgery for hepatic hydatid cysts. *N. Engl. J. Med.* **337:**881–887.

101. **Klaasen, H. L., M. J. Molkenboer, M. P. Vrijenhoek, and M. J. Kaashoek.** 2003. Duration of immunity in dogs vaccinated against leptospirosis with a bivalent inactivated vaccine. *Vet. Microbiol.* **95:**121–132.

102. **Knauer, K. W.** 1998. Human dirofilariasis. *Clin. Tech. Small Anim. Pract.* **13:**96–98.

103. **Koene, M. G., D. J. Houwers, J. R. Dijkstra, B. Duim, and J. A. Wagenaar.** 2004. Simultaneous presence of multiple *Campylobacter* species in dogs. *J. Clin. Microbiol.* **42:**918–821.

104. **Komnenou, A. A., M. E. Mylonakis, V. Kouti, L. Tendoma, L. Leontides, E. Skountzou, A. Dessiris, A. F. Koutinas, and R. Ofri.** 2007. Ocular manifestations of natural canine monocytic ehrlichiosis *(Ehrlichia canis):* a retrospective study of 90 cases. *Vet. Ophthalmol.* **10:**137–142.

105. **Kosunen, T. U., O. Kauranen, J. Martio, T. P. Aponka, L. Hortling, S. Aittoniemi, O. Penttila, and S. Koskimies.** 1980. Reactive arthritis after *Campylobacter jejuni* enteritis in patients with HLA-B27. *Lancet* **i:**1312–1313.

106. **Labarca, J. A., J. Sturgeon, L. Borenstein, N. Salem, S. M. Harvey, E. Lehnkering, R. Reporter, and L. Mascola.** 2002. *Campylobacter upsaliensis:* another pathogen for consideration in the United States. *Clin. Infect. Dis.* **34:**59–60.

107. **Lam, M. M., J. E. Clarridge III, E. J. Young, and S. Mizuki.** 2007. The other group G streptococcus: increased detection of *Streptococcus canis* ulcer infections in dog owners. *J. Clin. Microbiol.* **45:**2327–2329.

108. **Lauer, E. A., W. C. White, and B. A. Lauer.** 1982. Dog bites: a neglected problem in accident prevention. *Am. J. Dis. Child.* **136:**202–204.

109. **Le Moal, G., C. Landron, G. Grollier, R. Robert, and C. Burucoa.** 2003. Meningitis due to *Capnocytophaga canimorsus* after receipt of a dog bite: case report and review of the literature. *Clin. Infect. Dis.* **36:**e42–e46.

110. **Leoni, F., C. Amar, G. Nichols, S. Pedraza-Diaz, and J. McLauchlin.** 2006. Genetic analysis of *Cryptosporidium* from 2414 humans with diarrhoea in England between 1985 and 2000. *J. Med. Microbiol.* **55:**703–707.

111. **Levett, P. N.** 2001. Leptospirosis. *Clin. Microbiol. Rev.* **14:**296–326.

112. **Lindsay, D. S., J. P. Dubey, and B. L. Blagburn.** 1997. Biology of *Isospora* spp. from humans, nonhuman primates, and domestic animals. *Clin. Microbiol. Rev.* **10:**19–34.

113. **Liu, L. X., and P. F. Weller.** 1998. Trichinosis and infections with other tissue nematodes, p. 1206–1208. *In* A. S. Fauci, E. Braunwald, K. J. Isselbacher, J. D. Wilson, J. B. Martin, D. L. Kasper, S. L. Hauser, and D. L. Longo (ed.), *Harrison's Principles of Internal Medicine.* McGraw-Hill, New York, NY.

114. **Lorenzo, C., H. B. Ferreira, K. M. Monteiro, M. Rosenzvit, L. Kamenetzky, H. H. Garcia, Y. Vasquez, C. Naquira, E. Sanchez, M. Lorca, M. Contreras, J. A. Last, and G. G. Gonzalez-Sapienza.** 2005. Comparative analysis of the diagnostic performance of six major *Echinococcus granulosus* antigens assessed in a double-blind randomized multicenter study. *J. Clin. Microbiol.* **43:**2764–2770.

115. **Magnaval, J. F., L. T. Glickman, P. Dorchies, and B. Morassin.** 2001. Highlights of human toxocariasis. *Korean J. Parasitol.* **39:**1–11.

116. **Maurin, M., and D. Raoult.** 1999. Q fever. *Clin. Microbiol. Rev.* **12:**518–553.

117. **Mayer, G., and S. VanOre.** 1983. Recurrent pharyngitis in family of four. *Postgrad. Med.* **74:**277–279.

118. **McManus, D. P., W. Zhang, J. Li, and P. D. Bartley.** 2003. Echinococcosis. *Lancet* **362:**1295–1304.

119. **Medeiros, I., and H. Saconato.** 2001. Antibiotic prophylaxis for mammalian bites. *Cochrane Database Syst. Rev.* **2:**CD001738.

120. **Merrill, J. R., J. Otis, W. D. Logan, Jr., and B. Davis.** 1980. The dog heartworm *(Dirofilaria immitis)* in man: an epidemic pending or in progress? *JAMA* **243:**1066–1068.

121. **Mitchell, I., N. McNellis, F. J. Bowden, and G. Nikolic.** 2002. Electrocardiographic myocardial infarction pattern in overwhelming post-splenectomy sepsis due to *Capnocytophaga canimorsus. Intern. Med. J.* **22:**415–418.

122. **Mohamed, A. E., M. I. Yasawy, and M. A. Al Karawi.** 1998. Combined albendazole and praziquantel versus albendazole alone in the treatment of hydatid disease. *Hepatogastroenterology* **45:**1690–1694.

123. **Molina, C. P., J. Ogburn, and P. Adegboyega.** 2003. Infection by *Dipylidium caninum* in an infant. *Arch. Pathol. Lab. Med.* **127:**e157–e159.

124. **Moro, P., and P. M. Schantz.** 2006. Cystic echinococcosis in the Americas. *Parasitol. Int.* **55:**S181–S186.

125. **Mulder, A. H., P. G. Gerlag, L. H. Verhoef, and A. W. van den Wall Bake.** 2001. Hemolytic uremic syndrome after *Capnocytophaga canimorsus* (DF-2) septicemia. *Clin. Nephrol.* **55:**167–170.

126. **Muro, A., C. Genchi, M. Cordero, and F. Simon.** 1999. Human dirofilariasis in the European Union. *Parasitol. Today* **15:**386–389.

127. **Nerad, J. L., and S. Black.** 2004. Miscellaneous gram negative bacilli: Acinetobacter, Cardiobacterium, Actinobacillus, Chromobacterium, Capnocytophaga, and others, p. 1751–1761. *In* S. L. Gorbach, J. G. Bartlett, and N. R. Blacklow (ed.), *Infectious Diseases,* 3rd ed. Lippincott, Williams, and Wilkins, Philadelphia, PA.

128. **Nicoletti, A., V. Sofia, A. Mantella, G. Vitale, D. Contrafatto, V. Sorbello, R. Biondi, P. M. Preux, H. H. Garcia, M. Zappia, and A. Bartoloni.** 2008. Epilepsy and toxocariasis: a case-control study in Italy. *Epilepsia* **49:**594–599.

129. **Olsen, S. J., E. E. DeBess, T. E. McGivern, N. Marano, T. Eby, S. Mauvais, V. K.**

Balan, G. Zirnstein, P. R. Cieslak, and F. J. Angulo. 2001. A nosocomial outbreak of fluoroquinolone-resistant *Salmonella* infection. *N. Engl. J. Med.* **344:**1572–1579.

130. Ortiz, J. J., A. Ayoub, and N. L. Gargala. 2001. Randomized clinical study of nitazoxanide compared to metronidazole in the treatment of symptomatic giardiasis in children from northern Peru. *Aliment. Pharmacol. Ther.* **15:** 1409–1415.

131. Paderes, C., C. Zanartu, and G. Castillo. 2001. Environmental contamination with *Toxocara* sp. eggs in public squares and parks from Santiago, Chile, 1999. *Bol. Chil. Parasitol.* **55:** 86–91.

132. Panaphut, T., S. Domrongkitchaiporn, A. Vibhagool, B. Thinkamrop, and W. Susaengrat. 2003. Ceftriaxone compared with sodium penicillin G for treatment of severe leptospirosis. *Clin. Infect. Dis.* **36:**1507–1513.

133. Pappas, G., N. Akritidis, M. Bosilkovski, and E. Tsianos. 2005. Brucellosis. *N. Engl. J. Med.* **352:**2325–2336.

134. Pawlowski, Z. S., J. Eckert, D. A. Vuitton, R. W. Ammann, P. Kern, P. S. Craig, F. K. Dar, F. De Rosa, C. Filice, B. Gottstein, F. Grimm, C. N. L. Macpherson, N. Sato, T. Todorov, J. Uchino, W. von Sinner, and H. Wen. 2001. Echinococcosis in humans: clinical aspects, diagnosis and treatment, p. 20–66. *In* J. Eckert, M. A. Gemmell, F. X. Meslin, and Z. S. Pawlowski (ed.), *WHO/OIE Manual on Echinococcosis in Humans and Animals: a Public Health Problem of Global Concern.* World Organization for Animal Health, Paris, France.

135. Perez, M., M. Bodor, C. Zhang, Q. Xiong, and Y. Rikihisa. 2006. Human infection with *Ehrlichia canis* accompanied by clinical signs in Venezuela. *Ann. N. Y. Acad. Sci.* **1087:**110–117.

136. Pers, C., B. Gahrn-Hansen, and W. Frederiksen. 1996. *Capnocytophaga canimorsus* septicemia in Denmark, 1982–1995: review of 39 cases. *Clin. Infect. Dis.* **23:**71–75.

137. Polizopoulou, Z. S., A. F. Koutinas, M. N. Saridomichelakis, M. N. Patsikas, L. S. Leontidis, N. A. Roubies, and A. K. Desiris. 2000. Clinical and laboratory observations in 91 dogs infected with *Dirofilaria immitis* in northern Greece. *Vet. Rec.* **146:**466–469.

138. Polt, S. S., W. E. Dismukes, A. Flint, and J. Schaefer. 1982. Human brucellosis caused by *Brucella canis*: clinical features and immune response. *Ann. Intern. Med.* **97:**717–719.

139. Puylaert, J. B., R. J. Vermeijden, S. D. van der Werf, L. Doornbos, and R. K. Koumans. 1989. Incidence and sonographic diagnosis of bacterial ileocaecitis masquerading as appendicitis. *Lancet* **ii:**84–86.

140. Rolando, I., L. Olarte, G. Vilchez, M. Lluncor, L. Otero, M. Paris, C. Carrillo, and E. Gotuzzo. 2008. Ocular manifestations associated with brucellosis: a 26-year experience in Peru. *Clin. Infect. Dis.* **46:**1338–1345.

141. Rossignol, J. F. 2006. Nitazoxanide in the treatment of acquired immune deficiency syndrome-related cryptosporidiosis: results of the United States compassionate use program in 365 patients. *Aliment. Pharmacol. Ther.* **24:**887–894.

142. Rossignol, J. F., A. Ayoub, and M. S. Ayers. 2001. Treatment of diarrhea caused by *Cryptosporidium parvum*: a prospective randomized, double-blind, placebo-controlled study of nitazoxanide. *J. Infect. Dis.* **184:**103–106.

143. Rubel, D., A. Seijo, B. Cernigoi, A. Viale, and C. Wisnivesky-Colli. 1997. *Leptospira interrogans* in a canine population of Greater Buenos Aires: variables associated with seropositivity. *Pan Am. J. Public Health* **2:**102–105.

144. Sakai, S., Y. Shida, N. Takahashi, H. Yabuuchi, H. Soeda, T. Okafuji, M. Hatakenaka, and H. Honda. 2006. Pulmonary lesions associated with visceral larva migrans due to *Ascaris suum* or *Toxocara canis*: imaging of six cases. *AJR Am. J. Roentgenol.* **186:**1697–1702.

145. Salfield, N. J., and E. J. Pugh. 1987. *Campylobacter* enteritis in young children living in households with puppies. *Br. Med. J.* **294:**21–22.

146. Sandoe, J. A. 2004. *Capnocytophaga canimorsus* endocarditis. *J. Med. Microbiol.* **53:**245–248.

147. Sauret, J. M., and N. Vilissova. 2002. Human brucellosis. *J. Am. Board Fam. Pract.* **15:** 401–406.

148. Scanziani, E., F. Origgi, A. M. Giusti, G. Iacchia, A. Vasino, G. Pirovano, P. Scarpa, and S. Tagliabue. 2002. Serological survey of leptospiral infection in kenneled dogs in Italy. *J. Small Anim. Pract.* **43:**154–157.

149. Schaefer, J. W., and Y. M. Khan. 1991. Echinococcus (hydatid disease): lessons from experience with 59 patients. *Rev. Infect. Dis.* **13:** 243–247.

150. Schantz, P. M., and L. T. Glickman. 1978. Toxocaral visceral larva migrans. *N. Engl. J. Med.* **298:**436–439.

151. Schieven, B. C., M. Brennan, and Z. Hussain. 1991. *Echinococcus granulosus* hydatid disease. *ASM News* **57:**407–410.

152. Schmidt, D. R., R. E. Winn, and T. J. Keefe. 1989. Leptospirosis: epidemiologic features of a sporadic case. *Arch. Intern. Med.* **149:** 1878–1880.

153. Scott, D. W., and R. T. Horn, Jr. 1987. Zoonotic dermatoses of dogs and cats. *Vet. Clin. N. Am. Small Anim. Pract.* **17:**117–144.

154. Scully, R., E. J. Mark, W. F. McNeely, and B. U. McNeely. 1987. Case records of the Massachusetts General Hospital, case 45-1987. *N. Engl. J. Med.* **317:**1209–1218.

155. Shetty, A. K., and D. H. Aviles. 1999. Nephrotic syndrome associated with *Toxocara canis* infection. *Ann. Trop. Paediatr.* **19:**297–300.

156. Simon, F., J. Lopez-Belmonte, C. Marcos-Atxutegi, R. Morchon, and J. R. Martin-Pacho. 2005. What is happening outside North America regarding human dirofilariasis? *Vet. Parasitol.* **133:**181–189.

157. Simon, F., L. H. Kramer, A. Roman, W. Blasini, R. Morchon, C. Marcos-Atxutegi, G. Grandi, and C. Genchi. 2007. Immunopathology of *Dirofilaria immitis* infection. *Vet. Res. Commun.* **31:**161–171.

158. Singer, A. J., and A. B. Dagum. 2008. Current management of acute cutaneous wounds. *N. Engl. J. Med.* **359:**1037–1046.

159. Smith, F. B., and T. F. Claypoole. 1967. Canine scabies in dogs and in humans. *JAMA* **199:**95–100.

160. Smith, H. V., and G. D. Corcoran. 2004. New drugs and treatment for cryptosporidiosis. *Curr. Opin. Infect. Dis.* **17:**557–564.

161. Solera, J., E. Martinez-Alfaro, and L. Saez. 1994. Meta-analysis of the efficacy of rifampicin and doxycycline in the treatment of human brucellosis. *Med. Clin.* (Barcelona) **102:**731–738.

162. Spielman, A., and M. Wachtel. 1998. Arthropods, p. 2499–2513. *In* S. L. Gorbach, J. G. Bartlett, and N. R. Blacklow (ed.), *Infectious Diseases,* 2nd ed. W. B. Saunders Company, Philadelphia, PA.

163. Stasi, M. F., D. Amati, C. Costa, D. Resta, G. Senepa, C. Scarafioti, N. Aimonino, and M. Molaschi. 2004. Pet-therapy: a trial for institutionalized frail elderly patients. *Arch. Gerontol. Geriatr.* **9:**407–412.

164. Stehr-Green, J. K., G. Murray, P. M. Schantz, and S. P. Wahlquist. 1987. Intestinal parasites in pet store puppies in Atlanta. *Am. J. Public Health* **77:**345–346.

165. Sunnotel, O., C. J. Lowery, J. E. Moore, J. S. G. Dooley, L. Xiao, B. C. Millar, P. J. Rooney, and W. J. Snelling. 2006. *Cryptosporidium. Lett. Appl. Microbiol.* **43:**7–16.

166. Supputtamongkol, Y., K. Niwattayakul, C. Suttinont, K. Losuwanaluk, R. Limpaiboon, W. Chierakul, V. Wuthiekanum, S. Triengrim, M. Chenchittikul, and N. J. White. 2004. An open, randomized, controlled trial of penicillin, doxycycline, and cefotaxime for patients with severe leptospirosis. *Clin. Infect. Dis.* **39:**1417–1424.

167. Takafuji, E. T., J. W. Kirkpatrick, R. N. Miller, J. J. Karwacki, P. W. Kelley, M. R. Gray, K. M. McNeil, H. L. Timboe, R. E. Kane, and J. L. Sanchez. 1984. An efficacy trial of doxycycline chemoprophylaxis against leptospirosis. *N. Engl. J. Med.* **310:**497–500.

168. Takeda, N., K. Kikuchi, R. Asano, T. Harada, K. Totsuka, T. Sumiyoshi, T. Uchiyama, and S. Hosoda. 2001. Recurrent septicemia caused by *Streptococcus canis* after a dog bite. *Scand. J. Infect. Dis.* **33:**927–928.

169. Talan, D. A., D. M. Citron, F. M. Abrahamian, G. J. Moran, E. J. C. Goldstein, and the Emergency Medicine Animal Bite Study Group. 1999. Bacteriologic analysis of infected dog and cat bites. *N. Engl. J. Med.* **34:**85–92.

170. Tan, J. S. 1997. Human zoonotic infections transmitted by dogs and cats. *Arch. Intern. Med.* **157:**1933–1943.

171. Taylor, D. H., and D. L. Morris. 1989. Combination chemotherapy is more effective in post spillage prophylaxis for hydatid disease than either albendazole or praziquantel alone. *Br. J. Surg.* **76:**954.

172. Tenkate, T. D., and R. J. Stafford. 2001. Risk factors for *Campylobacter* infection in infants and young children: a matched case-control study. *Epidemiol. Infect.* **127:**399–404.

173. Thompson, R. C. A., C. S. Palmer, and R. O'Handley. 2008. The public health and clinical significance of *Giardia* and *Cryptosporidium* in domestic animals. *Vet. J.* **177:**18–25.

174. Thomsett, L. R. 1968. Mite infestations of man contracted from dogs and cats. *Br. Med. J.* **3:**93–95.

175. Tierney, D. M., L. P. Strauus, and J. L. Sanchez. 2006. *Capnocytophaga canimorsus* mycotic abdominal aortic aneurysm: why the mailman is afraid of dogs. *J. Clin. Microbiol.* **44:**649–651.

176. Traub, R. J., I. D. Robertson, P. Irwin, N. Mencke, and R. C. Thompson. 2002. The role of dogs in transmission of gastrointestinal parasites in a remote tea-growing community in northeastern India. *Am. J. Trop. Med. Hyg.* **67:**539–545.

177. Traub, R. J., R. T. Monis, I. Robertson, P. Irwin, N. Mencke, and R. C. Thompson. 2004. Epidemiological and molecular evidence supports the zoonotic transmission of *Giardia* among humans and dogs living in the same community. *Parasitology* **128:**253–262.

178. Tsianakas, P., B. Polack, L. Pinquier, B. Levy Klotz, and C. Prost-Squarcioni. 2000.

Cheyletiella dermatitis: an uncommon cause of vesiculobullous eruption. *Ann. Dermatol. Venereol.* **127:**826–829.

179. **Tsung, S. H., J. I. Lin, and D. Han.** 1982. Pulmonary dirofilariasis in man. *Am. J. Med. Sci.* **283:**106–110.

180. **Turner, J. A.** 1962. Human dipylidiasis (dog tapeworm infection) in the United States. *J. Pediatr.* **61:**763–768.

181. **Tzipori, S., and I. Campbell.** 1981. Prevalence of *Cryptosporidium* antibodies in 10 animal species. *J. Clin. Microbiol.* **14:**455–456.

182. **Vinetz, J. M.** 2003. A mountain out of a molehill: do we treat acute leptospirosis, and if so, with what? *Clin. Infect. Dis.* **36:**1514–1515.

183. **Wanke, M. M.** 2004. Canine brucellosis. *Anim. Reprod. Sci.* **82–83:**195–207.

184. **Weber, D. J., and A. R. Hansen.** 1991. Infections resulting from animal bites. *Infect. Dis. Clin. N. Am.* **5:**663–680.

185. **Weiss, H. B., D. I. Friedman, and J. H. Coben.** 1998. Incidence of dog bite injuries treated in emergency departments. *JAMA* **279:**51–53.

186. **Willard, M. D., B. Sugarman, and R. D. Walker.** 1987. Gastrointestinal zoonoses. *Vet. Clin. N. Am. Small Anim. Pract.* **17:**145–178.

187. **Wilson, K. S., S. Antone, and R. M. Gander.** 1995. The family pet as an unlikely source of group A beta-hemolytic streptococcal infection in humans. *Pediatr. Infect. Dis. J.* **14:**372–375.

188. **Wolfs, T. F., B. Duim, S. P. Geelen, A. Ritger, F. Thomson-Carter, A. Fleer, and J. A. Wagenaar.** 2001. Neonatal sepsis by *Campylobacter jejuni:* genetically proven transmission from a household puppy. *Clin. Infect. Dis.* **32:**97–99.

189. **Woodruff, A. W., B. Bisseru, and J. C. Bowe.** 1966. Infection with animal helminthes

as a factor in causing poliomyelitis and epilepsy. *Br. Med. J.* **1:**1576–1579.

190. **World Health Organization.** 2001. PAIR: puncture, aspiration, injection, re-aspiration. An option for treatment of cystic echinococcosis. World Health Organization, Geneva, Switzerland. http://whqlibdoc.who.int/hq/2001/WHO_CDS_CSR_APH_2001.6.pdf. [Accessed 10 October 2008.]

191. **Wormser, G. P., R. J. Dattwyler, E. D. Shapiro, J. J. Halperin, A. C. Steere, M. S. Klempner, P. J. Krause, J. S. Bakken, F. Strle, G. Stanek, L. Bockenstedt, D. Fish, J. S. Dumler, and R. B. Nadelman.** 2006. The clinical assessment, treatment, and prevention of Lyme disease, human granulocytic anaplasmosis, and babesiosis: clinical practice guidelines by the Infectious Diseases Society of America. *Clin. Infect. Dis.* **43:**1089–1134.

192. **Xiao, L., R. Fayer, U. Ryan, and S. J. Upton.** 2004. *Cryptosporidium* taxonomy: recent advances and implications for public health. *Clin. Microbiol. Rev.* **17:**72–97.

193. **Xiao, L., and U. M. Ryan.** 2004. Cryptosporidiosis: an update in molecular epidemiology. *Curr. Opin. Infect. Dis.* **17:**483–490.

194. **Xiao, L., V. A. Cama, L. Cabrera, Y. Ortega, J. Pearson, and R. H. Gilman.** 2007. Possible transmission of *Cryptosporidium canis* among children and a dog in a household. *J. Clin. Microbiol.* **45:**2014–2016.

195. **Yoder, J. S., M. J. Beach, and the Centers for Disease Control and Prevention.** 2007. Cryptosporidiosis surveillance—United States, 2003–2005. *MMWR Surveill. Summ.* **56**(SS07):1–10.

196. **Yoder, J. S., M. J. Beach, and the Centers for Disease Control and Prevention.** 2007. Giardiasis surveillance—United States, 2003–2005. *MMWR Surveill. Summ.* **56**(SS07):11–18.

AROUND CATS

Ellie J. C. Goldstein and Craig E. Greene

6

The origins of the domestic cat are unknown. However, mummified cats have been found in the treasure rooms of the Egyptian pyramids, and their images are inscribed in the royal hieroglyphics. The genus *Felis* includes the modern domestic house cat as well as the puma (cougar), golden cats, jaguarundi, ocelot, serval, lynx, and bobcat. Today it is estimated that more than 88.3 million cats are kept as household pets in the United States and that 34% of households have cats (41). There are numerous diseases that may be transmitted from cats to humans or that cats and people acquire from common sources, some of which are described in this chapter (13, 32, 33, 47). However, it is likely that the domestic cat can act as a reservoir for many other zoonoses that are as yet unrecognized (33). The diseases discussed are arranged by the general method of transmission from cat to person, although more than one route is possible for certain infections.

Ellie J. C. Goldstein, R. M. Alden Research Laboratory, Santa Monica, CA 90404, and UCLA School of Medicine, Los Angeles, CA 90024. *Craig E. Greene*, Department of Small Animal Medicine, College of Veterinary Medicine, University of Georgia, Athens, GA 30602.

TRANSMISSION BY INHALATION

Bordetellosis

Bordetella bronchiseptica is a gram-negative coccobacillus that causes a pertussis-like illness (whooping cough) in humans, especially children. It can be found in the respiratory tracts of clinically healthy or ill animals, including laboratory and domestic cats. The prevalence rate is much higher in cats in congregated environments such as catteries or shelters. While a cough is common in dogs infected with *B. bronchiseptica* (kennel cough), it is usually much less prominent in infected cats, which manifest disease with fever, nasal discharge, sneezing, submandibular lymphadenomegaly, and lethargy. If a cat exhibits cough, it may be associated with pneumonia. In a study of 100 cats with upper respiratory tract disease, 26% had infection with *B. bronchiseptica* (26). Vaccines are available for protection of cats against this pathogen; an attenuated intranasal product has been licensed in the United States, and one genetically engineered product was once, but is no longer, available in Europe.

Humans, especially immunocompromised hosts, such as those with human immunodeficiency virus (HIV) infection (AIDS) and hematopoietic transplant and cystic fibrosis patients (76), may infrequently acquire disease from cats and may manifest illness from mild

Infections of Leisure, Fourth Edition, Edited by David Schlossberg,
© 2009 ASM Press, Washington, DC

upper respiratory tract symptoms to frank pneumonia (27). The organism is difficult to cultivate on routine media and may be misidentified by human clinical laboratories. By the time humans become adults, the possible cross-immunity that can be developed because of pertussis vaccination in childhood is most likely to have waned to nonprotective levels. Fluoroquinolones have in vitro susceptibility and have been used successfully for therapy (12, 76), while resistance to trimethoprim, chloramphenicol, and sulfonamides has been reported due to class 1 integrons (43).

Plague

Plague is caused by *Yersinia pestis,* a gramnegative coccobacillus. While cat fleas are considered poor vectors for transmission, domestic and wild cats may contract this disease, usually in the summer months (21). Cats are exposed via ingestion of an infected rodent or by their fleas. Cats manifest plague in the same way as humans, with either the bubonic, septicemic, or pneumonic form. In 1996, there were five human cases of plague reported in the United States, two of which were fatal; for one, there was exposure to an infected pet cat (13). Between 1970 and 1995, five persons infected by inhalation were known to be exposed to infected domestic cats (13). The CDC has suggested that "the risk of cat-associated human plague is likely to increase" (31). In 2006, there were 17 cases of plague reported (14). Due to climate change, the incidence of plague is increasing, as is the expansion of its northern and southern limits. (63) This illness is covered further in chapter 9.

Q Fever

Cats may be infected with *Coxiella burnetii* (a class B bioterrorism agent), the rickettsia that causes Q fever. Cat infection may ensue from a tick bite, ingestion of infected body tissues, or inhalation of organisms in a contaminated environment. Most cats are asymptomatic, although in pregnant queens, abortion or birth of stillborn or weak kittens has been observed.

Experimentally infected cats maintained *C. burnetii* in their blood for 1 month and excreted it in their urine for 2 months (32). *C. burnetii* has also been isolated from infected cat uteri postpartum. Seroprevalence studies in various parts of the world have shown exposure to *C. burnetii* in 15 to 20% of cats. Humans may occasionally become infected from cats by direct exposure to or inhalation of infected material from parturient or aborted tissue from infected cats. In 2006, the CDC reported 169 cases in the United States (14). Oral doxycycline (100 mg every 12 h for 14 days) is the treatment of choice for acute disease (36). Although fluoroquinolones are used, there is limited supportive clinical data, and macrolides have been shown to be unreliable (36).

VECTOR-BORNE SPREAD

Ehrlichiosis and Anaplasmosis

Ehrlichiae are obligate, intracellular, rickettsial organisms causing tick-borne disease in many animals and in humans. At least two species of *Ehrlichia (E. chaffeensis* and *E. ewingii)* and *Anaplasma phagocytophilum* cause diseases in humans, and historically these diseases have collectively been referred to as "human ehrlichiosis." Some *Ehrlichia* species cross-infect mammalian hosts, so cats may serve as reservoirs or sentinels for human infection. Cats can be infected experimentally by inoculation with *E. chaffeensis* (22). Experimental and natural *A. phagocytophilum* infection in cats has been described previously (10, 11, 29, 50, 64). This organism can cause a febrile illness. Routes of transmission between cats are unknown, and transmission from cats to humans has not (as yet) been documented.

Cat Scratch Disease

Cat scratch disease (CSD) is worldwide in distribution, and in temperate climates, there are fall and winter prevalences (2, 71). A prospective population-based study in Connecticut in 1992 to 1993 found a statewide annual incidence of 3.7/100,000 persons (35). It often affects children (median age, 14 years) and persons <21 years old (80% of cases). In the Connecticut study, the age-specific attack rate was highest for persons <10 years old (9.3/100,000) and decreased with increasing age (35). Exposure was usually associated with a young newly acquired or stray cat and not usually with longtime pets. Injury has occurred as a bite or scratch or from licks. Approximately 1 week after injury (range, 3 to 10 days), a primary inoculation papule or pustule (0.5 to 1 cm), which often goes unnoticed, may appear at the site of injury in 25 to 60% of patients. The papule may become vesicular and may crust. Subsequent to the inoculation papule, 5 to 120 days later (average, 2 weeks), tender, regional adenopathy may develop. Adenopathy, which often lasts >3 weeks, may be the only symptom in half the cases and suppurates in approximately 15% of cases. Since this is usually a benign and self-limiting disease (6 to 12 weeks) in immunocompetent individuals, it often goes unnoticed or unreported. Some healthy patients experience a "flu-like" illness. Most patients who seek medical attention present because of the adenopathy, especially if it involves the head and neck area and/or fever (low grade, 50% of patients). Consequently, the differential diagnosis often centers on these problems. Depending on the area of the adenopathy, various diseases should be excluded, including streptococcal pharyngitis, infectious mononucleosis, toxoplasmosis, cytomegalovirus infection, syphilis, lymphogranuloma venereum, cellulitis, Hodgkin's disease, dental abscess, etc.

Accompanying symptoms include fatigue and malaise (28%), fever (101 to 106°F) (31%), splenomegaly (12%), musculoskeletal manifestations (arthropathy, myalgia, tendonitis) (11%) (56), exanthema (4%), parotid swelling (2%), and seizures (1 to 2%). Other syndromes include ocular granuloma (Perinaud's oculoglandular syndrome—conjunctival granuloma, periauricular adenopathy, and nonsuppurative conjunctivitis), erythema nodosum, thrombocytopenic purpura, figurate erythema, os-

teomyelitis, pneumonia, and liver abscesses. The most serious complication is the development of acute encephalopathy and altered consciousness. Spontaneous recovery is usual with encephalopathy as well, usually within 2 weeks. Endocarditis due to *Bartonella quintana* has been reported for homeless men and those exposed to cats and their fleas; *Bartonella henselae* has also been reported as an unusual cause of endocarditis in humans, especially the elderly (9, 17, 18, 69). In the elderly, lymphadenopathy is often absent (9). In human bartonellosis, atypical cases can occur, and immunocompromised patients may have diverse and unusual manifestations (5) [see "Bacillary (Epithelioid) Angiomatosis" below].

Cats are the natural reservoir host for *B. henselae,* and it produces an intraerythrocytic subclinical bacteremia. The organism was isolated from the blood of 40% of the cats in a covenant in San Francisco, CA (16). Naturally infected cats can maintain subclinical bacteremia for several months, although the organism can cause endocarditis (18). Impounded or formerly stray cats are more likely to be bacteremic than long-term domestic pet cats. Other factors associated with bacteremia are the presence of fleas (which can readily transmit *Bartonella* from one cat to another) and the age of the cat being less than 1 year. Cats develop increasing immunity to infection with age, which may occur from natural exposure to the organism. Limited trials have shown that cats can be treated for *Bartonella* infection with a variety of antimicrobials (tetracyclines, quinolones, etc.) similar to that used in humans (34).

Diagnosis is often made on clinical grounds. A history of feline contact (usually with an immature cat) and, if possible, the identification of an inoculation site should be sought. Other diagnostic possibilities should be excluded. If there is an unusual reason to pursue the diagnosis, then a lymph node biopsy sample showing granulomatous inflammation, preferably with stellate microabscesses, is supportive. A modified

Warthin-Starry stain of the node may show organisms, but this test is difficult to interpret in many pathology laboratories due to the infrequency of its use, the unavailability of positive controls, and a variety of other technical factors. Isolation of the organism from human specimens is ideal but is also technically difficult for most laboratories, even with the correct media. In contrast, isolation from infected cats is quite rewarding due to the high numbers of organisms. The organism is a slow-growing (2 to 3 weeks), fastidious, gram-negative bacterium. It grows on chocolate agar as well as CDC agar. The colonies are small, nonhemolytic, rough, dry, and yellow to gray. Growth on human blood agar is superior to that on horse or sheep blood agar. It is oxidase and catalase negative and is X factor dependent.

Serologic evidence of recent infection with *B. henselae* is also helpful, but the tests are often either unavailable or not standardized. A new, modified immunofluorescent-antibody assay has been noted (59) to have a sensitivity of 85% and a specificity of 98% for both immunoglobulin G (IgG) and IgM components. The IgM remained positive for less than 3 months, and the IgG decreased over time, with 25% of patients remaining seropositive for >1 year; no association was found between titers and clinical manifestations or duration of disease.

Therapy at this time is supportive (72). Aspiration of a necrotic node is preferable to excision and may be necessary in some cases. Chronically draining sinus tracts can develop. The role of antimicrobial therapy remains undetermined (58, 62). Recent data suggest that bacillary angiomatosis and hepatosplenic disease respond more favorably (rapidly and consistently) than typical CSD to antimicrobial therapy for unclear reasons. Organisms in granulomas may be "walled off" from penetration by antibacterials. Rifampin has been used successfully, and with a rapid rate of response, in hepatosplenic cases (5). The combination of doxycycline and rifampin has been used successfully to treat CSD-associated retinitis (70). *Bartonella* organisms are noted to be macrolide susceptible, and reports have noted the clinical success of azithromycin in treating typical CSD (7). Susceptibility studies have suggested that isolates may be variously susceptible to other antibiotics, with much strain-to-strain variation (58). Clinical success and failure have been attributed to the same antimicrobial agents, including gentamicin, tetracyclines, ciprofloxacin, and sulfamethoxazole-trimethoprim (39, 62, 85). In vitro resistance of *B. henselae* to broad-spectrum cephalosporins correlates with clinical therapeutic failure.

Prevention is accomplished by control of fleas in pets and discussion with a veterinarian about pet health, especially for immunocompromised prospective pet owners. No vaccine exists for cats. Blood culture of a prospective pet cat and, if indicated, subsequent antimicrobial therapy may be prudent for certain household situations.

Bacillary (Epithelioid) Angiomatosis

Patients with HIV infection may develop Kaposi's sarcoma-like papular lesions after a cat scratch or contact with a cat (45, 46, 78, 83). Lesions may also be found in immunocompetent patients as well. Lesions may be nodular, subcutaneous, or even polypoid and may be pigmented or nonpigmented. Lesions contain a distinctive pattern of vascular proliferation on histopathological sections. CSD and bacillary angiomatosis have organisms that appear similar upon Warthin-Starry staining. Lesions are often multiple and appear on a variety of body surfaces. Lesions may also be osseous and appear in the fibula, radius, femur, and tibia, as well as present as hepatic abscesses, splenic involvement, colonic mucosal lesions, and even as extensive bone marrow infiltration. Systemic symptoms, including fever, night sweats, and weight loss, may also be associated with disease. This disease was originally thought to be a variant of CSD in an immunocompromised patient population and is difficult to differentiate from it on clinical grounds. *B. henselae* and *B. quintana* have been isolated from patients with bacillary angiomatosis and bacillary peliosis and have been shown to be the etiologic agents of these diseases. Host immunoincompetency, as opposed to lymphatic containment of the organisms, is likely responsible for the systemic spread.

Rickettsia felis ("Flea-Borne Spotted Fever") and *Rickettsia typhi* (Murine Typhus)

Rickettsia typhi, the causative agent of murine typhus, is of worldwide distribution and classically associated with urban rat fleas. Humans acquire disease via flea bites and inoculation of flea feces into the wound during feeding. A newly described rickettsial organism, *R. felis,* is transmitted to humans, who are incidental hosts, by the cat flea *(Ctenocephalides felis),* which can become infected transovarially and transstadially. Opossums and cats are reservoirs. The clinical diseases in humans are similar for these organisms. Human cases have been reported globally (44, 65). *R. felis* DNA was detected in 25% of Hawaiian rat fleas, while *R. typhi* was detected in only 2% (28). In California, murine typhus has become a suburban disease, especially linked to opossums and cat fleas rather than cats (19). The human illness, manifested as a febrile exanthema, is probably more widespread than generally appreciated. The exanthema may be easily missed; patients often have headache (40 to 90%) and elevated liver enzymes and may have cough (15 to 40%).

Leishmaniasis

Leishmaniasis is caused by parasitic protozoans of the genus *Leishmania* and can be a cat-associated zoonosis (23, 53). The parasites live in dogs, foxes, rodents, and humans. More than 40 cases of feline leishmaniasis have been reported (57). In a recent Portuguese study, *Leishmania* DNA was detected in the blood of 30% of stray cats, and it was suggested that cats may act as a "habitual reservoir" of *Leishmania infantum* (53). Leishmaniasis is usually trans-

mitted by the bites of sand flies. There are two forms of leishmaniasis. The more serious, called kala-azar or visceral leishmaniasis, affects the internal organs, causing fever, anemia, splenomegaly, and discoloration of the skin. Untreated, it can be fatal. The second form, which is cutaneous, may leave deep scars at the site of the bite.

FECAL-ORAL TRANSMISSION

Campylobacteriosis

Campylobacter jejuni has emerged as one of the most frequent bacterial causes of diarrheal diseases in the United States. The organism is a motile, curved, microaerophilic, gram-negative rod that inhabits the gastrointestinal tracts of clinically healthy and diarrheic animals and has been isolated from cat feces. Newly acquired, young cats are more likely to be carriers. Those cats with diarrhea pose a greater zoonotic risk. Most cases of human infection are acquired from contaminated food, especially undercooked poultry, and water.

In humans, a flu-like illness with fever, malaise, etc. precedes the development of cramping diarrhea. Infection is usually self-limiting; however, colitis, bacteremia, and metastatic infections may result. A reactive arthritis or Guillain-Barré syndrome may also occur after resolution of the diarrheal illness. *# 75*

Prevention of infection by hand washing after cat contact and prior to eating should be common sense. Cats should also not be fed raw or poorly cooked meat. Therapy consists of symptomatic treatment. Antimicrobial agents, such as erythromycin or the fluoroquinolones (norfloxacin, ciprofloxacin, levofloxacin, moxifloxacin, etc.), have proven effective in decreasing diarrhea when begun early. While resistance is less frequent in the United States, increasing numbers of strains from Europe and Southeast Asia have been reported to be resistant to quinolones and/or to macrolides. The use of antimicrobials in feed, as a growth promoter for food-producing animals, is suspected of being re-

#76

sponsible for this resistance. Some companies and countries have encouraged the use of these agents in pet or food-producing animals only for therapeutic purposes and not for prophylaxis or growth enhancement.

Helicobacteriosis

An increasing number of *Helicobacter* species, including *H. canis, H. felis, H. bilis, H. cinaedi, H. baculiformis,* and "*H. heilmannii,*" have been isolated from cats' gastric mucosae (6). *Helicobacter bizzozeronii ("Helicobacter heilmannii")* has been isolated from a few people with gastritis; in some reports, cats have been associated with disease (51), and one was considered causally related to human disease (82). In addition, it was reported that a researcher exposed to cat stomachs developed gastritis, which was attributed to infection with *Helicobacter felis* (33). *Helicobacter felis* caused a bacteremia in a 7-month-old and was associated with cats (67). *Helicobacter pylori* has also been demonstrated in the gastric mucosae of cats in research colonies; the presumed source of infection was animal caretakers. Further genetic comparisons of human and feline isolates will determine the extent of feline-associated human disease. Most of the feline isolates are susceptible to ampicillin, clarithromycin, and tetracycline, while two *H. felis* strains have shown resistance to metronidazole (81).

Cryptosporidiosis

Human cryptosporidiosis was first reported in 1976 and has become recognized as an important cause of gastrointestinal illness (42). National reporting began in the United States in 1995, with 2,972 human cases (13), and in 2006, there were 6,071 reported cases, which represents a continued annual increase (14). Outbreaks linked to the water supplies of urban cities (>400,000 cases in Milwaukee, WI) have generated public concern and awareness as well as "made-for-TV" movies. The disease is particularly problematic in AIDS patients, in whom it causes not only diarrhea but also cholecystitis. The diarrhea is often profuse and watery and is associated with cramping, abdominal pain, fever, and emesis. Immunocompetent patients sometimes have a mild and self-limiting form of illness, while immunocompromised patients have prolonged and severe courses that warrant attempts at therapeutic intervention. Weight loss and volume depletion, with electrolyte imbalance, may even require hospitalization. Infection is often in the small intestine (ileum) and may be focal in nature. Cryptosporidial cholecystitis may be manifested by upper-right-quadrant pain, emesis, and a thickened gallbladder wall and dilated ducts on ultrasound. In AIDS patients, it must also be differentiated from cytomegalovirus acalculous cholecystitis. Cryptosporidia have also been isolated from sputum and lung tissue from immunocompromised hosts, although its role in pulmonary disease is less well defined.

Cats and many other species of mammals, birds, and reptiles may act as definitive hosts for cryptosporidia. Experimental infection in healthy cats and young kittens resulted in nonsymptomatic infections and colonization. In naturally infected cats, watery diarrhea may be self-limiting. Immunocompromised cats have more symptoms, including chronic, large-volume, watery diarrhea; anorexia; and weight loss. In cats, infection with feline leukemia or immunodeficiency virus or the presence of other intestinal pathogens is associated with more-severe disease and increased shedding.

Infection has been transmitted between species, such as from animals to humans, as well as from humans to humans. *Cryptosporidium parvum* genospecies subtype 1 infects only people, while subtype 2 is adapted to cows but infects a wide variety of mammalian hosts, including cats and people. Cats have their own genospecies, which also infects people. Cat-to-human transmission has been reported; however, cattle are thought to be the main source of animal-related human infections. After ingestion, the sporozoite excysts and enters the villous intestinal border. Several asexual developmental forms ensue. Ultimately, thin-walled oocysts may invade other cells, while thick-walled oocysts are excreted into the feces. These oocysts are quite hardy and difficult to destroy. Crowding of either animals or humans (e.g., as occurs in day care centers or underdeveloped countries) and unsanitary practices are associated with an increased risk of acquiring cryptosporidiosis.

Diagnosis is made by demonstrating the organism in stool specimens or tissue biopsy samples. Routine ova-and-parasite examination of stool specimens fails to identify this pathogen, as it is extremely small and special stains or immunodiagnostic tests are required for identification. Consequently, a cryptosporidium exam must be specifically ordered; cryptosporidiosis is probably underdiagnosed and underreported. For cats, a positive test may not be associated with active infection. Definitive therapy remains imperfect. Nitazoxanide is effective in immunocompetent hosts but not in HIV-infected patients (3, 4).

Toxoplasmosis

Toxoplasma gondii, the causative agent of toxoplasmosis, is a ubiquitous, obligate intracellular protozoan that can affect almost all warm-blooded animals, including humans. Domestic cats and their relatives are definitive hosts of *T. gondii.* Millions of oocysts are excreted in the feces daily, and ingestion of infested food or water may cause disease in cats. Cat excretion of oocysts is self-limiting and occurs for only 1 to 3 weeks after initial infection. However, approximately 1% of cats in the United States (~560,000) are thought to be infected and excreting oocysts on any given day. Congenital or lactational transmission in cats (tachyzoites) and ingestion of tissue cysts (bradyzoites) in contaminated meats (most common) can also lead to feline disease.

Following ingestion, bradyzoites are released from the infected muscle and penetrate the epithelium of the cat small intestine. Subsequently, the parasite develops within the intestinal epithelium and disseminates into tissues while also going through a variety of stages until it forms unsporulated and uninfective oocysts, which are passed in the feces. This process may take between 3 days and 3 weeks to be completed. As soon as 2 to 3 days after being shed, uninfective oocysts begin to sporulate, depending on climate and temperature, and they may remain infective and viable for 1 year in the soil. Sporulation does not occur at <4 or >37°C; consequently, the disease is less prevalent in cold and arid climates.

Human infection may occur after ingestion of uncooked or undercooked meat of livestock (especially pork or goat) that contains tissue cysts; ingestion is probably the most usual method of zoonotic transmission. Single tissue cysts, which may contain thousands of organisms, are common in skeletal muscle, heart muscle, and brain tissue. However, infection may develop from exposure to sporulated fecal oocysts when humans change cat litter boxes or garden in areas where cat feces have been deposited.

The clinical spectrum of human disease is varied and includes asymptomatic forms (common) and acute or chronic symptomatic forms. Human congenital transmission occurs when a woman becomes acutely infected, usually asymptomatically, during pregnancy. This may result in spontaneous abortion or stillbirth. While congenital toxoplasmosis is currently rare in the United States, no statistical correlation between disease and cat ownership has been proven (66). Variable percentages of infants born after such exposure may develop a wide variety of sequelae, including mental and psychomotor retardation, cerebral calcifications, chorioretinitis, jaundice, hepatosplenomegaly, anemia, and pneumonia. "The incidence of transplacental transmission and severity of congenital disease depend on gestational age at which maternal seroconversion occurs" (66). Each presentation must be differentiated from other causes of similar problems, such as the other etiologic agents of the TORCH syndrome complex (toxoplasmosis, other [syphilis, sepsis, listeriosis, etc.], rubella, cytomegalovirus, herpes-virus). The management of toxoplasmosis in pregnancy has recently been reviewed (60).

Approximately 10 to 20% of immunocompetent individuals manifest symptomatic toxoplasmosis, usually with cervical adenopathy that does not require therapy. This regional adenopathy needs to be differentiated from that due to streptococcal pharyngitis, infectious mononucleosis, Hodgkin's disease, CSD, sarcoidosis, and cytomegalovirus infection. The disease manifestations are both protean and nonspecific. Other symptoms may include fever, malaise, fatigue, myalgias, sore throat, and rash. While most cases of disease are self-limiting, rarely lasting more than 3 to 6 months, some patients have prolonged symptoms, including depression, and some infections disseminate, with development of myocarditis, pneumonia, retinal disease, or encephalitis. A disseminated form of acute cutaneous toxoplasmosis may occur. Patients with disseminated disease often benefit from therapy. Immunocompromised hosts, including AIDS patients, HIV-infected patients, and cancer patients (especially those on chemotherapy), may develop more-serious disease manifestations, including brain abscess, retinitis, encephalopathy, pneumonia, and hepatitis. Immunocompromised patients always require therapy for acute toxoplasmosis or any complication of recurrent (reactivated) disease.

Diagnosis is made by serologic studies or by isolation or cytologic demonstration of the organism from blood or body fluids or by histologic demonstration of the trophozoite. Most cases are diagnosed by serologic means. However, a high prevalence of *T. gondii*-specific antibodies, sometimes even at high levels (>1:512), in the general population may make this difficult. Both false-positive and false-negative tests can occur. However, a negative serologic test result virtually excludes the diagnosis in an immunocompetent individual. In cats, a positive serotest result measuring IgG indicates that the cat is not an exposure risk, as the oocyst shedding phase has already occurred during prior exposure.

The need for therapy depends on the immune status of the host, host defenses, and location of infection. The standard therapy has been sulfadiazine and pyrimethamine. The duration of therapy depends on specific host factors and the site of infection. Prevention of disease in AIDS patients may be accomplished with the use of sulfonamide-based compounds used for the prevention of *Pneumocystis carinii* pneumonia. If an AIDS patient does develop cerebral toxoplasmosis, he or she will require prolonged therapy. Trimethoprim-sulfamethoxazole has been used instead of sulfadiazine. Alternative therapy with clindamycin plus pyrimethamine has been advocated for sulfonamide-allergic patients. Spiramycin has been used in therapy of pregnant women and infants with congenital infection.

Prevention of infection should be advocated for immunocompromised patients at risk for disease. They should be instructed not to change cat litter boxes or to do so daily so that the oocysts do not have a chance to sporulate prior to exposure. In addition, they should not garden in areas where cats may have defecated, nor should they beat-clean rugs, which may be contaminated by cat feces.

Salmonellosis

There has been a continual increase in the number of cases of human salmonellosis reported in the United States (13). A small number of these approximately 50,000 annual cases may come from exposure to household pets, usually reptiles or amphibians. In these instances, the victims are usually children who acquire infection from direct fecal-oral exposure. Cats may acquire infection from infected foods, especially offal, live prey, uncooked meat or fish meal, or contaminated water. If one feeds his or her cat any of these potentially contaminated products, good hand washing is in order. However, handling of manufacturer-contaminated commercial pet food has also been a risk factor (15). The prevalence of infection in cats being exclusively fed commercial rations is very low; however, up to 18% of healthy and healthy-appearing cats may be

80

infected or carriers when foodstuffs are not restricted. Cats may also pick up salmonellosis from staying in a contaminated kennel. Cats may acquire infection, often *Salmonella enterica* serovar Typhimurium, from ingestion of birds, which occurs in association with the seasonal songbird migration in the northeastern United States.

Infected cats can shed organisms orally and conjunctivally as well as fecally. Their fur may become contaminated, as may their water dishes. They may manifest illness as a gastroenterologic disease, with diarrhea, excessive salivation, or emesis or as a systemic illness with fevers, etc. In utero infection may occur. Kittens less than 7 weeks old may not manifest symptoms even if bacteremic.

The characteristics of human salmonellosis can be divided into an asymptomatic state (most usual), enterocolitis, enteric fever with bacteremia, metastatic complications, and a chronic carrier state. The enterocolitis must be differentiated from other infectious diarrheal illnesses, such as campylobacteriosis, shigellosis, and viral disease, and noninfectious diarrheal diseases. The incubation period is 6 to 48 h. Cramping, abdominal pain, emesis, nausea, and diarrhea are common. Occasionally, salmonellosis must be differentiated from appendicitis and other surgical causes of the acute abdomen.

Diagnosis is made by isolation of the organism from stool cultures or blood cultures. Most infections are asymptomatic or mild and self-limiting and do not require antimicrobial therapy. However, for patients with serious infection, such as enteric fever, bacteremia, or metastatic complications, or for immunocompromised hosts, antimicrobial therapy is advocated. The choice of antimicrobial must be determined by considering local resistance patterns for empirical therapy. There has been an increasing incidence of multidrug resistance in *Salmonella* species worldwide (48, 73, 84). This includes resistance to ampicillin, chloramphenicol, trimethoprim-sulfamethoxazole, cephalosporins, and the fluoroquinolones. Empirical therapy should be based on local

susceptibility patterns. Prevention by practicing good hand washing after petting cats, changing litter boxes, or feeding cats raw fish or meat products is prudent.

Anaerobiospirillum Diarrhea

Anaerobiospirillum species are anaerobic spiral bacteria with bipolar tufts of flagella that have been associated with cases of human diarrhea (54). Two species, *Anaerobiospirillum succiniciproducens* and *Anaerobiospirillum thomasii,* have been isolated from cats with diarrhea (55). *A. succiniciproducens* has been implicated as a cause of human bacteremia and sepsis. *A. thomasii* has been implicated as a cause of human diarrhea. Human disease included 3 to 7 days of diarrhea, fever, abdominal pain, and emesis. Malnick et al. (54) developed a selective medium that allowed its detection in the feces of 7 of 10 asymptomatic cats sampled during elective surgery. Consequently, cats may act as a vector in human disease.

Yersinia pseudotuberculosis Gastroenteritis

Y. pseudotuberculosis is a well-established cause of human diarrheal disease, diffuse abdominal illness sometimes mimicking acute appendicitis, and sepsis. Serotyping and endonuclease restriction analysis proved that two young children had become infected and symptomatic after having ingested water from puddles in a garden that was contaminated by feces from cats. Cats may be asymptomatic carriers but may also exhibit clinical infection, with anorexia, vomiting, and severe diarrhea, which are most likely to occur in the winter and spring (30).

Toxocariasis

Toxocara cati is a helminthic parasite that affects cats and may incidentally infect humans. Cats may be infected transplacentally or may become infected via oral intake of infected feces (25). After ingestion, the ova hatch in the small intestine and migrate to other body organs, including the liver and lungs. Organisms that are coughed up or subsequently swallowed will then mature in the small intestinal lumen. Excreted ova subsequently develop in the soil, taking weeks to mature. Human infection results from ingestion of infected soil or animal feces and is most usual in toddlers with pica and toddlers playing in areas where cats defecate.

Most human infection is asymptomatic. Some patients develop a cough, wheezing, or asthma from the parasites' pulmonary migration. Some patients present with hepatomegaly, abdominal pain, and eosinophilia. This must be differentiated from other parasitic diseases, such as strongyloidiasis, trichinosis, ascariasis, anisakiasis, schistosomiasis, and echinococcosis. The organism may migrate to any part of the body and may localize in the retina, causing blindness.

Diagnosis is usually made on clinical grounds. Serologic studies are available but are not specific. The organism is occasionally found incidentally in tissue biopsy specimens. Therapy for this form of disease is usually symptomatic, as the disease is usually self-limiting.

Occasionally, *T. cati* can cause cutaneous larva migrans or the creeping eruption. More commonly, cats are infected with *Ancylostoma braziliense* and subsequently shed ova. This is also a disease of children who play in areas where cats defecate. It is more common in the southeastern United States and in areas with a temperate climate and sandy or shady soil. Larvae come into contact with human skin and burrow under it, causing itching and paresthesias. The lesion can become erythematous along a serpiginous tract. Eosinophilia may be present. Disease is usually self-limiting but may be treated with thiabendazole, orally or topically.

Opisthorchiasis

Opisthorchis felineus is a common liver fluke of cats that can occasionally be transmitted to humans. It is a disease of fish-eating mammals, such as cats, and is endemic in Southeast Asia and Eastern Europe but not the United States. Embryonated eggs are excreted in the feces by the definitive host. The eggs are ingested by

specific snail species and develop until they are released as cercariae into freshwater, where they penetrate into the intermediate fish host. Human infection comes from ingestion of rare or raw infected fish. The parasites mature into adults in the bile ducts. Most patients are asymptomatic; however, signs of cholangitis and hepatitis may develop. Diagnosis is made by finding eggs in a fecal sample. Praziquantel is used for therapy.

Dipylidiasis

Dipylidium caninum is a common cat tapeworm that may infect humans, usually children. Fleas ingest eggs, which then develop into the cysticercus stage. When fleas are ingested, the tapeworm subsequently develops in the intestinal tract; humans become infected when they ingest fleas. The patient may develop eosinophilia and mild gastrointestinal discomfort. Diagnosis is made by demonstration of proglottids in a stool sample. Praziquantel is used for therapy, with niclosamide as an alternative. This disease needs to be distinguished from other parasitic causes of eosinophilia.

TRANSMISSION VIA BITE, SCRATCH, OR PUNCTURE

Rabies

Approximately 6,000 animals per year are proven positive for rabies in the United States (14). While domestic animals account for less than 10% of all rabid animals, over the past 10 years, rabid cats have been more common than rabid dogs. Vaccination of cats is not legally mandated in all areas as it is for dogs, making them more susceptible to infection. Cats acquire rabies from exposure to infected wildlife and a "spillover effect." Rabid cats may develop frenzied rabies but more often become reclusive. Rabies is covered in chapter 10.

Erysipelothrix Infection

Erysipelothrix rhusiopathiae is a geographically widespread, facultative, gram-positive rod that may be isolated from soil, water, and animals. Human disease is usually associated with cellulitis acquired by animal contact and occurs usually in slaughterhouse workers. *E. rhusiopathiae* has been isolated from two infected wounds secondary to cat bites (77). Human disease may be manifested by a painful, ulcerating, and progressive papular skin lesion that is associated with pain or stiffness in the local joint. Disease may be self-limiting and disappear in approximately 3 weeks. A human-disseminated form which may include a vasculitic rash and endocarditis can also occur. The source animals are often not clinically ill. A new species, *Erysipelothrix tonsillarum,* has been shown to cause septicemia and endocarditis in dogs but has not yet been associated with human illness. Therapy with penicillin or a cephalosporin may be useful in localized cases as well as for disseminated disease.

Anthrax

Anthrax is caused by *Bacillus anthracis,* a large, gram-positive, spore-forming rod. Infections in humans are almost always the result of contact with infected animals or their by-products (especially goat hair). The alkaline soil of many tropical and subtropical regions allows vegetative spore growth, resulting in a soil-borne systemic disease of domestic animals. Domestic herbivores have the highest prevalence of infection, and cats are uncommonly affected. Soil may remain contaminated for many years. In cats, anthrax is manifested by inflammation, edema, and necrosis of the upper gastrointestinal tract. Spread to regional lymph nodes, liver, and spleen is frequent. Human infection usually results from handling infected tissues, carcasses, or animal skin. Inhalation anthrax is a rare phenomenon in humans in the United States but has recently gained attention because of potential threats of bioterrorism. Before the autumn of 2001, the last case of inhalation anthrax reported in the United States was in 1992; in the 1960s and 1970s, there were an average of one or two cases (range, zero to six) reported annually in the United States (13).

In humans, cutaneous lesions account for >95% of cases. One to five days after exposure, a small and often pruritic papule may form at the inoculation site. The area, although painless, develops a brawny edema; the lesion enlarges, and the center becomes necrotic. Regional adenopathy and lymphangitis may be associated with the skin lesion. The lesion of anthrax should be covered. The differential diagnosis includes brown recluse spider bite, orf, CSD, erythema gangrenosum, tularemia, and plague.

Diagnosis is achieved by Gram staining of the exudate and isolation of the organism. The laboratory should be warned if the diagnosis is suspected. Several serologic tests are available but are not of help in rapidly progressive cases. Therapy with intravenous penicillin G and subsequent oral penicillin for 7 to 10 days is generally effective for cutaneous disease. There are rare reports of penicillin-resistant *B. anthracis.* Inhalation anthrax is difficult to diagnose and is therefore usually fatal.

Pasteurella multocida Infection

P. multocida has been commonly associated with infected dog and cat bite wounds in people (32); indeed, almost all feline species commonly carry this organism in their oropharynx as part of their normal flora. Additionally, when cats lick their paws, they are in effect inoculating *P. multocida* onto their claws.

It is estimated that 400,000 persons are bitten or severely scratched by cats annually in the United States. Many of these wounds never become infected and are trivial in severity. However, infection resulting from cat bites and scratches is an important and frequent medical problem. Most people are bitten or scratched by cats they know, and these injuries occur while handling the cat. Cat bites become infected more frequently than do dog bites. Cat's teeth are small but sharp, and when the bite is to the hand, it can easily penetrate the joints, bones, and tendons. Infections following cat bites are usually cellulitis, often with a gray malodorous discharge but without lymphangitis or regional adenopathy, but may also be septic arthritis, tenosynovitis, and osteomyelitis. Consequently, the use of antimicrobial therapy as prophylactic therapy in cases of moderate-to-severe wounds, such as those to the hands (especially those that have come near a joint) or those causing pain, is warranted to reduce the prevalence of infection. Other organisms, in both aerobic and anaerobic feline oral floras, can be cultured from many wounds.

Pasteurella infection in humans has also been associated both with general animal contact and, in approximately 15 to 20% of cases, such as respiratory infection, without known animal contact. The possibility of more-remote contact and persistence of the isolate on the skin or mucous membranes has been entertained.

In 1992, Holst et al. (40) characterized 159 strains of *Pasteurella* recovered from human infections and studied their distribution, which was as follows: *Pasteurella multocida* subsp. *multocida,* 60%; *Pasteurella multocida* subsp. *septica,* 13%; *Pasteurella canis,* 18%; *Pasteurella stomatis,* 6%; and *Pasteurella dagmatis,* 3%. They did not fully differentiate the distribution of species in the 87 of 159 cases associated with cat bites and contact. However, they did note different ecological niches for the different species and subspecies and slightly different pathogenic potentials. *P. multocida* subsp. *multocida* and *P. multocida* subsp. *septica* were usually associated with more-severe infections; the former was associated with almost all bacteremic cases, and the latter was associated with several cases of central nervous system infection.

The bacteriology of 57 infected cat bite wounds has recently been studied in a prospective, multicenter project, which shows the great diversity of isolates (77). Women accounted for 72% of cat bite victims, compared to 38% of dog bite victims. Cat bites presented as abscesses 19% of the time, as purulent wounds 39% of the time, and as nonpurulent cellulitis 42% of the time. A median of six bacterial isolates were found per cat bite wound, and these isolates were mixed cultures (both aerobes and anaerobes) 63% of the time. The prevalences and distributions of *Pasteurella* species are different for dog and cat bites. Surprisingly, *Pasteurella* species were present in 75% of cat bite wounds in the following dis-

tribution: *P. multocida* subsp. *multocida,* 54%; *P. multocida* subsp. *septica,* 28%; *P. dagmatis,* 7%; *P. stomatis,* 4%; and *P. canis,* 2%.

Most wounds can be treated with outpatient management. If there is any edema, then the affected body part should be elevated. Failure to adequately elevate the injured part is one of the most common causes of therapeutic failure. The location of punctures, especially in relation to the bones and joints of the hand, should be noted. Prophylactic therapy with an antimicrobial agent such as penicillin or amoxicillin-clavulanic acid is inexpensive and prudent. Alternative agents could include trimethoprim-sulfamethoxazole, doxycycline, fluoroquinolones (ciprofloxacin, levofloxacin, moxifloxacin, etc.), and possibly cefuroxime axetil. The duration of therapy for prophylaxis is 3 to 5 days, while therapy for an established infection, such as cellulitis, often requires 10 to 14 days. More-serious complications such as septic arthritis and osteomyelitis require prolonged courses of antimicrobials. Occasionally, anti-inflammatory agents reduce the posttraumatic arthritis that subsequently develops in a minority of cases. In some areas, rabies prophylaxis may be considered (see chapter 10). Tetanus toxoid should be administered if the patient is not current on his or her immunizations.

Mixed Aerobic and Anaerobic Bacterial Infections

There are approximately 400,000 infected cat bite wounds annually in the United States and an even greater number of cat scratches that get infected. Cat claws become infected when cats are grooming and inoculate normal flora onto their claws. Cat bites are most often to the hand (63%) and upper extremity (23%), and a few (9%) are to the lower extremities. Most victims are women (72%), with a median age of 39 years (77). Presentation to an emergency department for medical help is usually associated with a nonpurulent but infected wound (42%), while 39% have purulent wounds and 19% have abscesses. The wounds grow 2 to 13 isolates, with 63% having both aerobic and anaerobic bacteria cultured from the wounds. A plethora of different bacteria may be cultured from these wounds, as noted by Talan et al. (77), and include not only *P. multocida* and other *Pasteurella* species (75%) but also numerous other bacteria, including streptococci (46%), staphylococci (35%), *Neisseria* spp. (19%), *Corynebacterium* spp. (28%), *Moraxella* spp. (35%), *Bacteroides* spp. (especially *Bacteroides tectus*) (28%), *Fusobacterium* spp. (33%), and *Porphyromonas* spp. (30%). Conrads et al. recently reported a new species of fusobacterium, *Fusobacterium canifelinum*, that is associated with cat and dog bites and is resistant to fluoroquinolones (20). Almost all isolates come from the normal flora of the biting cat.

Sporotrichosis

Sporothrix schenckii is an endemic, dimorphic fungus that can cause ulcerated, verrucous, or erythematous and nodular skin infection after direct inoculation by cat bite or scratch (24). On cats, lesions are seen on the head, limbs, or tail base and are often draining puncture wounds similar to fight wound abscesses. Cats have been reported to be bacteremic from naturally acquired infection (74). Cats may further spread disease by licking and grooming. In humans, sporotrichosis may also cause nodular pulmonary lesions after inhalation of infected soil. Cutaneous sporotrichosis is more common in the cooler, distal extremities, with painless, smooth or verrucous lesions that may ulcerate and have raised erythematous borders. Lesions may have a deep-red or purplish coloration. Secondary lesions may occur along lymphatic channels and in lymph nodes. Osteoarticular disease also occurs and may affect the hands, elbows, ankles, and knees. AIDS patients may develop disseminated disease, including meningitis and parenchymal brain lesions.

Diagnosis is made by culture of tissue or blood. Biopsy samples reveal granulomatous changes, but the organism is often difficult to identify in specimens. Therapy with a saturated solution of potassium iodide has been previously employed. Patients started off with 5 to 10 drops of solution thrice daily, increasing to up to 40 to 50 drops thrice daily or until side effects, such as nausea, diarrhea, anorexia, and parotid enlargement, limited therapy. de Lima Barros et al. (24) described 24 human cases related to transmission by domestic cats; all patients responded to itraconazole therapy.

Feline Orthopox

Infection with cowpox virus (an orthopoxvirus) is the most common poxvirus infection in cats. Infection is more common in Europe than in the United States, and cats, usually rural cats that hunt rodents, are usually incidental hosts. Cats often start with a single lesion on the head, neck, or forelimb that occurs from a bite or skin wound inoculation. Dissemination occurs, with the cats manifesting coryza and diarrhea; secondary bacterial infections also occur. Both cat-to-cat transmission and cat-to-human transmission have been reported (8, 37). Cat-to-human transmission is unlikely when basic hygiene is followed after contact.

Tularemia

Tularemia is caused by a small, gram-negative coccobacillus, *Francisella tularensis,* that grows poorly on routine culture media. It is ubiquitous and most often found in wild mammals, such as rabbits, but may affect cats. Four subspecies are recognized; the different subspecies are associated with different geographic locations worldwide. *F. tularensis* subsp. *tularensis* is found predominantly in the United States; *F. tularensis* subsp. *holarctica* is found in Europe, the former Soviet Union, and Japan; *F. tularensis* subsp. *mediasiatica* is found in Kazakhstan and Uzbekistan; and "*F. tularensis* subsp. *novicida*" is found in North America (79). *F. tularensis* survives in amoebae and is therefore associated with waterways (79). Cat infection usually results from a bite by an infected tick, which may serve as both reservoir and vector, or by hunting or ingestion of infected rabbits. Young cats may die from disseminated infection. Older cats may develop draining abscesses as well as fever and adenopathy. Cat-associated human tularemia has occurred in conjunction with bite wounds. The organism is highly virulent and has an infectious dose of 10 to 50 CFU. Consequently, the local prevalence of infected animals and appropriate vectors should alert the physician to this possibility. A study of the epidemiology of tularemia in the southwestern and central United States showed that 17 of 1,041 (1.6%) human cases diagnosed between 1981 and 1987 were associated with cat scratches or bites (13).

The ulceroglandular form of tularemia is most common and causes regional adenopathy and ulcerative skin lesions. This manifestation must be differentiated from other skin infections, including staphylococcal or streptococcal infection, bite wound infection due to *P. multocida,* and CSD. Pneumonia, without sputum production, may develop in 15% of patients with ulceroglandular disease. Most cases are diagnosed by a compatible clinical picture and antibody titers, since isolation of the organism is difficult and, if accomplished, may pose health risks to the laboratory technologists.

Standard therapy consists of streptomycin (10 to 20 mg/kg of body weight/day intramuscularly for 7 to 14 days). Tetracyclines and chloramphenicol have been used successfully but may be associated with increased rates of relapse. Fluoroquinolones and some cephalosporins, such as ceftriaxone, have in vitro activity against *F. tularensis* (80), but more studies documenting clinical efficacy are required.

SOILBORNE SPREAD

Histoplasmosis

Histoplasma capsulatum is an imperfect dimorphic fungus that is endemic in the central United States and may be found in other temperate and tropical climates. The free-living mycelial stage of *H. capsulatum* grows in the soil and produces both micro- and macroconidia. Inhalation of microconidia leads to conversion to the yeast phase in the body and subsequent pulmonary infection, which in turn may lead to dissemination. Soil, organi-

cally enriched by bird droppings, is the most frequent source of human exposure. Cats are also susceptible to histoplasmosis, and common-source outbreaks involving animals and people have occurred. As with most systemic fungal infections, direct animal-to-animal or animal-to-human spread is unlikely. Cats <4 years old and female cats seem to be more prone to developing histoplasmosis. There is no breed predilection. Infected cats that develop disseminated disease usually die but may also develop ulcerated skin lesions. Direct cat-to-human transmission has not been reported. Histoplasmosis in cats can be treated with itraconazole (38). Human disease may be treated with itraconazole or amphotericin B.

DIRECT-CONTACT TRANSMISSION

Methicillin-Resistant
Staphylococcus aureus

Community-acquired methicillin-resistant *S. aureus* (MRSA) has become known as the "most common identifiable cause" of skin and soft tissue infection across the United States (61). It has also been cultured from a variety of companion animals, including cats, and has been documented to be transmitted from a healthy pet cat to humans (75). The human strains and feline strains are indistinguishable (52). However, *Staphylococcus aureus* is a human commensal organism, while cats generally have their own species of staphylococci (1). Animals can become colonized with MRSA strains from human contact. MRSA infection in cats is considered a reverse zoonosis; however, once colonized, these cats serve as a potential reservoir for human infection. Consequently, hand decontamination after petting cats should be considered in appropriate clinical situations, such as pet visitation in schools, nursing homes, or hospital wards.

Dermatophilosis

Cats may become infected with *Dermatophilus congolensis,* an actinomycete that causes abscesses in muscles and lymph nodes and fis-

#82

tulous tracts. Humans handling infected cats may become accidentally infected. Human infection is manifested by an exudative, pustular dermatitis at the site of contact. The lesions spontaneously resolve within 2 weeks and do not usually require antimicrobial therapy. In cats, the hair should be clipped around the lesion and kept dry. Repeated bathing, application of iodine solutions, and in some cases the use of penicillin-related compounds are therapeutic.

Scabies

Sarcoptes scabiei, which causes a condition known as the "seven-year itch," can infect cats and be transmitted to humans. Scabies mites cause hypersensitivity in human hosts often manifested by pruritic, papular lesions at areas where they burrow into the skin. The itching increases at night. Cat scabies mites are unable to burrow into human skin to complete their life cycle, so a cutaneous scraping test is not diagnostic. Rather, diagnosis is made by clinical presentation. Therapy consists of ridding the affected pet of mites and laundering clothes and bedding.

Cheyletiella Mite Infestation

Cheyletiella species are animal mites, some of which can infest cats and may occasionally cause human infestation.

Dermatophytosis

Domestic cats can harbor a wide variety of molds and yeasts in the fur of their coats and on their skin. Both symptomatic disease and asymptomatic carriage may occur. These organisms include *Epidermophyton floccosum, Microsporum* species, and *Trichophyton* species. These dermatophytes spread between animals, potentially from animals to humans, and also from humans to animals. Infections often involve the hair shaft and follicle, from which infectious arthrospores are disseminated to the local environment and remain viable for months. Up to 89% of cats may harbor dermatophytes, of which *Microsporum canis* is the most common. Fomites contaminated by cat

#83

hair can also act as a vector. The incubation period is often 1 to 3 weeks.

In cats, the most common manifestation is a patchy alopecia but may include a scaling or granulomatous dermatitis. A variety of lesions that mimic other skin conditions have been observed. Since transmission is possible and cats can be subclinical carriers, they are often treated with clipping of the hair and with topical antifungal bathing over their entire body, and some may require oral antifungal agents as well. Additionally, the environment must be cleaned of hairs and dander to stop transmission. Approximately 50% of humans exposed to cat dermatophytes develop symptomatic infection, including ringworm and tinea capitis. In humans, the infection can manifest as alopecia, scaling or crusting lesions, and ulcers and nodules. Secondary bacterial infection may also occur.

Diagnosis is made by culture of skin scrapings and examination of scrapings using potassium hydroxide digestion or by using a Wood's lamp. As for cats, human therapy usually consists of topical antifungals such as clotrimazole, miconazole, etc., or in severe cases oral agents such as fluconazole or itraconazole. Again, cleaning the environment of cat hairs and dander from carpets, bedding, clothing, etc. is essential for control. Air conditioning and heating filters must also be changed regularly. Pets may need to be restricted from bedrooms. Cats may be treated with topical agents such as lime sulfur dip or miconazole shampoo with or without chlorhexidine. The same products in lotions are less effective in penetrating cat hair. Oral agents such as itraconazole are of the most benefit with the fewest side effects.

Uncertain Associations

HEPATITIS E

Hepatitis E virus is present in Southeast and Central Asia and the Middle East but rare in the United States; it is thought to be enterically transmitted. Transmission from humans to nonhuman primates has been reported as well as infection in swine and rodents (68).

The case for cat-to-human infection is uncertain. Kuno et al. (49) reported a case of hepatitis E virus infection in a 47-year-old Japanese man whose pet cat had antibody to hepatitis E virus.

PRACTICAL TIPS

- In patients with cat bites, when the bite is in proximity to a bone or a joint and the immediate pain is out of proportion to the injury, consider periosteal penetration.
- Murine typhus is increasingly associated with opossums infected with cat fleas in a suburban setting.
- Rescue and stray cats are very frequently infected with *Bartonella henselae* and may have prolonged and persistent bacteremia.

REFERENCES

1. **Abraham, J. L., D. O. Morris, G. C. Griffeth, F. S. Shofer, and S. C. Rankin.** 2007. Surveillance of healthy cats and cats with inflammatory skin disease for colonization of the skin by methicillin-resistant coagulase-positive staphylococci and *Staphylococcus schleiferi* ssp. *schleiferi. Vet. Dermatol.* **18:**252–259.
2. **Adal, K. A., C. J. Cockerell, and W. A. Petri, Jr.** 1994. Cat scratch disease, bacillary angiomatosis, and other infections due to *Rochalimaea. N. Engl. J. Med.* **330:**1509–1515.
3. **Amadi, B., M. Mwyla, J. Musuku, A. Watuka, S. Sianoga, A. Ayoub, and P. Kelly.** 2002. Effect of nitazoxanide on morbidity and mortality in Zambian children with cryptosporidiosis: a randomized controlled trial. *Lancet* **360:**1375–1380.
4. **Anderson, V. R., and M. P. Curran.** 2007. Nitazoxanide: a review of its use in the treatment of gastrointestinal infections. *Drugs* **67:**1947–1967.
5. **Arisoy, E. S., A. G. Correa, M. L. Wagner, and S. L. Kaplan.** 1999. Hepatosplenic cat-scratch disease in children: selected clinical features and treatment. *Clin. Infect. Dis.* **28:**778–784.
6. **Baele, H., A. Decostere, P. Vandamme, K. van den Bulck, I. Gruntar, J. Mehle, J. Mast, R. Ducatelle, and P. Haesebrouch.** 2008. *Helicobacter baculiformis* sp. nov., isolated from feline stomach mucosa. *Int. J. Syst. Evol. Microbiol.* **58:**357–364.
7. **Bass, J. W., B. C. Freitas, A. D. Freitas, C. L. Sisler, D. S. Chan, J. M. Vincent, D. A. Person, J. R. Claybaugh, R. R. Whitter, M. E. Weisse, R. L. Regnery, and L. N. Slater.** 1998. Prospective randomized double blind placebo-controlled evaluation of azithromycin for treatment of cat-scratch disease. *Pediatr. Infect. Dis. J.* **17:**447–452.
8. **Baxby, D., M. Bennett, and B. Getty.** 1994. Human cowpox: a review based on 54 cases, 1969–1993. *Br. J. Dermatol.* **131:**598–607.
9. **Ben-Ami, R., M. Ephros, B. Avidor, E. Katchman, M. Varon, C. Leibowitz, D. Comaneshter, and M. Giladi.** 2005. Cat-scratch disease in the elderly. *Clin. Infect. Dis.* **41:**969–974.
10. **Billeter, S. A., J. A. Spenser, B. Griffin, C. C. Dykstra, and B. L. Blagburn.** 2007. Prevalence of *Anaplasma phagocytophilum* in domestic felines in the United States. *Vet. Parasitol.* **147:**194–198.
11. **Bjoersdorff, A., L. Svendenius, J. H. Owens, and R. F. Massung.** 1999. Feline granulocytic ehrlichiosis—a report of a new clinical entity and characterization of the infectious agent. *J. Small Anim. Pract.* **40:**20–24.
12. **Carbone, M., M. T. Fera, M. G. Pennisi, M. Masucci, A. De Sarro, and C. Marci.** 1999. Activity of nine fluoroquinolones against strains of *Bordetella bronchiseptica. Int. J. Antimicrob. Agents* **12:**355–358.
13. **Centers for Disease Control and Prevention.** 1997. Summary of notifiable diseases, United States, 1996. *MMWR Morb. Mortal. Wkly. Rep.* **45**(53):1–103.
14. **Centers for Disease Control and Prevention.** 2008. Summary of notifiable diseases, United States, 2006. *MMWR Morb. Mortal. Wkly. Rep.* **55:**1–94.
15. **Centers for Disease Control and Prevention.** 2008. Update: recall of dry dog and cat food products associated with human *Salmonella* Schwarzengrund infections—United States, 2008. *MMWR Morb. Mortal. Wkly. Rep.* **57:**1200–1202.
16. **Chomel, B. B., R. C. Abbott, R. W. Kasten, K. A. Floyd-Hawkins, P. H. Kass, C. A. Glaser, N. C. Pedersen, and J. E. Koehler.** 1995. *Bartonella henselae* prevalence in domestic cats in California: risk factors and association between bacteremia and antibody titers. *J. Clin. Microbiol.* **33:**2445–2450.
17. **Chomel, B. B., R. W. Kasten, J. E. Sykes, H. J. Boulouis, and E. B. Breitschwerdt.** 2003. Clinical impact of persistent *Bartonella* bacteremia in humans and animals. *Ann. N. Y. Acad. Sci.* **990:**267–278.
18. **Chomel, B. B., A. C. Wey, R. W. Kasten, B. A. Stacy, and P. Labelle.** 2003. Fatal case

of endocarditis associated with *Bartonella henselae* infection in a domestic cat. *J. Clin. Microbiol.* **41:** 5337–5339.

19. **Civen, R., and V. Ngo.** 2008. Murine typhus: an unrecognized suburban vectorborne disease. *Clin. Infect. Dis.* **46:**913–918.

20. **Conrads, G., D. M. Citron, S. Jang, and E. J. C. Goldstein.** 2004. *Fusobacterium canifelinum* sp. *novum* from the oral cavity of cats and dogs. *Syst. Appl. Microbiol.* **27:**407–413.

21. **Craven, R. B., and A. M. Barnes.** 1991. Plague and tularemia. *Infect. Dis. Clin. N. Am.* **5:** 165–175.

22. **Dawson, J. E., I. Abeygunawardena, C. J. Holland, M. M. Buese, and M. Ristic.** 1988. Susceptibility of cats to infection with *Ehrlichia risticii*, causative agent of equine monocytic ehrlichiosis. *Am. J. Vet. Res.* **49:**2096–2100.

23. **del Giudice, P., and P. Marty.** 2003. Cat-associated zoonosis: don't forget rabies and leishmaniasis. *Arch. Intern. Med.* **163:**1238.

24. **de Lima Barros, M. B., A. de Oliveira Schubach, M. C. Galhardo, T. M. Schubach, R. S. dos Reis, M. J. Conceicao, and A. C. do Valle.** 2003. Sporotrichosis with widespread cutaneous lesions: report of 24 cases related to transmission by domestic cats in Rio de Janeiro, Brazil. *Int. J. Dermatol.* **42:**677–681.

25. **Despommier, D.** 2003. Toxocariasis: clinical aspects, epidemiology, medical ecology, and molecular aspects. *Clin. Microbiol. Rev.* **16:**265–272.

26. **Di Martino, B., C. E. Di Francesco, I. Meridiani, and F. Marsillo.** 2007. Ecological investigation of multiple respiratory infections in cats. *New Microbiol.* **30:**455–461.

27. **Dworkin, M. S., P. S. Sullivan, S. E. Buskin, R. D. Harrington, J. Olliffe, R. D. MacArthur, and C. E. Lopez.** 1999. *Bordetella bronchiseptica* infection in human immunodeficiency virus-infected patients. *Clin. Infect. Dis.* **28:**1095–1099.

28. **Eremeeva, M. E., W. R. Warashina, M. M. Sturgeon, A. E. Buchholz, G. K. Olmsted, S. Y. Park, P. V. Effler, and S. E. Karpathy.** 2008. *Rickettsia typhi* and *R. felis* in rat fleas (*Xenopsylla cheopis*), Oahu, Hawaii. *Emerg. Infect. Dis.* **14:**1613–1615.

29. **Foley, J. E., C. M. Leutenegger, J. S. Dumler, N. C. Pedersen, and J. E. Madigan.** 2003. Evidence for modulated immune response to *Anaplasma phagocytophila* sensu lato in cats with FIV-induced immunosuppression. *Comp. Immunol. Microbiol. Infect. Dis.* **26:**103–113.

30. **Fukushima, H., M. Gomyoda, S. Ishikura, T. Nishio, S. Moriki, J. Endo, S. Kaneko, and M. Tsubokura.** 1989. Cat-contaminated environmental substances lead to *Yersinia pseudo-*

tuberculosis infection in children. *J. Clin. Microbiol.* **27:**2706–2709.

31. **Gage, K. L., D. T. Dennis, K. A. Orloski, P. Ettestad, T. L. Brown, P. J. Reynolds, W. J. Pape, C. L. Fritz, L. G. Carter, and J. D. Stein.** 2000. Cases of cat associated human plague in the western US, 1977–1998. *Clin. Infect. Dis.* **30:**893–900.

32. **Goldstein, E. J. C., D. M. Citron, B. Wield, U. Blachman, V. L. Sutter, T. A. Miller, and S. M. Finegold.** 1978. Bacteriology of human and animal bite wounds. *J. Clin. Microbiol.* **8:**667–672.

33. **Greene, C. E. (ed.).** 2006. *Infectious Diseases of the Dog and Cat*, 3rd ed. The W. B. Saunders Co., Philadelphia, PA.

34. **Greene, C. E., R. McDermott, P. H. Jameson, and A. M. Marks.** 1996. *Bartonella henselae* infection in cats: evaluation during primary infection, treatment, and rechallenge infection. *J. Clin. Microbiol.* **34:**1682–1685.

35. **Hamilton, D. H., K. M. Zangwill, J. L. Hadler, and M. L. Cartter.** 1995. Cat-scratch disease—Connecticut, 1992–1993. *J. Infect. Dis.* **172:**570–573.

36. **Hartzell, J. D., R. N. Wood-Morris, L. J. Martinez, and R. F. Trotta.** 2008. Q fever: epidemiology, diagnosis and treatment. *Mayo Clin. Proc.* **83:**574–579.

37. **Hawranek, T., M. Tritscher, W. H. Muss, J. Jecel, N. Nowotny, J. Kolodziejek, M. Emberger, H. Schaeppi, and H. Hintner.** 2003. Feline orthopoxvirus infection transmitted from cat to human. *J. Am. Acad. Dermatol.* **49:**513–518.

38. **Hodges, R. D., A. M. Legendre, L. G. Adams, M. D. Willard, R. P. Pitts, K. Monce, C. C. Needles, and H. Ward.** 1994. Itraconazole for the treatment of histoplasmosis in cats. *J. Vet. Intern. Med.* **8:**409–413.

39. **Holley, H. P., Jr.** 1991. Successful treatment of cat-scratch disease with ciprofloxacin. *JAMA* **265:**1563–1565.

40. **Holst, E., J. Rolof, L. Larsson, and J. P. Nielsen.** 1992. Characterization and distribution of *Pasteurella* species recovered from infected humans. *J. Clin. Microbiol.* **30:**2984–2987.

41. **The Humane Society of the United States.** American Pet Products Manufacturers Association (APPMA) 2007–2008 National Pet Owners Survey. http://www.hsus.org/pets/issues_affecting_our_pets/pet_overpopulation_and_ownership_statistics/us_pet_ownership_statistics.html. (Accessed 5 May 2009.)

42. **Juranek, D. D.** 1995. Cryptosporidiosis: sources of infection and guidelines for prevention. *Clin. Infect. Dis.* **21**(Suppl. 1):57–61.

43. **Kadlek, K., C. Kehrenberg, and S. Schwarz.** 2005. Molecular basis of resistance to trimetho-

prim, chloramphenicol and sulphonamides in *Bordetella bronchiseptica*. *J. Antimicrob. Chemother.* **56:**485–490.

44. **Kenny, M. J., R. J. Birtles, M. J. Day, and S. E. Shaw.** 2003. *Rickettsia felis* in the United Kingdom. *Emerg. Infect. Dis.* **9:**1023–1024.

45. **Koehler, J. E., and J. W. Tappero.** 1993. Bacillary angiomatosis and bacillary peliosis in patients infected with human immunodeficiency virus. *Clin. Infect. Dis.* **17:**612–624.

46. **Koehler, J. E., F. D. Quinn, T. G. Berger, P. E. LeBoit, and J. W. Tappero.** 1992. Isolation of Rochalimaea species from cutaneous and osseous lesions of bacillary angiomatosis. *N. Engl. J. Med.* **327:**1625–1631.

47. **Kravetz, J. D., and D. G. Federman.** 2002. Cat-associated zoonoses. *Arch. Intern. Med.* **162:**1945–1952.

48. **Kumar, S., M. Rizvi, and N. Berry.** 2008. Rising prevalence of enteric fever due to multidrug-resistant Salmonella: an epidemiological study. *J. Med. Microbiol.* **57:**1247–1250.

49. **Kuno, A., K. Ido, N. Isoda, Y. Satoh, K. Ono, S. Satoh, H. Inamori, K. Sugano, N. Kanai, T. Nishizawa, and H. Okamoto.** 2003. Sporadic acute hepatitis E of a 47-year-old man whose pet cat was positive for antibody to hepatitis E virus. *Hepatol. Res.* **26:**237–242.

50. **Lappin, M. R., E. B. Breitschwerdt, W. A. Jensen, B. Dunnigan, J.-Y. Rha, R. Williams, M. Brewer, and M. Fall.** 2004. Molecular and serologic evidence of *Anaplasma phagocytophilum* infection in cats in North America. *J. Am. Vet. Med. Assoc.* **225:**893–896.

51. **Lee, A.** 1992. Helicobacter pylori and Helicobacter-like organisms in animals: overview of mucus-colonizing organisms, p. 259–275. *In* B. J. Rathbone and R. U. Heatley (ed.), *Helicobacter pylori and Gastroduodenal Disease,* 2nd ed. Blackwell Scientific, London, England.

52. **Leonard, F. C., and B. K. Markey.** 2008. Methicillin-resistant *Staphylococcus aureus* in animals: a review. *Vet. J.* **175:**27–36.

53. **Maia, C., M. Nunez, and L. Campino.** 2008. Importance of cats in zoonotic leishmaniasis in Portugal. *Vector Borne Zoonotic Dis.* **8:**555–560.

54. **Malnick, H., K. Williams, J. Phil-Ebosie, and A. S. Levy.** 1990. Description of a medium for isolating *Anaerobiospirillum* spp., a possible cause of zoonotic disease, from diarrheal feces and blood of humans and use of the medium in a survey of human, canine, and feline feces. *J. Clin. Microbiol.* **28:**1380–1384.

55. **Malnick, H.** 1997. *Anaerobiospirillum thomasii* sp. nov., an anaerobic spiral bacterium isolated from the feces of cats and dogs and from diarrheal feces of humans, and emendation of the genus *Anaerobiospirillum*. *Int. J. Syst. Bacteriol.* **47:**381–384.

56. **Maman, E., J. Bickets, M. Ephros, D. Paran, D. Comaneshter, E. Metzkor-Cotter, B. Avigdor, M. Varon-Graidy, S. Weintroub, and M. Giladi.** 2007. Musculoskeletal manifestations of cat scratch disease. *Clin. Infect. Dis.* **45:**1535–1540.

57. **Martin-Sanchez, J., C. Acedo, M. Munoz-Perez, B. Pesson, O. Marchal, and F. Morillas-Marquez.** 2007. Infection by *Leishmania infantum* in cats: epidemiological study in Spain. *Vet. Parasitol.* **145:**267–273.

58. **Maurin, M., S. Gasquet, C. Ducco, and D. Raoult.** 1995. MICs of 28 antibiotic compounds for 14 *Bartonella* (formerly *Rochalimaea*) isolates. *Antimicrob. Agents Chemother.* **39:**2387–2391.

59. **Metzkor-Cotter, E., Y. Kletter, B. Avidor, M. Varon, Y. Golan, M. Ephros, and M. Giladi.** 2003. Long-term serological analysis and clinical follow-up of patients with cat scratch disease. *Clin. Infect. Dis.* **37:**1149–1154.

60. **Montoya, J. G., and J. S. Remmington.** 2008. Management of Toxoplasmosis gondii infection during pregnancy. *Clin. Infect. Dis.* **47:**554–566.

61. **Moran, G. J., A. Krishnadasan, R. J. Horowitz, G. F. Fosheim, L. K. McDougal, R. R. Carey, and D. A. Talan.** 2006. Methicillin-resistant *S. aureus* infections among patients in emergency departments. *N. Engl. J. Med.* **355:**666–674.

62. **Mui, B. S. K., M. E. Mulligan, and W. L. George.** 1990. Response of HIV-associated disseminated cat scratch disease to treatment with doxycycline. *Am. J. Med.* **89:**229–231.

63. **Nakazawa, Y., R. Williams, A. T. Peterson, A. T. Mead, E. Staples, and K. L. Gage.** 2007. Climate change on plague and tularemia in the United States. *Vector Borne Zoonotic Dis.* **7:**529–540.

64. **Ortuno, A., C. B. Gauss, F. Garcia, and J. F. Gutierrez.** 2005. Serological evidence of Ehrlichia spp. exposure in cats from northeastern Spain. *J. Vet. Med. B* **52:**246–248.

65. **Perez-Osorio, C. E., J. E. Zavala-Velasquez, J. J. A. Leon, and J. E. Zavala-Castro.** 2008. Riskettsia felis as emergent global threat for humans. *Emerg. Infect. Dis.* **14:**1019–1023.

66. **Pinard, J. A., N. S. Leslie, and P. J. Irvine.** 2003. Maternal serologic screening for toxoplasmosis. *J. Midwifery Womens Health* **48:**308–316.

67. **Prag, J., J. Blom, and K. A. Korogfelt.** 2007. Helicobacter canis bacteremia in a 7-month-old child. *FEMS Immunol. Med. Microbiol.* **50:**264–267.

68. **Purcell, R. H., and S. U. Emerson.** 2000. Hepatitis E virus, p. 1958–1970. *In* G. L. Man-

dell, J. E. Bennett, and R. Dolin (ed.), *Principles and Practice of Infectious Diseases,* 5th ed. Churchill Livingstone, Philadelphia, PA.

69. **Raoult, D., P. E. Fournier, M. Drancourt, T. J. Marrie, J. Etienne, J. Cosserat, P. Cacoub, Y. Poinsignon, P. Leclerq, and A. M. Sefton.** 1996. Diagnosis of 22 new cases of Bartonella endocarditis. *Ann. Intern. Med.* **125:**646–652.

70. **Reed, J. B., D. K. Scales, M. T. Wong, and C. P. Lattuada, Jr.** 1998. Cat scratch disease retinitis, therapy. *Ophthalmology* **105:**459–466.

71. **Regnery, R., and J. Tappero.** 1997. Unraveling mysteries associated with cat-scratch disease, bacillary angiomatosis, and related syndromes. *Emerg. Infect. Dis.* **1:**16–21.

72. **Rolain, J. M., P. Brouqui, J. E. Koehler, C. Maguina, M. J. Dolan, and D. Raoult.** 2004. Recommendations for treatment of human infections caused by *Bartonella* species. *Antimicrob. Agents Chemother.* **48:**1921–1933.

73. **Rotami, V. O., W. Jamal, T. Pal, A. Sovenned and M. J. Albert.** 2008. Emergence of CTX-M-15 type extended-spectrum beta-lactamase-producing Salmonella spp. in Kuwait and the United Arab Emirates. *J. Med. Microbiol.* **57:**881–886.

74. **Schubach, T. M., A. Schubach, T. Okamoto, I. V. Pellon, P. C. Fialho-Monteiro, R. S. Reis, M. B. Barros, M. Andrade-Perez, and B. Wanke.** 2003. Haematogenous spread of *Sporothrix schenckii* in cats with naturally acquired sporotrichosis. *J. Small Anim. Pract.* **44:**395–398.

75. **Singh, A., C. Tuschak, and S. Hormansdorfer.** 2008. Methicillin-resistant *Staphylococcus aureus* in a family and its pet cat. *N. Engl. J. Med.* **358:**1200–1201.

76. **Spilker, T., A. A. Liwienski, and J. J. Li Puma.** 2008. Identification of Bordetella spp. in respiratory specimens from individuals with cystic fibrosis. *Clin. Microbiol. Infect.* **14:**504–506.

77. **Talan, D. A., D. M. Citron, F. A. Abrahamian, G. J. Moran, E. J. C. Goldstein, and the Emergency Medicine Animal Bite Infection Study Group.** 1999. The bacteriology and management of dog and cat bite wound infections presenting to emergency departments. *N. Engl. J. Med.* **340:**85–92.

78. **Tappero, J. W., J. Mohle-Boetani, J. E. Koehler, B. Swaminathan, T. G. Berger, P. E. LeBoit, L. L. Smith, J. D. Wenger, R. W. Pinner, C. A. Kemper, and A. L. Reingold.** 1993. The epidemiology of bacillary angiomatosis and bacillary peliosis. *J. Am. Med. Assoc.* **269:**770–775.

79. **Titball, R. W., and A. Sjostedt.** 2003. Francisella tularensis: an overview. *ASM News* **69:**558–563.

80. **Urich, S. K., and J. M. Petersen.** 2008. In vitro susceptibility of isolates of *Francisella tularensis* types A and B from North America. *Antimicrob. Agents Chemother.* **52:**2276–2278.

81. **Van den Bulck, K., A. Decostere, I. Gruntar, M. Baele, B. Krt, R. Ducatelle, and F. Haesebrouck.** 2005. In vitro antimicrobial susceptibility testing of *Helicobacter felis, H. bizzozeronii,* and *H. salomonis. Antimicrob. Agents Chemother.* **49:**2997–3000.

82. **van Loon, S., A. Bart, E. J. den Hertog, P. G. Nikkels, R. H. Houwen, J. E. De Schryver, and J. H. Oudshoorn.** 2003. *Helicobacter heilmannii* gastritis caused by cat to child transmission. *J. Pediatr. Gastroenterol. Nutr.* **36:**407–409.

83. **Welch, D. F., D. A. Pickett, L. N. Slater, A. G. Steigerwalt, and D. J. Brenner.** 1992. *Rochalimaea henselae* sp. nov., a cause of septicemia, bacillary angiomatosis, and parenchymal bacillary peliosis. *J. Clin. Microbiol.* **30:**275–280.

84. **Whichard, J. M., K. Gay, J. E. Stevenson, K. J. Joyce, K. L. Cooper, M. Omondi, F. Medalla, G. A. Jacoby and T. J. Barrett.** 2007. Human Salmonella and concurrent decreased susceptibility to quinolones and extended-spectrum cephalosporins. *Emerg. Infect. Dis.* **13:**1681–1688.

85. **Wolfson, C., J. Branley, and T. Gottlieb.** 1996. The Etest for antimicrobial susceptibility testing of Bartonella henselae. *J. Antimicrob. Chemother.* **38:**963–968.

FEATHERED FRIENDS

Matthew E. Levison

7

Although many people these days actually work very hard at leisure time activities, diseases are most commonly acquired from birds during the course of work in the usual sense of the term, not leisure. However, travel for pleasure to areas where the diseases are highly endemic puts people at risk of acquiring some of these bird-related diseases (for example, histoplasmosis and arbovirus infections), as does ownership of birds as pets (psittacosis).

Infectious diseases can be transmitted to humans from birds by one of several mechanisms (Table 1). In group 1 infections, birds are the natural reservoirs for the infectious agent, which causes illness among them. The diseased birds then disseminate the infectious agent into the environment, and humans become infected as accidental hosts. Examples of such infections include psittacosis, Newcastle disease, avian influenza, and yersiniosis. In group 2 and 3 infections, birds are the natural reservoirs for the infectious agent but do not become ill themselves. The infectious agents of group 2 infections (for example, salmonel-

losis and mite infections) disseminate from the colonized birds into the environment directly, and the agents of group 3 infections (for example, eastern equine encephalitis [EEE], western equine encephalitis [WEE], St. Louis encephalitis [SLE], and Japanese B encephalitis [JE]) disseminate by means of arthropod vectors and involve humans as accidental hosts. With group 4 infections, birds are not the natural reservoirs, but they facilitate growth of the organisms in the environment by means of their fecal matter. Examples of infections of the last category include the fungal diseases histoplasmosis and cryptococcosis (1).

GROUP 1

Psittacosis

PATHOGEN
Chlamydophila (formerly Chlamydia) psittaci is an obligate intracellular bacterial parasite that hijacks the host cell's carbon and energy production intermediates for its own purposes.

SOURCE OF INFECTION
The natural reservoirs of *C. psittaci* are wild and domestic birds. Many types of birds are susceptible to *C. psittaci* infection, but most

Matthew E. Levison, Drexel University College of Medicine and Drexel University School of Public Health, Philadelphia, PA 19102.

Infections of Leisure, Fourth Edition, Edited by David Schlossberg,
© 2009 ASM Press, Washington, DC

TABLE 1 Bird-related diseases

| Natural reservoir(s) | Disease | Illness(es) in: | | Mode(s) of spread |
		Birds	Humans	
Group 1				
Birds	Psittacosis	Intestinal, respiratory	Respiratory	Aerosolized bird feces
Domestic and wild fowl	Newcastle disease	Respiratory, neurological	Conjunctivitis	Aerosols, contaminated hands
	Influenza	Respiratory, intestinal, neurological	Respiratory	Aerosols, droplets, contaminated hands
Domestic and wild turkeys	Yersiniosis	Intestinal	Intestinal	Contaminated food
Group 2				
Domestic and wild birds	Mite infestation	None	Pruritic rash	Indirect and direct contact
Domestic fowl	Salmonellosis	None	Diarrhea	Contaminated food
Group 3				
Domestic and wild birds	Arbovirus infections	None	Encephalitis, polyarthritis, rash	Insect vector
Group 4				
Soil fertilized by bird droppings	Histoplasmosis	None	Respiratory	Aerosols
	Cryptococcosis	None	Respiratory, neurological	Aerosols

human cases are acquired from infected cockatiels, parakeets, parrots, and macaws. *C. psittaci* infection in birds is usually latent but may become apparent when resistance is compromised by conditions such as crowding, prolonged transport, or nutritional deficiencies. The infection in birds is primarily gastrointestinal and respiratory and results in diarrhea, fever, conjunctival congestion, and respiratory distress. The agent is shed in the liquid feces, contaminating the environment and the bird's feathers. As the fecal matter dries, the chlamydiae become airborne, which is facilitated by the motion of the feathers. The dried organisms can remain viable for months at room temperature.

In addition to coprophagy and cannibalism, birds acquire the disease by inhalation of infectious aerosols, i.e., airborne particles less than 5 μm in diameter. Airborne particles of this size do not readily settle out by gravity but remain suspended for prolonged periods and are disseminated in the environment by prevailing air currents; only ventilation, filtration by the lungs, and, eventually, gravity remove these particles from the atmosphere. Humans acquire the disease by inhalation of infectious aerosols of bird feces. Person-to-person transmission is so unusual that isolation of the *C. psittaci*-infected patient is thought to be unnecessary.

HUMAN ACTIVITY

Psittacosis is mainly an occupational disease among workers in turkey-processing plants (8, 9), duck or goose pluckers, pigeon breeders, and pet store employees. ProMED recently reported (23) an outbreak at a bird show in The Netherlands that involved 19 of 49 bird handlers, 7 of whom required hospitalization, but the outbreak involved only 6 of the more than 150 spectators, who undoubtedly had much less intense bird exposure than the bird handlers. Inhalation of infectious aerosols generated by mowing lawns has also been noted to be a risk factor.

#84

HUMAN DISEASE

Psittacosis is rare in humans; the U.S. Centers for Disease Control and Prevention recorded 813 cases of psittacosis between 1988 and 1998. The incubation period generally is 5 to 14 days following exposure. From experimental studies of monkeys exposed to infectious aerosols, the earliest lesion is thought to be a respiratory bronchiolitis, followed by centrifugal spread that results in a lobular pneumonia (20). The organisms are also thought to spread systemically via the bloodstream and cause on occasion a typhoid-like syndrome, hepatitis, myocarditis, pericarditis, endocarditis, neurologic involvement, or nephritis.

The illness in humans presents as atypical pneumonia, that is, pneumonia characterized by an insidious, rather than an abrupt, onset; a predominance of constitutional symptoms (such as fever, headache, and myalgias); shortness of breath; and a nonproductive hacking cough. Chest X rays show focal infiltrates, usually at the lung bases. More-severe illness may be accompanied by nausea, vomiting, diarrhea, delirium, and hepatosplenomegaly.

The untreated illness usually lasts 1 to 2 weeks, but the course can be shortened by the use of antibiotic therapy, e.g., doxycycline. The mortality rate prior to the advent of antimicrobial treatment was approximately 15 to 20% and is now less than 1% with appropriate antibiotic therapy. The disease has been noted to be more severe, with high mortality, in the rare instances in which the infection is acquired from another person.

The diagnosis is suspected on the basis of an atypical pneumonia presentation that follows exposure to birds and is usually confirmed serologically by a fourfold rise in serum complement-fixing antibody titers between onset and convalescence or by means of a culture or PCR of respiratory secretions. The organisms can also be cultured from blood. Isolation of the organism should be attempted only in laboratories that use strict isolation techniques.

 # 85

Treatment for adults consists of 2 weeks of doxycycline at 100 mg orally every 12 h. The macrolide azithromycin achieves high intracellular concentrations, is bactericidal, has a long half-life that allows single daily dosing, is well tolerated after oral administration, and may prove to be as or more efficacious than doxycycline.

CONTROL

The U.S. Department of Agriculture (USDA) requires veterinary inspection of birds at the first port of entry into the United States and *# 86* quarantine for a minimum of 30 days at a USDA-approved facility to determine if the birds are free of evidence of communicable diseases of poultry. In addition, during U.S. quarantine, psittacine birds receive medicated feed containing chlortetracycline for the entire quarantine period as a precautionary measure against avian chlamydiosis (3). The USDA recommends that importers continue antibiotic prophylactic treatment of psittacine birds for an additional 15 days (i.e., for 45 continuous days). However, because birds may not eat the feed containing chlortetracycline or the incubation period exceeds the 30 to 45 days of quarantine, these importation measures do not guarantee that all birds entering the United States will not develop avian chlamydiosis. In addition, because smugglers evade importation measures, it is recommended that birds be purchased only from reputable sources.

Newcastle Disease

PATHOGEN

The Newcastle disease agent is a paramyxovirus that is related to the mumps virus. In birds, infection due to Newcastle virus usually produces respiratory and neurological findings, the severity of which varies with the strain of virus and the species of bird. More-virulent strains produce hemorrhagic lesions in the digestive tract, associated with high mortality. More-susceptible species of birds include chickens. A carrier state may exist in psittacines and some other wild birds.

SOURCE OF INFECTION

Domestic fowl, especially poultry, and wild fowl are the natural reservoirs of the virus. Sources of the virus include respiratory secretions, carcasses, and feces of infected birds. Transmission among birds occurs by aerosol inhalation; the ingestion of secretions, especially feces, of an infected bird; or contact with contaminated water, feed, implements, premises, or human clothing.

HUMAN ACTIVITY

Human disease occurs primarily in poultry slaughterhouse workers, laboratory personnel, and vaccinators of the live Newcastle disease virus vaccines. It is transmitted by rubbing the eyes with contaminated hands or by inhalation of infectious aerosols (5).

HUMAN DISEASE

After an incubation period of several days, patients usually develop conjunctivitis, with minimal constitutional symptoms; rarely, some patients develop an influenza-like illness, thought to be the consequence of aerosol exposure (13).

CONTROL

The disease has been controlled by the routine use of Newcastle disease virus vaccines in the poultry industry.

Avian Influenza

PATHOGEN

Influenza viruses are divided into three genera (A, B, and C) determined by the viral ribonucleoprotein antigen. Influenza is caused by influenza A and B viruses. Of the two, influenza A virus is the more important and the cause of regional seasonal outbreaks and pandemics of influenza in humans. Influenza B virus causes seasonal outbreaks only in hu-

mans, whereas influenza A viruses circulate in humans as well as other animals (30).

The antigenic specificities of the two surface proteins hemagglutinin (H) and neuraminidase (N), which function, respectively, to bind the virus to and release it from the host cell, determine influenza virus type. There are 16 known types of H (1 to 16) and 9 types of N (1 to 9). The H type determines the host ranges of influenza A viruses. For example, only types H1, H2, and H3 commonly cause human infection, but all 16 influenza A virus types infect wild waterfowl, usually causing only localized intestinal infection and fecal shedding of large numbers of virions, without causing illness (22). Strains called low-pathogenicity avian influenza (LPAI) viruses lack molecular traits that facilitate systemic spread in poultry and cause localized intestinal infection and fecal shedding in these animals. Wild waterfowl and poultry infected with LPAI viruses act as "silent" reservoirs of the virus, perpetuating transmission to other birds. LPAI H5 and H7 viruses, unlike other LPAI H types, however, can mutate to highly pathogenic avian influenza (HPAI) viruses, which have molecular traits that allow HPAI H5 and H7 viruses to spread very rapidly through poultry flocks, to cause systemic disease affecting multiple internal organs, and to kill up to 100% of infected animals, often within 48 h (11, 22).

HPAI virus subtype H5N1 in poultry and humans was first reported in Hong Kong in 1997, when 18 people were infected, of whom 6 died (26, 27). This outbreak ceased after the slaughter of all of Hong Kong's 1.4 million chickens. HPAI virus H5N1 reappeared in 2003 in Hong Kong. By 2004, the disease had spread to Southeast Asia and by 2005 to Central Asia, Russia, and Eastern Europe. The disease continued to escalate into a global problem in 2006, when it reached Africa, the Middle East, and Western Europe. By early 2008, 61 countries or territories reported the occurrence of HPAI H5N1, and hundreds of millions of poultry were culled or died of

#89

the disease. As of May 2009, 423 human cases of HPAI H5N1 were reported, with 258 deaths in 15 countries (Azerbaijan, Bangladesh, Cambodia, China, Djibouti, Egypt, Indonesia, Iraq, Laos, Myanmar, Nigeria, Pakistan, Thailand, Turkey, and Vietnam). Indonesia accounts for the most cases (33%) and deaths (45%) (35).

As HPAI H5N1 virus continues to spread, its genetic diversity has increased because of mutations, which arise continuously in the infected host and may become predominant by circumventing the host immune response that suppresses the wild-type organism but allows the mutant to propagate. The result of this so-called antigenic drift is not sufficient to compromise immunity completely.

It is thought that antigenic drift, which usually results in regional outbreaks, may also result in a pandemic by allowing, for example, an avian strain to adapt to a human host. In addition, the segmented genomes of influenza viruses allow for genetic reassortment to occur when two different influenza A viruses, e.g., an avian and a human influenza virus, infect the same cell. This provides influenza viruses a powerful option for the generation of genetic diversity to evade host immune responses through a major antigenic change (antigenic shift) and has resulted in pandemics in the past.

H5N1 virus variants are classified on the basis of their H genetic sequence into 10 distinct branches of the virus's family tree or phylogenetic clades; the viral subgroups are named according to their position in the tree (34). Four clades or subclades have been linked to human cases. Clade 1 includes human and bird isolates from Hong Kong, Vietnam, Thailand, and Cambodia and bird isolates from Laos and Malaysia. Most currently circulating H5N1 viruses belong to clade 2, and isolates of this clade were first identified in birds from China, Indonesia, Japan, and South Korea before spreading westward to the Middle East, Europe, and Africa. Genetic analysis has identified six subclades of clade 2,

three of which (2.1, 2.2, and 2.3.4) have distinct geographic distributions and have been implicated in human infections; clade 2.2 viruses have the largest geographical spread, causing bird outbreaks in more than 60 countries and human infections in 8 countries in Africa, Asia, the Middle East and Europe.

The relative importance of the migration of wild birds versus commerce of infected poultry to explain the regional spread of HPAI H5N1 virus is the subject of ongoing debate (11). Global expansion of the commercialized large-scale poultry industry, with an estimated 16 billion chickens and 1 billion ducks worldwide, is associated with the movement of live poultry and poultry products across international borders and over long distances. Traffic in birds used as pets or for cockfighting is an additional problem. Infected live poultry are potential agents for the introduction of HPAI either when the birds (i) are in the incubation period of HPAI virus, (ii) are infected with LPAI virus capable of mutating to HPAI virus, or (iii) are a species that sheds HPAI virus but does not show overt clinical signs (such as seems to be the case for some duck species). Importation and quarantine provisions for captive wild birds are now restricted to birds bred in captivity from approved breeding establishments from a limited list of countries, although illegal importations pose a continued risk.

Wild waterfowl are capable of shedding HPAI H5N1 virus in feces while remaining healthy. Transmission of HPAI H5N1 virus is thought to occur mainly via the fecal-oral route, with virus being shed into ponds, which act as vehicles for dissemination to domestic poultry holdings that share the ponds with wild waterfowl as a consequence of the pond's location under migratory flyways or in close proximity to wild-bird breeding or resting sites. Subsequent reinfection of wild birds may complement the transmission from wild bird species to domestic poultry. Additional mechanisms for transmission of HPAI H5N1 virus among birds include transfer of infected respiratory secretions and eating of infected flesh by carrion birds.

SOURCES OF HUMAN INFECTION AND HUMAN ACTIVITY

Before 1997, strains infecting domestic birds were not known to produce disease by direct transfer to humans, although seroprevalence studies in southern China did reveal that inapparent infection with avian strains had occurred in up to 38% of the local human population.

Since then, most human cases of H5N1 virus infection have been associated with the direct handling of infected poultry; slaughtering or preparing of sick poultry for consumption; consumption of uncooked poultry products, such as raw blood; or close contact with live poultry. Contact with a contaminated environment, such as water and poultry feces used as fertilizer or fish feed, has been suspected of being a source of infection in human H5N1 cases who had no direct exposure to poultry. In bird-to-human transmission, the likely portals of HPAI H5N1 virus entry are either the respiratory tract, as occurs for seasonal influenza, or the gastrointestinal tract. The relative importance of each of these modes of transmission of avian influenza viruses is unknown.

Person-to-person transmission of HPAI H5N1 has rarely occurred, and when it has, it has usually occurred among family members, suggesting to some that there may be a genetic predisposition for acquiring HPAI H5N1. A genetic predisposition may also explain the fact that only relatively few cases of HPAI H5N1 have occurred despite possibly very large numbers of people exposed to the virus worldwide. The relative importance of possible modes of person-to-person transmission of HPAI H5N1 is unknown; inhalation of aerosols or droplets of respiratory secretions and direct contact with respiratory secretions or fomites are possible. In addition, fecal-oral spread is suggested by the prominent gastrointestinal involvement and diarrhea with a high fecal viral load in some patients infected by HPAI H5N1 virus. Several domestic animals, including pigs, cats, and dogs, are susceptible to H5N1 HPAI virus under natural and experimental conditions. Dogs in Southeast Asia exposed to avian influenza have developed asymptomatic infection. However, H5N1 virus has failed to spread between mammalian species, which makes the chance for virus transmission to humans low.

From 2002 to 2004, H7 viruses also caused several disease outbreaks in poultry in Europe and North America and occasionally infected humans, typically causing only mild conjunctivitis, but in 2003, the National Influenza Center in The Netherlands reported 83 confirmed human cases of H7N7 infection among poultry workers, with person-to-person spread to their families and with one fatality, in a veterinarian.

The systemic nature of HPAI virus in poultry suggests that if avian influenza virus is present, fresh poultry products carry a risk of containing viable virus. In nonoutbreak areas, the likelihood of infected poultry being marketed and eventually handled by a consumer or a restaurant worker is considered to be very low.

In areas affected by HPAI H5N1 virus, handling of frozen or thawed, raw, infected poultry meat prior to cooking may be hazardous if good hygienic practices are not observed, and contaminated kitchen equipment, packaging materials, and trays may represent a source of viable virus. Standard hygienic handling practices should be used to prevent cross-contamination. Because there have been reports of only a few human cases of avian influenza potentially linked to the consumption of raw poultry parts (e.g., raw-blood-based dishes) in areas experiencing outbreaks of avian influenza, poultry and poultry products can safely be consumed provided these items are properly cooked and properly handled during food preparation. The virus is inactivated at temperatures reached during conventional cooking (70°C in all parts of the food, i.e., with no "pink" parts of meat). Eggs for consumption may be infected with avian influenza virus. However, cooking egg products should inactivate the virus.

As of February 2008, one report of potential transmission of HPAI H5N1 from wild birds to humans has been made, in which case infection from wild swans being defeathered in Azerbaijan was the most likely source of human infection. Because HPAI H5N1 has not as yet arrived in North America, hunters there do not need to be overly concerned at this time about avian influenza, but all hunters should practice good hygiene in the field when handling any wild bird or mammal. Birds that are obviously sick or birds found dead should not be handled. To be safe, hunters in regions of HPAI endemicity should wash hands frequently and avoid letting hunting dogs lick the hunters' hands or faces.

HUMAN DISEASE

Direct transmission of H7 viruses to humans has caused mainly conjunctivitis and, in a few cases, a febrile flu-like illness (22). However, a veterinarian who had visited an affected farm subsequently developed pneumonia due to HPAI H7N7 virus complicated by acute respiratory distress syndrome and ultimately fatal multiorgan failure. In contrast, direct transmission of HPAI H5N1 to humans has caused, usually within 2 to 4 days of the last exposure to sick poultry, fever, cough, shortness of breath, and radiological evidence of pneumonia that progressed rapidly to acute respiratory distress syndrome requiring mechanical ventilation within days of hospitalization (33). The pneumonia usually seemed to be of primary viral origin, with no evidence of bacterial superinfection in most cases. Unlike with human infections with H7 viruses, conjunctivitis or upper respiratory tract symptoms did not seem to be prominent in H5N1 virus-infected patients. Diarrhea though was common. Other reported complications included multiorgan failure with disseminated intravascular coagulopathy, renal and cardiac dysfunction, Reye's syndrome, lymphopenia, leukopenia, thrombocytopenia, and pulmonary hemorrhage. Central nervous system involvement has rarely been observed in human H5N1 infection. Death supervened for the fatal cases usually within 9 days.

TREATMENT

Patients suspected of having HPAI H5N1 on the basis of a history of exposure to poultry in a region of endemicity should be hospitalized, receive proper infection control precautions (see below), and be treated with an antiviral drug active against avian influenza virus, plus broad-spectrum antibiotics, while awaiting confirmation of the diagnosis of H5N1 virus infection by serology or culture of a throat swab (which, unlike the situation for seasonal influenza, is superior to a nasal or nasopharyngeal swab) obtained prior to initiation of antiviral therapy. The use of aspirin in children and young adults with influenza is risky because of the possible development of Reye's syndrome.

Two classes of antiviral drugs, the M2 influenza virus A membrane protein channel inhibitors amantadine and rimantadine (the adamantanes) and the neuraminidase inhibitors oseltamivir and zanamivir are specifically active against influenza viruses. The neuraminidase inhibitors are effective for the treatment and prophylaxis of influenza A and B viruses, while the adamantanes are active only against influenza A viruses. Viral resistance to adamantanes can emerge rapidly during treatment because of a single point mutation at amino acid position 26, 27, 30, 31, or 34 of the M2 protein, which confers cross-resistance to both amantadine and rimantadine. The adamantane-resistant viruses that emerge soon after the start of adamantane therapy can readily be transmitted to contacts and are fully pathogenic.

A recent report showed a significant increase worldwide in the prevalence of adamantane-resistant seasonal influenza viruses. In the United States, the frequency of adamantane resistance increased from 1.9% in

2004 to 14.5% during the first 6 months of the 2004–2005 influenza season. For the 2005–2006 season, 91% of influenza A (H3N2) viruses, the predominant influenza A pathogen isolated from patients in 23 states in the United States contained an amino acid change at position 31 of the M2 protein which conferred resistance to amantadine and rimantadine.

Of the H5N1 viruses, clade 1 strains from Cambodia, Thailand, and Vietnam carry mutations in the M2 gene conferring high-level resistance to the adamantanes. This has precluded the use of this group of antiviral agents in the treatment and prevention of human infection due to these strains, although some H5N1 viruses isolated in other parts of Asia and Europe remain susceptible to the adamantanes.

As of 2009, a high proportion of nonavian seasonal influenza A H1N1 virus strains in the United States and Europe are resistant to oseltamivir but still fully susceptible to zanamivir. Resistance of H5N1 strains to neuraminidase inhibitors has been clinically negligible so far, although emergence of oseltamivir resistance on therapy has already been seen.

Oseltamivir is currently recommended for prophylaxis of human avian influenza and, when used to treat disease due to H5N1 virus, may improve prospects of survival. Data from the treatment of experimental infection and responses to the treatment of severely ill humans suggest that, to be effective, oseltamivir should be started early (within 48 h of the onset of symptoms) at an increased dosage for a duration that is more prolonged than usually recommended for seasonal influenza. However, clinical efficacy data are limited. Use of an inhaled drug, like zanamivir, or an oral drug, like oseltamivir, is problematic in patients with systemic infection and respiratory failure on mechanical ventilation. In these situations, antiviral strategies ideally should include intravenous therapy (e.g., intravenous zanamivir and peramivir, which are not as yet clinically available) or the use of combined antiviral treatment (adamantanes and neuraminidase inhibitors, oseltamivir plus ribavirin, or two neuraminidase inhibitors) to minimize the emergence of drug resistance (7). Coadministering probenecid with oseltamivir to increase levels of oseltamivir in plasma has also been suggested (16).

CONTROL

Although at present the HPAI H5N1 virus is poorly transmissible from birds to humans and from person to person, because of the uncertainty about the modes of person-to-person transmission, the high lethality of human disease, and the possibility that the virus may change to a strain capable of more-efficient person-to-person transmission, full-barrier precautions (i.e., standard, contact, and airborne precautions) should be used when working in direct contact with suspected or confirmed H5N1 virus-infected patients (27a). These precautions include hand hygiene, gowns, gloves, face shields or goggles, a particulate respirator (N95 level), and negative-pressure isolation rooms. Under resource-poor circumstances, standard and droplet (surgical mask and gown) precautions with gloves and eye protection seem to be the minimal infection control practice for managing these patients.

Culling, biosafety on poultry farms, and safe disposal of poultry carcasses have been among the most effective measures limiting the spread of virus (11). H5N1 vaccines for poultry have also been used as part of a comprehensive control strategy. A human H5N1 vaccine is anticipated to provide some protection for critical portions of the population in the early stages of a pandemic, should the H5N1 virus evolve into a pandemic strain. Because of the anticipated delay required to produce a vaccine that is closely matched to the pandemic strain, the U.S. Department of Health and Human Services has stockpiled several H5N1 virus variants out of concern that a vaccine based on one strain will not work well against a pandemic virus stemming from a different strain.

Yersiniosis

PATHOGEN

Yersinia spp. are enteric, facultative anaerobic, gram-negative bacilli in the family *Enterobacteriaceae,* like *Escherichia coli, Proteus mirabilis, Klebsiella pneumoniae,* etc. Yersiniae grow well at refrigerator temperatures, unlike other enteric pathogens, and also at 37°C on routine media. So-called cold enrichment is used to isolate *Yersinia* from clinical material. *Yersinia pseudotuberculosis* is the least common of the three main *Yersinia* species to cause infections in humans. The other two more common *Yersinia* pathogens in humans are *Y. pestis,* which causes plague, and *Y. enterocolitica,* which causes an illness similar to the one caused by *Y. pseudotuberculosis.*

SOURCE OF INFECTION

Y. pseudotuberculosis, unlike *Y. enterocolitica,* is rarely isolated from soil, water, and foods. The natural reservoirs for *Y. pseudotuberculosis* are believed to be domestic and wild animals, including turkeys, guinea pigs, sheep, cats, and rabbits (31, 36).

HUMAN ACTIVITY

The mechanisms by which the disease is transmitted to humans are unknown, but fecal contamination of food from the animal reservoir is thought to be an important factor.

HUMAN DISEASE

Yersiniosis presents as an acute abdominal infection that simulates acute appendicitis, with fever, lower-right-quadrant pain, and, in some patients, mucous membrane rash, strawberry tongue (Izumi fever), and a scarlet fever-like rash involving the head, neck, and upper and lower extremities (3a, 24a).

The course is usually benign and lasts for about 1 week unless interrupted by surgery for suspected acute appendicitis (28). Late complications of yersinia infection also include reactive arthritis and erythema nodosum. Ophthalmic findings include uveitis and conjunctivitis. Rarely, septic complications, which occur in patients with chronic liver diseases, may be associated with a >75% mortality in these patients.

Although it has not been subjected to critical analysis, treatment consisting of a 2-week course of either doxycycline or a fluoroquinolone, e.g., ciprofloxacin (750 mg every 12 h) is thought to be effective.

CONTROL

In view of the obscure modes of transmission to humans, control of yersiniosis is problematic, but it should involve protection of food and water against fecal contamination by fowl and other animals.

GROUP 2

Mites

PATHOGEN

Mites that infest wild and domestic birds have four stages (egg, larva, nymph, and adult) in their life cycles, which can be completed within 1 week under favorable circumstances.

SOURCE OF INFECTION

The natural reservoirs for these mites are birds. Humans are accidental hosts. The adults of the species *Dermanyssus gallinae* feed on birds at night. During the day these mites infest the buildings that house the birds, where the female mites lay eggs after feeding on the host's blood. Two other species of mites, *Ornithonyssus bursa* and *Ornithonyssus sylviarum,* complete their entire life cycles on birds.

HUMAN ACTIVITY

People who work during the day in buildings that house mite infested birds can become accidental hosts of *D. gallinae,* whereas human infestation by *Ornithonyssus* occurs mainly from handling mite-infested birds.

HUMAN DISEASE

Intensely pruritic papular urticaria develops at sites on the skin where the mites have bitten.

#92

CONTROL

The most effective method to control mite bites is spraying clothing with insect repellent, such as products that contain dimethyl phthalate.

Salmonellosis

PATHOGEN

Non-Typhi salmonellae are enteric facultative anaerobic gram-negative bacilli in the family *Enterobacteriaceae*. Over 1,000 serotypes are known to infect humans. The majority of these strains can be grouped with polyvalent antisera into groups A to E. Definitive identification of a serotype depends on reactivity to antisera directed against somatic O and flagellar H antigens. The relative frequencies at which specific serotypes are isolated vary among different geographic areas. *Salmonella enterica* serovar Typhimurium is the most frequent salmonella serotype isolated in the United States.

SOURCE OF INFECTION

Whereas serovar Typhi is specific for humans, the natural reservoirs of non-Typhi salmonellae are a large variety of both wild and domestic animals (6). Animal-to-animal transmission can be facilitated by contamination of animal feed whose main ingredients are meal made from bone and meat. The most common sources of human disease are poultry products, such as eggs and the meat of chicken, turkey, and ducks, but meat from other animals is also involved. Salmonellae on raw meat can contaminate utensils and surfaces where food is prepared and then be transferred to previously uncontaminated food. Cooking temperatures may not be high enough to lower the bacterial count sufficiently, and in fact, the cooking temperatures, for example, in the center of a stuffed turkey or a soft-boiled or quick-scrambled egg, may actually foster bacterial growth.

HUMAN ACTIVITY

Salmonellosis is acquired by ingestion of food or water contaminated by large numbers of organisms, e.g., >10^5 CFU/ml. Traveler's diarrhea can occasionally be caused by non-Typhi *Salmonella* but is most commonly caused by enteropathogenic *E. coli*. Direct transmission from person to person without food or water as the intervening vehicle does occur, usually by means of the fecal-oral route during male homosexual activity. Person-to-person spread has also been implicated in nursery and hospital outbreaks, which involve patients in whom host defenses in the gastrointestinal tract, such as gastric acidity, small intestinal motility, and colonic bacterial flora, are compromised so that lower inoculum concentrations, i.e., <10^5 CFU/ml, are able to colonize the bowel and subsequently induce disease. Gastrointestinal defenses may be compromised by antacids, gastrectomy, agents that slow intestinal motility, and antibiotics. Some diseases, such as cirrhosis, lymphoma, and human immunodeficiency virus (HIV) infection, which impair systemic host defenses, also increase susceptibility to salmonellosis.

Salmonella colonizes and invades the intestinal mucosa and then may gain access to the bloodstream to produce transient bacteremia. Metastatic infection, usually in tissues that are previously diseased, such as hematomas, neoplasms, bone infarcts, areas of degenerative arthritis, or even atherosclerotic abdominal aneurysms, may follow episodes of transient bacteremia. Control of *Salmonella* bacteremia is impaired in patients with HIV infection and in patients with an underlying hemolytic condition, such as sickle-cell anemia. In fact, in patients with sickle-cell anemia, *Salmonella* rather than *Staphylococcus aureus* is the most common cause of osteomyelitis in areas of bone compromised by ischemia or necrosis.

HUMAN DISEASE

Non-Typhi *Salmonella* causes an acute, self-limited, febrile, diarrheal disease of about 1 week's duration. Patients can carry *Salmonella* in their intestinal tracts for several weeks or, more rarely, for up to several months during convalescence. Transient bacteremia is unusually detected in adult patients but is more frequently detected in infants (up to 50% of patients during the first week of life), in elderly patients, in patients with HIV infection, and in patients with an underlying hemolytic condition, and it is more common with some *Salmonella* species, such as *Salmonella enterica* serovar Choleraesuis.

CONTROL

Control is currently based on the education of cooks at home and in commercial establishments about appropriate methods to reduce contamination of food. Antibiotic therapy of infected patients, even with new potent agents, such as the fluoroquinolones, does not shorten the course of the illness or ameliorate the symptoms and fails to shorten the duration of the convalescent carrier state (21). The methods recommended for the prevention of traveler's diarrhea apply to the prevention of salmonellosis for travelers to areas where hygiene and sanitation are inadequate: use no ice in drinks; drink only bottled water, canned or bottled carbonated beverages, hot tea or coffee, or beer; brush teeth with any of the aforementioned liquids; eat only cooked, hot food; and eat no raw vegetables (e.g., salads), undercooked meats or fish, or unpeeled fruits (see chapter 13 for more on travel-related illnesses).

GROUP 3

Arthropod-Borne Viruses

PATHOGENS

Arthropod-borne viruses (also called arboviruses) are a heterogeneous group of RNA viruses that have a common mode of vector-borne transmission. These species belong to either the alphaviruses *(Togaviridae)* or flaviviruses. EEE, WEE, and Sindbis viruses are alphaviruses, and SLE (10, 19), JE (12, 24), Murray Valley encephalitis (MVE), West Nile encephalitis, Central Europe encephalitis, and Russian spring-summer encephalitis viruses are flaviviruses.

SOURCE OF INFECTION

The geographic distributions of EEE, WEE, and SLE viruses overlap extensively. For example, EEE virus has been isolated from eastern Canada, the Gulf and Atlantic coasts of the United States, the Caribbean islands, and Central and South America. WEE and SLE viruses also are distributed from Canada to Argentina. JE virus is found in most countries of the Far East and in India. Sindbis virus is found in Africa, Scandinavia, countries of the former Soviet Union, and Asia, and MVE virus is found in northern Australia and New Guinea.

The natural reservoirs of most arboviruses are various native wild-bird species. Once infected by an arthropod bite, the reservoir species is usually not seriously affected but will, at least for a time, produce enough virus in its blood to infect other arthropods. In this manner, arthropods pick up the virus and become vectors that transmit the disease to vertebrate hosts, such as other birds, horses, or humans. Arboviruses persistently infect the epithelial cells of the vector's salivary gland, thus permitting the life-long ability to transmit virus to vertebrate hosts during their acquisition of blood meals.

Mosquitoes (in particular, *Culex* spp.) are the vectors for most arboviruses, but ticks (arachnids) transmit a few (Central European encephalitis and Russian spring-summer encephalitis viruses). Viral amplification in other vertebrate species may lead to epidemic outbreaks that involve domestic animals and humans, who are accidental hosts. Horses and humans are generally thought to be "dead-end" hosts because they do not produce enough virus in their blood to infect insects and thereby spread the disease.

HUMAN ACTIVITY

Habitation or travel in an area where arboviruses are endemic places a person at risk of infection.

HUMAN DISEASE

All of these viruses, except Sindbis virus, produce an acute illness, characterized by sudden onset of fever, headache, decreased sensorium, and stiff neck. More-severe cases are complicated by progressive delirium, convulsions, coma, and death or residual neurological deficits in those who recover. EEE, JE, and MVE, in particular, are associated with great morbidity and mortality. SLE and West Nile virus (WNV) infection are most severe in patients >60 years of age. Sindbis virus produces a mild illness characterized by fever, polyarthritis, jaundice, and a maculopapular or vesicular rash (29).

CONTROL

Effective vaccines are available against JE, tick-borne encephalitis, WEE, and EEE. However, only the vaccines for tick-borne encephalitis and JE have been extensively used in humans. Mass vaccination programs against JE have been carried out in several countries in the Far East, including Japan, Korea, and China, with good results in Japan. The vaccine is now available in the United States for travelers who plan prolonged stays in regions where the disease is endemic.

Prevention of arbovirus infections in general includes avoidance of mosquito bites through the use of protective clothing, insect repellents on the body (such as products containing 30% DEET [*N,N*-diethyl-*m*-toluamide]) and on clothing (such as permethrin), and mosquito netting in dwellings in areas where the diseases are endemic. These efforts are especially important at dusk and during the night, because *Culex* mosquitoes, the predominant vector of arboviruses, are night biters and readily enter homes and bite indoors. Because these vectors mature only in stagnant water, elimination of stagnant water and sites in which stagnant water accumulates are major control measures. Larvicides, such as methoprene, "*Bacillus thuringiensis* subsp. *israelensis,*" or *Bacillus sphaericus,* can be applied to water where mosquito larvae develop. The toxicity of these larvicides is quite low, and they are considered safe to use in water containing fish. Goldfish (*Carassius* spp.) can be used in ornamental ponds as a larvicide as well. Other types of larvicides include those that cover the surface of the water with a thin film of liquid, such as oil, designed to prevent larvae from obtaining oxygen at the water's surface.

Killing adult mosquitoes is a supplement to larvicide use and is used when mosquitoes become too numerous or when high levels of virus activity in mosquitoes threaten populated areas with disease. Control of adult mosquitoes usually involves fogging, i.e., application of fine droplets of pesticides released from specialized trucks or aerial equipment. Fogging is more expensive than larviciding and to be effective requires selection of the appropriate insecticide and equipment, accurate application, and favorable environmental conditions (generally used in the evening when mosquitoes are active, when the temperature is between 60°F and 85°F, and when there is little wind). Application of coarse spray of some insecticides to surfaces where mosquitoes rest, such as vegetation and the exterior walls of buildings, is less demanding of environmental conditions and is less expensive than fogging.

WEST NILE VIRUS

Of special note is WNV. WNV was first isolated in Uganda in 1937 and first isolated in the United States in 1999. WNV is now seen throughout the United States, in Canada, and in the Caribbean basin. The 2002 WNV epidemic in the United States was the largest arboviral meningoencephalitis outbreak ever documented in the Western Hemisphere and the largest reported meningoencephalitis epidemic. As a newly introduced species, WNV is having a major effect on the North American ecosystem. WNV and SLE virus are closely related; both are transmitted by *Culex* mosquitoes and amplified in birds, but unlike SLE virus, WNV is an avian neuropathogen and causes high mortality in many avian species, including crows (which have the highest rate of WNV infection), blue jays, ravens, and raptors, such as eagles, hawks, and owls. In addition, WNV is a neuropathogen in other

#96

vertebrate species, such as horses, rabbits, squirrels, chipmunks, goats, and reptiles.

A major die-off due to WNV infection is reported for many species of birds, mammals, and reptiles, although over time species are expected to adapt. The usual sentinel event that signals WNV activity in a region is the sighting of dead crows. WNV infection in birds is characterized by high-level viremia of sufficient magnitude to maintain a reservoir of infected mosquitoes. WNV can also pass transovarially from adult mosquitoes to their eggs, so that larvae are hatched already infected, and WNV probably can also survive winter in other unknown hosts. Although many species of mosquito are vectors of WNV, *Culex* species are the most common. WNV can also be found in bird feces and saliva, and perhaps birds of prey can acquire the infection by eating infected prey or by having contact with their droppings or pass the virus to their chicks transovarially.

Most human WNV infections are acquired by a bite of an infected mosquito, but a few patients have become infected by accidental percutaneous inoculation in the laboratory, by administration of blood and blood products from infected donors, by transplantation of organs from infected donors, possibly by breast-feeding, and by transplacental transmission, with evidence of congenital severe central nervous system damage in the child. WNV causes illness in humans from June to November in southern states and from July to October in northern states, with peak activity in late August.

The incubation period is 2 to 14 days. Infected patients are usually asymptomatic, but a few develop a nonspecific acute febrile illness, with headache, myalgias, swollen lymph nodes, and back pain, that resolves rapidly (West Nile fever). Fewer than 1% of patients develop meningitis, encephalitis, or acute flaccid paralysis after an initial mild febrile illness. Severe neurological illness and neurological residua, e.g., oculomotor palsies, muscle weakness, and movement disorders, which may mimic stroke, Parkinsonism, or polio-myelitis, are seen most frequently in older or immunocompromised patients, and relatively higher mortality rates occur in these groups. For example, WNV-infected transplant patients have an estimated 40-fold-greater risk for developing neuroinvasive disease than the general population, and, similar to SLE virus, WNV causes more-severe illness; neuroinvasive disease likely results in a prolonged recuperation and rehabilitation period in persons over 65 years of age (18). The overall mortality rate for WNV infection is 6 to 7%.

Infection is thought to confer immunity against subsequent exposure. No antiviral drugs are known to be effective in the prevention or treatment of WNV infection. Control of WNV includes spraying with insecticide for control of adult mosquitoes and use of larvicides in the summertime, draining or treating stagnant water in urban and suburban areas during the mosquito season (mosquitoes lay their eggs in standing water), and using personal protective measures to reduce mosquito exposure (e.g., using DEET on exposed skin, using permethrin or DEET on clothing, wearing clothing that minimizes exposed skin, sleeping under mosquito nets impregnated with permethrin, and limiting outdoor exposure at dawn and dusk, when mosquito biting is most intense). Bird-based surveillance is used to monitor regional WNV activity in an area before the recognition of human cases.

Although mosquito-borne transmission is the major mode of WNV transmission, transfusion-associated transmission has also been identified. In June 2003, the blood supply of the United States was screened for WNV RNA by testing pooled samples from 6 to 16 donors, using investigational nucleic acid amplification tests. Such pooling dilutes viremic plasma by 6- to 16-fold and potentially reduces the assay's sensitivity compared with that of screening each donor's plasma individually. About 4.5 million people receive blood or blood products annually. Between June and December 2003, 818 WNV-positive donations in the United States that could have

#97

#98

potentially transmitted WNV to recipients if transfused were interdicted by the nucleic acid amplification tests. However, six cases of WNV infection have been attributed to transfusion of blood that had been screened by testing pooled samples and had been found to be negative for WNV RNA, presumably because of very low levels of WNV. Individual donor testing for WNV RNA has been implemented since 2004 in regions with high WNV infection rates. Individual donor testing for WNV is especially important for the elderly and immunosuppressed recipients, because elderly individuals or people with weakened immune systems are more likely to develop severe diseases, such as encephalitis or meningitis, if they become infected. Diagnosis of WNV infection is based on serologic tests and detection of WNV RNA by nucleic acid amplification. The viremia is typically of a low level and of short duration during the incubation period. Viremia has usually resolved by the time of onset of symptoms. WNV can be detected in the cerebrospinal fluid, and immunoglobulin M antibody specific for WNV can be detected in cerebrospinal fluid within 3 to 5 days of the onset of clinical disease and in serum by day 6. Immunoglobulin G antibody appears several days later, and acute- and convalescent-phase serum samples, collected at least 2 weeks apart, can be run simultaneously to assess for a fourfold or greater rise in antibody titer. Antibodies against other flaviviruses can cross-react in serologic tests for WNV.

GROUP 4

Histoplasmosis

PATHOGEN

Histoplasma capsulatum is a dimorphic fungus. The yeast form grows in vitro at 37°C and in tissues; the mycelial form grows in vitro at room temperature. One variety of the organism (*H. capsulatum* var. *duboisii*) has been isolated only in central Africa. The other variety is distributed worldwide, usually in major river valleys. In the United States, infection is concentrated in the Mississippi, Missouri, and Ohio river valleys (2, 14). Histoplasmosis is also endemic in most of Latin America.

SOURCE OF INFECTION

The natural reservoir is soil, especially soils fertilized by bird or bat guano. Unlike birds, bats shed the fungus from their gastrointestinal tracts in their droppings. When contaminated soil is disturbed, for example, by bulldozing or razing old buildings, infectious aerosols of microconidia may be created. Similarly, in poorly ventilated caves, tunnels, and mines inhabited by bats, the air may become heavily laden with infectious aerosols when the ground is disturbed by human activity (15, 25).

HUMAN ACTIVITY

Infection occurs in humans when they inhale infectious aerosols while working at construction sites or when visiting caves, tunnels, and abandoned mines in which bat droppings have accumulated.

HUMAN DISEASE

In areas where the disease is endemic, infection is common, although the precise prevalence may vary from area to area. From 20 to over 80% of the population in areas of endemicity have positive reactions to the histoplasmin skin test, which indicates past or current infection with *H. capsulatum*. The pathogenesis of histoplasmosis is thought to be identical to that of tuberculosis. The inhaled aerosols, particles less than 3 μm in diameter, which may consist of only one or two infectious microconidia, easily bypass defense mechanisms in the upper respiratory tract and airways to lodge in the alveoli. In the lung, the microconidia may begin to grow and divide. Some particles may be engulfed by macrophages, which are eventually carried to regional lymph nodes. From there the intracellular pathogens disseminate via the lymphatics into the bloodstream and then throughout the body to lodge in other reticuloendothelial organs, such as the bone marrow, liver, and spleen during the first

2 weeks of infection before specific immunity has developed. (This process is called primary lymphohematogenous dissemination.) Acute pulmonary histoplasmosis resembles atypical pneumonia, the severity of which depends on the number of infectious particles inhaled. Asymptomatic infection or mild pulmonary disease follows low intensity exposure in healthy individuals, whereas heavy exposure may cause severe diffuse pulmonary infection. Fever, headache, myalgias, and a dry, hacking cough develop initially. Several weeks after exposure to the infectious aerosol, some patients develop erythema nodosum and arthralgias, probably when the immune response first develops. With the onset of the immune response, the balance between the patient and the fungus then temporarily shifts in favor of the patient; hematogenous dissemination fails to progress, and further growth of the organisms is curtailed. Not all the organisms are killed, however; residual foci of latent infection remain, which can reactivate at any time in the future if host defenses should fail. In most patients, acute pulmonary histoplasmosis is a self-limiting process, and the only residual signs of this initial encounter with histoplasma microconidia are diffusely scattered foci of fine pulmonary or splenic calcifications.

Primary progressive pulmonary disease develops in a few patients, especially those with underlying centrilobular emphysema. The initial pulmonary infiltrates develop into a fibronodular pattern, and cavities enlarge over months to years. Progressive dissemination with involvement primarily of the lung, liver, and bone marrow occurs rarely. Most of these patients have defects in cell-mediated immunity, e.g., patients with AIDS or severe debility, the very young, or the very old. The tempo of the illness may be acute or chronic, and it is invariably fatal if untreated. It is manifested by hepatosplenomegaly, fever, night sweats, and mucosal ulcerations. Involvement of the bone marrow may produce anemia, leukopenia, and thrombocytopenia.

H. capsulatum var. *duboisii* produces granulomatous lesions in skin, subcutaneous soft tissue, and bone in the form of abscesses and ulcerations.

A positive histoplasmin skin test indicates the presence of cellular immunity, but the test may be negative early in the course of disease or in patients with disseminated disease. It is used only for epidemiological purposes, not to diagnose a specific individual's illness. Indeed, the skin test may itself elicit an antibody response and confound the results of subsequent serologic testing. Testing of serologic response, sputum culture, and culture and histology of biopsied tissues, e.g., bone marrow, liver, and mucosal lesions, are the main diagnostic methods. Treatment is not indicated in the typical patient with acute pulmonary histoplasmosis because the illness is self-limited and associated with minimal morbidity (32). Treatment is reserved for those patients with severe acute pulmonary, chronic progressive, or disseminated disease. Itraconazole is the treatment of choice for patients who do not require hospitalization and for continuation of therapy in those with more-severe disease whose condition has improved in response to initial use of intravenously administered amphotericin B.

CONTROL
Control of the organism in the environment is difficult. Spraying the ground with 3% Formalin has been recommended, as has the use of face masks when dirt or buildings where birds have roosted are disturbed.

Cryptococcosis

PATHOGEN
Cryptococcus is a urease-positive yeast that has worldwide distribution. *Cryptococcus neoformans,* the only species that is pathogenic, has four serotypes (A to D), based on capsular polysaccharide, and two varieties: var. *neoformans* (serotypes A and D) and var. *gattii* (serotypes B and C).

The organism exists in tissues in an encapsulated form and in soil in an unencapsulated form. It reproduces both asexually as a yeast and sexually as a basidiomycete. The sexual reproductive phase of *Cryptococcus* constitutes the genus *Filobasidiella*, e.g., *Filobasidiella neoformans* var. *neoformans* for *C. neoformans* var. *neoformans* and *Filobasidiella neoformans* var. *bacillispora* for *C. neoformans* var. *gattii*. *Cryptococcus* is identified in clinical specimens by detection of its polysaccharide capsule by means of an India ink preparation in fluid specimens, mucicarmine staining of the polysaccharide capsule around the organism in tissue sections, or testing for an antibody to the capsular polysaccharide antigen in serum and other body fluids.

SOURCE OF INFECTION

Birds carry *C. neoformans* var. *neoformans* in their intestinal tracts without becoming ill. The organism is isolated from bird feces and soil contaminated with bird feces. The creatinine in the feces serves as a source of nitrogen for the organisms. Inhalation of an infectious aerosol, which is generated from contaminated dust or soil, is thought to be the mode of infection for humans. However, the exact form of the infectious agent is unknown. The size of the encapsulated yeast (4 to 7 μm in diameter) may be too large for it to be an efficient aerosol. However, the unencapsulated yeast or the basidiospore, which measures 2 μm in diameter, may be a more appropriate size for the infectious particle.

C. neoformans var. *gattii* infection is noted here only briefly, because in contrast to *C. neoformans* var. *neoformans,* var. *gattii* is not known to be bird associated. *C. neoformans* var. *gattii* is endemic in eucalyptus-growing regions of Australia and Papua New Guinea (the bark and leaves are an ecological habitat for var. *gattii*) and in parts of Africa, the Mediterranean region, India, Southeast Asia, Mexico, Brazil, and Paraguay. Its occurrence in the latter regions lacking eucalyptus trees suggests that additional environmental niches for this fungus are yet to be discovered (D. H. Ellis [University of Adelaide, Adelaide, Australia], personal communication, and reference 20a). Whereas cryptococcal infections among immunodeficient individuals are predominantly caused by *C. neoformans* var. *neoformans,* 70 to 80% of cryptococcal infections among immunocompetent hosts are caused by *C. neoformans* var. *gattii;* var. *gattii* infections are mainly pulmonary (75%), although neurologic (8%) and combined (9%) infections are seen.

C. neoformans var. *gattii* has caused a large-scale outbreak since 1999 that involved terrestrial and marine mammals and several hundred humans in British Columbia and the Pacific Northwest of the United States. The route by which *C. neoformans* var. *gattii* was introduced into North America has not been established, although importation of contaminated eucalyptus trees or wooden pallets or crates made from eucalyptus that are not routinely inspected for microbial contamination upon entry into Canada or the United States has been implicated, with subsequent spread possibly by human and other animal activity (17).

HUMAN ACTIVITY

Work in areas where pigeons roost or where soil is contaminated with pigeon feces poses a danger for exposure to *C. neoformans* var. *neoformans.* Transmission via organ transplantation has been reported when infected donor organs were used.

HUMAN DISEASE

The portal of infection is thought to be the respiratory tract, although only a minority of patients develop a respiratory illness following inhalation of aerosolized soil or dust contaminated with infected bird droppings.

At the time most patients present with clinical cryptococcosis due to *C. neoformans* var. *neoformans,* they have extrapulmonary involvement, usually of the central nervous system; the asymptomatic primary pulmonary infection has either resolved spontaneously or left a residual pulmonary nodule (cryptococcoma). For the few patients with symptomatic pulmonary infection, the patient complains of fever, chest pain, cough, and hemoptysis, and unless the patient is immunocompromised, the disease has not disseminated to extrapulmonary sites. Dissemination of *C. neoformans* var. *neoformans* is likely in patients with AIDS, lymphoma, diabetes mellitus, or cirrhosis or those being treated with corticosteroids.

Involvement of the central nervous system presents insidiously over weeks, with severe headache and progressive deterioration in mental status. The patient may have a stiff neck and focal cranial nerve signs. The cerebrospinal fluid has a lymphocytic pleocytosis (5 to 500 leukocytes/mm^3), low glucose concentration (<45 mg/100 ml), and high protein concentration (>45 mg/100 ml). In patients with AIDS, but less so in others, the organisms are so numerous in the cerebrospinal fluid that they are readily visible in the India ink preparation. In any case, the antibody test for capsular polysaccharide in the cerebrospinal fluid and serum is positive for over 95% of patients and is rarely falsely positive. In fact, the test with serum is more sensitive than that with cerebrospinal fluid for patients with AIDS. Patients may have focal neurological involvement as a consequence of cerebral cryptococcomas. Other sites for the development of disseminated disease include bone, skin, and the prostate gland. The prostate has been implicated as a frequent site for relapsing infection after a course of antimicrobial therapy.

Effective treatment for cryptococcal meningitis in patients without AIDS has been shown to be amphotericin B at a daily dose of 0.3 mg/kg of body weight intravenously combined with 5-flucytosine at 150 mg/kg daily in four divided oral doses for 6 weeks (4). In patients with AIDS, 5-flucytosine has been associated with an excessive bone marrow-suppressive effect, and amphotericin B alone fails to eradicate the disease. After an initial course of 0.4 to 0.6 mg of amphotericin B per kg for at least 6 weeks, relapse of cryptococcal meningitis can be prevented in most patients with AIDS by giving 0.6 mg/kg intravenously weekly. Almost equally effective is fluconazole at 200 to 400 mg daily for 10 to 12 weeks after the last positive cerebrospinal fluid culture. However, because of a slower initial response in the clearance of cryptococci from the cerebrospinal fluid and excessive early mortality with fluconazole compared to that with amphotericin B therapy, initial treatment with amphotericin B at 0.6 mg/kg intravenously daily for 2 weeks followed by fluconazole at 200 mg daily for the rest of the patient's life is recommended for patients with AIDS.

CONTROL

Control of pigeon populations in areas of human habitation has been attempted for aesthetic and health reasons, with varying success.

PRACTICAL TIPS

- Because smugglers evade importation measures imposed by the USDA aimed at the prevention of communicable avian diseases, it is recommended that pet birds be purchased only from reputable sources.
- Because HPAI H5N1 virus has not as yet arrived in North America, hunters there do not need to be overly concerned at this time about avian influenza, but all hunters should practice good hygiene in the field when handling any wild bird or mammal. Birds that are obviously sick or birds found dead should not be handled. To be safe, hunters in regions of HPAI endemicity should wash hands frequently and avoid letting hunting dogs lick their hands or face.
- In nonoutbreak areas, the likelihood of infected poultry being marketed and eventually handled by a consumer or a restaurant worker is considered to be very low. In areas affected by HPAI H5N1 virus, handling of frozen or thawed raw infected poultry meat prior to cooking may be hazardous if good hygienic practices are not observed, and contaminated kitchen equipment, packaging materials, and trays may represent a source of viable virus. Standard hygienic handling practices should be used to prevent cross-contamination. Because

there have been reports of a few human cases of avian influenza potentially linked to the consumption of raw poultry parts (e.g. raw-blood-based dishes), in areas experiencing outbreaks of avian influenza, poultry and poultry products can be safely consumed provided these items are properly cooked and properly handled during food preparation. The virus is inactivated at temperatures reached during conventional cooking (70°C in all parts of the food, i.e., with no "pink" parts of the meat). Eggs for consumption may be infected with avian influenza virus. However, cooking egg products should inactivate the virus.

• The methods recommended for prevention of traveler's diarrhea apply to prevention of salmonellosis for travelers in areas where hygiene and sanitation are inadequate: use no ice in drinks; drink only bottled water, canned or bottled carbonated beverages, hot tea or coffee, or beer; brush teeth with any of the aforementioned liquids; eat only cooked, hot food; and eat no raw vegetables (e.g., salads), undercooked meats or fish, or unpeeled fruits.

• JE virus vaccine is now available in the United States for travelers who plan prolonged stays in regions where the disease is endemic. Prevention of arbovirus infections in general includes avoidance of mosquito bites through the use of protective clothing and insect repellents on the body (such as products containing 30% DEET) and on clothing (such as permethrin) and the use of mosquito netting in dwellings in areas where the diseases are endemic. These efforts are especially important at dusk and during the night, because *Culex* mosquitoes, the predominant vector of arboviruses, are night biters and readily enter homes and bite indoors. Because these vectors mature only in stagnant water, elimination of stagnant water and of sites in which stagnant water accumulates is a major control measure. Larvicides, such as methoprene, "*Bacillus thuringiensis* subsp. *israelensis,*" or *B. sphaericus,* can be applied to water where mosquito larvae develop. The toxicity of these larvicides is quite low, and they are considered safe to use in water containing fish. Goldfish *(Carassius)* can be used in ornamental ponds as a larvicide as well.

REFERENCES

1. **Acha, P. N., and B. Szyfres.** 1987. *Zoonoses and Communicable Diseases Common to Man and Animals,* 2nd ed. Pan American Health Organization, Washington, DC.
2. **Ajello, L.** 1967. Comparative ecology of respiratory mycotic disease agents. *Bacteriol. Rev.* **31:** 6–24.
3. **Armstein, P., B. Eddie, and K. F. Meyer.** 1968. Control of psittacosis by group chemotherapy of infected parrots. *Am. J. Vet. Res.* **29:** 2213–2227.
3a. **Baba, K., N. Takeda, and M. Tanaka.** 1991. Cases of *Yersinia pseudotuberculosis* infection having diagnostic criteria of Kawasaki disease. *Contrib. Microbiol. Immunol.* **12:**292–296
4. **Bennett, J. E., W. E. Dismukes, R. J. Duma, G. Medoff, M. A. Sande, H. Gallis, J. Leonard, B. T. Fields, M. Bradshaw, H. Haywood, Z. A. McGee, T. R. Cate, C. G. Cobbs, J. F. Warner, and D. W. Alling.** 1979. A comparison of amphotericin B alone and combined with flucytosine in the treatment of cryptococcal meningitis. *N. Engl. J. Med.* **301:** 126–131.
5. **Brandly, C. A.** 1964. The occupational hazard of Newcastle disease to man. *Lab. Anim. Care* **14:** 433–440.
6. **Bryan, F. L.** 1981. Current trends in food-borne salmonellosis in the United States and Canada. *J. Food Prot.* **44:**394–402.
7. **Calfee, D. P., A. W. Peng, L. M. Cass, M. Lobo, and F. G. Hayden.** 1999. Safety and efficacy of intravenous zanamivir in preventing experimental human influenza A virus infection. *Antimicrob. Agents Chemother.* **43:**1616–1620.
8. **Center for Disease Control.** 1974. Follow-up on turkey-associated psittacosis. *Morb. Mortal. Wkly. Rep.* **23:**309–310.
9. **Centers for Disease Control.** 1982. Psittacosis associated with turkey processing—Ohio. *Morb. Mortal. Wkly. Rep.* **30:**638–640.
10. **Centers for Disease Control.** 1987. Arboviral infections of the central nervous system—United

States, 1986. *Morb. Mortal. Wkly. Rep.* **36:**450–455.

11. **European Food Safety Authority.** 2008. Scientific opinions, question no. EFSA-Q-2007-179, adopted 7 May 2008. http://www.efsa.europa.eu/EFSA/efsa_locale-1178620753812_1178713016506.htm.

12. **Gatus, B. J., and M. R. Rose.** 1983. Japanese B encephalitis; epidemiology, clinical and pathologic aspects. *J. Infect.* **6:**213–218.

13. **Goebel, S. J., J. Taylor, J. C. Barr, H. R. Castro-Malaspina, C. V. Hedvat, K. A. Rush-Wilson, C. D. Kelly, S. W. Davis, W. A. Samsonoff, K. R. Hurst, M. J. Behr, and P. S. Masters.** 2007. Isolation of avian paramyxovirus 1 from a human case of pneumonia. *J. Virol.* **81:**12709–12714.

14. **Goodwin, R. A., and R. M. DesPrez.** 1978. State of the art. Histoplasmosis. *Am. Rev. Respir. Dis.* **117:**929–956.

15. **Hoff, G. L., and W. J. Bigler.** 1981. The role of bats in the propagation and spread of histoplasmosis: a review. *J. Wildl. Dis.* **17:**191–196.

16. **Holodniy, M., S. R. Penzak, T. M. Straight, R. T. Davey, K. K. Lee, M. B. Goetz, D. W. Raisch, F. Cunningham, E. T. Lin, N. Olivo, and L. R. Deyton.** 2008. Pharmacokinetics and tolerability of oseltamivir combined with probenecid. *Antimicrob. Agents Chemother.* **52:**3013–3021.

17. **Kidd, S. E., P. J. Bach, A. O. Hingston, S. Mak, Y. Chow, L. MacDougall, J. W. Kronstad, and K. H. Bartlett.** 2007. *Cryptococcus gattii* dispersal mechanisms, British Columbia, Canada. *Emerg. Infect. Dis.* **13:**51–57.

18. **Klee, A. L., B. Maldin, B. Ewin, I. Poshni, F. Mostashari, A. Fine, M. Layton, and D. Nash.** 2004. Long-term prognosis for clinical West Nile virus infection. *Emerg. Infect. Dis.* **10:**1405–1411.

19. **Luby, J. P., S. E. Sulkin, and J. P. Sanford.** 1969. The epidemiology of St. Louis encephalitis: a review. *Annu. Rev. Med.* **20:**329–350.

20. **McGavran, M. H., C. W. Beard, R. F. Berendt, and R. M. Nakamura.** 1962. The pathogenesis of psittacosis. Serial studies on rhesus monkeys exposed to a small-particle aerosol of the Borg strain. *Am. J. Pathol.* **40:**653–670.

20a.**Mycology Online.** http://www.mycology.adelaide.edu.au/Fungal_Descriptions/Yeasts/Cryptococcus/C_gattii.html.

21. **Neill, M. A., S. M. Opal, J. Heelan, R. Giusti, J. E. Cassidy, R. White, and K. H. Mayer.** 1991. Failure of ciprofloxacin to eradicate convalescent fecal excretion after acute salmonellosis: experience during an outbreak in

healthcare workers. *Ann. Intern. Med.* **114:**195–199.

22. **Peiris, J. S. M., M. D. de Jong, and Y. Guan.** 2007. Avian influenza virus (H5N1): a threat to human health. *Clin. Microbiol. Rev.* **20:**243–267. doi:10.1128/CMR.00037-06.

23. **ProMED-mail.** 2007. Psittacosis, bird show—Netherlands: (Gelderland) 20071203.3891. http://promedmail.org.

24. **Rosen, L.** 1986. The natural history of Japanese encephalitis virus. *Annu. Rev. Microbiol.* **40:**395–414.

24a.**Sato, K., K. Ouchi, and M. Taki.** 1983. *Yersinia pseudotuberculosis* infection in children, resembling Izumi fever and Kawasaki syndrome. *Pediatr. Infect. Dis.* **2:**123–126.

25. **Schech, W. F., L. J. Wheat, J. L. Ho, M. L. French, R. J. Weeks, R. B. Kohler, C. E. Deane, H. E. Eitzen, and J. D. Band.** 1983. Recurrent urban histoplasmosis, Indianapolis, Indiana, 1980–1981. *Am. J. Epidemiol.* **118:**301–312.

26. **Snacken, R., A. P. Kendal, L. R. Haaheim, and J. M. Wood.** 1999. The next influenza pandemic: lessons from Hong Kong, 1997. *Emerg. Infect. Dis.* **5:**195–203.

27. **Subbarao, K., A. Klimov, J. Katz, H. Regnery, W. Lim, H. Hall, M. Perdue, D. Swayne, C. Bender, J. Huang, M. Hemphill, T. Rowe, M. Shaw, X. Xu, K. Fukuda, and N. Cox.** 1998. Characterization of an avian influenza (H5N1) virus isolated from a child with a fatal respiratory illness. *Science* **279:**393–396.

27a.**Tellier, R.** 2006. Review of aerosol transmission of influenza A virus. *Emerg. Infect. Dis.* **12:**1657–1662.

28. **Tertti, R., K. Granfors, O.-P. Lehtonen, J. Mertsola, A. L. Makela, I. Valimaki, P. Hanninen, and A. Toivanen.** 1984. An outbreak of *Yersinia pseudotuberculosis* infection. *J. Infect. Dis.* **149:**245–250.

29. **Tesh, R. B.** 1982. Arthritides caused by mosquito-borne viruses. *Annu. Rev. Med.* **33:**31–40.

30. **Treanor, J. J.** 2000. Influenza virus, p. 1823–1848. *In* G. L. Mandell, J. E. Bennett, and R. Dolin (ed.), *Principles and Practice of Infectious Diseases*, 5th ed. Churchill Livingstone, New York, NY.

31. **Wallner-Pendleton, E., and G. Cooper.** 1983. Several outbreaks of *Yersinia pseudotuberculosis* in California turkey flocks. *Avian Dis.* **27:**524–526.

32. **Wheat, J., G. Sarosi, D. McKinsey, R. Hamill, R. Bradsher, P. Johnson, J. Loyd, and C. Kauffman.** 2000. Practice guidelines for the management of patients with histoplasmosis. *Clin. Infect. Dis.* **30:**688–695.

33. **Wong, S. S. Y., and K.-Y. Yuen.** 2006. Avian influenza virus infections in humans. *Chest* **129:** 156–168.

34. **World Health Organization.** 2008. Antigenic and genetic characteristics of H5N1 viruses and candidate H5N1 vaccine viruses developed for potential use as human vaccines. February 2008. World Health Organization, Geneva, Switzerland. http://www.who.int/csr/disease/avian_influenza / guidelines / H5VaccineVirusUpdate 20080214.pdf.

35. **World Health Organization.** 2009. Cumulative number of confirmed human cases of avian influenza reported to WHO: 6 May 2009. World Health Organization, Geneva, Switzerland. http://www.who.int / csr / disease / avian_influenza / country / cases_table_2009_05_06 / en / index.html.

36. **World Health Organization Scientific Working Group.** 1980. Enteric infections due to Campylobacter, Yersinia, Salmonella and Shigella. *Bull. W. H. O.* **58:**519–537.

LESS COMMON HOUSE PETS

Bruno B. Chomel

8

Many infectious diseases in humans can be acquired through contact with pets. Dogs and cats may be the most common pets around the world, but there are also many other vertebrates that share our household environment. Approximately 60% of all households in the United States have at least one pet, and 5% have pet birds, but the pet population also includes several million rodents and rabbits (9.5 million), reptiles (13.4 million), and aquarium fish (freshwater, 142 million; saltwater, 9.6 million), not to mention less common species (e.g., miniature pigs) and exotic species, including wild carnivores, wild rodents, and pet monkeys (6, 153). It is estimated that 20 million American homes have aquariums at any given time (6). Pet rabbits are among the most common specialty and exotic pets, accounting for almost 5 million animals present in approximately 2% of the households (6). Specialty or exotic pet ownership had increased from 6.7% of all households in 1991 to 10.7% in 1996, and the number of households with exotic pets was similar in 2006 to that in 1996 after a decrease in

2001 (6). It is estimated that between 1996 and 2001, the number of pet ferrets increased by 25.3%, with an estimated 1 million ferrets present in 0.5% of all households (6). A 12.6% increase in pet turtle ownership was also reported for the same time period (6). Similarly, the estimated number of households with reptiles doubled from approximately 850,000 to 1.7 million from 1991 to 2001 (37).

The objective of this chapter is not to cover every species that can be kept as pets and every disease, especially the rare and exotic ones, that they can transmit to us but rather to focus on the other most common "house pets" and the major health threats that they can represent. Only a brief discussion at the end of this chapter is devoted to more uncommon pets, especially ferrets and primates. However, because of the outbreak of monkeypox in prairie dogs and humans which occurred in the spring of 2003 in the United States, a few words are devoted to the risk of ownership of exotic pets.

PET RABBITS AND RODENTS

Zoonoses transmitted by pet rabbits and pet rodents are quite rare (Table 1). Most of the health problems encountered with these animals are related to allergies or bites. A major distinction should be made between domes-

Bruno B. Chomel, Department of Population Health and Reproduction, School of Veterinary Medicine, University of California, Davis, Davis, CA 95616.

Infections of Leisure, Fourth Edition, Edited by David Schlossberg,
© 2009 ASM Press, Washington, DC

TABLE 1 Zoonoses potentially transmitted by pet rabbits and rodents

Animal	Zoonosis (pathogen)[a]			
	Viral	Bacterial	Parasitic	Mycotic
Rabbit	[Rabies] [Monkeypox]	**Pasteurellosis** **Salmonellosis** Yersiniosis [Listeriosis] [Tuberculosis] [Tularemia]	**Cheyletiellosis** [*Baylisascaris* infection] [*Encephalitozoon cuniculi*	**Dermatophytosis** (*T. mentagrophytes, Microsporum*)
Mouse	**LCM** [HFRS]	**Salmonellosis** Pasteurellosis Yersiniosis Mycoplasmosis [RBF] [Leptospirosis]	**Taeniasis** (*H. nana, H. diminuta*)	**Dermatophytosis** (*T. mentagrophytes*)
Rat, Gambian rat	**HFRS** **Monkeypox** **Encephalomyocarditis** [Rabies] [Cowpox] **Hepatitis E?**	**Salmonellosis** **Pasteurellosis** Yersiniosis **RBF** [Leptospirosis] [Tularemia?] [Plague?]	**Taeniasis** (*H. nana, H. diminuta*) Acariasis (*Trixacarus diversus*)	**Dermatophytosis** (*T. mentagrophytes* var. *quinckeanum*) [Sporotrichosis]
Guinea pig	LCM?	**Salmonellosis** **Yersiniosis** Campylobacteriosis **Pasteurellosis** Plague	**Acariasis** (*T. caviae*)	**Dermatophytosis** (*T. mentagrophytes*)
Hamster	**LCM**	**Campylobacteriosis** **Salmonellosis** Yersiniosis **Pasteurellosis**	**Acariasis** **Taeniasis** (*H. nana*)	**Dermatophytosis**
Gerbil	None	**Salmonellosis**	**Taeniasis** (*H. nana*)	None
Prairie dog	**Monkeypox**	**Plague**	None	None
Squirrel	**Monkeypox**	**Pasteurellosis** **RBF** **Tularemia** [Relapsing fever] [Rocky Mountain spotted fever] [Epidemic typhus]	None	None

[a]Boldface indicates the most common zoonoses; brackets indicate rare zoonoses.

ticated pets (rabbits, guinea pigs, hamsters, mice, or rats) and wild or exotic rodents kept as pets. Although the first group is rarely involved in transmitting zoonoses, a special warning should be given for wild animals and exotic pets. As a general rule, wildlife and exotic animals should not be sold or kept as pets. Examples of potential zoonotic risks are that woodchucks may transmit rabies, as 46 wild woodchucks (*Marmota monax*) were diagnosed as rabid in 2007 in the United States (18), and squirrels may transmit tularemia, rat-bite fever (RBF), or leptospirosis. However, a recent trend in pet ownership has emerged, especially in developed countries, namely, the purchase of exotic or nonconventional pets captured locally or imported from various parts of the world, where many zoonoses are endemic, or ownership of unconventional pets. This danger is well illustrated by an outbreak of tularemia which was identified among commercially distributed prairie dogs *(Cynomys ludovicianus)* at a commercial exotic-animal distribution facility in Texas (34); approximately 250 of an estimated 3,600 prairie dogs caught in South Dakota and transported to Texas died at this facility. Potentially infected rodents were distributed to wholesalers, retailers, and persons in several states or exported to Belgium, the Czech Republic, Japan, The Netherlands, and Thailand. An unusually high number of sick or dead prairie dogs were reported from Texas and the Czech Republic (34). Prairie dogs have been documented to also be infected with other human pathogens (e.g., *Yersinia pestis,* the agent of plague). In May 1998, a heavy die-off among prairie dogs at a Texan exotic-animal retailer led to a positive diagnosis of plague in that colony (10). Any wild animal should be handled with caution and referred to wildlife specialists. The May 2003 outbreak of monkeypox in the midwestern United States (36) is also a reminder that exotic pets can be a source of infection of native species in that they are highly susceptible to infections that they have never encountered before and can be a very effective source of human infection.

Rabbits

The domestic or European rabbit *(Oryctolagus cuniculus),* which can be housed indoors or outdoors and fed a readily available pelleted feed, makes a good pet that can be housetrained. The rabbit is certainly an excellent pet for children, as diseases of major public health importance are rarely encountered in domestic rabbits. Biting is uncommon, but rabbits can inflict painful scratches with their rear limbs if improperly restrained (83).

INFECTIOUS ZOONOSES
Among the organisms causing infectious diseases in rabbits, *Pasteurella multocida* may cause cutaneous infection in susceptible persons (82). Other diseases to which rabbits are susceptible, e.g., salmonellosis and tularemia, are extremely rare and are more commonly transmitted to humans by wild animals. Cases of listeriosis have been reported to occur in farm rabbitries but do not seem to be of concern from pet rabbits. On the other hand, direct zoonotic transmission of *Yersinia pseudotuberculosis* infection from domestic rabbits has been documented (73). A recent study of pet rabbits in southern Italy investigated the presence of *Encephalitozoon cuniculi* antibodies (57). Overall, antibodies to *E. cuniculi* were found in 84 (67.2%) of the 125 pet rabbits tested. The results of that survey reinforced the assumption that rabbits may be the main reservoir of *E. cuniculi*; therefore, routine screening examinations of pet rabbits are strongly advised, considering the zoonotic potential of this parasite. Cerebral larva migrans caused by *Baylisascaris procyonis* was reported to occur in pet rabbits infected by bedding straw contaminated with raccoon feces, but human contamination from these pets is very unlikely (54). Rabies and tuberculosis have infrequently been diagnosed in pet rabbits. For example, rabies virus infection (raccoon variant) was reported in 2005 in seven pet rabbits and one pet guinea pig in New York State, and postexposure treatment was required for several adults and children. These pets were caged outdoors unsupervised (63)

More commonly, some external parasites of the rabbit may be transmitted to humans and cause infections, including fur mite *(Cheyletiella parasitivorax)* acariasis and dermatophytosis *(Trichophyton mentagrophytes).*

Cheyletiella (Rabbit Fur Mite) Infestation.
The rabbit fur mite, *C. parasitivorax,* is uncommon in the domestic rabbit. It is an external parasite of the skin and hair that does not excavate tunnels or furrows in the skin. The life cycle is completed in about 35 days. Adult females and eggs can survive for 10 days off the animal's body, but the larvae, nymphs, and adult males are not very resistant and die in about 2 days in the environment (2). Lesions in rabbits involve hair loss and a mild,

scaly, oily dermatitis. In humans, the disease consists of a papular and pruritic eruption on the arms, thorax, waist, and thighs. Human infestation is transitory, as the mites do not reproduce on human skin. In a recent human case, treatment with benzyl benzoate (Ascabiol) resolved all the patient's symptoms (160). To prevent human infestation, infested rabbits should be treated with insecticides (e.g., methyl carbamate) once a week for 3 to 4 weeks.

Dermatophytosis. Fungal skin infections (ringworm) due to *T. mentagrophytes* are relatively rare. A few recent cases related to rabbit exposure have been reported in the scientific literature. Two human cases of tinea corporis due to *Arthroderma benhamiae* (teleomorph of *T. mentagrophytes*) were described for the first time in Japan (123). The two persons acquired the infection from their crossbred rabbit. Similarly, two cases of tinea gladiatorum due to *T. mentagrophytes* var. *quinckeanum* were described. A pet rabbit was probably the primary source of infection, which was then spread further by human-to-human contact to four other members of the same wrestling team, who were affected by tinea corporis (150). In rabbits, irritation and inflammation of skin areas occur, with crusts, scabs, and hair loss. Some rabbits (about 4%) are asymptomatic carriers (22). Affected animals should be isolated. Antifungal treatment with topical or systemic griseofulvin (25 mg/ kg of body weight) for 4 weeks is effective. The spectrum of ringworm in humans varies from subclinical colonization to an inflammatory scaly eruption that spreads peripherally and causes localized alopecia. Diagnosis is made by identifying hyphae in skin scrapings on a potassium hydroxide slide or by isolation in fungal culture media, the only method that allows identification of the species. In humans, topical treatment with clotrimazole (Lotrimin or Mycelex) or miconazole (Monistat-derm) twice a day for 2 to 4 weeks is usually sufficient. Application of ketoconazole cream twice daily for 2 months was used for the two

Japanese patients (123). When extensive lesions are observed, oral griseofulvin (Fulvicin, Grifulvin V, or Grisactin) should be used. For adults, the dosage is 500 mg twice a day for at least 4 weeks (48). For children, the usual dose of oral microcrystalline griseofulvin is 10 to 15 mg/kg (up to 500 mg) given in one or two doses, preferably with fatty food, such as ice cream or whole milk. Treatment should be continued for 4 to 8 weeks.

Rodents

Although rodents, especially mice and rats, are definitively associated with transmission to humans of major fatal diseases, such as plague, typhus, and leptospirosis, they can be very good pets. The albino rat, the domestic variety of the brown rat *(Rattus norvegicus),* and the albino domestic mouse *(Mus musculus)* are kept by many people. However, guinea pigs, hamsters, and gerbils are the most common house pets among rodents. It should be noted that introduction and ownership of gerbils are illegal in California. Furthermore, following the monkeypox outbreak in prairie dogs, restrictions on African rodents, prairie dogs, and certain other animals were recently set by the U.S. government (38). New World flying squirrels (mainly *Glaucomys volans* and *Glaucomys sabrinus*) have also gained some popularity as household pets, with an estimated 5,000 to 8,000 owners in the United States (137).

As mentioned by Wagner and Farrar (162), the most important concerns about rodents for pet owners are bites and allergies. Human allergies to rodent dander are common. Symptoms are characterized by cutaneous (reddening, itching, and hives) and respiratory problems.

Zoonotic diseases from pet rodents are relatively rare. Among these, salmonellosis, lymphocytic choriomeningitis (LCM), and, more recently, monkeypox virus infection are of major concern. Rodent-borne zoonotic diseases are presented below in the following order: viral zoonoses, bacterial zoonoses, parasitic zoonoses, and fungal zoonoses.

VIRAL ZOONOSES

#1

LCM. LCM virus (LCMV) is found in many rodent species and spreads to humans through contact with infected aerosols, direct animal contact, or rodent bites. The natural reservoir of the disease is the domestic mouse (*Mus musculus*), which usually does not present any symptoms (2, 48, 77, 83).

Epidemiology. First described in 1933, LCM is a rodent-borne zoonosis associated with the common house mouse (*M. musculus*). LCMV (an RNA virus of the family *Arenaviridae*) is transmitted horizontally among rodents through secretions (urine, saliva, and feces) and vertically to the embryos, especially in mice. Infected offspring develop a persistent infection and shed the virus during most of their life spans. Outbreaks have been reported to occur in laboratory mice, and cases have occurred in humans in houses where infected mice were caught. In humans, the disease is sporadic, but outbreaks may occasionally occur.

Since 1960, three epidemics of LCMV infection involving at least 236 human cases have occurred in the United States (71). Such outbreaks of LCMV infection occurred in the late 1960s and early 1970s in Germany and the United States, related to the use of hamsters as pets. In Germany, 47 cases in humans associated with pet hamsters were reported within a 2-year period (3). In the United States, a nationwide epidemic occurred in late 1973 and early 1974 totaling at least 181 cases in 12 states, with 57 cases in New York State (16) and California. All were associated with pet hamsters from a single breeder in Birmingham, AL. This breeder was an employee of a biological-product firm whose tumor cell lines were found to be positive for LCMV. The same cell source was also incriminated in a prior outbreak at the University of Rochester Medical Center, Rochester, NY (79). Since the suspension of the sale of pet hamsters by the Birmingham breeder and of the distribution of positive tumor cell lines by the biological-product firm, no further major outbreaks have been reported in the United States. In southern France, four human cases of acute meningitis due to LCMV occurred in 1993 after close contact with pet Syrian hamsters (138). More recently (2005), four human cases, of which three were fatal, were acquired in the United States following organ transplantation from a donor whose household had recently acquired a pet hamster (42, 68). Viral sequences from the organ recipients were identical to those from the pet hamster acquired by the donor's household 17 days before organ donation (7). The hamster was traced back through a Rhode Island pet store to a distribution center in Ohio, and more LCMV-infected hamsters were discovered in both. Rodents from the Ohio facility and its parent facility in Arkansas were tested for the same LCMV strain as that involved in the transplant-associated deaths. Phylogenetic analysis of virus sequences linked the rodents from the Ohio facility to the Rhode Island pet store, the index hamster, and the transplant recipients (7). The seroprevalence of LCMV in rodents in surveys has been reported to be between 2.5% (California) and 21% (Washington, DC), but serology is not very reliable (46). In the investigation of a human case in Michigan, 22 (96%) of 23 mice captured were viremic but none were seropositive (71)! Serologic studies conducted in urban areas of the United States have indicated that the prevalence of LCMV infection among humans is approximately 5% (42). Human-to-human transmission of LCMV has not been reported, except in a case of vertical transmission from an infected mother to her fetus (42).

Symptoms. In hamsters, LCMV infection is usually not associated with signs of illness (56) and can be detected only by laboratory tests. In humans, the course of infection varies from being clinically unapparent to a flu-like infection, with fever, headache, and severe myalgia, occurring 5 to 10 days after infection. A small number of patients progress to aseptic meningitis, which is characterized by a very high lymphocyte count in the cerebrospinal fluid. On rare occasions, there may be meningoencephalitis. Chronic sequelae are not common, and fatal cases are rare.

Diagnosis. Diagnosis of infection in humans is based on isolation of the virus from the blood or from nasopharyngeal or cerebrospinal fluid samples taken early in the attack and inoculated onto tissue cultures or injected intracerebrally into LCMV-free adult mice. LCMV testing also includes assays such as immunohistochemistry, reverse transcription-PCR, and TaqMan real-time PRC (7). Serodiagnostic tests include enzyme-linked immunosorbent assay (ELISA), indirect immunofluorescence assay, and immunoglobulin G (IgG) Western blotting. Serum screening is performed by indirect immunofluorescence assay and titration of IgM and IgG antibodies by ELISA (68, 138).

Treatment. Since the disease is self-limiting, treatment is for symptomatic relief only.

Monkeypox. The first outbreak of human monkeypox infection in the Western Hemisphere began in May 2003 in the midwestern United States and was attributed to contact with infected exotic pets. Seventy-one suspected cases of monkeypox were investigated, primarily in Wisconsin, Indiana, and Illinois (36). Most of the affected people reported close contact with ill prairie dogs, although at least one case is thought to be related to an ill rabbit (which had contact with a sick prairie dog). No patients have been confirmed to have had exposure to persons with monkeypox as their only possible exposure. In a follow-up study, case patients were more likely than controls to have had daily exposure to a sick animal (odds ratio [OR] 4.0; 95% confidence interval [CI], 1.2 to 13.4), to have cleaned cages or removed bedding of a sick animal (OR, 5.3; 95% CI, 1.4 to 20.7), or to have touched a sick animal (OR, 4.0; 95% CI, 1.2 to 13.4) (133). These findings showed that

human infection was associated with handling of monkeypox virus-infected animals and suggested that exposure to excretions and secretions of infected animals can result in infection. Prairie dogs appear to have been infected through contact with Gambian giant rats and dormice that originated in Ghana. Trace-back investigations to identify the source of introduction of monkeypox into the United States identified a Texas animal distributor who had imported a shipment of approximately 800 small mammals from Ghana on 9 April 2003 that contained 762 African rodents, including rope squirrels (*Funisciurus* spp.), tree squirrels (*Heliosciurus* spp.), Gambian giant rats (*Cricetomys* spp.), brush-tailed porcupines (*Atherurus* spp.), dormice (*Graphiurus* spp.), and striped mice (*Hybomys* spp.) (36). The U.S. Department of Health and Human Services issued an embargo order on the import of rodents from Africa, effective 11 June 2003. In addition, the U.S. Department of Health and Human Services has also prohibited the distribution, sale, transport, or intentional release into the wild of prairie dogs and six African rodent species (38).

In humans, the signs and symptoms of monkeypox are characterized, after an incubation period of approximately 12 days, by fever, headache, muscle aches, backache, swollen lymph nodes, a general feeling of discomfort, and exhaustion. Within 1 to 3 days after the onset of fever, the patient develops a papular rash, often first on the face but sometimes initially on other parts of the body. The lesions usually develop through several stages before crusting and falling off. The illness typically lasts for 2 to 4 weeks. No specific treatment is available, but smallpox vaccination has been used in people in contact with infected humans and people exposed to infected rodents (36).

Cowpox. Human cowpox is a relatively rare zoonosis which occurs sporadically in the United Kingdom and across Europe and in some western states of the former Soviet Union. The virus circulates in wild rodents, mainly field and bank voles and wood mice in the United Kingdom (13). A young boy was bitten by a rodent when swimming in a Dutch canal and developed cowpox (129). More recently, a cowpox virus was isolated from the ulcerative eyelid lesions of a young Dutch girl who owned many pets (turtles, hamsters, guinea pigs, birds, ducks, cats, and a dog) and had cared for a clinically ill wild rat that later died (167).

Rabies. Because bites from pet rodents are frequent events, one must be concerned with rabies. No case of rabies has ever been reported from bites by pet rodents. However, one should be very careful any time a wild rodent kept as a pet has bitten a person. Cases of rabies have been reported to occur in woodchucks, squirrels, and even a rat (18, 121).

HFRS, or Korean Hemorrhagic Fever, and Hantavirus Pulmonary Syndrome (HPS). Hemorrhagic fever with renal syndrome (HFRS) describes a group of rodent-borne viral diseases (hantaviruses) that are endemic or occur as focal epidemics on the Eurasian continent and in Japan. In general, hantavirus isolates from Asia or eastern Europe (Hantaan, Dobrava, and Seoul viruses) are considered more pathogenic to humans than the northern European strains (Puumala virus). Wild rodents in rural areas or wild rats in cities (36) are the reservoirs of the virus, and they can shed the virus for several weeks. Several outbreaks involving laboratory personnel (104) infected by laboratory rats have been reported in Japan and Europe. Hantaviruses cause chronic, apparently asymptomatic infections of their rodent hosts, but associated cases in humans may reveal the animal infection. The disease in laboratory personnel has been characterized by fever and a flu-like syndrome, with fever, myalgia, and, a few days later, oliguria, proteinuria, and hematuria. Usually, patients recover without sequelae. The infection is contracted by handling in-

fected animals or from contaminated aerosols. Most laboratory rat suppliers employ a screening test and destroy infected colonies. The diagnosis of infection is based on viral isolation and, more often, on serodiagnosis by indirect immunofluorescence or ELISA.

In the United States, HPS was first reported in the spring of 1993 and was caused by a virus called Sin Nombre virus. There were 465 reported human cases by the end of March 2007 (http://www.cdc.gov/ncidod/diseases/hanta/hps/noframes/caseinfo.htm), with a fatality rate of 35%. Most of the cases have been reported in the western states, especially New Mexico, Arizona, and Colorado. The reservoir of Sin Nombre virus is *Peromyscus maniculatus,* the deer mouse. Other hantaviruses have been identified in humans and various rodent species in North America, such as Black Creek Canal virus, which has been identified in Florida, with the cotton rat *(Sigmodon hispidus)* as the reservoir (94). Other viruses, such as Monongahela, New York, and Bayou viruses, also cause HPS and are found in eastern Canada and the eastern and southeastern United States. In South and Central America, several hantaviruses have been identified as causing HPS, including Andes virus in Argentina and Chile; Andes-like viruses, including Oran, Lechiguanas, and Hu39694 viruses in Argentina; Laguna Negra virus in Bolivia and Paraguay; Bermejo virus in Argentina; Juquitiba virus in Brazil; and Choclo virus in Panama (94, 155). No cases in humans acquired by contact with pet rodents have been reported.

Encephalomyocarditis. Encephalomyocarditis is a rare disease in humans caused by an RNA virus of the family *Picornaviridae.* Sporadic cases have been reported, and the virus has been isolated from children in Germany and The Netherlands; in the United States, epizootics have occurred in pigs (2). Rodents, especially of the genus *Rattus,* have been considered the main reservoirs of the virus, and they transmit the virus to rats and

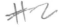

other species through bites. However, no case from a rodent source has been identified in humans.

Hepatitis E. Hepatitis E virus (HEV) is an important cause of enterically transmitted human hepatitis in developing countries. However, autochthonous cases of hepatitis E have been reported in the United States and other industrialized countries. The source of HEV infection in these cases is unknown, but zoonotic transmission has been suggested. Recent cases from consumption of raw deer or wild boar meat have been reported from Japan (114, 157). Antibodies to HEV have been detected in many animals in areas where HEV is endemic and in domestic swine and rats in the United States (67, 86). In the United States, an antibody prevalence of almost 60% was reported for rats, with higher prevalence in rodents from urban habitats than in animals captured from rural areas (67). A 12% seroprevalence of HEV antibodies was reported for rats trapped in a valley in Nepal where HEV was hyperendemic, and HEV RNA was detected in four animals (86). Phylogenetic analysis of the four genome sequences showed that they were identical and closely related to two human isolates from Nepal and distinct from the sequences of HEV isolated elsewhere (86). Similarly, in Japan, 114 of 362 (31.5%) Norway rats *(R. norvegicus)* and 12 of 90 (13.3%) black rats *(Rattus rattus)* were positive for anti-HEV IgG (89). Rats may play a role as a potential reservoir of HEV, but no cases of human infection from a pet rat have yet been reported.

BACTERIAL ZOONOSES

Pasteurellosis. Among bite-transmitted zoonoses, infection by *P. multocida* is certainly the most common in domestic pets. Although most of the cases occur from cat and dog bites, rodents nevertheless harbor *P. multocida* in their oral cavities and can at times transmit the organism through a bite wound. *P. multocida* is likely to be the pathogen if cellulitis devel-

ops within a few hours after the bite (2). Swelling, reddening, and intense pain in the region are the main signs and symptoms. If the incubation period is longer, staphylococcal or streptococcal infection is more likely. A case of *Pasteurella pneumotropica* peritonitis was reported in a child maintained on peritoneal dialysis following contamination of the dialysis tube by a pet hamster (21). *P. pneumotropica* has been isolated primarily from rodents. The patient responded well to intraperitoneal tobramycin and vancomycin. Cultures of samples from infected bite wounds should always be performed in order to administer the appropriate antibiotics. Treatment should be carried out with amoxicillin-clavulanate potassium (Augmentin), 500 mg three times daily for 5 to 7 days, or doxycycline, 100 mg orally twice a day.

RBF. RBF is a rare disease that can be transmitted by rats, which are healthy carriers of *Streptobacillus moniliformis* or "*Spirillum minus*" in the nasopharynx. Streptobacillary RBF is a rare disease in the United States. Of 14 cases on record since 1958, 7 originated from the bites of laboratory rats (9, 25). Bites by wild rodents (rats and squirrels) can also transmit the infectious agent (25). Infection has also followed consumption of contaminated raw milk (9). According to a case report from New Mexico, a 15-year-old boy was infected after he drank water from an open irrigation ditch next to a baseball field (32). In Europe, a case of septic arthritis of the hip due to *S. moniliformis* after a bite on the finger of a 14-year-old boy from a rat for sale in a pet shop was also reported (60). The case was successfully treated by arthrotomy, drainage, and joint lavage followed by administration of penicillin. In The Netherlands, a 43-year-old woman presented, after being bitten by a pet rat, with a generalized febrile illness; an exanthema with mixed maculopapular and pustular eruptions on the lower halves of the extremities, elbows, knees, palms, and soles; and severe arthralgia and asymmetric arthritis (145). In France, a case of septic arthritis following a pet rat bite was described in 2007 (119). *Streptobacillus moniliformis* was detected in the knee synovial fluid and identified by 16S rRNA sequencing. The patient was cured by an amoxicillin treatment. A few fatal cases of RBF in pet shop employees have been reported in the United States (39, 149). A 24-year-old male pet shop employee contracted the disease through a minor superficial finger wound on a contaminated rat cage. The disease progressed from a flu-like illness to a severe endocarditis and sepsis, leading to death less than 60 days after the initial injury (149). A 52-year-old woman who was a pet store employee and had been bitten by a pet rat developed a severe disease and died of *S. bacilliformis* septicemia (39). These cases highlight a possible danger of keeping rats as pets. Streptobacillary RBF has an incubation period of 2 to 10 days, a rapidly healing point of inoculation, and abrupt onset of irregularly relapsing fever, asymmetric polyarthritis, shaking chills, vomiting, headache, arthralgia, myalgia, and regional lymphadenopathy. Two to four days after onset, a maculopapular rash appears on the extremities. Endocarditis is a possible complication. Diagnosis of RBF is made by culture of the organism from the blood or joint fluid (48). Recommended therapy for RBF is penicillin G, amoxicillin, or tetracycline (25). Clindamycin can also be effective.

Spirillary RBF is an even less common disease, with an incubation period of 1 to 6 weeks (2, 8). Clinically, "*S. minus*" infection differs from streptobacillary fever in the rarity of arthritic symptoms, a distinctive rash, and a common reactivation of the healed wound when symptoms appear.

Tularemia. Tularemia, also known as "rabbit fever," is an acute febrile illness caused by *Francisella tularensis*. Rodents are very susceptible to the disease, which usually culminates in a fatal septicemia. Because the disease is transmitted mainly from rodent to rodent by ticks and fleas, having pet rabbits or rodents should not be a major risk for the transmission of tularemia. There have been documented cases of transmission from domestic cats and, more recently, from the bite of a squirrel kept as a household pet, which died minutes after biting a child (111). Cases among commercially distributed prairie dogs from Texas raised concerns about the human risk of contamination in the United States and abroad (34). A case of tularemia was reported in Colorado in April 2004 in a 3-year-old boy who had been bitten by a pet hamster on the left fourth finger just before it died (40). The boy had been exposed to six pet hamsters purchased in Denver. Each hamster had died of diarrhea within a week of purchase. The boy had a painful enlarged lymph node, fever, malaise, and skin sloughing at the bite site.

Plague. Plague is endemic in many wild rodents in the western United States. Although several cases in humans have been associated with pets, especially cats (64), there are no reports in the literature of transmission to humans from pet rodents. The potential commercial distribution of plague-infected prairie dogs in Texas in 1998 should remind people of the danger of keeping wild animals as pets (10). Recurrent outbreaks of plague in Peru were also associated with the indoor presence of infected guinea pigs, used as both pets and sources of food by the natives (P. Arambulo, personal communication).

Epidemic Typhus. Epidemic typhus is caused by *Rickettsia prowazekii* and is usually transmitted from person to person by the human body louse. Sporadic cases have been reported in the United States for people living in rural areas after contacts with flying squirrels (61, 134, 137). From 1976 to 2001, approximately one-third of the 39 *R. prowazekii* infections documented in the United States occurred after contact with flying squirrels or their nests (134).

Leptospirosis. Although rodents, especially rats, are known to harbor and shed various *Leptospira interrogans* serovars for long periods, very few cases of human infection from pet rodents have been reported. In one instance, *L. interrogans* serovar Ballum was contracted from a pet mouse (75). More recently, leptospirosis was diagnosed in an HIV-infected patient in Germany who likely acquired his infection from his pet rats (81). The infection was due to *L. interrogans* serogroup Icterohaemorrhagiae or serovar Icterohaemorrhagiae or Copenhageni isolates originating from the patient's rats. Outbreaks in personnel working with laboratory rats and mice have been documented in Europe and the United States (73).

Salmonellosis. Guinea pigs are highly susceptible to salmonella infection and develop severe clinical disease (septicemia). In guinea pigs, high mortality is the rule. Fish et al. (69) reported a family outbreak of salmonellosis due to contact with guinea pigs raised on a commercial ranch in Canada. An outbreak of multidrug-resistant *Salmonella enterica* serovar Typhimurium associated with hamsters purchased at retail pet stores in Minnesota occurred in 2004 (41, 154). Thirteen (59%) of 22 patients in 10 states reported exposure to pet hamsters, mice, or rats, and 2 (9%) had secondary infections. High mortality after showing signs of diarrhea was reported from several hamsters. The outbreak strain of *S. enterica* serotype Typhimurium was cultured from a patient's pet mouse and from seven hamsters from pet stores. Human, rodent, and environmental isolates were resistant to ampicillin, chloramphenicol, streptomycin, sulfisoxazole, and tetracycline. Therefore, pet rodents probably are an underrecognized source of human salmonella infection. Mice and rats are also very susceptible and may carry subclinical infections for long periods. These infections are usually caused by *Salmonella enterica* serovar Typhimurium or *S. enterica* serovar Enteritidis. If salmonellosis occurs in a child who has a pet rodent, the pet's feces should be cultured for *Salmonella*. However, shedding may be only intermittent.

Yersiniosis. Infections with *Yersinia pseudotuberculosis* and *Yersinia enterocolitica* may be contracted from pet rodents. Guinea pigs are very commonly infected with *Y. pseudotuberculosis* (8, 65). The course of the disease in these animals is usually subacute. Loss of weight and diarrhea are often the only clinical signs. Healthy carriers are common. In rats and mice, the infection is common, but usually without any symptoms. Children can be infected by fecal-oral contamination. In humans, the disease is observed mainly in children, adolescents, and young adults. The most common clinical form, after 1 to 3 weeks of incubation, is mesenteric adenitis or pseudoappendicitis with acute abdominal pain in the right iliac fossa, fever, and vomiting. The disease is usually more common in young males. Diagnosis requires the isolation and identification of the etiologic agent. Serologic tests by ELISA are also available. When the disease is mild (uncomplicated pseudoappendicular syndrome), antimicrobial chemotherapy is not useful (23). *Y. pseudotuberculosis* is usually sensitive to ampicillin, aminoglycosides, or tetracycline (88). *Y. enterocolitica* is also found in rodents, which are usually healthy carriers (146). Chinchillas are very susceptible to the infection, and several epizootics have occurred in Europe and the United States (2). Guinea pigs also are commonly infected by *Y. enterocolitica,* but serotypes found in rodents usually do not affect humans. *Y. enterocolitica* affects mainly young children. The main symptom is an acute enteritis with watery diarrhea, sometimes bloody, lasting 3 to 14 days, and abdominal pain. Diagnosis is based on isolation of the agent from the feces of patients. Serodiagnosis by ELISA on paired sera is also useful to determine infection. Aminoglycosides and trimethoprim-sulfamethoxazole are the most appropriate antibiotics (88).

Campylobacteriosis. *Campylobacter* species infection can occur in some rodent species. Proliferative ileitis, a specific enteric syndrome of hamsters, is probably caused by a strain of *Campylobacter.* Hamsters certainly represent a potential source of human infection, but no hamster-associated cases have been reported (77). In humans, campylobacter infection is characterized by diarrhea, abdominal pain, cramps, fever, and vomiting. The diarrhea is frequently bloody. The incubation period is 2 to 5 days, and the disease usually does not last more than a week. Usually treatment is limited to fluid replacement therapy.

PARASITIC ZOONOSES

Cestodiasis or Taeniasis (Tapeworm). Cestodes, or tapeworms, infect a wide range of species, including rabbits and rodents (2). *Hymenolepis nana,* the dwarf tapeworm, is found in rodents, especially hamsters. *Hymenolepis diminuta* is the rat tapeworm, but it may also be found in other rodents. Hymenolepiasis occurs primarily in children. The prepatent period is 15 to 30 days. Usually, the infestation is asymptomatic in humans, but if parasites are present in large numbers, gastrointestinal disorders, such as abdominal pain, nausea, vomiting, and diarrhea, may occur. Eggs of some *Hymenolepis* spp. are infective to the definitive host when passed in the feces. Humans may acquire the infection from infected rodents either by ingestion of eggs from fecally contaminated fingers or from contaminated food or water. When eggs of the directly transmitted *Hymenolepis* spp. are ingested, they hatch in the intestine, liberating an oncosphere that enters a mucosal villus and develops into a cysticercoid larva within 5 days. The cysticercoid ruptures the villus, travels into the lumen, and attaches to the lower small intestine. It reaches the adult phase in 2 weeks and starts to release eggs. Diagnosis of infection is made by microscopic identification of the eggs in the feces. Praziquantel (Biltricide) and niclosamide (Yomesan or Niclocide) are effective for treatment of *Hymenolepis* infection (2, 82, 83, 88). Treatment of infected rodents can be done with 1 mg of niclosamide per 10 g of body weight

given at 7-day intervals or with 0.3% active ingredient in the feed for 7 days (162).

Acariasis (*Trixacarus caviae*). Several external parasites can infest rodents. Among these, *T. caviae,* a parasite found mainly in guinea pigs, can be transmitted to humans. In guinea pigs, the infection is usually asymptomatic. Stress and/or poor care can lead to severe alopecia, dermatitis, and pruritus on the body and legs. The skin is thickened, dry, and scaly. Flaky, thickened, pruritic skin lesions caused by *T. caviae* in a 3-year-old male pet guinea pig that presented for agitation and itching were recently reported in Germany (14). Treatment is based on a solution of 1:40 lime sulfur in water applied to the skin and repeated weekly for 6 weeks or a once-a-week application of 10% lindane for 3 weeks. Ivermectin injected subcutaneously at 200 mg/kg is a useful treatment for ectoparasitism (5). Treatment of the infected guinea pig includes spot-on dermal treatment every 30 days on days 0, 30, and 60 with a topical 10% imidacloprid–1% moxidectin solution (14). In humans, pruritic skin lesions on the hands, arms, or neck can be observed in children. Diagnosis may be established by recovering the mite from its burrow and identifying it microscopically. For infected children, crotamiton (Eurax) in one application per day for 2 to 5 days is the most common treatment; lindane (1% γ-benzene hexachloride) (Kwell) may also be used (83, 88).

FUNGAL ZOONOSES

Dermatophytosis. Tinea favus of rats and mice, caused by *T. mentagrophytes* var. *quinckeanum,* is widespread (83). Mice and guinea pigs are the important sources of human infection with *T. mentagrophytes* var. *mentagrophytes* or *Microsporum gypseum* (128).

In 2002 in a Slovakian family, dermatomycosis caused by *T. mentagrophytes* var. *quinckeanum,* the source of which was a pet guinea pig, was confirmed in the father and son (17). Rats, chinchillas, and hamsters are much less common sources of ringworm in humans (128). The lesion, localized on the head or trunk, is white and scabby, but rodents often have no noticeable lesions. The infection is transmitted to humans and dogs. (For diagnosis and treatment, see "Dermatophytosis" under "Rabbits" above.) In rodents, oral griseofulvin at 15 to 25 mg/kg orally once daily for 3 to 5 weeks is the recommended treatment (128).

Sporotrichosis. A few human cases of lymphocutaneous sporotrichosis caused by *Sporothrix schenckii* have been associated with rodent bite accidents (128).

HEDGEHOGS

It is estimated that about 40,000 households own a pet hedgehog in the United States (135, 137). Salmonellosis has been diagnosed in patients who own hedgehogs as pets (30). The African pygmy hedgehog *(Atelerix albiventris)* has been associated with cases of *S. enterica* serovar Tilene infection in children in the United States and Canada (109, 168). It is estimated that 40,000 households own such a

pet in the United States (137). Ringworm cases (inflammatory tinea corporis) caused by *T. mentagrophytes* var. *erinacei* have been reported from owners of pet African pygmy hedgehogs (136). Recently, an outbreak among hedgehog owners was reported in Germany (142). Eight hedgehog caretakers from Göttingen and the surrounding area developed dermatophytosis caused by *Trichophyton erinacei*. Four patients who handled the animals without gloves developed lesions on their hands that looked like hand eczema, whereas the other caretakers who wore gloves presented with typical ringworm on their arms, big toes, back, abdomen, and thighs. Human cases are easily treated with oral itraconazole (200 mg daily for 7 days). The hedgehog can be treated by application of a miconazole-containing veterinary lotion. The African pygmy hedgehog (Fig. 1) has not yet been documented to carry any mycobacterial diseases; however, infection by various *Mycobacterium* species *(Mycobacterium marinum* and *Mycobacterium avium)* has been reported for the European hedgehog (137). Therefore, hedgehogs are not recommended pets for patients with HIV infection (135).

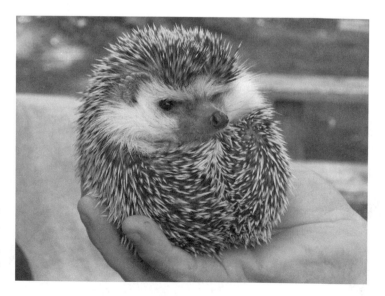

FIGURE 1 A pet African pygmy hedgehog (source: http://www.farscapeweekly.com/weblog/archive/2008_08_01_archive.html). Photo credit: Joan O. Hedman (with permission).

REPTILES AND AMPHIBIANS

Reptiles (Fig. 2) are increasingly popular pets in the United States, as an estimated 13 million pet reptiles were owned by approximately 3% of households in 2007 (http://exoticpets.about.com/cs/resourcesgeneral/a/petstates.htm). During the period from 2001 to 2006, the number of turtles kept as pets in the United States increased 86% to nearly 2 million turtles (43). There is a large international trade of live reptiles, with the United States accounting for 80% of this trade. Over 10,000 green iguanas were imported annually in the United Kingdom during the 1990s (131), and the British Federation of Herpetologists estimates that there are 7 million to 8 million reptiles and amphibians being kept as pets in the United Kingdom (http://exoticpets.about.com/b/2008/11/25/more-pet-reptiles-than-dogs-in-uk.htm). More than half a million reptiles were imported in Germany in 2007 through the Frankfurt am Main airport (66). Table 2 lists the major zoonoses transmitted by reptiles and amphibians.

Bacterial Zoonoses

SALMONELLOSIS

Salmonellosis is certainly the most frequent and major zoonosis transmitted by reptiles, especially turtles (26, 102), iguanas and lizards (29), and snakes (37, 70). Increasing evidence suggests that amphibians (e.g., frogs, toads, newts, and salamanders) also can pose risks for salmonellosis in humans. The U.S. Centers for Disease Control and Prevention has empha-

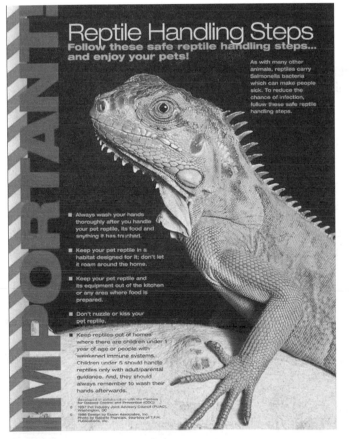

FIGURE 2 Poster from the California Department of Health Services on safe handling of pet reptiles. (Source: Ben Sun, Veterinary Public Health Unit.)

TABLE 2 Major zoonoses potentially transmitted by reptiles and aquarium fishes

Animal	Zoonosis (pathogen)[a]			
	Viral	Bacterial	Parasitic	Mycotic
Turtle	None	**Salmonellosis**	*Cryptosporidium*	[Dermatophytosis]
		Yersiniosis		
		Campylobacteriosis		
		[*Aeromonas* infection]		
Lizard, snake	None	**Salmonellosis**	Pentastomiasis	[Dermatophytosis]
		Yersiniosis	[*Mesocestoides* infection]	
		[*E. tarda* infection]		
		[*Plesiomonas* infection]		
		[*S. marcescens* infection]		
Frog	None	**Salmonellosis**	None	[Dermatophytosis]
Fish	None	**Mycobacteriosis**		None
		[*Erysipelothrix* infection]		
		[*A. hydrophila* infection]		
		Comamonas infection		
		[Melioidosis *(B. pseudomallei)*]		
		[*S. iniae* infection]		
		[*Vibrio* infection]		
		[*Y. enterocolitica* infection]		

[a]Boldface indicates the most common zoonoses; brackets indicate rare zoonoses.

sized the risk associated with ownership of reptiles and amphibians (37), as they are a well-established source of human salmonellosis. A study conducted in 1996 and 1997 attributed an estimated 6% of all human, laboratory-confirmed, sporadic *Salmonella* infections in the United States (and 11% of infections among persons aged <21 years) to contact with reptiles and amphibians (117, 118). *Salmonella* infections present the most significant hazard to children, who are at greater risk of disease than adults because they are frequently in close contact with animals and their hand-washing practices are often not well developed (5). In a case-control study of sporadic *Salmonella* infection in infants, exposure to reptiles was among the main risk factors (OR, 5.2; 95% CI, 3.4 to 7.9), with cases exposed mainly to iguanas and lizards (25 cases each), snakes (20 cases), and turtles or tortoises (14 cases) (95). For instance, in 1994, 413 (81%) of 513 *S. enterica* serovar Marina cases occurred in children aged 1 year (33).

Pet turtles have been recognized as a major source of human salmonellosis since Hershey and Mason isolated *S. enterica* serovar Hartford from the pet turtle of a 7-month-old infant with serovar Hartford gastroenteritis (24). Subsequent investigations established that 14% of the estimated 2 million cases of human salmonellosis in the United States in 1970 and 1971 were linked to pet turtles, mainly the red-eared turtle *(Pseudemys scripta elegans)* (47).

With annual sales of 15 million turtles, zoonotic salmonellosis was a growing problem. By 1975, commercial distribution of turtles less than 4 inches long was banned within the United States by the Food and Drug Administration. A 77% decrease in turtle-associated salmonellosis was noted following enactment of the ban (49, 52). Despite this prohibition, small turtles remain available to the public from various sources, including pet shops, flea markets, street vendors, and Internet websites (43). During the period from 2001 to 2006, the number of turtles kept as pets in the United States increased 86% to nearly 2 million turtles (6), suggesting that this exception might provide a mechanism by which small turtles become household pets. A multistate outbreak of *Salmonella* Paratyphi B var. Java infections related to pet turtles between 2007 and 2008 was reported in the United States (43). Furthermore, an estimated 3 to 4 million turtles are shipped annually from the United States and sold around the world. Consequently, several outbreaks of salmonellosis have been reported in Japan (76), the United Kingdom (19), Puerto Rico (156), Israel (45), and France (140). For instance, an outbreak caused by *S. enterica* serovar Tel-el-kebir was reported in Ireland among owners of terrapin turtles (109). In a study of salmonellosis in people from southwestern Germany, owners of puppies, kittens, or turtles were almost seven times more likely to have *Salmonella* infection than were healthy controls (99). Turtles are usually healthy carriers of salmonellae, and shedding is very irregular, but they may shed salmonellae for up to 11 months. The problem of *Salmonella* infection in turtles arises from the widespread contamination and persistence of the microorganisms in turtle breeding ponds and nesting areas. Turtles can acquire the organisms in ovo or after hatching (97). The pattern of *Salmonella* excretion in amphibians and reptiles was studied in a vivarium over a 3-year period (127). *Salmonella* could be isolated about twice as often from animals kept under arid or mesic conditions as from animals living in humid or aquatic environments. Animals feeding on mice ($P = 0.04$) and reptiles in general ($P = 0.04$) more commonly excreted *Salmonella*. Use of antibiotics for attempted control of salmonellae in pet turtle husbandry has been widely practiced. In their attempt to eradicate salmonellae with gentamicin sulfate, turtle farmers have created an even greater health hazard through selection of antibiotic-resistant strains (51). Treatment of pet turtles is not recommended, and infected reptiles should be destroyed. However, knowledge of the potential health hazards, along with proper sanitation, is usually sufficient to prevent human infection. Pet turtles should not be displayed in classrooms where children can handle them or have contact with their containers. Identifi-

cation of the microorganism from stool culture and an antibiogram should be performed any time salmonellosis is suspected. Similarly, culture should be performed from the pet reptile or from its aquarium. In humans, primary treatment of salmonellosis consists of fluid and electrolyte replacement. Antibiotics are not recommended, except in severe forms, as they not only fail to shorten the duration of the illness but also may prolong the carrier state.

Salmonella infection can also be acquired from other reptiles, such as lizards or snakes (70), chameleons (166), and amphibians (12, 37). The 1990s were characterized by an explosion in pet reptile ownership in the United States. Because the most popular reptile species (iguanas, for example) do not breed if closely confined, most reptiles are captured in the wild and imported. From 1989 through 1993, reptile imports to the United States increased by 82%, from 1.1 million to 2.1 million, with iguana imports increasing by 431%, from 143,000 to 760,000 animals (4). Pet iguana-associated salmonellosis cases in two infants residing in Indiana were reported in 1990 (27), and many other cases have been reported from several states (27, 28, 37, 50, 117) since then, underscoring the important role played by reptiles, particularly pet lizards, in the transmission of zoonoses. In several cases, a rare *S. enterica* serotype, Marina, was involved, and there was no direct contact between the pet iguana and the infant (27, 28). These cases demonstrate that direct contact between the reptile and the infant is not necessary for transmission to occur. Similarly, a human case of salmonellosis acquired through a platelet transfusion from a donor with a boa constrictor was reported (92). Isolation of rare serotypes of *Salmonella* spp. often alerts public health staff about possible transmission of infection from reptiles to humans. For instance, isolations of *Salmonella* serovars Marina and Poona from humans increased, respectively, from 2 and 199 in 1989 to 47 and 341 in 1998 (33). Similarly, cases caused by a rare serotype, Poona, were associated with savanna monitor lizards (*Varanus exanthematicus*) imported as

#5

pets from Ghana and Togo (117). An outbreak of salmonellosis among children attending a Komodo dragon exhibit at a zoo was the cause of at least 65 cases of serovar Enteritidis infection (74). In 1995 there were as many as 6,700 reptile-caused salmonella infections in the United States, but the incidence may be closer to 80,000 cases per year, 80% of them in children. In Canada, an estimated 3 to 5% of all cases of salmonellosis in humans are associated with exposure to exotic pets (168). A high proportion of reptiles (more than 90%) are asymptomatic carriers of *Salmonella*. Reptiles can become infected through transovarial transmission or direct contact with other infected reptiles or contaminated reptile feces. High rates of fecal carriage of *Salmonella* organisms can be related to the eating of feces by hatchlings, a behavior typical of iguanas and other lizards. In a cohort study of 12 captive iguanas, fecal shedding of *Salmonella* organisms was monitored for 10 weeks (20). All 12 iguanas were found to shed *Salmonella* organisms at least once, and multiple serotypes were isolated from 7/12 animals. Salmonellae were isolated from 83% of the fecal samples tested. In a limited survey in a green-iguana farm in El Salvador to identify sources of *Salmonella* in green iguanas and their environment, *Salmonella* spp. were isolated from the intestines of both adult (3/20) and hatchling (8/20) iguanas and from the surfaces of 40% (7/16) of the egg surfaces tested (120). Soil samples from a breeding pen and a nest in that farm were positive for *Salmonella* spp.

EDWARDSIELLA INFECTION

Human infection with *Edwardsiella tarda* is uncommon. This organism can be found in cold-blooded animals, reptiles, and fish (goldfish, catfish, and bass). In humans, the organism may cause gastroenteritis resembling *Salmonella* infections. Wound infections, such as cellulitis or gas gangrene associated with trauma to mucosal surfaces, and systemic disease, such as septicemia, meningitis, cholecystitis, and osteomyelitis, have been reported. At least one case associated with a pet turtle was reported in the United States (122). This bac-

terium is susceptible to most commonly prescribed antibiotics, but fatal gastrointestinal and extraintestinal infections have been described (93).

PLESIOMONAS INFECTION

Plesiomonas (Aeromonas) shigelloides is a gram-negative rod that causes progressive ulcerative stomatitis in snakes ("mouth rot disease"). It may cause gastroenteritis in humans. A case of acute gastroenteritis in a zoo animal keeper infected by handling a sick boa constrictor has been reported (53). Diagnosis is made by stool culture. Treatment with trimethoprim-sulfamethoxazole (Bactrim or Septra) for 5 days is usually effective.

YERSINIA INFECTION

Y. enterocolitica has been found in water and on cold-blooded animals, such as frogs and fish (85, 169). However, the serotypes involved are not usually found in humans.

CAMPYLOBACTER FETUS

During the course of a *Salmonella enterica* serovar Agona case investigation, *Campylobacter fetus* was isolated for the first time from a pet turtle (84). This suggests that turtles, in addition to being reservoirs for *Salmonella* species, may also be reservoirs for *C. fetus*.

SERRATIA MARCESCENS CELLULITIS

A case of cellulitis caused by *S. marcescens* was reported to have occurred in an 8-year-old boy who was bitten by a pet iguana on his left index finger (91). The *Serratia* isolate was resistant to ampicillin and cefazolin but was susceptible to ampicillin-sulbactam and gentamicin.

Parasitic Zoonoses of Reptiles

PENTASTOMIASIS

Pentastomes (*Armillifer* spp.) are annulate metazoa that are almost exclusively parasites of the reptilian respiratory system. Pentastomiasis is endemic to western and central Africa (62). Snakes are the definitive hosts, and many wild rodents, on which snakes feed, are the intermediate hosts. The female parasite deposits eggs in the respiratory cavities of the reptiles. The eggs are expectorated or swallowed and then eliminated with the feces. Most cases of human pentastomiasis are caused by two species of pentastomids, both of which have characteristics of arthropods and annelids, viz., *Armillifer armillatus* and *Linguatula serrata* (62). Humans can become accidental hosts by handling infected reptiles and placing contaminated hands to the mouth. In humans, the infection is usually asymptomatic. The encapsulated larvae may be found during laparotomies or can be diagnosed by radiographic examination (2, 87). A few cases of infected patients presenting with abdominal discomfort, a patient presenting with an acute abdominal emergency, two isolated cases of lethal infection, and infection of the human eye have been reported (62).

MESOCESTOIDES (CESTODA) INFECTION

Infections with *Mesocestoides* spp., cestodes of mammals and birds, occur infrequently in humans (143). One case occurred in California in 1990 in a child who was exposed to a large variety of animals in a day care center. That case was unique in that the day care facility housed all the animals necessary for the complete life cycle of this cestode. Niclosamide was used to treat this child, with apparent success.

CRYPTOSPORIDIUM SPP.

Tortoises, including pet tortoises, may disseminate *Cryptosporidium* oocysts in the environment. The identification of a zoonotic genotype in the feces of captive European tortoises indicates a potential risk for humans within the household (159).

Fungal Zoonoses of Reptiles and Amphibians

Very limited information is available on fungal diseases of reptiles and amphibians. It does not appear that reptiles and amphibians are a major source of fungal zoonoses. Dermatophytosis caused by *Trichophyton* and *Microsporum* species

in reptilian species has rarely been reported (144). Treatment of these infections in reptiles is based mainly on the use of itraconazole and ketoconazole (15 to 30 mg/kg orally once daily for at least 2 weeks) or amphotericin B and nystatin.

ORNAMENTAL (AQUARIUM) FISH

Over 1 billion ornamental fish comprising more than 4,000 freshwater and 1,400 marine species are traded internationally each year, with 8 million to 10 million imported into Australia alone (165). In Australia, it is estimated that 12 to 14% of the population keep ornamental fish as pets (105). In the United States, about 20 million household aquariums are maintained, accommodating an estimated 169 million pet fish (148; http://www.mapsofworld.com/world-top-ten/countries-with-most-pet-fish-population.html), mostly from foreign countries (in Southeast Asia and South America) and from Florida. There are about 24 million pet fish in the United Kingdom (http://www.ornamentalfish.org/aquanautmarket/number.php). However, very few cases of zoonosis are reported (Table 2), and no major outbreaks of human disease for which diseased fish were directly responsible have been reported recently (147, 148). The main pathogens acquired topically from fish (through spine puncture or open wounds) are *Aeromonas hydrophila*, *Edwardsiella tarda*, *Erysipelothrix rhusiopathiae*, *M. marinum*, *Streptococcus iniae*, *Vibrio vulnificus*, and *Vibrio damsela* (105, 108). *S. iniae* has recently emerged as a public health hazard associated with aquaculture, and *M. marinum* often infects home aquarium hobbyists. With the expansion of aquaculture and the popularity of recreational fishing, medical practitioners can expect to see more infections of this nature. Among these bacterial diseases of fish, mycobacteriosis is certainly of major concern.

MYCOBACTERIOSIS

Mycobacterial infections are certainly among the major zoonoses that can be transmitted by aquarium fish (55, 105, 158). Mycobacterial infections are increasingly reported for fish fanciers who keep an aquarium (98). *Mycobacterium marinum, Mycobacterium fortuitum,* and *"Mycobacterium platypoecilus"* have been associated with both fish and human disease for many years. Skin ulcers due to *M. marinum,* contracted from fish tanks, have been reported. In two cases, a cut on the hand had preceded the cleaning of a home fish aquarium (100). Infection by *M. marinum,* also known as "swimming pool granuloma" or "fish tank granuloma," is characterized, after inoculation on an abraded skin and an incubation period of 2 to 3 weeks, by papulonodules, ulcers, or verrucous plaques. These may progress into sporotrichoid lesions or into deeper infections involving tendons and bone.

In infected fish, granulomatous lesions are usually observed. A diagnosis can be made by isolating and identifying the organism. Histopathological examination shows a nonspecific inflammatory infiltrate in the acute phase. In chronic lesions the histopathological pattern is a tubercle-like granuloma. Infected fish should be destroyed, and the aquarium should be disinfected (with 5% calcium hypochlorite solution) before other fish are added (106). In humans, infection resolves following treatment with minocycline (Minocin), 100 mg twice daily orally for 6 to 8 weeks (48). Use of rifampin (Rifadin or Rimactane) has also been very successful (59), although indications for therapy are controversial.

MELIOIDOSIS AND EXOTIC FISH

Melioidosis is an uncommon disease in humans caused by *Burkholderia* (previously *Pseudomonas*) *pseudomallei,* with a wide range of clinical manifestations from unapparent infection to a rapid fatal septicemia. The infectious agent is endemic in Southeast Asia, where it is saprophytic in certain soils and waters. Studies have shown that the water of tanks in which exotic aquarium fishes were imported was contaminated with this bacillus. Disinfection of aquariums with bleach between water changes should be recommended in pet stores to prevent the spread of infection (58).

ERYSIPELOTHRIX INFECTION

Erysipelothrix insidiosa infection has been reported to occur in humans contaminated by handling fish (105, 130). It is an occupational disease affecting mainly fishermen. The organism can be found on the surface of the fish and produces skin lesions known as "fish roses" in humans. *Erysipelothrix* infection is almost invariably introduced through minor skin wounds. Local erysipeloid most commonly occurs on the hands, with the occasional complication of local lymphangitis and lymphadenitis. As reported by Lehane and Rawlin (105), 11 of 49 recorded cases of *E. insidiosa* septicemia in the United States between 1912 and 1988 were associated with fish. According to Lowry and Smith (108), 22% of infected humans contract the disease from fish or shellfish and 38% are likely to die. Despite the potential of this organism to infect aquarium owners, no cases have been reported to occur in humans as a result of aquarium fish contamination. Penicillin is the appropriate treatment for erysipeloid (148), as are cephalosporins (105).

S. INIAE INFECTION

S. iniae is a pathogen of fish capable of causing invasive disease and outbreaks in aquaculture farms (164). It can also produce invasive infection, characterized mainly by cellulitis but also by sepsis, endocarditis, meningitis, and arthritis, after skin injuries during handling of whole fresh fish. In 1995 and 1996, nine Asian patients in Toronto, Canada, had invasive *S. iniae* infections (31). Eight of the nine patients had bacteremic cellulitis (164). No cases associated with aquarium fish owners have been reported. More recently, two cases (one case of cellulitis and one case of osteomyelitis) were reported for two Chinese patients after they handled fresh fish for cooking (103). Most of the human cases have been reported in Asia and were related to fish preparation. Older age and underlying conditions were also identified as risk factors for developing invasive infection (103).

E. TARDA AND ORNAMENTAL FISH

Protracted diarrhea in a 2-month-old Belgian infant was associated with *E. tarda,* and the same organism was isolated from a tropical aquarium fish in the home of the patient (161). Similarly, fibrinopurulent arthritis in a young man who had his knee punctured by a silver cobbler *(Arius midgleyi)* was reported in Australia (105). He recovered after treatment, which included intravenous gentamicin.

AEROMONAS AND COMAMONAS BACTEREMIA

A case of *Comamonas* bacteremia that could be related to tropical fish exposure has been described. The patient was treated successfully with levofloxacin (151). *Comamonas* species are environmental gram-negative rods that rarely cause human infection (151). *Aeromonas hydrophila* infection in a wound can lead to cellulitis, muscle necrosis, or septicemia (105). It is commonly acquired by contact with mucus or tissues from infected freshwater fish, especially when hands have cuts or abrasions (108).

VIBRIO VULNIFICUS AND VIBRIO DAMSELA

Vibriosis is an infection often acquired from saltwater fish. Wound infection by these bacteria may be mild or self-limiting or lead to severe cellulitis and myositis, sometimes mimicking gas gangrene (105). In Australia, *V. vulnificus* infection occurred in a 68-year-old man who was spiked in the buttock by the dorsal spine of a flathead. He had acute septicemia associated with cellulitis, skin necrosis, necrotizing fasciitis, and myositis, which resolved after administration of doxycycline (115). Similarly, a few cases of wound infections caused by *V. damsela* were reported in Australia, with one fatal case in a 61-year-old man who received a puncture wound from a catfish spine (105).

WILD CARNIVORES: FERRETS

Among the large variety of house pets, wild carnivores, especially ferrets, have experienced increasing popularity; an estimated 6,000 ferrets are sold annually (15). There are approximately 12 to 17 million pet ferrets in about 4 million households (3 to 4 ferrets per owner) in the United States (124). Despite the fact that ferrets are enjoyable pets, much concern has been raised following severe injuries to children by ferrets kept as house pets. The state of California does not allow ferrets or several other exotic animals as house pets (139). As pets, ferrets can also represent a health hazard by transmitting several zoonoses to humans (Table 3).

Rabies

Like other carnivores, ferrets are susceptible to rabies. In the United States, fewer than 30 cases of rabies in domestic ferrets have been reported since 1958, most often from pet ferrets, some of which were acquired from pet shops (124, 139). Rabies immunization of ferrets with an inactivated vaccine has been shown to be effective for at least a year (139). The U.S. Department of Agriculture granted approval on 8 February 1990 for the use of this vaccine in ferrets 3 months of age or older. Annual booster vaccinations are re-

TABLE 3 Major zoonoses transmitted by ferrets[a]

Viral	Bacterial	Parasitic	Mycotic
Influenza	**Campylobacteriosis**	Cryptosporidiosis	Dermatophytosis
Rabies	**Salmonellosis**	Toxocariasis	
SARS CoV	Tuberculosis	Giardiasis	
	Leptospirosis		
	Listeriosis		

[a]Boldface indicates the most common zoonoses.

quired. Since 1998, the National Association of State Public Health Veterinarians has recommended in its compendium of animal rabies control that ferrets be treated like dogs and cats for postexposure management. Therefore, the previous requirements that all ferrets that have bitten human beings be killed and their brains be examined for rabies are no longer applicable (44).

Influenza

Ferrets are very susceptible to influenza viruses and have served for years as animal models in the laboratory (15, 112). In ferrets, influenza is characterized by sneezing, fever, lethargy, mucoserous nasal discharge, conjunctivitis, and photophobia. The course of the influenza infection usually lasts less than a week. The disease can be severe in young ferrets. Cases of influenza in humans have occurred from contamination by aerosols from infected ferrets (112). Similarly, ferrets can be infected by humans shedding the virus.

Severe Acute Respiratory Syndrome

An acute and often severe respiratory illness emerged in the southern part of the People's Republic of China in late 2002 and rapidly spread to different areas of Asia as well as several countries around the world. When the outbreak of this apparently novel infectious disease, termed severe acute respiratory syndrome (SARS), came to an end in July 2003, it had caused over 8,000 probable cases worldwide and more than 700 deaths. A novel coronavirus (CoV) was identified as the cause of the 2003 global outbreak of SARS (101). Genetic analysis and epidemiological studies suggest that the SARS CoV was introduced into humans not long ago, and SARS CoV-like viruses were isolated in Himalayan palm civets (*Paguma larvata*) and raccoon dogs (*Nyctereutes procyonoides*) in a retail live-animal market in Guangdong Province, southern China (80). Furthermore, a higher seroprevalence (13%) of SARS CoV IgG antibody in workers in live-animal markets in Guangzhou, Guangdong Province, than in persons in control groups (1

to 3%) was reported, suggesting indirect support for the hypothesis of an animal origin for SARS CoV (35). Finally, ferrets and domestic cats were shown to be experimentally susceptible to the SARS CoV, and it was also shown that they could efficiently transmit the virus to previously uninfected animals that were housed with them (113). It is noteworthy that only the ferrets developed clinical signs (lethargy, conjunctivitis) after infection and that some of them died of their infection. Therefore, owners of pet ferrets should be concerned about the risk of infection of their pets by a SARS or SARS-related virus and the possible transmission to humans. However, the natural reservoirs of CoVs related to SARS were shown to be bats, civets being amplifiers of the virus (107, 163).

Other Potential Zoonotic Pathogens

Ferrets can harbor several pathogenic microorganisms in their digestive tracts, especially *Salmonella* and *Campylobacter*. In a 9-month survey of ferrets used in biomedical research, 4% had *Salmonella* and 18% had *Campylobacter jejuni* or *Campylobacter coli* organisms isolated from their feces (72). Although no cases have been reported to occur in humans from ferret contamination, ferrets must be considered possible reservoirs for *Campylobacter* and *Salmonella* organisms. Ferrets should not be allowed to roam freely, and their feces should be discarded in a hygienic manner (112). Ferrets can harbor many other zoonoses, such as cryptosporidiosis (*Cryptosporidium* causes ill thrift and mucoid diarrhea), tuberculosis, and listeriosis. A case of zoonotic *Giardia intestinalis* was detected in a ferret exhibited at a pet shop (1). Ferrets share many parasites with dogs and cats (e.g., *Toxocara* and *Ancylostoma* spp.) as well as dermatophytes (*Microsporum canis* and *T. mentagrophytes*). However, fungal diseases are uncommon in the domestic ferret. A few cases of disseminated coccidioidomycosis have been reported from ferrets from the southwestern United States, and all cases of dermatophytosis reported from ferrets occurred in animals that had been exposed to cats (78).

Ferrets respond poorly to treatment compared with dogs and cats (78). A complete description of these infections has been published by Marini et al. (112).

PET BATS

Among the uncommon exotic pet species, bats may represent a major public health issue, as bats can be infected with various lethal viruses, such as rabies, Hendra, and Nipah viruses (90, 110). A case of rabies-associated virus infection was diagnosed in France in 1999 in a pet African bat (*Rousettus* sp.), imported from either Togo or Egypt and sold by a Belgian exotic-pet dealer to another pet dealer in Bordeaux, France, where the owner, who was from Nîmes, France, bought it (11). The virus was identified to be a Lagos bat lyssavirus (lyssavirus genotype 2). Cases of rabies have also been reported to occur in bats belonging to the same species kept in a zoological garden collection in Denmark (11). The incriminated virus was European bat lyssavirus 1a. Similarly, rabies is of major concern for people working in animal rehabilitation centers. The first human case of Australian bat lyssavirus was reported to occur in a 39-year-old female animal handler from Queensland, in November 1996, within 5 weeks after she was scratched and possibly bitten by a yellow-bellied, sheath-tailed bat *(Saccolaimus flaviventris)* (116).

NONHUMAN PRIMATES

During the last 35 years, laws restricting importation of nonhuman primates into the United States have considerably reduced the number of primates appearing in the pet trade. However, nonhuman primates sometimes find their way into the hands of pet owners. Until the 1974 prohibition, New World primates, especially the squirrel monkey, were used extensively in the pet trade (132). Because of close phylogenetic ties between humans and nonhuman primates, zoonoses transmitted by monkeys are numerous, some of them being particularly severe in humans. For public health reasons, as well as for animal welfare and environmental protection, I strongly support the policy that monkeys should not be kept as pets. It is not my purpose to present all the zoonoses that can be transmitted by primates, as excellent reviews have been published (126, 132, 141, 152). A short table of the major and most severe zoonoses is included for information (Table 4).

Among the major zoonoses, salmonellosis and shigellosis are certainly the most frequent in monkeys, as gastrointestinal illnesses are very common. Nonhuman primates are also very susceptible to respiratory infections, and tuberculosis must be considered a major risk for monkeys and their owners or caretakers. Monkeys are very susceptible to *Mycobacterium tuberculosis, Mycobacterium bovis,* and *M. avium,* and suspect animals should not be treated. Monkeys are also very susceptible to some viral diseases, such as measles. Infected children can easily transmit the virus to pet monkeys. Some viral diseases of nonhuman primates may be deadly to humans who are infected. An example is herpes B virus, which may be shed by healthy Asian monkeys (mainly ma-

TABLE 4 Major zoonoses transmitted by nonhuman primates[a]

Viral	Bacterial	Parasitic	Mycotic
Hepatitis A	**Salmonellosis**	**Amoebiasis**	Dermatophytosis
Measles	**Shigellosis**	**Balantidosis**	(*T. mentagrophytes,*
Herpes B	**Tuberculosis**	*Hymenolepis* infection	*Microsporum* spp.)
[Rabies]	Campylobacteriosis	*Strongyloides* infection	
[Ebola and Marburg virus infections]	Yersiniosis	Giardias	
[Monkeypox]	Klebsiellosis		
SFV	[Tularemia]		

[a]Boldface indicates the most common zoonoses; brackets indicate rare zoonoses.

caques) in their saliva. In a recent study of non-occupational-exposure incidents involving macaques in the United States, children were more than three times as likely to be bitten as adults. Herpes B virus must be assumed to be a potential health hazard from macaque bite wounds; this risk makes macaques unsuitable as pets (125). In monkeys, rabies is a rare disease, but cases have been reported to occur in pet monkeys vaccinated with live modified strains; thus, only inactivated rabies vaccines should be used to immunize monkeys. Simian foamy viruses (SFVs) are retroviruses that are prevalent in all species of nonhuman primates. Among 305 persons who lived or worked around nonhuman primates in several southern Asian and Southeast Asian countries and who were tested for SFVs, 8 (2.6%) were confirmed to be SFV positive by Western blotting and, for some, by PCR (96). The interspecies interactions that likely resulted in virus transmission were diverse; five macaque taxa were implicated as potential sources of infection. Phylogenetic analysis showed that SFV from three infected persons was similar to that from the nonhuman primate populations with which the infected persons reported contact. Thus, SFV infections are likely to be prevalent among persons who live or work near nonhuman primates in Asia.

ADDENDUM IN PROOF

Two outbreaks of cowpox after exposure to pet rodents were reported in early 2009 in Germany and France (H. Campe, P. Zimmermann, K. Glos, M. Bayer, H. Bergemann, C. Dreweck, P. Graf, B. K. Weber, H. Meyer, M. Büttner, U. Busch, and A. Sing, *Emerg. Infect. Dis.* **15**:777–780, 2009; L. Ninove, Y. Domart, C. Vervel, C. Voinot, N. Salez, D. Raoult, H. Meyer, I. Capek, C. Zandotti, and R. N. Charrel, *Emerg. Infect. Dis.* **15**:781–784, 2009). A cluster of five epidemiologically linked cases of human cowpox virus infection caused by contact with a litter of pet rats *(R. norvegicus)* was identified in Bavaria (greater Munich area) (Campe et al., 2009). In northern France, another cluster of four human cases of cowpox virus cutaneous infection, resulting from direct contact with infected pet rats *(R. norvegicus),* was reported. The pet rats, which originated from the same pet store, were shown to be infected by a unique virus strain and transmitted the infection to humans who purchased or had contact with the rats (Ninove et al., 2009).

PRACTICAL TIPS

- Zoonotic diseases transmitted by domestic pets are quite uncommon events but should be systematically considered when disease occurs in both animals and humans or in the pet's household. Regular veterinary care is strongly suggested to keep pets healthy and prevent any human infection.
- Animals acquired or rescued from the wild as well as exotic "pets" can carry a wide range of pathogens and should not be adopted as pets.
- Ownership of reptiles and amphibians is not recommended for families with young children (especially toddlers) or for people who are immunocompromised (including organ transplant recipients or people having immunosuppressive therapy).

REFERENCES

1. **Abe, N., C. Read, R. C. Thompson, and M. Iseki.** 2005. Zoonotic genotype of *Giardia intestinalis* detected in a ferret. *J. Parasitol.* **91**:179–182.
2. **Acha, P., and B. Szyfres.** 2001–2003. *Zoonoses and Communicable Diseases Common to Man and Animals,* 3rd ed. Publication 580. Pan American Health Organization, Washington, DC.
3. **Ackermann, R., W. Stille, W. Blumenthal, E. B. Helm, K. Keller, and O. Baldus.** 1972. Syrische Goldhamster als Übertrager von lymphozytarer Choriomeningitis. *Dtsch. Med. Wochenschr.* **97**:1725–1731.
4. **Ackman, D. M., P. Drabkin, G. Birkhead, and P. Cieslak.** 1995. Reptile-associated salmonellosis in New York State. *Pediatr. Infect. Dis. J.* **14**:955–959.
5. **Altman, R., J. C. Gorman, L. L. Bernhardt, and M. Goldfield.** 1972. Turtle-associated salmonellosis. II. The relationship of pet turtles to salmonellosis in children in New Jersey. *Am. J. Epidemiol.* **95**:518–520.

6. **American Veterinary Medical Association.** 2008. Results of the 2006 AVMA survey of companion animal ownership in US pet-owning households. *J. Am. Vet. Med. Assoc.* **232:**695–696.

7. **Amman, B. R., B. I. Pavlin, C. G. Albariño, J. A. Comer, B. R. Erickson, et al.** 2007. Pet rodents and fatal lymphocytic choriomeningitis in transplant patients. *Emerg. Infect. Dis.* **13:**719–725.

8. **Anderson, L. C.** 1987. Guinea pig husbandry and medicine. *Vet. Clin. N. Am. Small Anim. Pract.* **17:**1045–1060.

9. **Anderson, L. C., S. L. Leary, and P. J. Manning.** 1983. Rat-bite fever in animal research laboratory personnel. *Lab. Anim. Sci.* **33:**292–294.

10. **Anonymous.** Accessed 15 March 2009. ProMED-mail, archive no. 19980710.1303. International Society for Infectious Diseases. http://www.promedmail.org / pls / otn / wwv _ flow.accept.

11. **Aubert, M., O. Lemarignier, C. Gibon, M. B. Alvado-Brette, P. Brie, and F. Rosenthal.** 1999. Un cas de rage dans le Gard sur une rousette d'Egypte considérée comme animal familier. *Bull. Epidemiol. Mens. Rage Anim. France* **29**(4–6):1–4.

12. **Bartlett, K. H., T. J. Trust, and H. Lior.** 1977. Small pet aquarium frogs as a source of *Salmonella. Appl. Environ. Microbiol.* **33:**1026–1029.

13. **Baxby, D., and M. Bennett.** 1997. Poxvirus zoonoses. *J. Med. Microbiol.* **46:**17–20.

14. **Beck, W., F. Buck, and N. Pantchev.** 2007. What is your diagnosis? Mange due to *Trixacarus caviae* infestation. *Lab. Anim.* (New York) **36:**17–19.

15. **Besch-Williford, C. L.** 1987. Biology and medicine of the ferret. *Vet. Clin. N. Am. Small Anim. Pract.* **17:**1155–1183.

16. **Biggar, R. J., J. P. Woodall, P. D. Walter, and G. E. Haughie.** 1975. Lymphocytic choriomeningitis outbreak associated with pet hamsters. Fifty-seven cases from New York State. *JAMA* **232:**494–500.

17. **Bilek, J., Z. Baranova, M. Kozak, M. Fialkovicova, T. Weissova, and E. Sesztakova.** 2005. *Trichophyton mentagrophytes* var. *quinckeanum* as a cause of zoophilic dermatomycosis in a human family. *Bratisl. Lek. Listy* **106:**383–385.

18. **Blanton, J. D., D. Palmer, K. A. Christian, and C. E. Rupprecht.** 2008. Rabies surveillance in the United States during 2007. *J. Am. Vet. Med. Assoc.* **233:**884–897.

19. **Borland, E. D.** 1975. *Salmonella* infection in dogs, cats, tortoises and terrapins. *Vet. Rec.* **96:**401–402.

20. **Burnham, B. R., D. H. Atchley, R. P. DeFusco, K. E. Ferris, J. C. Zicarelli, J. H. Lee, and F. J. Angulo.** 1998. Prevalence of fecal shedding of *Salmonella* organisms among captive green iguanas and potential public health implications. *J. Am. Vet. Med. Assoc.* **213:**48–50.

21. **Campos, A., J. H. Taylor, and M. Campbell.** 2000. Hamster-bite peritonitis: *Pasteurella pneumotropica* peritonitis in a dialysis patient. *Pediatr. Nephrol.* **15:**31–32.

22. **Canny, C. J., and C. S. Gamble.** 2003. Fungal diseases of rabbits. *Vet. Clin. Exot. Anim.* **6:**429–433.

23. **Carniel, E., and H. H. Mollaret.** 1990. Yersiniosis. *Comp. Immunol. Microbiol. Infect. Dis.* **13:**51–58.

24. **Center for Disease Control.** 1963. Salmonella *Surveillance Report no. 10,* p. 22–24. Center for Disease Control, Atlanta, GA.

25. **Centers for Disease Control.** 1984. Rat-bite fever in a college student, California. *MMWR Morb. Mortal. Wkly. Rep.* **33:**318–320.

26. **Centers for Disease Control.** 1986. Turtle-associated salmonellosis—Ohio. *MMWR Morb. Mortal. Wkly. Rep.* **35:**733–734, 739.

27. **Centers for Disease Control.** 1992. Iguana-associated salmonellosis—Indiana, 1990. *MMWR Morb. Mortal. Wkly. Rep.* **41:**38–39.

28. **Centers for Disease Control.** 1992. Lizard-associated salmonellosis—Utah. *MMWR Morb. Mortal. Wkly. Rep.* **41:**610–611.

29. **Centers for Disease Control and Prevention.** 1995. Reptile-associated salmonellosis—selected states, 1994–1995. *MMWR Morb. Mortal. Wkly. Rep.* **44:**347–350.

30. **Centers for Disease Control and Prevention.** 1995. African pygmy hedgehog-associated salmonellosis—Washington, 1994. *MMWR Morb. Mortal. Wkly. Rep.* **44:**462–463.

31. **Centers for Disease Control and Prevention.** 1996. Invasive infection due to *Streptococcus iniae*—Ontario, 1995–1996. *MMWR Morb. Mortal. Wkly. Rep.* **45:**650–653.

32. **Centers for Disease Control and Prevention.** 1998. Rat-bite fever—New Mexico, 1996. *MMWR Morb. Mortal. Wkly. Rep.* **47:**89–91.

33. **Centers for Disease Control and Prevention.** 1999. Reptile-associated salmonellosis—selected states, 1996–1998. *MMWR Morb. Mortal. Wkly. Rep.* **48:**1009–1013.

34. **Centers for Disease Control and Prevention.** 2002. Outbreak of tularemia among commercially distributed prairie dogs, 2002. *MMWR Morb. Mortal. Wkly. Rep.* **51:**688, 699.

35. **Centers for Disease Control and Prevention.** 2003. Prevalence of IgG antibody to SARS-associated coronavirus in animal traders

Guangdong Province, China, 2003. *MMWR Morb. Mortal. Wkly. Rep.* **52:**986–987.

36. **Centers for Disease Control and Prevention.** 2003. Update: multistate outbreak of monkeypox—Illinois, Indiana, Kansas, Missouri, Ohio, and Wisconsin, 2003. *MMWR Morb. Mortal. Wkly. Rep.* **52:**642–646.

37. **Centers for Disease Control and Prevention.** 2003. Reptile-associated salmonellosis—selected states, 1998–2002. *MMWR Morb. Mortal. Wkly. Rep.* **52:**1206–1209.

38. **Centers for Disease Control and Prevention.** 2003. Control of communicable diseases; restrictions on African rodents, prairie dogs, and certain other animals. Interim final rule; opportunity for public comment. *Fed. Regist.* **68:**62353–62369.

39. **Centers for Disease Control and Prevention.** 2005. Fatal rat-bite fever—Florida and Washington, 2003. *MMWR Morb. Mortal. Wkly. Rep.* **53:**1198–1202.

40. **Centers for Disease Control and Prevention.** 2005. Tularemia associated with a hamster bite—Colorado, 2004. *MMWR Morb. Mortal. Wkly. Rep.* **53:**1202–1203.

41. **Centers for Disease Control and Prevention.** 2005. Outbreak of multidrug-resistant *Salmonella typhimurium* associated with rodents purchased at retail pet stores—United States, December 2003–October 2004. *MMWR Morb. Mortal. Wkly. Rep.* **54:**429–433.

42. **Centers for Disease Control and Prevention.** 2005. Lymphocytic choriomeningitis virus infection in organ transplant recipients—Massachusetts, Rhode Island, 2005. *MMWR Morb. Mortal. Wkly. Rep.* **54:**537–539.

43. **Centers for Disease Control and Prevention.** 2008. Multistate outbreak of human *Salmonella* infections associated with exposure to turtles—United States, 2007–2008. *MMWR Morb. Mortal. Wkly. Rep.* **57:**69–72.

44. **Centers for Disease Control and Prevention and National Association of State Public Health Veterinarians.** 2008. Compendium of animal rabies prevention and control, 2008. *MMWR Recommend. Rep.* **57**(RR-2):1–12.

45. **Chassis, G., E. M. Gross, Z. Greenberg, M. Tokar, N. Platzner, R. Mizrachi, and A. Wolff.** 1986. *Salmonella* in turtles imported to Israel from Louisiana. *JAMA* **256:**1003.

46. **Childs, J. E., G. E. Glass, T. G. Ksiazek, C. A. Rossi, J. G. Oro, and J. W. Leduc.** 1991. Human-rodent contact and infection with lymphocytic choriomeningitis and Seoul viruses in an inner-city population. *Am. J. Trop. Med. Hyg.* **44:**117–121.

47. **Chiodini, R. J., and J. P. Sundberg.** 1981. Salmonellosis in reptiles: a review. *Am. J. Epidemiol.* **113:**494–499.

48. **Chretien, J. H., and V. F. Garagusi.** 1990. Infections associated with pets. *Am. Fam. Pract.* **41:**831–845.

49. **Cohen, M. L., M. Potter, R. Pollard, and R. A. Feldman.** 1980. Turtle-associated salmonellosis in the United States. Effect of public health action, 1970–1976. *JAMA* **243:**1247–1249.

50. **Dalton, C., R. Hoffman, and J. Pape.** 1995. Iguana-associated salmonellosis in children. *Pediatr. Infect. Dis. J.* **14:**319–320.

51. **D'Aoust, J. Y., E. Daley, M. Crozier, and A. M. Sewell.** 1990. Pet turtles: a continuing international threat to public health. *Am. J. Epidemiol.* **132:**233–238.

52. **D'Aoust, J. Y., and H. Lior.** 1978. Pet turtle regulations and abatement of human salmonellosis. *Can. J. Public Health* **69:**107–108.

53. **Davis, W. A., II, J. H. Chretien, V. F. Garagusi, and M. A. Goldstein.** 1978. Snake-to-human transmission of *Aeromonas* (Pl) *shigelloides* resulting in gastroenteritis. *South. Med. J.* **71:**474–476.

54. **Deeb, B. J., and R. F. DiGiacomo.** 1994. Cerebral larva migrans caused by *Baylisascaris* sp. in pet rabbits. *J. Am. Vet. Med. Assoc.* **205:**1744–1747.

55. **De Guzman, E., and E. B. Shotts.** 1988. Bacterial culture and evaluation of diseases of fish. *Vet. Clin. N. Am. Small Anim. Pract.* **18:**365–374.

56. **Deibel, R., J. P. Woodall, W. J. Decher, and G. D. Schryver.** 1975. Lymphocytic choriomeningitis virus in man. Serologic evidence of association with pet hamsters. *JAMA* **232:**501–504.

57. **Dipineto, L., L. Rinaldi, A. Santaniello, M. Sensale, A. Cuomo, M. Calabria, L. F. Menna, and A. Fioretti.** 2008. Serological survey for antibodies to *Encephalitozoon cuniculi* in pet rabbits in Italy. *Zoonoses Public Health* **55:**173–175.

58. **Dodin, A., and M. Galimand.** 1981. La mélioidose: maladie de pathologie comparée. *Bull. Soc. Sci. Vet. Med. Comp.* **83:**255–258.

59. **Donta, S. T., P. W. Smith, R. E. Levitz, and R. Quintiliani.** 1986. Therapy of *Mycobacterium marinum* infections. Use of tetracyclines vs. rifampin. *Arch. Intern. Med.* **146:**902–904.

60. **Downing, N. D., G. D. Dewnany, and P. J. Radford.** 2001. A rare and serious consequence of a rat bite. *Ann. R. Coll. Surg. Engl.* **83:**279–280.

61. **Duma, R. J., D. E. Sonenshine, F. M. Bozeman, J. M. Veazey, Jr., B. L. Elisberg, D. P. Chadwick, N. I. Stocks, T. M. McGill, G. B. Miller, Jr., and J. N. MacCormack.** 1981. Epidemic typhus in the United States associated with flying squirrels. *JAMA* **245:**2318–2323.

62. **Du Plessis, V., A. J. Birnie, I. Eloff, H. Reuter, and S. Andronikou.** 2007. Pentastomiasis (*Armillifer armillatus* infestation). *S. Afr. Med. J.* **97:**928, 930.

63. **Eidson, M., S. D. Matthews, A. L. Willsey, B. Cherry, R. J. Rudd, and C. V. Trimarchi.** 2005. Rabies virus infection in a pet guinea pig and seven pet rabbits. *J. Am. Vet. Med. Assoc.* **227:**932–935.

64. **Eidson, M., J. P. Thilsted, and O. J. Rollag.** 1991. Clinical, clinicopathologic, and pathologic features of plague in cats: 119 cases (1977–1988). *J. Am. Vet. Med. Assoc.* **199:**1191–1197.

65. **Enriquez, C., N. Nwachuku, and C. P. Gerba.** 2001. Direct exposure to animal enteric pathogens. *Rev. Environ. Health* **16:**117–131.

66. **Eurosurveillance Editorial Team, S. Bertrand, R. Rimhanen-Finne, F. X. Weill, W. Rabsch, L. Thornton, J. Perevoscikovs, W. van Pelt, and M. Heck.** 2008. *Salmonella* infections associated with reptiles: the current situation in Europe. *Euro. Surveill.* **13**(24). http://www.eurosurveillance.org/ViewArticle.aspx?ArticleId=18902.

67. **Favorov, M. O., M. Y. Kosoy, S. A. Tsarev, J. E. Childs, and H. S. Margolis.** 2000. Prevalence of antibody to hepatitis E virus among rodents in the United States. *J. Infect. Dis.* **181:**449–455.

68. **Fischer, S. A., M. B. Graham, M. J. Kuehnert, C. N. Kotton, A. Srinivasan, et al.** 2006. Transmission of lymphocytic choriomeningitis virus by organ transplantation. *N. Engl. J. Med.* **354:**2235–2249.

69. **Fish, N. A., A. L. Fletch, and W. E. Butler.** 1968. Family outbreak of salmonellosis due to contact with guinea pigs. *Can. Med. Assoc. J.* **99:**418–420.

70. **Fonseca, R. J., and L. M. Dubey.** 1994. *Salmonella montevideo* sepsis from a pet snake. *Pediatr. Infect. Dis. J.* **13:**550.

71. **Foster, E. S., K. A. Signs, D. R. Marks, H. Kapoor, M. Casey, M. G. Stobierski, and E. D. Walker.** 2006. Lymphocytic choriomeningitis in Michigan. *Emerg. Infect. Dis.* **12:**851–853.

72. **Fox, J. G., J. A. Adkins, and K. O. Maxwell.** 1988. Zoonoses in ferrets. *Lab. Anim. Sci.* **38:**500–501.

73. **Fox, J. G., C. E. Newcomer, and H. Rozmiarek.** 1984. Selected zoonoses and other health hazards, p. 613–648. *In* J. G. Fox, B. J. Cohen, and F. M. Loew (ed.), *Laboratory Animal Medicine.* Academic Press, New York, NY.

74. **Friedman, C. R., C. Torigian, P. J. Shillam, R. E. Hoffman, D. Heltzel, J. L. Beebe, G. Malcolm, W. de Witt, L. Hutwagner, and P. M. Griffin.** 1998. An outbreak of salmonellosis among children attending a reptile exhibit at a zoo. *J. Pediatr.* **132:**802–807.

75. **Friedmann, C. T. H., E. L. Spiegel, E. Aaron, and R. McIntyre.** 1973. *Leptospira ballum* contracted from pet mice. *Calif. Med.* **118:**51–52.

76. **Fujita, K., K. I. Murono, and H. Yoshioka.** 1981. Pet-linked salmonellosis. *Lancet* **ii:**525.

77. **Goscienski, P. J.** 1983. Zoonoses. *Pediatr. Infect. Dis. J.* **2:**69–81.

78. **Greenacre, C. B.** 2003. Fungal diseases of ferrets. *Vet. Clin. Exot. Anim.* **6:**435–448.

79. **Gregg, M. B.** 1975. Recent outbreaks of lymphocytic choriomeningitis in the United States of America. *Bull. W. H. O.* **52:**549–553.

80. **Guan, Y., B. J. Zheng, Y. Q. He, X. L. Liu, Z. X. Zhuang, C. L. Cheung, S. W. Luo, P. H. Li, L. J. Zhang, Y. J. Guan, K. M. Butt, K. L. Wong, K. W. Chan, W. Lim, K. F. Shortridge, K. Y. Yuen, J. S. Peiris, and L. L. Poon.** 2003. Isolation and characterization of viruses related to the SARS coronavirus from animals in southern China. *Science* **302:**276–278.

81. **Guerra, B., T. Schneider, E. Luge, A. Draeger, V. Moos, C. Loddenkemper, A. Jansen, and K. Nöckler.** 2008. Detection and characterization of *Leptospira interrogans* isolates from pet rats belonging to a human immunodeficiency virus-positive patient with leptospirosis. *J. Med. Microbiol.* **57:**133–135.

82. **Harkness, J. E.** 1987. Rabbit husbandry and medicine. *Vet. Clin. N. Am. Small Anim. Pract.* **17:**1019–1044.

83. **Harkness, J. E., and J. E. Wagner.** 1983. *The Biology and Medicine of Rabbits and Rodents,* 2nd ed., p. 2104. Lea & Febiger, Philadelphia, PA.

84. **Harvey, S., and J. R. Greenwood.** 1985. Isolation of *Campylobacter fetus* from a pet turtle. *J. Clin. Microbiol.* **21:**260–261.

85. **Harvey, S., R. Greenwood, M. J. Pickett, and R. H. Mah.** 1976. Recovery of *Yersinia enterocolitica* from streams and lakes of California. *Appl. Environ. Microbiol.* **32:**352–354.

86. **He, J., B. L. Innis, M. P. Shrestha, E. T. Clayson, R. M. Scott, K. J. Linthicum, G. G. Musser, S. C. Gigliotti, L. N. Binn, R. A. Kuschner, and D. W. Vaughn.** 2002. Evidence that rodents are a reservoir of hepatitis E virus for humans in Nepal. *J. Clin. Microbiol.* **40:**4493–4498.

87. **Hendrix, C. M., and B. L. Blagburn.** 1988. Reptilian pentastomiasis: a possible emerging zoonosis. *Compend. Small Anim.* **10:**46–51.

88. **Heymann, D. L.** 2004. *Control of Communicable Diseases in Man,* 18th ed., p. 702. American Public Health Association, Washington, DC.

89. **Hirano, M., X. Ding, T. C. Li, N. Takeda, H. Kawabata, N. Koizumi, T. Kadosaka, I. Goto, T. Masuzawa, M. Nakamura, K. Taira, T. Kuroki, T. Tanikawa, H. Watanabe, and K. Abe.** 2003. Evidence for widespread infection of hepatitis E virus among wild rats in Japan. *Hepatol. Res.* **27:**1–5.

90. **Hoar, B. R., B. B. Chomel, F. J. Argaz Rodriguez, and P. A. Colley.** 1998. Zoonoses and potential zoonoses transmitted by bats. *J. Am. Vet. Med. Assoc.* **212:**1714–1720.

91. **Hsieh, S., and F. E. Balb.** 1999. *Serratia marcescens* cellulitis following an iguana bite. *Clin. Infect. Dis.* **28:**1181–1182.

92. **Jafari, M., J. Forsberg, R. O. Gilcher, J. W. Smith, J. M. Crutcher, M. McDermott, B. R. Brown, and J. N. George.** 2002. *Salmonella* sepsis caused by a platelet transfusion from a donor with a pet snake. *N. Engl. J. Med.* **347:**1075–1078.

93. **Janda, J. M., and S. L. Abbott.** 1993. Infections associated with the genus *Edwardsiella*: the role of *Edwardsiella tarda* in human disease. *Clin. Infect. Dis.* **17:**742–748.

94. **Jay, M., M. S. Ascher, B. B. Chomel, M. Madon, D. Sesline, B. A. Enge, B. Hjelle, T. G. Ksiazek, P. E. Rollin, P. H. Kass, and K. Reilly.** 1997. Seroepidemiologic studies of hantavirus infection among wild rodents in California. *Emerg. Infect. Dis.* **3:**183–190.

95. **Jones, T. F., L. A. Ingram, K. E. Fullerton, R. Marcus, B. J. Anderson, P. V. McCarthy, D. Vugia, B. Shiferaw, N. Haubert, S. Wedel, and F. J. Angulo.** 2006. A case-control study of the epidemiology of sporadic *Salmonella* infection in infants. *Pediatrics* **118:**2380–2387.

96. **Jones-Engel, L., C. C. May, G. A. Engel, K. A. Steinkraus, M. A. Schillaci, et al.** 2008. Diverse contexts of zoonotic transmission of simian foamy viruses in Asia. *Emerg. Infect. Dis.* **14:**1200–1208.

97. **Kaufmann, A. F., M. D. Fox, G. K. Morris, B. T. Wood, J. C. Feeley, and M. K. Frix.** 1972. Turtle-associated salmonellosis. III. The effects of environmental salmonellae in commercial turtle breeding ponds. *Am. J. Epidemiol.* **95:**521–528.

98. **Kiesch, N.** 2000. Aquariums and mycobacterioses. *Rev. Med. Brux.* **21:**A255–A256.

99. **Kist, M. J., and S. Freitag.** 2000. Serovar specific risk factors and clinical features of *Salmonella enterica* ssp. enterica serovar Enteritidis: a study in South-West Germany. *Epidemiol. Infect.* **124:**383–392.

100. **Kleeburg, H. H.** 1975. Tuberculosis and other mycobacterioses, p. 303–360. *In* W. T. Hub-

bert, W. F. McCulloch, and P. R. Schnurrenberger (ed.), *Diseases Transmitted from Animals to Man,* 6th ed. Charles C. Thomas, Publisher, Springfield, IL.

101. **Ksiazek, T. G., D. Erdman, C. Goldsmith, S. R. Zaki, T. Peret, S. Emery, et al.** 2003. A novel coronavirus associated with severe acute respiratory syndrome. *N. Engl. J. Med.* **348:**1953–1966.

102. **Lamm, S. H., A. Taylor, Jr., E. J. Gangarosa, H. W. Anderson, W. Young, M. H. Clark, and A. R. Bruce.** 1972. Turtle associated salmonellosis. I. An estimation of the magnitude of the problem in the United States, 1970–1971. *Am. J. Epidemiol.* **95:**511–517.

103. **Lau, S. K., P. C. Woo, H. Tse, K. W. Leung, S. S. Wong, and K. Y. Yuen.** 2003. Invasive *Streptococcus iniae* infections outside North America. *J. Clin. Microbiol.* **41:**1004–1009.

104. **LeDuc, J. W.** 1987. Epidemiology of Hantaan and related viruses. *Lab. Anim. Sci.* **37:**413–418.

105. **Lehane, L., and G. T. Rawlin.** 2000. Topically acquired bacterial zoonoses from fish: a review. *Med. J. Aust.* **173:**256–259.

106. **Leibovitz, L.** 1980. Fish tuberculosis (mycobacteriosis). *J. Am. Vet. Med. Assoc.* **176:**415.

107. **Li, W., Z. Shi, M. Yu, W. Ren, C. Smith, J. H. Epstein, et al.** 2005. Bats are natural reservoirs of SARS-like coronaviruses. *Science* **310**(5748)**:**676–679.

108. **Lowry, T., and S. A. Smith.** 2007. Aquatic zoonoses associated with food, bait, ornamental, and tropical fish. *J. Am. Vet. Med. Assoc.* **231:**876–880.

109. **Lynch, M., M. Daly, B. O'Brien, F. Morrison, B. Cryan, and S. Fanning.** 1999. *Salmonella tel-el-kebir* and terrapins. *J. Infect.* **38:**182–184.

110. **Mackenzie, J. S., H. E. Field, and K. J. Guyatt.** 2003. Managing emerging diseases borne by fruit bats (flying foxes), with particular reference to henipaviruses and Australian bat lyssavirus. *J. Appl. Microbiol.* **94**(Suppl.)**:**59S–69S.

111. **Magee, J. S., R. W. Steele, N. R. Kelly, and R. F. Jacobs.** 1989. Tularemia transmitted by a squirrel bite. *Pediatr. Infect. Dis. J.* **8:**123–125.

112. **Marini, R. P., J. A. Adkins, and J. G. Fox.** 1989. Proven or potential zoonotic diseases of ferrets. *J. Am. Vet. Med. Assoc.* **195:**990–994.

113. **Martina, B. E., B. L. Haagmans, T. Kuiken, R. A. Fouchier, G. F. Rimmelzwaan, G. Van Amerongen, J. S. Peiris, W. Lim, and A. D. Osterhaus.** 2003. SARS virus infection of cats and ferrets. *Nature* **425:**915.

114. **Matsuda, H., K. Okada, K. Takahashi, and S. Mishiro.** 2003. Severe hepatitis E virus in-

fection after ingestion of uncooked liver from a wild boar. *J. Infect. Dis.* **188**:944.

115. **Maxwell, E. L., B. C. Mayall, S. R. Pearson, and P. A. Stanley.** 1991. A case of *Vibrio vulnificus* septicaemia acquired in Victoria. *Med. J. Aust.* **154**:214–215.

116. **McCall, B. J., J. H. Epstein, A. S. Neill, K. Heel, H. Field, J. Barrett, G. A. Smith, L. A. Selvey, B. Rodwell, and R. Lunt.** 2000. Potential human exposure to Australian bat lyssavirus, Queensland, 1996–1999. *Emerg. Infect. Dis.* **6**:259–264.

117. **Mermin, J., B. Hoar, and F. J. Angulo.** 1997. Iguanas and Salmonella marina infection in children: a reflection of the increasing incidence of reptile-associated salmonellosis in the United States. *Pediatrics* **99**:399–402.

118. **Mermin, J., L. Hutwagner, D. Vugia, S. Shallow, P. Daily, et al.** 2004. Reptiles, amphibians, and human *Salmonella* infection: a population-based, case-control study. *Clin. Infect. Dis.* **38**(Suppl. 3):S253–S261.

119. **Mignard, S., B. Aubry-Rozier, M. de Montclos, G. Llorca, and G. Carret.** 2007. Pet-rat bite fever and septic arthritis: molecular identification of *Streptobacillus moniliformis. Med. Mal. Infect.* **37**:293–294. (In French.)

120. **Mitchell, M. A., and S. M. Shane.** 2000. Preliminary findings of *Salmonella* spp. in captive green iguanas *(Iguana iguana)* and their environment. *Prev. Vet. Med.* **45**:297–304.

121. **Moro, M. H., J. T. Horman, H. R. Fischman, J. K. Grigor, and E. Israel.** 1991. The epidemiology of rodent and lagomorph rabies in Maryland, 1981 to 1986. *J. Wildl. Dis.* **27**:452–456.

122. **Nagel, P., A. Serritella, and T. J. Layden.** 1982. *Edwardsiella tarda* gastroenteritis associated with a pet turtle. *Gastroenterology* **82**:1436–1437.

123. **Nakamura, Y., R. Kano, E. Nakamura, K. Saito, S. Watanabe, and A. Hasegawa.** 2002. Case report. First report on human ringworm caused by *Arthroderma benhamiae* in Japan transmitted from a rabbit. *Mycoses* **45**:129–131.

124. **Niezgoda, M., D. J. Briggs, J. Shaddock, D. W. Dreesen, and C. E. Rupprecht.** 1997. Pathogenesis of experimentally induced rabies in domestic ferrets. *Am. J. Vet. Res.* **58**:1327–1331.

125. **Ostrowski, S. R., M. J. Leslie, T. Parrott, S. Abelt, and P. E. Piercy.** 1998. B-virus from pet macaque monkeys: an emerging threat in the United States? *Emerg. Infect. Dis.* **4**:117–121.

126. **Parrott, T. Y.** 1986. An introduction to diseases of non-human primates. *Compend. Small Anim.* **8**:733–738.

127. **Pfleger, S., G. Benyr, R. Sommer, and A. Hassl.** 2003. Pattern of *Salmonella* excretion in amphibians and reptiles in a vivarium. *Int. J. Hyg. Environ. Health* **206**:53–59.

128. **Pollock, C.** 2003. Fungal diseases of laboratory rodents. *Vet. Clin. Exot. Anim.* **6**:401–413.

129. **Postma, B. H., R. J. A. Dierpersloot, G. J. C. M. Niessen, and R. P. Droog.** 1991. Cowpox-virus-like infection associated with rat bite. *Lancet* **337**:733–734.

130. **Reboli, A., and E. Farrar.** 1989. *Erysipelothrix rhusiopathiae:* an occupational pathogen. *Clin. Microbiol. Rev.* **2**:354–359.

131. **Redrobe, S.** 2002. Reptiles and disease—keeping the risks to a minimum. *J. Small Anim. Pract.* **43**:471–472.

132. **Renquist, D. M., and R. A. Whitney.** 1987. Zoonoses acquired from pet primates. *Vet. Clin. N. Am. Small Anim. Pract.* **17**:219–240.

133. **Reynolds, M. G., W. B. Davidson, A. T. Curns, C. S. Conover, G. Huhn, et al.** 2007. Spectrum of infection and risk factors for human monkeypox, United States, 2003. *Emerg. Infect. Dis.* **13**:1332–1339.

134. **Reynolds, M. G., J. S. Krebs, J. A. Comer, J. W. Sumner, T. C. Rushton, C. E. Lopez, W. L. Nicholson, J. A. Rooney, S. E. Lance-Parker, J. H. McQuiston, C. D. Paddock, and J. E. Childs.** 2003. Flying squirrel-associated typhus, United States. *Emerg. Infect. Dis.* **9**:1341–1343.

135. **Riley, P. Y., and B. B. Chomel.** 2005. Hedgehog zoonoses. *Emerg. Infect. Dis.* **11**:1–5.

136. **Rosen, T.** 2000. Hazardous hedgehogs. *South. Med. J.* **93**:936–938.

137. **Rosen, T., and J. Jablon.** 2003. Infectious threats from exotic pets: dermatological implications. *Dermatol. Clin.* **21**:229–236.

138. **Rousseau, M. C., M. F. Saron, P. Brouqui, and A. Bourgeade.** 1997. Lymphocytic choriomeningitis virus in southern France: four case reports and review of the literature. *Eur. J. Epidemiol.* **13**:817–823.

139. **Rupprecht, C. E., J. Gilbert, R. Pitts, K. R. Marshall, and H. Koprowski.** 1990. Evaluation of an inactivated rabies virus vaccine in domestic ferrets. *J. Am. Vet. Med. Assoc.* **196**:1614–1616.

140. **Sanchez, R., A. Martin, A. Bailly, and M. F. Dirat.** 1988. Salmonellose digestive associée à une tortue domestique. A propos d'un cas. *Med. Mal. Infect.* **18**:458–459.

141. **Satterfield, W. C., and W. R. Voss.** 1987. Nonhuman primates and the practitioner. *Vet. Clin. N. Am. Small Anim. Pract.* **17**:1185–1202.

142. **Schauder, S., M. Kirsch-Nietzki, S. Wegener, E. Switzer, and S. A. Qadripur.**

2007. From hedgehogs to men. Zoophilic dermatophytosis caused by *Trichophyton erinacei* in eight patients. *Hautarzt* **58**:62–67. (In German.)

143. **Schultz, L. J., R. R. Roberto, G. W. Rutherford, B. Hummert, and I. Lubell.** 1992. *Mesocestoides* (Cestoda) infection in a California child. *Pediatr. Infect. Dis. J.* **11**:332–334.

144. **Schumacher, J.** 2003. Fungal diseases of reptiles. *Vet. Clin. Exot. Anim.* **6**:327–335.

145. **Schuurman, B., A. J. van Griethuysen, J. H. Marcelis, and A. M. Nijs.** 1998. Rat-bite fever after a bite from a tame pet rat. *Ned. Tijdschr. Geneeskd.* **142**:2006–2009.

146. **Seguin, B., Y. Boucaud-Maitre, P. Quenin, and G. Lorgue.** 1986. Recherche de *Yersinia enterocolitica* et des espèces apparentées chez le rat d'égout: présence d'une souche pathogène humaine. *Med. Mal. Infect.* **16**:28–30.

147. **Shotts, E. B.** 1980. Bacteria associated with fish and their relative importance, p. 517–525. *In* J. H. Steele (ed.), *CRC Handbook Series in Zoonoses,* section A, vol. II. CRC Press, Boca Raton, FL.

148. **Shotts, E. B.** 1987. Bacterial diseases of fish associated with human health. *Vet. Clin. N. Am. Small Anim. Pract.* **17**:241–247.

149. **Shvartsblat, S., M. Kochie, P. Harber, and J. Howard.** 2004. Fatal rat-bite fever in a pet shop employee. *Am. J. Ind. Med.* **45**:357–360.

150. **Skorepova, M., J. Stork, and J. Hrabakova.** 2002. Case reports. *Tinea gladiatorum* due to *Trichophyton mentagrophytes. Mycoses* **45**:431–433.

151. **Smith, M. D., and J. D. Gradon.** 2003. Bacteremia due to *Comamonas* species possibly associated with exposure to tropical fish. *South. Med. J.* **96**:815–817.

152. **Soave, O.** 1981. Viral infections common to human and non-human primates. *J. Am. Vet. Med. Assoc.* **179**:1385–1388.

153. **Stehr-Green, J. K., and P. Schantz.** 1987. The impact of zoonotic diseases transmitted by pets on human health and the economy. *Vet. Clin. N. Am. Small Anim. Pract.* **17**:1–15.

154. **Swanson, S. J., C. Snider, C. R. Braden, D. Boxrud, A. Wünschmann, J. A. Rudroff, J. Lockett, and K. E. Smith.** 2007. Multidrug-resistant *Salmonella enterica* serotype Typhimurium associated with pet rodents. *N. Engl. J. Med.* **356**:21–28.

155. **Tager-Frey, M., P. C. Vial, C. H. Castillo, P. M. Godoy, B. Hjelle, and M. G. Ferres.** 2003. Hantavirus prevalence in the IX Region of Chile. *Emerg. Infect. Dis.* **9**:827–832.

156. **Tauxe, R. V., J. G. Rigau-Pérez, J. G. Wells, and P. A. Blake.** 1985. Turtle-associated salmonellosis in Puerto Rico. *JAMA* **254**:237–239.

157. **Tei, S., N. Kitajima, K. Takahashi, and S. Mishiro.** 2003. Zoonotic transmission of hepatitis E virus from deer to human beings. *Lancet* **362**:371–373.

158. **Thoen, C. O., A. G. Karlson, and E. M. Himes.** 1981. Mycobacterial infections in animals. *Rev. Infect. Dis.* **3**:960–972.

159. **Traversa, D., R. Iorio, D. Otranto, D. Modrý, and J. Slapeta.** 2008. *Cryptosporidium* from tortoises: genetic characterisation, phylogeny and zoonotic implications. *Mol. Cell. Probes* **22**:122–128.

160. **Tsianakas, P., B. Polack, L. Pinquier, B. Levy Klotz, and C. Prost-Squarcioni.** 2000. *Cheyletiella* dermatitis: an uncommon cause of vesiculobullous eruption. *Ann. Dermatol. Venereol.* **127**:826–829.

161. **Vandepitte, J., P. Lemmens, and L. de Swert.** 1983. Human edwardsiellosis traced to ornamental fish. *J. Clin. Microbiol.* **17**:165–167.

162. **Wagner, J. E., and P. L. Farrar.** 1987. Husbandry and medicine of small rodents. *Vet. Clin. N. Am. Small Anim. Pract.* **17**:1061–1087.

163. **Wang, L. F., Z. Shi, S. Zhang, H. Field, P. Daszak, and B. T. Eaton.** 2006. Review of bats and SARS. *Emerg. Infect. Dis.* **12**:1834–1840.

164. **Weinstein, M. R., M. Litt, D. A. Kertesz, P. Wyper, D. Rose, M. Coulter, A. McGeer, R. Facklam, C. Ostach, B. M. Willey, A. Borczyk, and D. E. Low.** 1997. Invasive infections due to a fish pathogen, *Streptococcus iniae. N. Engl. J. Med.* **337**:589–594.

165. **Whittington, R. J., and R. Chong.** 2007. Global trade in ornamental fish from an Australian perspective: the case for revised import risk analysis and management strategies. *Prev. Vet. Med.* **81**:92–116.

166. **Willis, C., T. Wilson, M. Greenwood, and L. Ward.** 2002. Pet reptiles associated with a case of salmonellosis in an infant were carrying multiple strains of *Salmonella. J. Clin. Microbiol.* **40**:4802–4803.

167. **Wolfs, T. F., J. A. Wagenaar, H. G. Niesters, and A. D. Osterhaus.** 2002. Rat-to-human transmission of cowpox infection. *Emerg. Infect. Dis.* **8**:1495–1496.

168. **Woodward, D. L., R. Khakhria, and W. M. Johnson.** 1997. Human salmonellosis associated with exotic pets. *J. Clin. Microbiol.* **35**:2786–2790.

169. **Zamora, J., and R. Enriquez.** 1987. *Yersinia enterocolitica, Y. frederiksenii* and *Y. intermedia* in *Cyprinus carpio* (Linneo 1758). *Zentralbl. Vetmed. Reihe B* **34**:155–159.

WITH MAN'S WORST FRIEND (THE RAT)

James G. Fox

9

Historically, the rat has been considered a scourge to mankind. For example, the rat is a reservoir for the plague bacillus that caused the Black Death, which accounted for millions of deaths in Europe during the Middle Ages. At least three pandemics (in the 5th and 6th, 8th through 14th, and 19th through 21st centuries) of plague ravaged civilizations, and the disease undoubtedly "plagued" humankind prior to recorded history. Also, numerous other diseases are spread to humans by rats; thus, a quote from Hans Zinsser's text *Rats, Lice, and History,* "Man and rat will always be pitted against each other as implacable enemies," conveys the general revulsion that society holds for the wild rat (187).

Numerous methods have been used by countless countries attempting to eradicate the rat, but it continues to successfully colonize both urban and rural settings on a global level. One novel approach first introduced in Asia and Europe and then in the United States was the use of domestic ferrets for rodent control.

Because the life cycle and transmission of *Yersinia pestis* are closely linked to rats and their fleas, tremendous efforts were mounted to eradicate the rat host and its flea, *Xenopsylla cheopis*. For example, in the Philippines, rat catcher groups of 300 men were assigned the formidable task of eliminating the omnipotent pest (76). When rats were encountered, they were killed immediately. Some of these work forces had fox terriers imported especially from Australia, because of their agility and quickness. Others utilized trained ferrets, which responded to their masters' calls, like dogs. The ferrets were even more effective than dogs in killing rats. A ferret would grasp a rat in its jaws, and the ferret's teeth would then sever the rat's spinal column (76). Undoubtedly, ferrets served similar roles in differing locales throughout the world to control rat infestations and hence to reduce the likelihood of further spread of the dreaded pestilence.

One author recommended that, when rats are hunted in plague agent-infested areas, the rats and the sack containing the dead rats be submerged in a germicidal solution as soon as they are killed (86). It was strongly urged that rats in plague areas, as well as the bag containing the rats, be incinerated. Even though attention was given to treating rat bite wound infection in ferrets, discussions on ferrets hunting *Y. pestis*-infected rats becoming infected with the plague bacillus were not found.

James G. Fox, Division of Comparative Medicine, Massachusetts Institute of Technology, 77 Massachusetts Avenue, Bldg. 16 825C, Cambridge, MA 02139.

Infections of Leisure, Fourth Edition, Edited by David Schlossberg,
© 2009 ASM Press, Washington, DC

The practice of using ferrets to control wild rodents also became popular in the United States during the early part of the 20th century, and tens of thousands of ferrets were raised and sold for this purpose. The Department of Agriculture distributed bulletins announcing the use of ferrets for rodent abatement (57). Because rodents are extremely fearful of ferrets and flee even their scent, only a few ferrets were needed to disperse literally hundreds of rodents from granaries, barns, and warehouses. A "ferretmeister" would deploy his ferrets on an infested farm or granary, and the animal would then "ferret out" the rodents from their hiding places and nests. Men and terrier dogs, strategically located, would eradicate the rodents as they emerged from hiding. Alternatively, small farms or granaries would maintain ferrets and allow the territorial imperative for up to about 650 ft (200 m)—considered to be the ranging domain of a ferret—with an adequate food source. The availability of commercially available rodenticides, however, has dramatically reduced the need of ferrets as rodent exterminators (57).

During the early 1900s, rodenticides containing live cultures of *Salmonella enteritidis* were distributed on a large-scale basis by commercial and public health organizations in an attempt to eliminate feral rats. These cultures were known as "rat viruses" and widely used in Europe, England, and the United States as "rat poisons" (178). However, the enthusiasm for their use waned when it was discovered that the spread of the organisms could not be limited; predictably, the baiting program was implicated in several epidemics among exposed human populations (178). Surprisingly, as late as the 1950s in England, *S. enteritidis* (serovar Danzy) was isolated from adults living 4 miles apart. The source of infection was traced to contaminated cakes from a local bakery. Mice which had acquired the infection from living *S. enteritidis* serovar Danzy cultures in rodenticide baits had infected food in the bakery (22).

On a global scale, there has been a dramatic increase in the number of feral cats. During the last decade, it is estimated that 50 million to 60 million feral cats inhabit the United States. This tremendous number raises the question as to whether they are playing a role in controlling the wild rat population in both rural and urban settings. Though feral cats' predatory habits have a profound effect on reducing the number of wild bird species and small rodents and reptiles, they supposedly do not kill rats over 200 g.

The black roof rat *(Rattus rattus),* which coexisted with humans in the small, crowded, unsanitary environs of the medieval era, has been largely displaced by the more aggressive, larger brown Norway rat *(Rattus norvegicus)* (35, 126, 147). This species of rat lives farther from contemporary, better-constructed urban domiciles by taking up residence in backyards, sewers, industrial buildings, dumps, or granaries. In this environment, the rat often competes for food and territory with other wild rodents and therefore can share zoonotically transmitted diseases. Fortunately, human fleas, which accounted for widespread human-to-human transmission of plague, have almost been eliminated from cities in the United States, and thus the likelihood of epidemics initiated by rat zoonoses has been reduced. Nevertheless, zoonotic transmission of rat diseases still occurs, and as major cities suffer from overcrowding, structural decay, and inadequate waste removal, the rat population will increase and the probability of transmission of these diseases to the homeless or underprivileged correspondingly increases.

Contrary to the image of the rat depicted by Zinsser, the laboratory rat, *Rattus norvegicus,* used extensively for decades in biomedical research, has provided immeasurable benefit to humankind's understanding of disease processes, their control, and elimination. However, the use of rats in research and the current popularity of rats as "pocket pets" also afford the opportunity for this segment of the population to become infected with rat-borne diseases. The purpose of this chapter, therefore, is to highlight those zoonotic diseases of rats, and in certain cases the same diseases in other rodents, which have clinical relevance in the United States and its territories (60).

RAT BITES

Relapsing fevers following rat bites have been noted clinically for over 2,000 years, being first recognized in India. Early recorded descriptions of the disease are found in the Yale medical archives of the 19th century. The term *Rattenbisskrankheit,* or rat-bite fever, was coined (100).

Approximately 40,000 rat bites are reported annually, according to one carefully researched report (35). In another report, the authors estimated that 1% of the 2 million animal bites that occur annually are rat bites (70). Several studies indicate that over two-thirds of the rat bites occur in children under 10 years of age. Adults attacked are usually debilitated or otherwise helpless. Most bites occur on the hands and feet, but bites may also be present on the heads and faces of infants, sometimes with disfiguring consequences. However, rat bites also occur in personnel using these animals for research or providing for their care in pet stores and, increasingly, in household members who have pet rats. Occasionally, deaths due to rat bites have been recorded for infants or debilitated adults (126). It has been estimated in one study that 2% of rodent bites in humans become infected (118). Several bacterial pathogens have been isolated from rat bites, including *Leptospira interrogans, Pasteurella multocida,* and *Staphylococcus species;* however, the most commonly isolated microorganisms are *Streptobacillus moniliformis* and *Spirillum minus* (175, 176).

BACTERIAL DISEASES

Rat-Bite Fever

Rat-bite fever can be caused by either of two microorganisms: *Streptobacillus moniliformis* or *Spirillum minus. Streptobacillus moniliformis* causes the diseases known as streptobacillary fever, streptobacillary rat-bite fever, and streptobacillosis. Haverhill fever and epidemic arthritic erythema are diseases associated with

ingestion of water, food, or raw milk contaminated with *S. moniliformis.* Sodoku (derived from the Japanese words for rat [*so*] and poison [*doku*]), spirillosis, and spirillary rat-bite fever are caused by another bacterium, *Spirillum minus,* which is commonly isolated from rat bites of humans residing in Asia. The bite of an infected rat is the usual source of infection. In some cases, bites of other animals, including mice, gerbils, squirrels, weasels, ferrets, dogs, and cats, or rare traumatic injuries unassociated with animal contact cause the infection (49). Exposure to cats and dogs that prey on wild rodents may also be the source of the organisms.

These organisms are present in the oral cavities and upper respiratory passages of asymptomatic rodents, usually rats, and exposure to rat saliva without an overt bite can transmit the organism to humans (180). In one study, *Streptobacillus moniliformis* was isolated as the predominant microorganism from the upper tracheas of laboratory rats (120). Other small surveys indicate isolation of the organism in 0 of 15, 7 of 10, 2 of 20, and 7 of 14 laboratory rats and in 4 of 6 wild rats (67). Presumably, the incidence of *S. moniliformis* is now lower in high-quality, commercially reared, specific-pathogen-free rats. Surveys of wild rats indicate 0 to 25% infection with *Spirillum minus* (87). *Spirillum minus* does not grow in vitro and historically has required inoculation of culture specimens into laboratory animals, with subsequent identification of the bacteria by dark-field microscopy. *Streptobacillus moniliformis* grows slowly on artificial media but only in the presence of 15% blood and sera, usually 10% to 20% rabbit or horse serum incubated at reduced partial pressures of oxygen (56). Sodium polyanethol sulfonate sometimes found in blood-based media because of its properties as a bacterial growth promoter should not be used due to its inhibitory effects on *S. moniliformis.* Growth on agar consists of 1- to 2-mm, gray, glistening colonies. The API ZYM diagnostic system can be used for rapid biochemical analysis and diagnosis. Specific PCR assays have also been used to diagnose the presence of the bacteria in both humans and rats (174). Fatty acid analysis can also be employed in cultured organisms.

Rat-bite fever is not a reportable disease, which makes its prevalence, geographic location, racial data, and source of infection in humans difficult to assess. The disease, though uncommon in humans, has nonetheless appeared among researchers or students working with laboratory rodents, particularly rats (6). Historically, wild-rat bites and subsequent illness (usually in small children) relate to poor sanitation and overcrowding (87). One survey of rat bites in Baltimore, MD, tabulated rat-bite fever in 11 of 87 cases (21). The disease can also occur in individuals who have no history of rat bites but reside or work in rat-infested areas. Acute febrile diseases, especially if associated with animal bites, are routinely treated with penicillin or other antibiotics. Therefore, accurate data regarding prevalence are usually not provided.

Streptobacillus moniliformis incubation varies from a few hours to 2 to 10 days, whereas *Spirillum minus* incubation ranges from 1 to 6 weeks (Table 1). Fever is present in either form. Inflammation associated with the bite and lymphadenopathies are frequently accompanied by headache, general malaise, myalgia, and chills (7, 34, 68, 109). The discrete macular rash that often appears on the extremities may generalize into pustular or petechial se-

quelae. Arthritis occurs in 50% of all cases of *Streptobacillus moniliformis* but is less common in *Spirillum minus*. *Streptobacillus moniliformis*, which has a predilection for synovial and serosal surfaces, may be cultured from serous-to-purulent effusion recovered from affected larger joints. The organism should be considered in the list of differential diagnoses for cases of septic arthritis, particularly with synovial fluid with high inflammatory cell counts (41).

Rat-bite fever has a mortality rate of approximately 13% when untreated. If antibiotic treatment, usually penicillin at doses of 400,000 to 600,000 units daily for 7 days, is not instituted early, complications such as pneumonia, hepatitis, pyelonephritis, enteritis, and endocarditis may develop (6, 7, 34, 68, 109, 131, 134, 142, 159). If endocarditis is present, the penicillin should be given parenterally at doses of 15 million to 20 million units daily for 4 for 6 weeks. Streptomycin and tetracyclines are also effective antibiotics for those individuals with penicillin-associated allergies. Death has occurred in cases of *Streptobacillus moniliformis* involving preexistent valvular disease. The recent reports of fatalities due to *S. moniliformis* in adults working in a pet store and having rats as pets highlight the need to be vigilant in recognizing the clinical manifestations of rat-bite fever in patients with

TABLE 1 Clinical signs of rat-bite fever[a]

Clinical feature(s)	Streptobacillary fever (*Streptobacillus moniliformis*)	Spirillosis (*Spirillum minus*)
Incubation period	2–10 days	1–6 wk
Fever	+++	+++
Chills	+++	+++
Myalgia	+++	+++
Rash	++; morbilliform, petechial	++; maculopapular
Lymphadenitis	+	++
Arthralgia, arthritis	++	+−
Indurated bite wound	−	+++
Recurrent fever, constitutional signs (untreated)	Irregular periodicity	Regular periodicity

[a]Modified from reference 100. Symbols: +, positive clinical sign, with increasing numbers of plus signs indicating increasing severity; −, clinical sign is not present.

a history of rat bites or intimate exposure to rats (24).

Plague

"The houses were filled with dead bodies and the streets with funerals; neither age or sex was exempt; slaves and plebeians were suddenly taken off amidst the lamentations of their wives and children, who, while they assisted the sick and mourned the dead, were seized with disease and, perishing, were burned on the same funeral pyre. To the knights and senators, the disease was less mortal though these also suffered in the common calamity" (76). This graphic account of the dreaded disease, the bubonic plague, was recorded in imperial Rome in the second century C.E. This pestilence occurred again and again during the ensuing centuries. By the 14th century, the disease appeared in the Far East, spread to Asia Minor, and followed the trade routes to Europe. It did not make its arrival in the United States until the early 1900s, when the disease appeared in California, where it still exists endemically in the ground squirrel and chipmunk.

Human infections due to *Yersinia pestis,* a gram-negative coccobacillus, in the United States are sporadic and limited, usually resulting from infected-flea or -rodent contact. Since 1924–1925, when a plague epidemic ravaged Los Angeles, neither urban plague nor rat-borne plague has been diagnosed in the United States (37). All reported cases since then have been reported in states located west of the 101st meridian.

Although wild rat populations are still the primary reservoirs of the plague bacillus in many parts of the world (with transmission of *Y. pestis* to humans via fleas, particularly *Xenopsylla cheopis*) and remain a continued threat in the United States, sciurid rodents (rock squirrels, California ground squirrels, chipmunks, and prairie dogs) are the primary plague bacillus reservoirs in the western part of the United States (92, 105, 141). Cricetid rodents, such as the wood rat, are occasionally cited as reservoirs. The oriental rat flea, *X.*

cheopis, the common vector of the plague bacillus, is well established throughout the United States, particularly in the southern part of the country and in southern California. It is important to remember that more than 1,500 species of fleas and 230 species of rodents are infected with *Y. pestis.* Only 30 to 40 rodent species, however, are permanent reservoirs of the infection (104). Plague is infrequently reported in the United States, with a low incidence of 1 case in 1972 and a high incidence of 40 cases in 1983 (37). Ninety percent of the cases have been diagnosed in New Mexico, Colorado, and California. Urban development (particularly in New Mexico) encroached into rodent habitats, where plague is enzootic, placing these populations at increased risk of contracting the disease. In addition to rodents, dogs and, increasingly, cats either have served as passive transporters of the disease or have been actively infected (137, 141). The disease occurs seasonally, with the highest proportion of cases occurring between May and September.

Transmission of *Y. pestis* via fleas to humans involves a complex interaction of the bacterium with the flea. Fleas become infected with *Y. pestis* after engorging blood from a bacteremic animal or human. Some fleas clear the bacteria even though they have ingested large numbers of yersiniae. However, *Y. pestis* most often replicates to large numbers in the midgut of the flea, which is normally sterile (122). Interestingly, the organisms do not invade cells or tissues of the flea, but after 72 h they aggregate into clumps in the midgut or attach to the proventriculus of the flea. The proventriculus, a valve-like chamber between the flea's esophagus and midgut, is lined with spine-like structures, and these structures mechanically disrupt cells, allowing the blood to enter the midgut. After a week, the yersiniae grow to large numbers and block the proventriculus. Once the proventriculus is blocked, the flea cannot ingest further blood into the midgut and starves to death (122). In an attempt to feed more often because of the blockage, the flea ingests the host's blood into

#12

its esophagus, where it mixes with yersiniae growing in this location and in the proventriculus. The blood now infected with *Yersinia* flows back into the wound inflicted by the flea, and the mammal becomes infected with *Y. pestis*. Experiments have shown that only blocked fleas can transmit *Y. pestis* to susceptible hosts. Interestingly, *Y. pestis* has evolved bacterial factors that allow it to invade the host by down-regulating immune responses (e.g., the Yop and LerV effector proteins) as well as growth factors that allow *Yersinia* to colonize and replicate in the flea. The hemin storage protein (Hms) is required by the yersiniae for colonization and blockage of the proventriculus by *Y. pestis* (81). A second virulence factor is *Yersinia* murine toxin (Ymt), so named because it is lethal when injected into mice. Its presence is essential to the survival of *Y. pestis* in fleas. Apparently, *ymt* acts from an intracellular level in *Y. pestis* and protects the bacterium from antibacterial activity normally present in the midguts of fleas (82). Clearly, these examples, among many, illustrate how the organism has evolved a genetic repertoire that has allowed it to survive not only in the mammalian host but also in the flea.

Human infection is usually the result of a bite from an infected flea but can also occur via cuts or abrasions in the skin or via infected aerosols coming in contact with the oropharyngeal mucous membrane. Although today the association with plague and rats seems obvious, it was not until the bacillus *Yersinia pestis* was isolated and cultured that this could be definitively proven. After discovery of the infectious nature of the disease, it was soon established that epidemics among human populations closely coincided with epizootics of the disease in rats, particularly *Rattus rattus*. It still was not apparent how the two diseases in the two hosts were linked. The hypothesis first conceived by P. L. Simond of Spain that the plague bacillus was transmitted by the rat flea, though first discounted, was proven to be correct (76).

Bubonic plague in humans is usually characterized by fever (2 to 7 days postexposure) and the formation of large, tender, swollen lymph nodes, or buboes. If untreated, the disease may progress to severe pneumonic or systemic plague. Inhaled infective particles, particularly from animals with plague pneumonia, may also result in the pneumonic form of the disease.

Primary pneumonic plague historically occurred by inhalation of infectious droplets from a pneumonic plague patient. However, in the last several decades, this form of the disease has occurred from exposure to infected animals (usually cats) which have developed secondary pneumonia due to septicemic spread of the organism (37, 137, 141). Owners or veterinarians attending these sick animals are then infected by inhaling aerosols containing the plague bacteria generated by the animals.

A presumptive diagnosis can be made by visualizing ovoid, gram-negative rods exhibiting bipolar staining upon microscopic examination of fluid from buboes, blood, sputum, or spinal fluid; confirmation can be made by culture. Complement fixation, passive hemagglutination, and immunofluorescence staining of specimens can be used for serologic confirmation.

Mortality without antibiotic therapy, particularly in cases of pneumonic plague, exceeds 50% in untreated patients. Although *Y. pestis* is susceptible to a wide variety of antibiotics, multiple-antibiotic-resistant strains are being isolated with increasing frequency (42). Aminoglycosides such as streptomycin and gentamicin are the most effective antibiotics in vivo against *Y. pestis*. Chloramphenicol is the drug of choice for treating plague meningitis and endophthalmitis (37, 114). In individuals exposed to *Y. pestis*, prophylactic therapy with tetracycline for a 7-day period is often prescribed.

An inactivated plague vaccine is available for laboratory personnel working with the organism and for high-risk individuals (e.g., wildlife management employees and Peace Corps volunteers) exposed to plague reservoirs in areas of endemicity. Rodent and flea control, particularly in areas of high endemicity, is an indispensable part of containing exposure to plague, as is restricting certain locales from recreational use.

Yersiniosis

Yersinia enterocolitica is now recognized as a cause of enteritis in humans. Cultural identification of the organism takes advantage of the fact that the bacterium replicates in culture media at refrigeration temperatures, which allows selective growth conditions to be utilized. Pigs and dogs are considered natural reservoirs for *Y. enterocolitica* serovar 3x biovar 4, a common cause of the disease in humans. This strain has also been isolated from *R. norvegicus* and *R. rattus* in Japan (91). It has been suggested that rats may play a role in the ecology of *Y. enterocolitica* in swine herds. Control of wild-rat populations in swine herds may reduce the potential transmission of this organism via pork products. More recently, another pathogenic strain, serovar O8, was isolated from wild rodents: wood mice, geisha mice, and a vole (89). This strain, however, was not evident in random samples of brown or black rats taken from select locales in Japan (89). Further epidemiological studies are needed in the United States to determine the importance of wild rats as reservoirs for *Y. enterocolitica*.

Leptospirosis

Leptospirosis is solely a zoonotic disease of livestock, pet and stray dogs, and wildlife, including wild rats. Rodent reservoir hosts of leptospires, besides rats, are mice, field moles, hedgehogs, gerbils, squirrels, rabbits, and hamsters (63, 164). Human-to-human transmission is extremely rare. *Leptospira interrogans* (comprising >200 serovars) has been isolated worldwide. Although particular serotypes usually have distinct host species, most serotypes can be carried by several hosts. *Leptospira* organisms are well adapted to a variety of mammals, particularly wild animals and rodents.

In the chronic form, the organism is carried and shed in the urine inconspicuously for long periods of time. Rodents are the only major

animal species that can shed leptospires throughout their life span without clinical manifestations (63, 164). Active shedding of leptospires by rodents can go unrecognized until personnel handling the animals become clinically infected or are infected by exposure to water or food contaminated by urine.

Leptospira interrogans serotype Icterohaemorrhagiae was first recovered in 1918 in the United States from wild rats sampled in New York City. In one recent study in Detroit, MI, more than 90% of adult brown Norway rats were infected with *L. interrogans* serotype Icterohaemorrhagiae (161). In an earlier study conducted in Baltimore, 45.5% of 1,643 rats were infected with *Leptospira;* higher prevalence rates occurred in older rats (~60%) (99). Other studies confirm the high prevalence of this organism in wild rats inhabiting cities in the United States (3, 143). Rats and mice are also common animal hosts for another serotype, *Leptospira interrogans* serovar Ballum, although it has been found in other wildlife as well. Water can often be contaminated with infected-rat urine. The infection can persist unnoticed in laboratory rodents, though the carrier rates for laboratory-maintained rodents in the United States are unknown but probably low (67). However, there has been a report of leptospirosis in a research colony of mice being housed in a large research institution in the United States (3).

Because leptospirosis in humans is often difficult to diagnose, the low incidence of reported infection in humans may be misleading. From 1974 to 1979, only 498 cases were reported, for an incidence of 0.05 per 100,000 people per year (143). Outbreaks have been documented in the United States from personnel working with laboratory mice (8, 152). In one study, 8 of 58 employees handling the infected laboratory mice (80% of breeding females were excreting *L. interrogans* serovar Ballum in their urine) contracted leptospirosis (152). In several European laboratories, personnel have been infected with leptospires from laboratory rats (67). Today, however, the routine availability of specific-pathogen-free rodents mitigates the likelihood of acquiring this infection from laboratory-maintained rats and mice.

Infection with leptospires most frequently results from handling infected animals (contaminating the hands with urine) or from aerosol exposure during cage cleaning (8, 64, 152). Skin abrasions or exposure to mucous membranes may serve as the portal of entry. All secretions and excretions from infected animals should be considered infective. In one instance, a father apparently was infected after his daughter used his toothbrush to clean a contaminated pet mouse cage (16). Handling infected wild rats also increases the risk of contracting leptospirosis (103). A young man died of acute leptospirosis by falling into a heavily polluted river contaminated with *L. interrogans* serotype Icterohaemorrhagiae (143). Rodent bites can also transmit the disease (102). In Detroit, children from the inner city had a significantly higher level of *L. interrogans* serotype Icterohaemorrhagiae antibody than children living in the Detroit suburbs. Therefore, children living in rat-infested tenements may be at increased risk of infection (40).

The disease may vary from unapparent infection to severe infection and death. Infected individuals experience a biphasic disease (52, 143, 152). They become suddenly ill, with weakness, headache, myalgia, malaise, chills, and fever, and usually exhibit leukocytosis. During the second phase of the disease, conjunctival suffusion and a rash may occur. Upon examination, renal, hepatic, pulmonary, and gastrointestinal findings may be abnormal. Penicillin is the drug of choice in treating early-onset leptospirosis (52, 158). Ampicillin and doxycycline also have been effective in treating people with leptospirosis. Tetracycline has been used successfully to eradicate *L. interrogans* serovar Ballum in a mouse colony (151).

Because of the variability in clinical symptoms and lack of pathognomonic pathologic findings for humans and animals, serologic diagnosis, use of molecularly based assays, or actual isolation of leptospires is imperative (52). As an aid to diagnosis, leptospires can some-times be observed by examination or direct staining of body fluids or fresh tissue suspensions (156). The definitive diagnosis for humans or animals is made by culturing the organisms from tissue or fluid samples or by inoculating animals (particularly 3- to 4-week-old hamsters), with subsequent culture and isolation. Culture media with long-chain fatty acids and 1% bovine serum albumin are routinely used as detoxicants (52). Serologic assessment is accomplished by indirect hemagglutination, agglutination analysis, complement fixation, microscopic agglutination, and fluorescent-antibody techniques (52). The serologic test most frequently used is the modified microtiter agglutination test. Titers of 1:100 or greater are considered significant.

Borrelia Species (TBRF)

Tick-borne relapsing fever (TBRF) is caused by at least 15 *Borrelia* sp. spirochetes and is transmitted through the painless and often unnoticed bites of *Ornithodoros* sp. ticks. Most cases are caused by *Borrelia hermsii,* which is transmitted by the tick *Ornithodoros hermsi* (48). The tick usually feeds on the host at night for less than 30 min. Rodents (i.e., squirrels, deer mice, rats, chipmunks, and prairie dogs) are vertebrate reservoirs for this spirochete. Rats and other rodents are also infected with several other *Borrelia* species, but the role for many of these *Borrelia* spp. in human disease is unknown (72). Rats have also been experimentally used to study the disease (156).

TBRF is a reportable disease in 11 western states, and approximately 25 cases are reported annually to the CDC. Symptoms occur 2 to 18 days after the bite of an infected tick and are characterized by the onset of lethargy, fever, myalgia, headache, and nausea. Typically, patients not treated with antimicrobials experience multiple episodes of similar clinical signs. Rarely, the patient presents with uveitis, myocarditis, cranial nerve palsy, or the Jarisch-Herxheimer reaction, which is attributed to decreasing bacterial numbers in the patient's blood and a massive cytokine release and occurs during initial treatment of the spirochetal infection with an effective antibiotic. Symptoms of this reaction include hypertension, tachycardia, chills, rigors, diaphoresis, fever, and acute respiratory distress syndrome (ARDS). It is now recognized that ARDS may occur more frequently in patients with TBRF than previously recognized. In a recent review of three patients with TBRF, all three patients had received antibiotics prior to the onset of ARDS (113). It is not known whether these patients had ARDS as a result of the Jarisch-Herxheimer reaction or as a result of an underlying sepsis. As such, optimal management for TBRF requires a prompt diagnosis and careful clinical observation during the initial treatment of the patient.

Diagnosis of the disease can presumptively be made by observations of spirochetes by dark-field microscopy or in Wright- or Giemsa-stained smears of peripheral blood collected during the febrile stage of the disease. Laboratory diagnosis is also made by culture, PCR, or serology at select reference laboratories. TBRF can be prevented by minimizing rodent infestation of homes and vacation sites (e.g., cabins), often located in coniferous forests 2,000 to 7,000 ft above sea level.

Salmonellosis

The genus *Salmonella* consists of gram-negative bacteria of approximately 2,500 serotypes or serovars. Salmonellae are flagellated nonsporulating, aerobic, gram-negative bacilli that can readily be isolated from feces on selective media designed to suppress bacterial growth of other enteric bacteria. *Salmonella* serotyping requires antigenic analysis (33). Nontyphoidal salmonellosis is caused by any of these serotypes. Except for infection with *Salmonella typhi*, the causative agent of typhoid fever, salmonellosis occurs worldwide and is important for humans and animals. There are five species of *Salmonella* recognized by the International Committee on Systematics of Prokaryotes, with *Salmonella choleraesuis* being the type species (19, 51). The other species

are *Salmonella enteritidis, Salmonella typhimurium, Salmonella typhi,* and *S. bongori.*

It is estimated that 1.4 million cases of salmonella infection occur annually in the United States (172), resulting in approximately 15,000 hospitalizations and 400 deaths. Although a high percentage of salmonellosis occurs via a food-borne route, it is becoming increasingly apparent that infections may be acquired through animal contact.

Rats are extremely susceptible to infection with *Salmonella* spp. In studies performed in the 1920s through 1940s, the prevalence of *Salmonella* in wild rats surveyed in the United States varied from 1 to 18%, compared to 19% in wild rats in Europe (3, 9, 67, 178). In experimental studies, when rats were dosed orally with salmonellae, 10% shed the organisms in the 2 months after inoculation, and a few remained carriers when examined 5 months after experimental challenge. These rats, when placed with other naive rats, were capable of initiating new epizootics (127). Fortunately, the disease in laboratory rats, though common prior to 1939, has rarely been isolated in U.S. commercially reared rats since that time. However, because rats are used experimentally to study salmonella pathogenesis, personnel working with these animals must take appropriate precautions to prevent zoonotic transmission.

Salmonellae are ubiquitous in nature and are routinely found in water or food contaminated with animal or human excreta. Fecal-oral transmission is the primary mode for the spread of infection from animal to animal or to humans. Rat feces can remain infective for 148 days when maintained at room temperature (179). Transmission is enhanced by crowding and poor sanitation.

As with other diseases transmitted by the fecal-oral route, control depends on eliminating contact with feces, food, or water contaminated with *Salmonella* or animal reservoirs excreting the organism. Salmonellae survive for months in feces and are readily cultured from sediments in ponds and streams previously contaminated with sewage or animal feces. Fat and moisture in food promote the survival of *Salmonella*. Pasteurization of milk and proper cooking of food (56°C for 10 to 20 min) effectively destroy *Salmonella* spp. Municipal water supplies should be routinely monitored for coliform contamination (121).

An outbreak of multidrug-resistant *Salmonella enterica* serotype Typhimurium associated with commercially distributed pet rodents, including rats, mice and hamsters, was recently reported (157). Twenty-eight matching isolates identified as *S. enterica* serotype Typhimurium by pulsed-field gel electrophoresis were identified from humans; 13 of the patients (59%) had previously had contact with rodents purchased from retail pet stores and 2 patients (9%) had secondarily acquired the infection from a patient who had been exposed to an infected rodent. These 15 patients, whose median age was 16 years (neonate to 43 years), resided in 10 different states. No single source of rodents was common among these cases, and every case household had purchased the rodents from different retail pet stores. It was ascertained that several of the rodent breeders and distributors routinely used antimicrobials (e.g., spectinomycin, leptomycin, tetracycline, and nitrofurazone) in the drinking water as a preventative measure for nonspecific rodent enteritis. Interestingly, all human animal and environmental samples of *S. enterica* serotype Typhimurium isolates tested in this outbreak were uniformly resistant to ampicillin, chloramphenicol, streptomycin, sulfisoxazole, and tetracycline (R-type ACSSuT). Patients infected with multiple-antibiotic-resistant strains of *S. enterica* serotype Typhimurium have higher hospitalization rates than patients infected with susceptible strains (106, 171). There are also reports of increased risk of septicemia, treatment failure, and mortality associated with multidrug-resistant *S. enterica* serotype Typhimurium (77). The spread of these multiple-antibiotic-resistant strains in rodents may have been facilitated by the widespread use of antibiotics as a prophylactic measure in the pocket pet retail industry. Indeed, treatment

with oral antibiotics may eliminate normal *Enterobacteriaceae* enteric flora and facilitate colonization with antibiotic-resistant salmonellae, as observed with mice treated with antimicrobials (128, 169, 170). The authors of the report of this outbreak urged heightened disease surveillance in pet retail facilities, as well as increased hygiene and husbandry practices, to minimize the need for prophylactic antimicrobial therapy. Individuals purchasing rodents as pets or for food consumption by reptiles should be alerted to the possibility that these animals' feces are potentially infectious. Recently, for example, additional outbreaks of salmonellosis were traced to households that had pet snakes. The source of human salmonella infection in these outbreaks was pet snakes, which, as part of their diet, were fed salmonella-infected frozen rats and mice sold commercially (65). The increased incidence of salmonella infections can be reduced by hand washing with soap and water after handling of rodents, their cages, and bedding.

Clinical signs of salmonellosis in humans include acute sudden gastroenteritis, abdominal pain, diarrhea, nausea, and fever. Diarrhea and anorexia may persist for several days. Although most cases are self-limiting, more-severe clinical disease has been documented; 40% of patients were hospitalized in a recently reported outbreak (157). For example, a mother and infant became infected after the mother had purchased live rats and mice from a local pet store to feed her ball python. The mother was hospitalized with diarrhea, fever, and abdominal pain. She had a laparotomy and subsequently delivered a preterm infant. Organisms invading the intestine may create septicemia without severe intestinal involvement; most clinical signs are attributed to hematogenous spread of the organisms. As with other microbial infections, the disease's severity relates to the organism's serotype, the number of bacteria ingested, and the host's susceptibility. In experimental studies with volunteers, several serovars induced a spectrum of clinical disease from brief enteritis to serious debilitation. Incubation varied from 7 to 72 h. Cases of asymptomatic carriers whose infection persisted for several weeks were common (87).

With careful management of fluid and electrolyte balance, antimicrobial therapy is not necessary. In humans, antimicrobial therapy may prolong rather than shorten the period that *Salmonella* spp. are shed in the feces (116, 121). In one double-blind placebo study of infants, oral antibiotics did not significantly effect the duration of salmonella carriage. Bacteriologic relapse after antibiotic treatment occurred in 53% of the patients, and 33% of these suffered a recurrence of diarrhea, whereas none of the placebo group relapsed (116).

Other Possible Bacterial Infections

Campylobacteriosis, a common diarrheal disease in humans caused by *Campylobacter jejuni* or *Campylobacter coli,* is isolated from a variety of animals, including rats. Animals can be responsible for the zoonotic spread of this organism; however, rats have not, to date, been incriminated (58, 185).

Helicobacter cinaedi (previously *Campylobacter cinaedi*) was first isolated from the lower bowels of homosexuals with proctitis and colitis. It has also been isolated from the blood of homosexual patients with human immunodeficiency virus, as well as children and adult women (32, 117, 119, 129, 130, 168). In a retrospective study of 23 patients with *H. cinaedi*-associated illness, 22 of the cases had the organism isolated from blood by an automated blood culture system, with which a slightly elevated growth index was noted (94). This study also described a new *H. cinaedi*-associated syndrome consisting of bacteremia and fever and accompanied by leukocytosis and thrombocytopenia. Recurrent cellulitis and/or arthritis is also noted in a high percentage of infected immunocompromised patients (23, 94). Although *H. cinaedi* is recovered primarily from immunocompromised individuals, the organism is also recovered from chronic alcoholics as well as immunocompetent men and women. It should be stressed that many hospital and veterinary laboratories have difficulty in isolating this organism. Because of the slow growth of *H. cinaedi,* laboratory diagnosis is unlikely if blood culture procedures that rely on visual detection of the culture media are used (23, 93, 94). Dark-field microscopy or use of acridine orange staining of blood culture media, rather than Gram staining, increases the likelihood of seeing the organism. Likewise, fecal isolation is difficult; selective antibiotic media are required, and recovery is facilitated by passing fecal homogenates through a 0.45-μm filter (66). Also, in a recent study, several strains of both *H. cinaedi* and *Helicobacter fennelliae* were inhibited by concentrations of cephalothin and cetazolin, used frequently in selective media for isolation of enteric microaerophilic bacteria. These organisms also require an environment rich in hydrogen for optimum in vitro growth.

The fastidious microaerophile *H. cinaedi* has also been recovered from blood and fecal specimens of children and a neonate with septicemia and meningitis. The mother of the neonate had cared for pet hamsters during the first two trimesters of her pregnancy (119). Because *H. cinaedi* has been isolated from the normal intestinal flora of hamsters, it was suggested that the pet hamsters served as a reservoir for transmission to the mother (66). The mother had a diarrheal illness during the third trimester of pregnancy; the newborn was likely to have been infected during the birthing process, although this was not proven (119). Further studies are needed to confirm the zoonotic risk of handling *H. cinaedi*-infected hamsters (66). Also of interest is the isolation, based on cellular fatty acid and identification analysis, of *H. cinaedi* from the feces of dogs and a cat (93). More recently, it was isolated from a macaque monkey with idiopathic colitis and hepatitis (62) as well as from asymptomatic macaques (62). Until diagnostic laboratories embark upon routine isolation attempts of *Helicobacter* spp. from feces, the extent of the presence of these organisms in companion and pocket pets and their zoonotic potential will be unknown.

Tetracycline and various aminoglycosides appear to be effective in treating infections with *H. cinaedi.* Apparent relapses of *H. cinaedi* bacteremia in patients treated with ciprofloxacin, despite its previous use to successfully treat *H. cinaedi* infection, and the occurrence of in vitro resistance of *H. cinaedi* isolates to ciprofloxacin suggest that this antibiotic should be used with caution (55, 93, 94).

Of recent interest are increasingly recognized enterohepatic *Helicobacter* spp. which cause both hepatic and intestinal disease in mice, rats, and hamsters (59, 115). One of these, *Helicobacter bilis,* has been found in Chilean patients with chronic cholecystitis and in patients with hepatocellular carcinoma and hepatobiliary carcinoma (61, 107). Given that these bacteria persist in the lower bowels of rodents and are shed in the feces of infected monkeys, it will be interesting to note after further studies are conducted whether these new helicobacters will be linked to zoonotic transmission from wild rodents.

Of the gastric helicobacters, *Helicobacter pylori* is the best known and the most important in terms of global impact on human disease. Another gastric helicobacter, *"Helicobacter heilmannii,"* is associated with gastric disease in humans and is worthy of discussion (75, 98).

A diagnosis of humans infected with *"H. heilmannii,"* first observed and reported to have occurred in three humans in 1987, has been made on morphological grounds by a variety of authors assessing human gastric biopsies (75, 80, 111, 112, 149, 154, 162). The frequency of occurrence is between 0.25 and 0.60%, depending on the study. However, as many as 6% of patients in Thailand and China have been reported to be infected with *"H. heilmannii"* (182, 184). *"H. heilmannii"*-infected patients have a chronic, active gastritis or chronic gastritis consisting of a lympho-plasmacytic inflammation. *"H. heilmannii"*-associated gastritis is considered milder than *H. pylori* gastritis (153). *"H. heilmannii"* has also been associated with primary gastric low-grade lymphoma in humans (111, 133). As with patients with *H. pylori*-associated lymphoma, clinical remission of the lymphoma was noted

for five patients after antibiotic eradication of the gastric helicobacter (88, 111, 136). These helicobacters can persist in humans for years, and presumably the same is true for other mammals. In addition to dogs and cats being potential zoonotic hosts of these gastric helicobacters, swine and wild rats may also be a source of infections for humans (69, 110).

Eradication of *"H. heilmannii"* by antimicrobial therapy also has resulted in the resolution of gastritis and peptic ulcer disease (71, 75, 80). *"H. heilmannii"* infections have been successfully treated with bismuth alone and with combination therapies that included metronidazole or amoxicillin (5, 75, 80).

Beta-hemolytic group G streptococci have been isolated from rats with cervical lymphadenitis, as well as from the pharynxes of normal laboratory rats (36). *Streptococcus* species group G causes a wide variety of clinical diseases in humans, including septicemia, pharyngitis, endocarditis, pneumonia, and meningitis. Asymptomatic carriage of group G streptococci is also common in humans. At present, however, there is no documented evidence that streptococci from rats are transmitted to, or acquired by, humans (139). Similarly, *Streptococcus pneumoniae* infection can be asymptomatic or cause systemic disease in both humans and rats, but zoonotic transmission of the organism between rats and humans has not been recognized to my knowledge.

Pathogenic *Staphylococcus aureus* of the human phage type can cause clinical disease in mice and rats. This organism has been introduced into specific-pathogen-free, barrier-maintained mouse colonies and specific-pathogen-free rats and guinea pigs; the same phage type was isolated from their animal caretakers (15, 38, 148). Colonization by normal *S. aureus* strains in the nasopharyngeal area of humans presumably minimizes the zoonotic potential of animal-origin *S. aureus*.

VIRAL DISEASES

HFRS and Nephropathia Epidemica (Hantaan Virus)

Hemorrhagic fever with renal syndrome (HFRS) and nephropathia epidemica are used to describe a group of rodent-borne diseases caused by several hantaviruses (family *Buny-aviridae*) (97, 183). In Southeast Asia, the disease is endemic, and focal epidemics throughout the Eurasian continent and Japan have been recorded. American soldiers became infected with the disease during the Korean War. The severity of the disease depends on the particular immunotype of the virus as well as the respective natural reservoir host.

Korean hemorrhagic fever in agricultural workers occurs seasonally with bimodal peaks in the populations of the reservoir host—the striped field mouse, *Apodemus agrarius*—and its ectoparasites. HFRS is characterized by fever, headache, myalgia, and hemorrhagic manifestations that may lead to shock from massive capillary leakage of plasma protein. Although previously significant, mortality has now been reduced to 6% with hospitalization and dialysis (165).

Nephropathia epidemica, a less severe form, is encountered in Scandinavia, the western Soviet Union, and several countries of Europe. The etiologic virus has been isolated and named Puumala virus by Finnish researchers. The natural reservoir is the bank vole, *Clethrionomys glareolus*. Infected persons, usually adult men with vole contact, exhibit a sudden onset of fever, abdominal or low back pain, elevated serum creatinine levels, and polyuria; fatalities are rare.

In the late 1970s, a disease resembling HFRS was reported to occur in laboratory workers of Japan, Belgium, and South Korea. Retrospective epidemiologic evaluation of the first laboratory-associated outbreak and additional urban outbreaks in Japan revealed that the reservoirs of the disease were laboratory and wild rats. Over 100 cases of HFRS in humans have been linked to exposure to laboratory rats infected with the virus (166, 167). Persons infected exhibited a range of illness, from a nonspecific influenza-like episode to acute renal insufficiency and hemorrhagic di athesis. The worldwide distribution of infected laboratory rats or their tissues has occurred. Transmission of hantavirus infection has been reported in Belgium and the United Kingdom as well as Japan (43, 101). One in-

dividual had serologic evidence of infection in the United States, and in Britain, a mild clinical case was diagnosed. Caesarian rederivation procedures employed for imported animals probably prevented or eliminated the spread of infection at most institutions.

Hantaan virus–related infection in wild rats, both *R. rattus* and *R. norvegicus*, raised concern regarding the potential spread of disease by international shipping. Seaports throughout the world, including many in the United States, harbor rats infected with Hantaan virus or a related virus. To date, serological evidence of disease in the United States has been noted, but no human clinical cases have been associated with this type of exposure (29).

The Prospect Hill virus, another hantavirus, has been isolated from meadow voles *(Microtus pennsylvanicus)* in Maryland; it has not been associated with human disease, although serologic surveys indicate inapparent infection throughout the United States, with the distribution of the virus being limited to the geographic distribution of the animal host.

Hantavirus Pulmonary Syndrome

In 1993, an outbreak of acute respiratory illness with significant mortality was linked to a newly recognized hantavirus (25). This zoonotic disease, now known as hantavirus pulmonary syndrome (HPS), was discovered in the southwestern part of the United States. This disease provided the first example of diseases now recognized as being caused by a complex of New World hantaviruses, each associated with a particular rodent species belonging to the subfamily Sigmodontinae, family Muridae. The prototype virus, *Sin Nombre* (SN) *virus*, which replicates in its natural host, the deer mouse *(Peromyscus maniculatus)* (150), causes more than 95% of the cases of HPS in North America, which are seen primarily in the southwestern part of the United States (83, 144).

Three other hantaviruses distinct from SN virus are also recognized as etiological agents of HPS in North America; their rodent reservoir hosts are the white-footed mouse, *Peromyscus leucopus*, which serves as the host for New York hantavirus (150); the cotton rat *(Sigmodon hispidus),* the reservoir host for Black Creek Canal virus (138); and the rice rat, *Oryzomys palustris,* the reservoir for Bayou virus (163). The last two viruses have been isolated in Florida, Louisiana, and eastern Texas.

A recently recognized hantavirus found in the pygmy rice rat *(Oligoryzomys microtis)* in Bolivia and Argentina has been linked to zoonotic HPS in humans residing in these countries (14). Serological tests to detect antibodies to hantavirus as well as confirmatory Western immunoblots are used to presumptively diagnose the disease in humans exposed to these various rodents (83). Reverse transcription-PCR with specific primers is used to definitely diagnose the virus in infected human or rodent biological and tissue samples (84).

Humans at risk are those that reside or work in areas heavily infested with reservoir hosts of hantavirus. Patients with HPS often present to emergency rooms with persistent and worsening dyspnea. Prodromal signs include fatigue and somnolence, with increasing shortness of breath and low-grade fever. Chest radiographs show interstitial and increasing bilateral interstitial alveolar infiltrates and pleural effusion. Patients often require 100% oxygen endotracheal intubation and positive and expiratory pressure support.

Elevation in creatine kinase, serum creatinine, and proteinuria can indicate renal insufficiency and myositis associated with HPS; the last two clinical manifestations are more commonly observed in cases of HPS caused by viruses of the oryzomine and sigmodon clades and much less frequently with SN virus infection (84, 144).

Hantaviruses do not cause disease in their respective rodent hosts, although virus can be detected in the salivary glands and numerous visceral organs of chronically infected animals. The virus is shed in the saliva, feces, and urine; transmission to humans is generally believed to be from aerosols generated from contaminated rodent excreta (165). There is also the potential that transmission can occur via ectoparasites. Detection of infected rodents or infected rodent tissue prior to entry of humans into laboratories is crucial in preventing zoonotic disease. Enzyme-linked immunosorbent assay, indirect immunofluorescence assay, and immunoblotting are available for serodiagnosis, in addition to PCR-based assays.

Monkeypox

Human monkeypox caused by an orthopoxvirus was first diagnosed in the Democratic Republic of the Congo in 1970, shortly after the eradication of smallpox in the United States in 1968. It is now recognized as a zoonotic disease that occurs primarily in the rain forest located in western and central Africa.

Besides zoonotic transmission, limited person-to-person transmission can also occur, especially where monkeypox is endemic. The first documented evidence of community-acquired monkeypox occurred in the United States in 2003 (26). The source of the two infections was identified as a common Illinois distributor where prairie dogs and Gambian rats were being housed together. The Gambian giant rats had been imported from Ghana in April 2003 by a Texas importer who subsequently sold them to the Illinois distributor. The diseased prairie dogs were then sold to pet stores in the region and were further disseminated at pet swaps. The shipment from Ghana contained approximately 800 small mammals of nine different species. The small actual source(s) could therefore have been multiple and highlights the serious public health hazard posed by the introduction of exotic species such as rodents from Africa. Because of this hazard and pursuant to 42 CFR 70.2 and 21 CFR 1240.30, the Communicable Disease Center and Food and Drug Administration have prohibited their transportation or importation into the United States. Since the original outbreak in 2003 and institution of strict importation guidelines, further monkeypox cases have not been diagnosed.

Although clinically similar in some ways to smallpox, monkeypox differs from it both biologically and epidemiologically (18). The disease has an incubation period of 7 to 17 days. The prodrome consists of a fever, backache, fatigue, and headache (132). In the large U.S. outbreak with 72 confirmed or suspected cases as of 30 July 2003, patients had a prodrome consisting of headaches, myalgias, chills, and drenching sweats. Over one-third of the patients had nonproductive coughs. The monkeypox rash occurring on the head, trunk, or extremities includes papules, vesicles, macules, and pustules that become encrusted over a 14- to 21-day period (90, 132). The major clinical difference between monkeypox and smallpox is the pronounced lymphadenopathy noted in the majority of patients infected with monkeypox virus (90) (Fig. 1). Mortality rates in areas of endemic monkeypox vary from 1 to 10%, with higher death rates for children. The outbreak in the United States which occurred in Illinois, Indiana, and Wisconsin (median age of patients, 26 years [range, 4 to 53 years]) affected more than 50 humans, 14 of whom required hospitalization.

Infected monkeypox patients or those suspected of having the disease should follow standard contact and airborne precautions. Appropriate diagnosis and management of exposed and ill pets should also be instituted to minimize the spread of the disease. Pet owners who suspect their animal of having a disease

compatible with monkeypox should isolate the animal from humans and other animals and contact their state and local health departments. They are also advised to wear a mask and gloves when handling the animal. In most instances, it is advisable for a veterinarian to examine the suspect animal. Illnesses noted in affected rodents include fever, cough, blepharoconjunctivitis, and lymphadenopathy, followed by a nodular rash. Mortality is varied. If animals are suspected of being infected with monkeypox virus, whole blood in EDTA or sera can be collected and refrigerated at 4°C before being shipped to a laboratory. If ill animals are euthanized, necropsy of these animals should be performed only in biosafety level 3 laboratories by personnel recently immunized with vaccine. Entire carcasses can be preserved for later viral isolation by freezing them at −70°C. Diagnosis of the disease in infected humans or animals is made by viral isolation from tissue culture, electron microscopy observation of the poxvirus, convalescence in infected tissues, and PCR-based assays. Sera also can be evaluated for antibodies to the virus.

Treatment of the disease is to provide supportive therapy if needed. No specific treatment has been recommended. In areas of endemicity, smallpox vaccine has been reported to reduce the risk of monkeypox among those

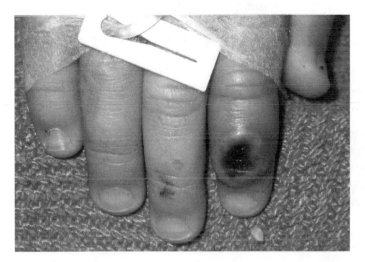

FIGURE 1 Infected finger of a child with monkeypox (Marshfield, WI, index case). The patient was bitten by a prairie dog on 27 May 2003; the primary inoculation site was the right index finger. The photo was taken 14 days after the prairie dog bite (11 days after the onset of febrile illness [hospital day 5]). (Courtesy of Kurt Reed, Marshfield Clinic, Marshfield, WI.)

individuals previously vaccinated. It is not known whether postexposure use of smallpox vaccine or antiviral therapy will be beneficial in treating monkeypox virus infection in humans.

Rabies

Rabies virus, a rhabdovirus, has been recognized as a clinical disease for centuries in both Europe and Asia. The virus when inoculated into animals, usually via a bite, produces with a high degree of probability a fatal disease in all warm-blooded species; rats should therefore be listed as a susceptible host.

Rabies occurs on all continents except Australia. Other islands, such as Hawaii, New Zealand, and Great Britain, are also fortunate in not having rabies virus in their domestic- or wild-animal population. Rabies occurs infrequently in humans, but its presence in natural reservoirs, such as wild carnivores, bats, and rarely certain rodents, such as squirrels, is endemic in certain parts of the United States as well as other parts of the world. Rabies in skunks, raccoons, and bats has increased markedly in the last several decades and now accounts for greater than 85% of all reported cases in the United States (108). From 1971 through 1989, woodchucks accounted for 68% of the 200 rodent cases reported in the United States (108). Other rodents, including rats, are almost never infected with rabies virus, and no human cases of rabies of rodent origin have been reported in the last 50 years. However, in the Federal Republic of Germany, from 1961 to 1967, nine Norway rats and eight muskrats were reportedly infected with rabies virus and had supposedly bitten humans (67).

RICKETTSIAL DISEASES

Murine Typhus (Endemic Typhus)

Murine typhus is caused by *Rickettsia typhi*. Although this disease has been recognized for centuries, it was not until the 1920s that it was distinguished from epidemic typhus. The absence of louse infestation in humans, the

seasonal occurrence of the disease, and its sporadic nature help differentiate it from louse-borne typhus (i.e., epidemic typhus). Epidemic typhus is seen only in the eastern United States in association with flying squirrels (47).

Murine typhus is primarily a disease of rats, with its principal vector being the oriental rat flea, *Xenopsylla cheopis,* and another flea, *Nosopsyllus fasciatus.* These fleas also naturally colonize the house mouse, *Mus musculus.* The cat flea, *Ctenocephalides felis* (as well as seven other species of fleas), has also been implicated in the spread of the disease. Rickettsias are ingested in a blood meal by the flea, where they multiply in the gut and are subsequently passed out in the dejecta of the flea. Infections in rats and humans are the result of contamination of the puncture wound by flea feces (53). Recent experimental evidence indicates that a flea bite also can directly transmit the infection (53). *R. typhi* is resistant to drying and remains infectious for up to 100 days in rat feces.

Murine typhus is worldwide, and in the United States, it is usually diagnosed in the southeastern or Gulf states, as well as in areas along the northern portion of the Mississippi River (20, 34). It also is associated with human populations subjected to areas of high-density wild-rat colonies, such as ports, granaries, farms, or rat-infested buildings in inner cities. Laboratory personnel have been infected with this agent when inoculating rodents and handling infected animals (20).

Since the 1970s, there has been a shift in the distribution of human cases of murine typhus to a more rural locale in southern California (Orange County) and central and southern Texas (2). The former was considered an unusual locale because Orange County was considered a wealthy area where rat infestation was uncommon. Epidemiologic studies indicated that opossums had a high seropositivity to murine typhus and that the cat fleas infesting the opossums were infected with either *R. typhi* or a newly recognized rickettsia first called the ELB agent and later named *Rickettsia felis* (1, 181). Findings extended to a survey of fleas on dogs, cats, and opossums in California, Texas, and Georgia also confirmed that fleas were infected with *R. typhi* or *R. felis,* helping to explain the spread of murine typhus into rural areas in the United States. Also, human cases of typhus caused by *R. felis* as determined by PCR have been recorded (145). It has not been possible to determine the exact taxonomic specifications of *R. felis* because no isolates have been obtained for detailed comparative analysis.

After humans are infected with the rickettsiae, the incubation period is 7 to 14 days. Because murine typhus is difficult to diagnose either clinically or anatomically from other rickettsial diseases, specific serologic tests are extremely important in making the correct diagnosis (53). The acute febrile disease is usually characterized by general malaise, headache, rash, and chills, with signs ranging from mild to severe. An encephalitic syndrome can also occur (114). In one report, 25% of 180 patients with the disease had delirium, stupor, or coma (155). Fortunately, these findings resolve with lowering of the febrile response. The fatality rate for all ages is about 2% but increases with age. In a recent study of 22 patients residing in the Canary Islands, murine typhus was diagnosed based on a titer of immunoglobulin M antibody to *R. typhi* of (1:40 or at least a fourfold increase in titers of immunoglobulin G against *R. typhi* as determined by direct immunofluorescence within 8 weeks after symptoms (78). These patients, in addition to having fevers of intermediate duration, had a distinct clinical presentation characterized by a higher incidence of complications, especially renal damage (including acute kidney failure and abnormal urinalysis). Interestingly, all had had contact with animals, most frequently dogs (78).

Recovery of rickettsial organisms or antigens from biological specimens is inconsistent and is not routinely done except in labs equipped to process and identify these samples. It must be remembered that rickettsiae are hazardous and have accounted for numerous infections of laboratory personnel. Currently, serological diagnosis is accomplished by enzyme-linked immunosorbent assay and radioimmunoprecipitation assay; however, the indirect immunofluorescence technique remains the most commonly used. Unfortunately, this test cannot distinguish epidemic from endemic typhus. The CDC considers a fourfold rise in titer detected by any technique (except the Weil-Felix technique) as evidence of rickettsial infection. A complement fixation titer of 1:16 or greater in a single serum sample from a patient with clinically compatible signs is also considered diagnostic (108).

Proper antibiotic therapy is the most effective measure to prevent morbidity or mortality due to rickettsial infections. Tetracycline and chloramphenicol have proven to be effective in hastening recovery and preventing neurologic sequelae, such as deafness due to involvement of cranial nerve VIII (114).

Fleas can be controlled by applying insecticides (organochlorines, as well as others) as residual powders or sprays in areas where rats nest or traverse. It is imperative that insecticides be applied prior to the use of rodenticides; this will prevent fleas from leaving the dead rodents and feeding on human hosts (11).

Rickettsialpox

A variety of rodents are infected with other rickettsial diseases. *Mus musculus* is the natural host for the causative agent of rickettsialpox, *Rickettsia akari,* a member of the spotted fever group of rickettsiae (13, 20). This organism is also isolated from *R. rattus* and *R. norvegicus,* and rats under certain circumstances may transmit the disease to humans. The disease is transmitted by the mite *Liponyssoides (Allodermanyssus) sanguineus.* The disease has been diagnosed in New York City and other eastern cities, as well as Russia, Egypt, and South Africa (13). The incubation period is approximately 10 to 24 days, and the clinical disease is similar to murine typhus. The rash of rickettsialpox commences as a discrete maculopapular rash, which then becomes vesicular.

The palms and soles are usually not involved. About 90% of affected persons develop an eschar, with a shallow ulcer covered by a brown scab (13, 53). Although headaches are common and may be accompanied by stiff necks, lumbar cerebrospinal fluid (CSF) samples are normal. Pulmonary and gastrointestinal involvement is almost never encountered. Diagnosis, treatment, and control are similar to those described for murine typhus and *Y. pestis.*

MYCOSES

Dermatophytes

In almost all rat- and mouse-associated ringworm infections in humans, *Trichophyton mentagrophytes* has been isolated as the etiological agent (4, 17, 27, 39, 44, 155). Classical murine ringworm, reportedly caused by *Trichophyton quinckeanum,* is usually restricted to feral rodents, but successful crossing of cultures of this strain with tester strains of perfect-state *T. mentagrophytes (Arthroderma benhamiae)* proves that *T. quinckeanum* is not a distinct species and is indistinguishable from *T. mentagrophytes* (125).

Dermatophytes are distributed worldwide, with some species reportedly being more common in certain geographic locations. From a study of 1,288 animals from 15 different species of small mammals in their natural habitats, 57 *T. mentagrophytes* strains were isolated, most commonly from the bank vole *(Clethrionomys glareolus),* followed by the common shrew *(Sorex araneus)* and house mouse *(M. musculus)* (30). Agricultural workers exposed to these mammals in granaries and barns risked contracting *T. mentagrophytes* infections; indeed, 77% of 137 agricultural workers were infected with ringworm. Only 23% of the workers showed signs of infection (30).

In laboratory mice and rats, ringworm infection is often asymptomatic, going unrecognized until personnel become infected (44). In one study, for the 8-month period before dermatophyte-infected mice were treated, almost half the people handling the mice developed ringworm, although less than 1% of the mice showed any signs of disease (39).

Transmission occurs via direct or indirect contact with asymptomatic carrier animals, skin lesions of infected rodents, contaminated grain, or animal bedding. Causal fungi present in air, in dust, or on surfaces of animal holding rooms are also transmittal sources (155).

Ringworm is in many cases nonfatal, usually self-limiting, and, because it is sometimes asymptomatic, often ignored by the affected person. The dermatophytes cause scaling, erythema, and occasionally vesicles and fissures; the fungi cause thickening and discoloration of the nails. On the skin of the trunk and extremities, lesions may be circular with a central clearing. The locations of the fungus signify the clinical categories, for example, tinea capitis or tinea unguium. When humans are infected by one of the dermatophytes recovered from mice, the fungus appears on the body and/or extremities, most commonly on the arms and hands.

Zoophilic *T. mentagrophytes* produces an acute inflammatory response which often undergoes rapid resolution; the infection may produce furunculosis, widespread tinea corporis, and deep involvement of the hair follicles.

Topical fungicides or griseofulvin per os is effective in eradicating dermatophytes from animals and humans. Strict environmental and personal hygiene helps lower the incidence of ringworm. Personnel should wear rubber gloves when touching infected rodents.

HELMINTH DISEASES

Roundworms

ANGIOSTRONGYLUS (PARASTRONGYLUS) CANTONENSIS: THE RAT LUNGWORM

A clinical syndrome known as eosinophilic meningitis is caused in humans who accidentally ingest raw aquatic animals, e.g., prawns (transport hosts) and snails or slugs (intermediate hosts) harboring infective larvae of the lungworm, or eat larvae which have contaminated vegetables. In humans, the infective larvae migrate to the central nervous system (CNS) and may undergo 1 to 2 molts but do not develop into an adult worms; thus, the human is a dead-end host. The rat serves as the reservoir host where the adult worm develops and passes infective eggs in their feces, which are then ingested by the intermediate host. Spread of the organism to rats has been linked to dispersal of the African land snail (*Achatina fulica*) (11, 96).

Historically, this disease was restricted to the Far East and the Pacific Rim, including Hawaii and Tahiti. Recently, the disease has been reported in Cuba, and the lungworm has been recovered from rats in Puerto Rico and New Orleans, LA (11, 96). It is therefore likely that the disease will be more commonly diagnosed in the Americas in the future.

The disease may often be subclinical or have an indistinct 2- to 4-month prepatent period. The distinguishing clinical feature of the disease is the presence of elevated eosinophils (>10%) of the leukocytes found in abnormal CSF. Other CNS signs can also be present, such as severe headache, meningeal irritation (nuchal rigidity), and increased intracranial pressure. Visual impairment may occur if there is ocular involvement. A febrile response is usually mild or absent. Only the most severe infections result in permanent impairment or in some cases death (95).

Occasionally (in <10% of the cases), larval or young-adult worms can be recovered from the CSF. The infection must be distinguished from other helminth CNS infections, such as paragonimiasis, fascioliasis, trichinosis, strongyloidiasis, cysticercosis, echinococcosis, and ascarids. A microenzyme-linked immunosorbent assay for antibodies directed against the antigens of the parasite in either serum or CSF has recently been developed and is helpful in confirming the diagnosis (96).

Effective anthelmintic regimens have not been developed (although ivermectin shows promise in animal trials), and potential therapeutic intervention designed to kill the parasite may indeed exacerbate the inflammatory response and clinical signs. Clinical treatment is usually supportive to relieve headache and nausea. In some cases, corticosteroids have been used. Thiabendazole has been used with some success during the first week of infection (95). Prevention of the infection is obviously preferred. This is accomplished by avoidance of eating raw vegetables and underwashed or unfrozen snails and aquatic crustaceans in areas of endemicity.

Tapeworms

RODENTOLEPIS (HYMENOLEPIS) NANA: THE DWARF TAPEWORM OF HUMANS

The dwarf tapeworm is a common parasite for both rats and mice. The infection in humans occurs most frequently in children who live in warm climates. Its presence in humans is noted worldwide, and it is the most frequently detected tapeworm in the United States (20). *Rodentolepis nana* is unique among tapeworms, because it does not require an intermediate host to complete its life cycle. The adult tapeworm develops after the egg is ingested; the hooked oncosphere invades the intestinal mucosa and develops into a cysticercoid larva, and 2 weeks later, the larva matures into an adult worm. The *Rodentolepis nana* eggs can contaminate hands, eating utensils, food, or aerosolized dust and then be accidentally ingested. Internal autoinfection may also occur. The tapeworm can also use fleas and beetles for the development of its life cycle; these in turn can then be ingested by humans. Personal hygiene, sanitation, and rodent control are important in preventing transmission. Humans with mild infection and in a good nutritional state usually have no symptoms, or the infection may cause diarrhea, anorexia, vomiting, pruritus of the nose and anus, or urticaria. In severe infections, signs are consistently present and include diarrhea, abdominal pain, anorexia, and CNS signs (20). Niclosamide for 5 to 7 days is the treatment of choice after demonstration of the characteristic eggs in the feces.

HYMENOLEPIS DIMINUTA: THE RAT TAPEWORM

This tapeworm, often described as the tapeworm of rats, is especially common in the Norway rat and the black rat; however, it is rarely diagnosed in humans (54), though it has been seen in patients from several parts of the United States (20).

The rat tapeworm requires an intermediate host for larval development. This is usually the larval stage of rat fleas, but other arthropods, such as many beetle species, earwigs, and meal moths, can serve as intermediate hosts.

Symptoms of the infection are usually not noted, and diagnosis is made by recovery of the eggs in feces. The eggs are distinguished from *Rodentolepis nana* by the lack of polar filaments.

Treatment with niclosamide, similar to the regimen used to treat *Rodentolepis nana,* is recommended. Control is dependent on elimination of rodents from the premises.

ARTHROPOD INFESTATIONS

Several arthropods found on rats, mice, and other wild rodents are vectors of human disease, and some cause allergic dermatitis as well (Table 2) (186). Fleas are seldom found in laboratory rodents but are common parasites of feral rodents. The oriental rat flea, *Xenopsylla cheopis,* and another flea, *Nosopsyllus fasciatus,* naturally infest both mice and rats; they are vectors for murine typhus and *Y. pestis.* That *X. cheopis* easily establishes itself in animal facilities can be demonstrated by the flea bites that two students received while working in animal rooms housing mice (186).

Mites

ORNITHONYSSUS BACOTI: THE TROPICAL RAT MITE

Ornithonyssus bacoti can be found on many rodents; the brown Norway rat and the black roof rat are probably the primary host species (11). Since the time of the first report of human *Ornithonyssus bacoti*-associated dermatitis in Australia in 1913 and a 1923 report on a human in the United States, many other cases have been described throughout the world (Table 3) (28, 45, 46, 60, 73, 79, 135, 160, 173, 177).

Ornithonyssus bacoti is an obligate bloodsucking parasite, usually tan but red when engorged with blood. Both the male and female feed on a rodent as their preferred host. The female is 700 μm to 1 mm in length; the male is smaller. Eggs are laid in bedding or wall crevices by the female, which survives for about 70 days and feeds about every 2 days during this period. The mite has five developmental stages: adult, egg, nonfeeding larva, bloodsucking protonymph, and nonfeeding deutonymph. After feeding, the adults and protonymphs leave their host and seek refuge in cracks and crevices. The life cycle from adult to egg requires 7 to 16 days at room temperature. Unfed protonymphs have survived for 43 days (20).

The mite often gains access to the premises on wild rodents and lives in crevices. If wild rodents are not readily available or are captured, the mite will seek blood elsewhere, either from a laboratory rodent (if in an animal research facility) or from a human. In some infestations, the rodent shows no clinical signs. However, in more-chronic cases, dermatitis and anemia may develop. In the past, this mite has been a troublesome parasite in certain laboratory animals, especially rats, mice, and hamsters (123).

Tropical rat mites produce painful, pruritic lesions on humans. Examination of patients often discloses papular lesions on the wrists, arms, abdomen, and chest. Raised erythematous papules and nodules several millimeters to more than 1 cm in size occur singly or in a linear configuration. Epidemiologically, cases usually occur in clusters that involve a common source of exposure to the mite. Experimentally, cases have been shown to be a vector of pathogens. In the laboratory, mite transmission of various rickettsial species, *Francisella tularensis,* and coxsackievirus between different laboratory animals has been shown (85, 123, 124, 146).

TABLE 2 Selected ectoparasites of rodents with zoonotic potential[a]

Species	Disease(s) in humans	Host(s)	Agent(s) transmitted
Mites			
Obligate skin mites *Sarcoptes scabiei* subspecies	Scabies	Mammals	
Trixacarus caviae	Dermatitis	Guinea pigs	
Nest-inhabiting parasites			
Ornithonyssus bacoti	Dermatitis, murine typhus, rickettsialpox	Rodents and other vertebrates	Coxsackie virus, WEE virus, SLE virus, *Rickettsia typhi*, *Rickettsia akari*, *Francisella tularensis*
Liponyssoides sanguineus	Dermatitis, rickettsialpox	Rodents, particularly *Mus musculus*	*Rickettsia akari*
Haemogamasus pontiger	Dermatitis	Rodents, insectivores, straw bedding	
Haemolaelaps casalis	Dermatitis	Birds, mammals, straw, hay	
Eulaelaps stabularis	Dermatitis, tularemia	Small mammals, straw bedding	*F. tularensis*
Ixodids (ticks)			
Dermacentor variabilis	Irritation, RMSF, tularemia, tick paralysis, other diseases	Wild rodents, cottontail rabbits, dogs from areas of endemicity	*Rickettsia rickettsii*, *F. tularensis*
Amblyomma americanum	Irritation, RMSF, tularemia	Wild rodents, dogs	
Ixodes scapularis	Irritation, possible tularemia	Dogs, wild rodents	
Ixodes dammini	Human babesiosis, Lyme disease	Wild rodents, especially *Peromyscus* sp.	*Borrelia burgdorferi*, *Babesia microti*
Ornithodoros spp.	TBRF	Wild rodents	*Borrelia* spp. (frequently *B. hermsii*)
Fleas			
Xenopsylla cheopis	Dermatitis, plague, murine typhus, *R. nana*, *H. diminuta*	Rat, mouse, wild rodents	Rodent tapeworms, *Yersinia pestis*, *Rickettsia typhi*
Nasopsyllus fasciatus	Dermatitis, plague, *R. nana*, *H. diminuta*, murine typhus	Rat, mouse, wild rodents	Rodent tapeworms, *Yersinia pestis*, *Rickettsia typhi*
Leptopsylla segnis	*H. diminuta*, *R. nana*, murine typhus	Rat	Rodent tapeworms, salmonellae, *Rickettsia typhi*

[a]Ectoparasites found in laboratory animals that cause allergic dermatitis or from which zoonotic agents have been recovered in nature (see reference 186). WEE, western equine encephalitis; SLE, St. Louis equine encephalitis; RMSF, Rocky Mountain spotted fever.

TABLE 3 Reports of *Ornithonyssus bacoti*-induced dermatitis in humans in the United States from 1931 through 2008

Host	Person(s) afflicted	Environment(s)	Lesions	Anatomical locations	Reference
Rat	200 adults and children	Residence, theater	Urticarial wheals and papules in adults; papules, urticarial wheals, and vesicles in children	Ankles, trunk, back, and neck in adults; beltline, upper part of shoulders in children	45
Rat	4 women, 1 man	Department store	Wheals, papules, a few wheals with central puncture	Arms and forearms in women; hands, ankles, legs, beltline, shoulders, and neck in man	177
Rat	Employees	Department store	Macular skin eruptions		135
Rat	Infants, adult occupants	Foundling home	Papular urticaria, grouping of bites		73
Rat	8-yr-old boy, with 5 siblings and both parents affected with milder symptoms	Residence	Excoriated urticarial papules	Trunk, upper parts of arms, buttocks	46
Norway rat	60-yr-old	Residence	1- to 4-mm papules, excoriated macules	Neck, shoulders, back, scalp, forearm, arms, abdomen	79
Rat	56-yr-old father and 2 sons; 73-yr-old woman	Residence (apartment over food store)	"Insect bites," papular excoriated dermatitis	Thorax, extremities, buttocks, genitalia, entire body	173
Rat	69-yr-old woman	Residence	Papules with erythema	Breast, shoulders, arm	28
Rat	3 female adults, 3 children	Residence	Papular urticaria (erythematous)	Neck, shoulders, arms, legs, abdomen, back	160
Mice	5 research personnel, 2 animal care technicians	Animal research laboratory	Raised erythematous papules and nodules (several mm to >1 cm)	Wrists, arm, abdomen, chest	60
Gerbils; rodents (species not specified)	3 children, 23-yr-old medical student	Residence; apartment above restaurant	Erythematous rash	Torso, arms	12
Rat	40 inhabitants 5 caretakers	Institution for disabled people	Pruritic red papules	Upper extremities, namely, neck, upper back, face	10
Rat	Male	Residence	Reddish papules, dermatitis	Arms, torso, back	140
Rodents	10 medical students (9 males, 1 female)	Library	Erythematous papules	Neck, axilla, abdomen, both extremities	31
Rodents	6 medical students	Residence in centuries-old house	Red papules and seropapules	Legs, arms, waist, laterally on the trunk	50

Affected individuals are treated with topical lindane. Papular dermatitis regresses 7 to 10 days posttherapy. Recurrence of *Ornithonyssus* infestations is common unless the premises and laboratory animals have been treated with an appropriate insecticide and any feral rodents eradicated. Lindane can also be used to eradicate the mites from research rodent colonies (74).

PRACTICAL TIPS
- Owners of pet snakes who feed their animals live or frozen rodents should be aware of the risk of acquiring infections of multiple-antibiotic-resistant *Salmonella*.
- Fatalities due to infections with *Streptobacillus moniliformis,* the causative agent of rat-bite fever, occur in previously healthy adults who acquire the infection from a bite or close contact with rats.
- Acute respiratory distress syndrome is now a recognized clinical sequela to infections with *Borrelia hermsii,* the causative agent of TBRF.
- The tropical rat mite *O. bacoti* causes dermatitis in persons living in residences infested with wild rats or mice, as well as in individuals with pet rodents or laboratory personnel handling rodents infested by the parasite.
- *Rodentolepis (Hymenolepis) nana* is a tapeworm with a direct life cycle; it can cause persistent diarrhea in patients with a heavy parasite burden. It is recognized as the most common tapeworm in humans residing in the United States.

REFERENCES
1. **Adams, J. R., E. T. Schmidtmann, and A. F. Azad.** 1990. Infection of colonized cat fleas, *Ctenocephalides felis* (Bouche), with a rickettsia-like microorganism. *Am. J. Trop. Med. Hyg.* **43**:400–409.
2. **Adams, W. H., R. W. Emmons, and J. E. Brooks.** 1970. The changing ecology of murine (endemic) typhus in Southern California. *Am. J. Trop. Med. Hyg.* **19**:311–318.
3. **Alexander, A. D.** 1984. Leptospirosis in laboratory mice. *Science* **224**:1158.
4. **Alteras, I.** 1965. Human infection from laboratory animals. *Sabouraudia* **3**:143–145.
5. **Andersen, L. P., A. Norgaard, S. Holck, J. Blom, and L. Elsborg.** 1996. Isolation of a "*Helicobacter heilmanii*"-like organism from the human stomach. *Eur. J. Clin. Microbiol. Infect. Dis.* **15**:95–96.
6. **Anderson, L. C., S. L. Leary, and P. J. Manning.** 1983. Rat-bite fever in animal research laboratory personnel. *Lab. Anim. Sci.* **33**:292–294.
7. **Arkless, H. A.** 1970. Rat-bite fever at Albert Einstein Medical Center. *Pa. Med.* **73**:49.
8. **Barkin, R. M., J. C. Guckian, and J. W. Glosser.** 1974. Infection by *Leptospira ballum:* a laboratory-associated case. *South. Med. J.* **67**:155, passim.
9. **Bartram, J. T., H. Welsh, and M. Ostroleur.** 1940. Incidence of members of the Salmonella group in rats. *J. Infect. Dis.* **67**:222–226.
10. **Baumstark, J., W. Beck, and H. Hofmann.** 2007. Outbreak of tropical rat mite (*Ornithonyssus bacoti*) dermatitis in a home for disabled persons. *Dermatology* **215**:66–68.
11. **Beaver, P. C., and R. C. Jung.** 1985. *Animal Agents and Vectors of Human Disease,* 5th ed. Lea & Febiger, Philadelphia, PA.
12. **Beck, W.** 2008. Occurrence of a house-infesting tropical rat mite (Ornithonyssus bacoti) on murides and human beings. *Travel Med. Infect. Dis.* **6**:245–249.
13. **Benenson, A. S. (ed.).** 1985. *Control of Communicable Disease in Man,* 14th ed. American Public Health Association, Washington, DC.
14. **Bharadwaj, M., J. Botten, N. Torrez-Martinez, and B. Hjelle.** 1997. Rio Mamore virus: genetic characterization of a newly recognized hantavirus of the pygmy rice rat, *Oligoryzomys microtis,* from Bolivia. *Am. J. Trop. Med. Hyg.* **57**:368–374.
15. **Blackmore, D. K., and R. A. Francis.** 1970. The apparent transmission of staphylococci of human origin to laboratory animals. *J. Comp. Pathol.* **80**:645–651.
16. **Boak, R. A., W. D. Linscott, and R. E. Bodfish.** 1960. A case of *Leptospirosis ballum* in California. *Calif. Med.* **93**:163–165.
17. **Booth, B. H.** 1952. Mouse ringworm. *Arch. Dermatol. Syphilol.* **66**:65–69.
18. **Breman, J.** 2000. Monkeypox: an emerging infection for humans?, p. 45–76. *In* W. Scheld, W. Craig, and J. Hughes (ed.), *Emerging Infections,* 4. ASM Press, Washington, DC.
19. **Brenner, F., R. Villar, F. Angulo, R. Tauxe, and B. Swaminathan.** 2000. *Salmonella* nomenclature. *J. Clin. Microbiol.* **38**:2465–2467.

20. **Brettman, L. R., S. Lewin, R. S. Holzman, W. D. Goldman, J. S. Marr, P. Kechijian, and R. Schinella.** 1981. Rickettsialpox: report of an outbreak and a contemporary review. *Medicine* (Baltimore) **60:**363–372.

21. **Brooks, J. E.** 1973. A review of commensal rodents and their control. *Crit. Rev. Environ. Control* **3:**405–453.

22. **Brown, C. M., and M. T. Parker.** 1957. Salmonella infection in rodents in Manchester. *Lancet* **273:**1277–1279.

23. **Burman, W. J., D. L. Cohn, R. R. Reves, and M. L. Wilson.** 1995. Multifocal cellulitis and monoarticular arthritis as manifestations of *Helicobacter cinaedi* bacteremia. *Clin. Infect. Dis.* **20:**564–570.

24. **Centers for Disease Control and Prevention.** 2005. Fatal rat-bite fever: Florida and Washington, 2003. *MMWR Morb. Mortal. Wkly. Rep.* **53:**1198–1202.

25. **Centers for Disease Control and Prevention.** 1993. Update: hantavirus disease—southwestern United States, 1993. *MMWR Morb. Mortal. Wkly. Rep.* **42:**570–572.

26. **Centers for Disease Control and Prevention.** 2003. Multistate outbreak of monkeypox—Illinois, Indiana, and Wisconsin, 2003. *MMWR Morb. Mortal. Wkly. Rep.* **52:**537–540.

27. **Cetin, E. T., M. Tahsinoglu, and S. Volkan.** 1965. Epizootic of Trichophyton mentagrophytes (interdigitale) in white mice. *Pathol. Microbiol.* **28:**839–846.

28. **Charlesworth, E. N., and R. W. Clegern.** 1977. Tropical rat mite dermatitis. *Arch. Dermatol.* **113:**937–938.

29. **Childs, J. E., G. E. Glass, G. W. Korch, R. R. Arthur, K. V. Shah, D. Glasser, C. Rossi, and J. W. Leduc.** 1988. Evidence of human infection with a rat-associated Hantavirus in Baltimore, Maryland. *Am. J. Epidemiol.* **127:**875–878.

30. **Chmel, L., L. Buchvald, and M. Valentova.** 1975. Spread of *Trichophyton mentagrophytes* var. gran. infection to man. *Int. J. Dermatol.* **14:**269–272.

31. **Chung, S., S. Hwang, S. Kwon, D. W. Kim, J. Jun, and B. Cho.** 1998. Outbreak of rat mite dermatitis in medical students. *Int. J. Dermatol.* **37:**591–594.

32. **Cimolai, N., M. J. Gill, A. Jones, B. Flores, W. E. Stamm, W. Laurie, B. Madden, and M. S. Shahrabadi.** 1987. ''*Campylobacter cinaedi*'' bacteremia: case report and laboratory findings. *J. Clin. Microbiol.* **25:**942–943.

33. **Coffey, E. M., and W. C. Eveland.** 1967. Experimental relapsing fever initiated by *Borrelia hermsi*. I. Identification of major serotypes by immunofluorescence. *J. Infect. Dis.* **117:**23–28.

34. **Cole, J. S., R. W. Stoll, and R. J. Bulger.** 1969. Rat-bite fever. Report of three cases. *Ann. Intern. Med.* **71:**979–981.

35. **Committee on Urban Pest Management.** 1980. *Urban Pest Management.* National Academy Press, Washington, DC.

36. **Corning, B. F., J. C. Murphy, and J. G. Fox.** 1991. Group G streptococcal lymphadenitis in rats. *J. Clin. Microbiol.* **29:**2720–2723.

37. **Craven, R. B., and A. M. Barnes.** 1991. Plague and tularemia in animal associated human infections. *Infect. Dis. Clin. N. Am.* **5:**165–175.

38. **Davey, D. G.** 1962. The use of pathogen free animals. *Proc. R. Soc. Med.* **55:**256–262.

39. **Davies, R. R., and J. Shewell.** 1964. Control of mouse ringworm. *Nature* **202:**406–407.

40. **Demers, R. Y., A. Thiermann, P. Demers, and R. Frank.** 1983. Exposure to Leptospira icterohaemorrhagiae in inner-city and suburban children: a serologic comparison. *J. Fam. Pract.* **17:**1007–1011.

41. **Dendle, G., et al.** 2006. Rat-bite fever septic arthritis: illustrative case and literature review. *Eur. J. Clin. Microbiol. Infect. Dis.* **25:**791–797.

42. **Dennis, D. T., and J. M. Hughes.** 1997. Multidrug resistance in plague. *N. Engl. J. Med.* **337:**702–704.

43. **Desmyter, J., C. van Ypersele de Strihou, and G. van der Groen.** 1984. Hantavirus disease. *Lancet* **ii:**158.

44. **Dolan, M. M., A. Klingman, and P. G. Kobylinski.** 1958. Ringworm epizootics in laboratory mice and rats: experimental and accidental transmission of infection. *J. Investig. Dermatol.* **30:**23–25.

45. **Dove, W. E., and B. Shelmire.** 1931. The tropical rat mite, *Liponyssus bacoti* Hirst 1914: the cause of a skin eruption of man, and a possible vector of endemic typhus fever. *JAMA* **96:**579–584.

46. **Dowlati, Y., and H. C. Maguire, Jr.** 1970. Rat mite dermatitis: a family affair. *Arch. Dermatol.* **101:**617–618.

47. **Duma, R. J., D. E. Sonenshine, F. M. Bozeman, J. M. Veazey, Jr., B. L. Elisberg, D. P. Chadwick, N. I. Stocks, T. M. McGill, G. B. Miller, Jr., and J. N. MacCormack.** 1981. Epidemic typhus in the United States associated with flying squirrels. *JAMA* **245:**2318–2323.

48. **Dworkin, M., and P. Shoemaker.** 2002. The epidemiology of tick-borne relapsing fever in the United States. *Am. J. Trop. Med. Hyg.* **60:**753–758.

49. **Elliott, S.** 2007. Rat bite fever and *Streptobacillus moniliformis.* *Clin. Microbiol. Rev.* **20:**13–22.

50. **Engle, P., J. Welzel, M. Maass, U. Schramm, and H. H. Wolff.** 1998. Tropical

rate mite dermatitis: case report and review. *Clin. Infect. Dis.* **27:**1465–1469.

51. **Ezaki, T., Y. Kawamura, and E. Yabuuchi.** 2000. Recognition of nomenclatural standing of *Salmonella typhi* (Approved Lists 1980) and *Salmonella typhimurium* (Approved Lists 1980), and conservation of the specific epithets *enteritidis* and *typhimurium.* Request for an opinion. *Int. J. Syst. Evol. Microbiol.* **50:**945–947.

52. **Faine, S.** 1991. Leptospirosis, p. 367–393. *In* A. Evans and P. S. Brachman (ed.), *Bacterial Infections in Humans.* Plenum Medical Book Co., New York, NY.

53. **Farhang-Azad, A., R. Traub, and S. Baqar.** 1985. Transovarial transmission of murine typhus rickettsiae in *Xenopsylla cheopis* fleas. *Science* **227:** 543–545.

54. **Faust, E. L., and P. F. Russel.** 1970. *Craig & Faust Clinical Parasitology,* 8th ed. Lea & Febiger, Philadelphia, PA.

55. **Flores, B. M., C. L. Fennell, K. K. Holmes, and W. E. Stamm.** 1985. In vitro susceptibilities of *Campylobacter*-like organisms to twenty antimicrobial agents. *Antimicrob. Agents Chemother.* **28:**188–191.

56. **Fox, J., C. Newcomer, and H. Rozmiarek.** 2002. Selected zoonoses, p. 1060–1128. *In* J. Fox, L. Anderson, F. Loew, and F. Quimby (ed.), *Laboratory Animal Medicine,* 2nd ed. Academic Press, Boston, MA.

57. **Fox, J. G. (ed.).** 1998. *Biology and Diseases of the Ferret,* 2nd ed. Williams and Wilkins, Baltimore, MD.

58. **Fox, J. G.** 1991. Campylobacter infections and salmonellosis. *Semin. Vet. Med. Surg. (Small Anim.)* **6:**212–218.

59. **Fox, J. G.** 2002. The non-*H. pylori* helicobacters: their expanding role in gastrointestinal and systemic diseases. *Gut* **50:**273–283.

60. **Fox, J. G., and J. B. Brayton.** 1982. Zoonoses and other human health hazards, p. 403–423. *In* H. L. Foster, J. D. Small, and J. G. Fox (ed.), *Biology of the Laboratory Mouse,* vol. II. Academic Press, New York, NY.

61. **Fox, J. G., F. E. Dewhirst, Z. Shen, Y. Feng, N. S. Taylor, B. J. Paster, R. L. Ericson, C. N. Lau, P. Correa, J. C. Araya, and I. Roa.** 1998. Hepatic *Helicobacter* species identified in bile and gallbladder tissue from Chileans with chronic cholecystitis. *Gastroenterology* **114:**755–763.

62. **Fox, J. G., L. Handt, B. J. Sheppard, S. Xu, F. E. Dewhirst, S. Motzel, and H. Klein.** 2001. Isolation of *Helicobacter cinaedi* from the colon, liver, and mesenteric lymph node of a rhesus monkey with chronic colitis and hepatitis. *J. Clin. Microbiol.* **39:**1580–1585.

63. **Fox, J. G., and N. S. Lipman.** 1991. Infections transmitted from large and small laboratory animals, p. 131–163. *In* A. Weinberg and D. Weber (ed.), *Infectious Diseases of North America.* W. B. Saunders, Philadelphia, PA.

64. **Friedmann, C. T., E. L. Spiegel, E. Aaron, and R. McIntyre.** 1973. *Leptospirosis ballum* contracted from pet mice. *Calif. Med.* **118:**51–52.

65. **Fuller, C.** 2008. A multi-state Salmonella typhimurium outbreak associated with frozen vacuum-packed rodents used to feed snakes. *Zoonoses Public Health* **55:**481–487.

66. **Gebhart, C. J., C. L. Fennell, M. P. Murtaugh, and W. E. Stamm.** 1989. *Campylobacter cinaedi* is normal intestinal flora in hamsters. *J. Clin. Microbiol.* **27:**1692–1694.

67. **Geller, E. H.** 1979. Health hazards for man. *In* H. J. Baker, J. R. Lindsey, and S. H. Weisbroth (ed.), *The Laboratory Rat,* vol. I. Academic Press, New York, NY.

68. **Gilbert, G. L., J. F. Cassidy, and N. M. Bennett.** 1971. Rat-bite fever. *Med. J. Aust.* **2:**1131–1134.

69. **Giusti, A. M., L. Crippa, O. Bellini, M. Luini, and E. Scanziani.** 1998. Gastric spiral bacteria in wild rats from Italy. *J. Wildl. Dis.* **34:** 168–172.

70. **Glaser, C., P. Lewis, and S. Wong.** 2000. Pet-, animal-, and vector-borne infections. *Pediatr. Rev.* **21:**219–232.

71. **Goddard, A. F., R. P. Logan, J. C. Atherton, D. Jenkins, and R. C. Spiller.** 1997. Healing of duodenal ulcer after eradication of *Helicobacter heilmannii. Lancet* **349:**1815–1816.

72. **Gundi, V. A. K. B., B. Davoust, A. Khamis, M. Boni, D. Raoult, and B. La Scola.** 2004. Isolation of *Bartonella rattimassiliensis* sp. nov. and *Bartonella phoceensis* sp. nov. from European *Rattus norvegicus. J. Clin. Microbiol.* **42:**3816–3818.

73. **Haggard, C. N.** 1955. Rat mite dermatitis in children. *Pediatrics* **15:**322–324.

74. **Harris, J. M., and J. J. Stockton.** 1960. Eradication of the tropical rat mite *Ornithonyssus bacoti* (Hirst 1913) from a colony of mice. *Am. J. Vet. Res.* **21:**316–318.

75. **Heilmann, K. L., and F. Borchard.** 1991. Gastritis due to spiral shaped bacteria other than *Helicobacter pylori:* clinical, histological, and ultrastructural findings. *Gut* **32:**137–140.

76. **Heiser, V.** 1936. *An American Doctor's Odyssey.* W. W. Norton Publishers, New York, NY.

77. **Helms, M., P. Vastrup, P. Gerner-Smidt, and K. Molbak.** 2002. Excess mortality associated with antimicrobial drug-resistant Salmonella typhimurium. *Emerg. Infect. Dis.* **8:**490–495.

78. **Hernandez-Cabrera, M., A. Angel-Moreno, E. Santana, M. Bolanos, A. Frances, A.**

Martin-Sanchez, and J. Perez-Arellano. 2004. Murine typhus with renal involvement in Canary Islands, Spain. *Emerg. Infect. Dis.* **10:**740–743.

79. Hetherington, G. W., W. R. Holder, and D. B. Smith. 1971. Rat mite dermatitis. *JAMA* **215:**1499–1500.

80. Hilzenrat, N., E. Lamoureux, I. Weintrub, E. Alpert, M. Lichter, and L. Alpert. 1995. *Helicobacter heilmannii*-like spiral bacteria in gastric mucosal biopsies. Prevalence and clinical significance. *Arch. Pathol. Lab. Med.* **119:**1149–1153.

81. Hinnebusch, B. J., R. D. Perry, and T. G. Schwan. 1996. Role of the *Yersinia pestis* hemin storage (hms) locus in the transmission of plague by fleas. *Science* **273:**367–370.

82. Hinnebusch, B. J., A. E. Rudolph, P. Cherepanov, J. E. Dixon, T. G. Schwan, and A. Forsberg. 2002. Role of *Yersinia* murine toxin in survival of *Yersinia pestis* in the midgut of the flea vector. *Science* **296:**733–735.

83. Hjelle, B., S. Jenison, N. Torrez-Martinez, B. Herring, S. Quan, A. Polito, S. Pichuantes, T. Yamada, C. Morris, F. Elgh, H. W. Lee, H. Artsob, and R. Dinello. 1997. Rapid and specific detection of Sin Nombre virus antibodies in patients with hantavirus pulmonary syndrome by a strip immunoblot assay suitable for field diagnosis. *J. Clin. Microbiol.* **35:**600–608.

84. Hjelle, B., N. Torrez-Martinez, F. T. Koster, M. Jay, M. S. Ascher, T. Brown, P. Reynolds, P. Ettestad, R. E. Voorhees, J. Sarisky, R. E. Enscore, L. Sands, D. G. Mosley, C. Kioski, R. T. Bryan, and C. M. Sewell. 1996. Epidemiologic linkage of rodent and human hantavirus genomic sequences in case investigations of hantavirus pulmonary syndrome. *J. Infect. Dis.* **173:**781–786.

85. Hopla, C. E. 1951. Experimental transmission of tularemia by the tropical rat mite. *Am. J. Trop. Hyg.* **31:**768–782.

86. Hovell, M. 1924. *Rats and How to Destroy Them.* John Bale, Sons & Danielson Ltd., London, United Kingdom.

87. Hull, T. G. 1955. *Diseases Transmitted from Animals to Man,* 4th ed. Charles C Thomas, Springfield, IL.

88. Hussell, T., P. G. Isaacson, J. E. Crabtree, and J. Spencer. 1996. *Helicobacter pylori*-specific tumour-infiltrating T cells provide contact dependent help for the growth of malignant B cells in low-grade gastric lymphoma of mucosa-associated lymphoid tissue. *J. Pathol.* **178:**122–127.

89. Iinuma, Y., H. Hayashidani, K. Kaneko, M. Ogawa, and S. Hamasaki. 1992. Isolation of *Yersinia enterocolitica* serovar O8 from free-living small rodents in Japan. *J. Clin. Microbiol.* **30:**240–242.

90. Jezek, Z., M. Szczeniowski, K. M. Paluku, and M. Mutombo. 1987. Human monkeypox: clinical features of 282 patients. *J. Infect. Dis.* **156:**293–298.

91. Kaneko, K. I., S. Hamada, Y. Kasai, and E. Kato. 1978. Occurrence of *Yersinia enterocolitica* in house rats. *Appl. Environ. Microbiol.* **36:**314–318.

92. Kaufman, A. F., J. M. Boyce, and W. J. Martone. 1980. Trends in human plague in the United States. *J. Infect. Dis.* **141:**522.

93. Kiehlbauch, J. A., D. J. Brenner, D. N. Cameron, A. G. Steigerwalt, J. M. Makowski, C. N. Baker, C. M. Patton, and I. K. Wachsmuth. 1995. Genotypic and phenotypic characterization of *Helicobacter cinaedi* and *Helicobacter fennelliae* strains isolated from humans and animals. *J. Clin. Microbiol.* **33:**2940–2947.

94. Kiehlbauch, J. A., R. V. Tauxe, C. N. Baker, and I. K. Wachsmuth. 1994. *Helicobacter cinaedi*-associated bacteremia and cellulitis in immunocompromised patients. *Ann. Intern. Med.* **121:**90–93.

95. Kliks, M. M., K. Kroenke, and J. M. Hardman. 1982. Eosinophilic radiculomyeloencephalitis: an angiostrongyliasis outbreak in American Samoa related to ingestion of *Achatina fulica* snails. *Am. J. Trop. Med. Hyg.* **31:**1114–1122.

96. Kliks, M. M., W. K. Lau, and N. E. Palumbo. 1988. Neurologic angiostrongyliasis: parasitic eosinophilic meningoencephalitis, p. 754–767. *In* A. Balows et al. (ed.), *Laboratory Diagnosis of Infectious Diseases: Principles and Practice,* vol. I. Springer-Verlag, New York, NY.

97. LeDuc, J. W. 1987. Epidemiology of Hantaan and related viruses. *Lab. Anim. Sci.* **37:**413–418.

98. Lee, A., S. L. Hazell, J. O'Rourke, and S. Kouprach. 1988. Isolation of a spiral-shaped bacterium from the cat stomach. *Infect. Immun.* **56:**2843–2850.

99. Li, H., and D. E. Davis. 1952. The prevalence of carriers of leptospira and salmonella in Norway rats of Baltimore. *Am. J. Hyg.* **56:**90–100.

100. Lipman, N. S. 1996. Rat bite fevers, p. 451–455. *In* D. Schlossberg (ed.), *Current Therapy of Infectious Diseases.* Mosby Yearbook, Inc., Philadelphia, PA.

101. Lloyd, G., E. T. Bowen, N. Jones, and A. Pendry. 1984. HFRS outbreak associated with laboratory rats in UK. *Lancet* **i:**1175–1176.

102. Looke, D. F. 1986. Weil's syndrome in a zoologist. *Med. J. Aust.* **144:**597, 600–601.

103. **Luzzi, G. A., L. M. Milne, and S. A. Waitkins.** 1987. Rat-bite acquired leptospirosis. *J. Infect.* **15:**57–60.

104. **Macy, D. W.** 1998. Plague. *In* C. E. Greene (ed.), *Infectious Diseases of the Dog and Cat,* 2nd ed. W. B. Saunders, Philadelphia, PA.

105. **Mann, J. M., W. J. Martone, J. M. Boyce, A. F. Kaufmann, A. M. Barnes, and N. S. Weber.** 1979. Endemic human plague in New Mexico: risk factors associated with infection. *J. Infect. Dis.* **140:**397–401.

106. **Martin, L. J., M. Fyfe, K. Doré, J. A. Buxton, F. Pollari, B. Henry, D. Middleton, R. Ahmed, F. Jamieson, B. Ciebin, S. A. McEwen, J. B. Wilson, and the Multi-Provincial *Salmonella* Typhimurium Case-Control Study Steering Committee.** 2004. Increased burden of illness associated with antimicrobial-resistant *Salmonella enterica* serotype Typhimurium infections. *J. Infect. Dis.* **189:** 377–384.

107. **Matsukura, N., S. Yokomuro, S. Yamada, T. Tajiri, T. Sundo, T. Hadama, S. Kamiya, Z. Naito, and J. G. Fox.** 2002. Association between *Helicobacter bilis* in bile and biliary tract malignancies: *H. bilis* in bile from Japanese and Thai patients with benign and malignant diseases in the biliary tract. *Jpn. J. Cancer Res.* **93:**842–847.

108. **McDade, J. E., and D. Fishbein.** 1988. *The Rickettsiae in Laboratory Diagnosis of Infectious Disease, Principles and Practice,* vol. II. Springer-Verlag, New York, NY.

109. **McGill, R. C., A. M. Martin, and P. N. Edmunds.** 1966. Rat-bite fever due to *Streptobacillus moniliformis. Br. Med. J.* **5497:**1213–1214.

110. **Mendes, E.** 1994. Are pigs a reservoir host for human Helicobacter infection?, abstr. 45. *Am. J. Gastroenterol.* **89:**1296.

111. **Morgner, A., N. Lehn, L. P. Andersen, C. Thiede, M. Bennedsen, K. Trebesius, B. Neubauer, A. Neubauer, M. Stolte, and E. Bayerdorffer.** 2000. Helicobacter heilmannii-associated primary gastric low-grade MALT lymphoma: complete remission after curing the infection. *Gastroenterology* **118:**821–828.

112. **Morris, A., M. R. Ali, L. Thomsen, and B. Hollis.** 1990. Tightly spiral shaped bacteria in the human stomach: another cause of active chronic gastritis? *Gut* **31:**139–143.

113. **Murphy, F. K.** 2007. Acute respiratory distress syndrome in persons with tickborne relapsing fever—three states, 2004–2005. *MMWR Morb. Mortal. Wkly. Rep.* **56:**1073–1076.

114. **Mushatt, D. M., and N. E. Hyslop, Jr.** 1991. Neurologic aspects of North American zoonoses. *Infect. Dis. Clin. North Am.* **5:**703–731.

115. **Nambiar, P., S. Kirchain, K. Courmier, and S. Xu.** 2006. Progressive proliferative and dysplastic typhlocolitis in aging Syrian hamsters naturally infected with Helicobacter spp.: a spontaneous model of inflammatory bowel disease. *Vet. Pathol.* **43:**2–14.

116. **Nelson, J. D., H. Kusmiesz, L. H. Jackson, and E. Woodman.** 1980. Treatment of Salmonella gastroenteritis with ampicillin, amoxicillin, or placebo. *Pediatrics* **65:**1125–1130.

117. **Ng, V. L., W. K. Hadley, C. L. Fennell, B. M. Flores, and W. E. Stamm.** 1987. Successive bacteremias with *"Campylobacter cinaedi"* and *"Campylobacter fennelliae"* in a bisexual male. *J. Clin. Microbiol.* **25:**2008–2009.

118. **Ordog, G. J., S. Balasubramanium, and J. Wasserberger.** 1985. Rat bites: fifty cases. *Ann. Emerg. Med.* **14:**126–130.

119. **Orlicek, S. L., D. F. Welch, and T. L. Kuhls.** 1993. Septicemia and meningitis caused by *Helicobacter cinaedi* in a neonate. *J. Clin. Microbiol.* **31:**569–571.

120. **Paegle, R. D., R. P. Tewari, W. N. Bernhard, and E. Peters.** 1976. Microbial flora of the larynx, trachea, and large intestine of the rat after long-term inhalation of 100 per cent oxygen. *Anesthesiology* **44:**287–290.

121. **Pavia, A. T., and R. V. Tauxe.** 1991. Salmonellosis: nontyphoidal, p. 573–592. *In* A. S. Evans and P. S. Brachman (ed.), *Bacterial Infections of Humans: Epidemiology and Control.* Plenum, New York, NY.

122. **Perry, R.** 2003. A plague of fleas—survival and transmission of *Yersinia pestis. ASM News* **69:** 336–338.

123. **Petrov, V. G.** 1971. On the role of the mite *Ornithonyssus bacoti* Hirst as a reservoir and vector of the agent of tularemia. *Parazitologiia* **1:**7–14.

124. **Philip, C. B., and L. E. Hughes.** 1948. The tropical rat mite, *Liponyssus bacoti,* as an experimental vector of rickettsial pox. *Am. J. Trop. Med. Hyg.* **28:**697–705.

125. **Povar, M. L.** 1965. Ringworm *(Trichophyton mentagrophytes)* infection in a colony of albino Norway rats. *Lab. Anim. Care* **15:**264–265.

126. **Pratt, H. D., B. F. Bjornson, and K. S. Littig.** 1976. *Control of Domestic Rats and Mice.* Publication no. (CDC) 76-8141. U.S. Department of Health, Education, and Welfare, Atlanta, GA.

127. **Price-Jones, C.** 1927. Infection of rats by Gartner's bacillus. *J. Pathol. Bacteriol.* **30:**45.

128. **Que, J., and D. Hentges.** 1985. Effect of streptomycin administration on colonization resistance to *Salmonella typhimurium* in mice. *Infect. Immun.* **48:**169–174.

129. Quinn, T. C., S. E. Goodell, C. Fennell, S. P. Wang, M. D. Schuffler, K. K. Holmes, and W. E. Stamm. 1984. Infections with *Campylobacter jejuni* and *Campylobacter*-like organisms in homosexual men. *Ann. Intern. Med.* **101:**187–192.

130. Quinn, T. C., W. E. Stamm, S. E. Goodell, E. Mkrtichian, J. Benedetti, L. Corey, M. D. Schuffler, and K. K. Holmes. 1983. The polymicrobial origin of intestinal infections in homosexual men. *N. Engl. J. Med.* **309:**576–582.

131. Raffin, B. J., and M. Freemark. 1979. Streptobacillary rat-bite fever: a pediatric problem. *Pediatrics* **64:**214–217.

132. Reed, K. D., J. W. Melski, M. B. Graham, R. L. Regnery, M. J. Sotir, M. V. Wegner, J. J. Kazmierczak, E. J. Stratman, Y. Li, J. A. Fairley, G. R. Swain, V. A. Olson, E. K. Sargent, S. C. Kehl, M. A. Frace, R. Kline, S. L. Foldy, J. P. Davis, and I. K. Damon. 2004. The detection of monkeypox in humans in the Western Hemisphere. *N. Engl. J. Med.* **350:**342–350.

133. Regimbeau, C., D. Karsenti, V. Durand, L. D'Alteroche, C. Copie-Bergman, E. H. Metman, and M. C. Machet. 1998. Low-grade gastric MALT lymphoma and *Helicobacter heilmannii* (*Gastrospirillum hominis*). *Gastroenterol. Clin. Biol.* **22:**720–723.

134. Richter, C. P. 1954. Incidence of rat bites and rat bite fever in Baltimore. *JAMA* **128:**324.

135. Riley, W. A. 1940. Rat mite dermatitis in Minnesota. *Minn. Med.* **23:**423–424.

136. Roggero, E., E. Zucca, G. Pinotti, A. Pascarella, C. Capella, A. Savio, E. Pedrinis, A. Paterlini, A. Venco, and F. Cavalli. 1995. Eradication of *Helicobacter pylori* infection in primary low-grade gastric lymphoma of mucosa-associated lymphoid tissue. *Ann. Intern. Med.* **122:**767–769.

137. Rollag, O. J., M. R. Skeels, L. J. Nims, J. P. Thilsted, and J. M. Mann. 1981. Feline plague in New Mexico: report of five cases. *J. Am. Vet. Med. Assoc.* **179:**1381–1383.

138. Rollin, P. E., T. G. Ksiazek, L. H. Elliott, E. V. Ravkov, M. L. Martin, S. Morzunov, W. Livingstone, M. Monroe, G. Glass, and S. Ruo. 1995. Isolation of black creek canal virus, a new hantavirus from *Sigmodon hispidus* in Florida. *J. Med. Virol.* **46:**35–39.

139. Rolston, K. V. 1986. Group G streptococcal infections. *Arch. Intern. Med.* **146:**857–858.

140. Rosen, S., I. Yeruham, and Y. Braveman. 2002. Dermatitis in humans associated with the mites Pyemotes tritici, Dermanyssus gallinae, Ornithonyssus bacoti and Androlaelaps casalis in Israel. *Med. Vet. Entomol.* **16:**442–444.

141. Rosner, W. W. 1987. Bubonic plague. *J. Am. Vet. Med. Assoc.* **191:**406–409.

142. Roughgarden, J. W. 1965. Antimicrobial therapy of rat bite fever. *Arch. Intern. Med.* **116:**39.

143. Sanger, J. G., and A. B. Thiermann. 1988. Leptospirosis. *J. Am. Vet. Med. Assoc.* **193:**1250–1254.

144. Schmaljohn, C., and B. Hjelle. 1997. Hantaviruses: a global disease problem. *Emerg. Infect. Dis.* **3:**95–104.

145. Schriefer, M. E., J. B. Sacci, Jr., J. S. Dumler, M. G. Bullen, and A. F. Azad. 1994. Identification of a novel rickettsial infection in a patient diagnosed with murine typhus. *J. Clin. Microbiol.* **32:**949–954.

146. Schwab, M. R., R. Allen, and S. E. Sulkin. 1952. The tropical rat mite (*Liponyssus bacoti*) as an experimental vector of coxsackie virus. *Am. J. Trop. Med. Hyg.* **1:**982–986.

147. Schwartz, E. 1942. Notes on commensal rats. *Am. J. Trop. Med.* **22:**577–579.

148. Shults, F. S., P. C. Estes, J. A. Franklin, and C. B. Richter. 1973. Staphylococcal botryomycosis in a specific-pathogen-free mouse colony. *Lab. Anim. Sci.* **23:**36–42.

149. Solnick, J. V., J. O'Rourke, A. Lee, B. J. Paster, F. E. Dewhirst, and L. S. Tompkins. 1993. An uncultured gastric spiral organism is a newly identified helicobacter in humans. *J. Infect. Dis.* **168:**379–385.

150. Song, J. W., L. J. Baek, D. C. Gajdusek, R. Yanagihara, I. Gavrilovskaya, B. J. Luft, E. R. Mackow, and B. Hjelle. 1994. Isolation of pathogenic hantavirus from white-footed mouse (*Peromyscus leucopus*). *Lancet* **344:**1637.

151. Stoenner, H. G., E. F. Grimes, F. B. Thraikill, and E. Davis. 1958. Elimination of *Leptospira ballum* from a colony of Swiss albino mice by use of chlortetracycline hydrochloride. *Am. J. Trop. Med. Hyg.* **7:**423–426.

152. Stoenner, H. G., and D. Maclean. 1958. Leptospirosis (balum) contracted from Swiss albino mice. *Arch. Intern. Med.* **101:**706–710.

153. Stolte, M., G. Kroher, A. Meining, A. Morgner, E. Bayerdorffer, and B. Bethke. 1997. A comparison of *Helicobacter pylori* and *H. heilmannii* gastritis. A matched control study involving 404 patients. *Scand. J. Gastroenterol.* **32:**28–33.

154. Stolte, M., E. Wellens, B. Bethke, M. Ritter, and H. Eidt. 1994. *Helicobacter heilmannii* (formerly *Gastrospirillum hominis*) gastritis: an infection transmitted by animals? *Scand. J. Gastroenterol.* **29:**1061–1064.

155. **Stuart, B. M., and R. L. Pullen.** 1945. Endemic (murine) typhus fever: clinical observations of 180 cases. *Ann. Int. Med.* **23:**520–525.

156. **Sulzer, C. R., T. W. Harvey, and M. M. Galton.** 1968. Comparison of diagnostic techniques for the detection of leptospirosis in rats. *Health Lab.* **5:**171–173.

157. **Swanson, S., C. Snider, R. Braden.** 2007. Multidrug-resistant Salmonella enterica serotype Typhimurium associated with pet rodents. *New Engl. J. Med.* **356:**21–28.

158. **Taber, E., and R. D. Feigin.** 1979. Spirochetal infections. *Pediatr. Clin. North Am.* **26:** 377.

159. **Taylor, A. F., T. G. Stephenson, and H. A. Giese.** 1984. Rat bite fever in a college student. *MMWR Morb. Mortal. Wkly. Rep.* **33:**318.

160. **Theis, J., M. M. Lavoipierre, R. LaPerriere, and H. Kroese.** 1981. Tropical rat mite dermatitis. Report of six cases and review of mite infestations. *Arch. Dermatol.* **117:**341–343.

161. **Thiermann, A. B.** 1977. Incidence of leptospirosis in the Detroit rat population. *Am. J. Trop. Med. Hyg.* **26:**970–974.

162. **Thomson, M. A., P. Storey, R. Greer, and G. J. Cleghorn.** 1994. Canine-human transmission of *Gastrospirillum hominis*. *Lancet* **343:** 1605–1607.

163. **Torrez-Martinez, N., M. Bharadwaj, D. Goade, J. Delury, P. Moran, B. Hicks, B. Nix, J. L. Davis, and B. Hjelle.** 1998. Bayou virus-associated hantavirus pulmonary syndrome in Eastern Texas: identification of the rice rat, Oryzomys palustris, as reservoir host. *Emerg. Infect. Dis.* **4:**105–111.

164. **Torten, M.** 1979. Leptospirosis, p. 363–421. *In* J. H. Steele (ed.), *CRC Handbook Series in Zoonoses*, vol. 1. CRC Press, Cleveland, OH.

165. **Tsai, T. F.** 1987. Hemorrhagic fever with renal syndrome: clinical aspects. *Lab. Anim. Sci.* **37:** 419–427.

166. **Tsai, T. F.** 1987. Hemorrhagic fever with renal syndrome: mode of transmission to humans. *Lab. Anim. Sci.* **37:**428–430.

167. **Umenai, T., H. W. Lee, P. W. Lee, T. Saito, T. Toyoda, M. Hongo, K. Yoshinaga, T. Nobunaga, T. Horiuchi, and N. Ishida.** 1979. Korean haemorrhagic fever in staff in an animal laboratory. *Lancet* **i:**1314–1316.

168. **Vandamme, P., E. Falsen, B. Pot, K. Kersters, and J. De Ley.** 1990. Identification of *Campylobacter cinaedi* isolated from blood and feces of children and adult females. *J. Clin. Microbiol.* **28:**1016–1020.

169. **van der Waaij, D.** 1968. The persistent absence of Enterobacteriaceae from the intestinal flora of mice following antibiotic treatment. *J. Infect. Dis.* **118:**32–38.

170. **van der Waaij, D., J. Berghuis-de Vries, and J. Lekkerkerk-van der Wees.** 1971. Colonization resistance of the digestive tract in conventional and antibiotic-treated mice. *J. Hyg.* (London) **69:**405–411.

171. **Varma, J. K., K. Molbak, et al.** 2005. Antimicrobial-resistant nontyphoidal Salmonella is associated with excess bloodstream infections and hospitalizations. *J. Infect. Dis.* **191:**554–561.

172. **Voetsch, A., T. Van Gilder, and F. Angulo.** 2004. FoodNet estimate of the burden of illness caused by nontyphoidal Salmonella infections in the United States. *Clin. Infect. Dis.* **38:**S127–S134.

173. **Wainschel, J.** 1971. Rat mite bite. *JAMA* **216:** 1964.

174. **Wallet, F., and C. E. A. Savage.** 2003. Molecular diagnosis of arthritis due to Streptobacillus moniliformis. *Diagn. Microbiol. Infect. Dis.* **47:** 623–624.

175. **Weber, D. J., and A. R. Hansen.** 1991. Infections resulting from animal bites. *Infect. Dis. Clin. North Am.* **5:**663–677.

176. **Weber, D. J., J. S. Wolfson, M. N. Swartz, and D. C. Hooper.** 1984. Pasteurella multocida infections. Report of 34 cases and review of the literature. *Medicine* (Baltimore) **63:**133–154.

177. **Weber, L. F.** 1940. Rat mite dermatitis. *JAMA* **114:**1442.

178. **Weisbroth, S.** 1979. Bacterial and mycotic diseases, p. 194–230. *In* H. Baker (ed.), *The Laboratory Rat*, vol. I. Academic Press, New York, NY.

179. **Welch, H., M. Ostrolenk, and M. T. Bartram.** 1941. Role of rats in the spread of food poisoning bacteria in Salmonella group. *Am. J. Public Health* **31:**332–340.

180. **Wilkins, E. G., J. G. Millar, P. M. Cockcroft, and O. A. Okubadejo.** 1988. Rat-bite fever in a gerbil breeder. *J. Infect.* **16:**177–180.

181. **Williams, S. G., J. B. Sacci, Jr., M. E. Schriefer, E. M. Andersen, K. K. Fujioka, F. J. Sorvillo, A. R. Barr, and A. F. Azad.** 1992. Typhus and typhuslike rickettsiae associated with opossums and their fleas in Los Angeles County, California. *J. Clin. Microbiol.* **30:** 1758–1762.

182. **Yali, Z., N. Yamada, M. Wen, T. Matsuhisa, and M. Miki.** 1998. Gastrospirillum hominis and Helicobacter pylori infection in Thai individuals: comparison of histopathological changes of gastric mucosa. *Pathol. Int.* **48:** 507–511.

183. **Yanagihara, R.** 1990. Hantavirus infection in the United States: epizootiology and epidemiology. *Rev. Infect. Dis.* **12:**449–457.

184. **Yang, H., J. A. Goliger, M. Song, and D. Zhou.** 1998. High prevalence of *Helicobacter heilmannii* infection in China. *Dig. Dis. Sci.* **43:** 1493.

185. **Young, V., D. Schauer, and J. Fox.** 2000. Animal models of Campylobacter infection, p. 287–301. *In* I. Nachamkin and M. Blaser (ed.), *Campylobacter,* 2nd ed. ASM Press, Washington, DC.

186. **Yunker, C. E.** 1964. Infections of laboratory animals potentially dangerous to man: ectoparasites and other arthropods, with emphasis on mites. *Lab. Anim. Care* **14:**455–465.

187. **Zinsser, H.** 1935. *Rats, Lice and History.* Little, Brown and Company, Boston, MA.

CLOSED DUE TO RABIES

Jesse D. Blanton and John W. Krebs

10

Rabies is one of the oldest recognized zoonotic diseases. The first recorded description of canine rabies was apparently made by Democritus around 500 B.C.E. Aristotle, writing of rabies in his *Natural History of Animals,* described dogs suffering from a madness causing irritability and noted that other animals became diseased after being bitten by these sick dogs. In most areas of the world where the disease is endemic, dogs and other carnivores remain the common sources of human rabies virus infection, resulting in little change over time in the epidemiology of the disease. However, ongoing discovery of new lyssaviruses and the epidemiology of human rabies in many developed countries continue to implicate bats as an important emerging rabies reservoir (9, 81).

Rabies has been enzootic or epizootic in domestic and wild animals in the United States since at least the 18th century; however, reported cases of rabies in humans have re-

mained rare in this country. During the first half of the 20th century, an average of about 50 cases of human rabies, most the result of infection spread by dogs, were reported each year (83). Following the control of canine rabies in the 1940s and 1950s, the number of indigenously acquired human rabies cases fell to an average of one to three cases per year during the 1960s and 1970s (2). Today, rabies is primarily a disease of wildlife in the United States, as it is in most developed countries. However, globally, an estimated 55,000 cases of human rabies are diagnosed each year, the majority in Asia and Africa, where rabies in domestic dogs remains the primary source of exposure (124). Between 1980 (when modern tissue culture-derived rabies vaccines were introduced in the United States) and 2008, 44 cases of human rabies were reported as acquired in the United States (an additional 19 imported human cases were reported during this time, one of which was from Puerto Rico). All but eight of these indigenously acquired cases (four cases due to organ transplantation from a donor infected with a bat variant of rabies virus) were attributed to insectivorous bats (9, 93, 104). Although the exact circumstances of the exposures were in most instances unknown, some of these infections may have been acquired during the pur-

#2 3

Jesse D. Blanton, Poxvirus and Rabies Branch, National Center for Zoonotic, Vector-Borne, and Enteric Diseases, Centers for Disease Control and Prevention, Atlanta, GA 30333. *John W. Krebs,* Rickettsial Zoonosis Branch, National Center for Zoonotic, Vector Borne, and Enteric Diseases, Centers for Disease Control and Prevention, Atlanta, GA 30333.

Infections of Leisure, Fourth Edition, Edited by David Schlossberg,
© 2009 ASM Press, Washington, DC

suit of leisure actives (17, 19–23, 27, 28, 31–35, 37, 39, 41–47, 59). In addition, the changing nature of human rabies exposure has increasingly involved mass exposures in public areas, such as at sporting events, exhibitions, and recreational facilities, or in some cases during the translocation of rabid animals in order to restock populations for hunting purposes (53–56, 60, 107).

Rabies in wildlife is now directly and indirectly responsible for most of the economic and public health burden of the disease in the United States; since 1960, more wild than domestic animals have been reported as rabid in this country. Annual expenditures for rabies prevention and control may exceed $1,000,000 per 100,000 people in the United States, with the principal components of these expenditures being the routine vaccination of pets against the disease (120). Ongoing analyses of possible savings via wildlife vaccination programs to control rabies have demonstrated the need for further research and evaluation of optimal bait distribution densities and strategies to better define costs and determine cost-saving ratios (78, 102).

In contrast to the situation in the United States, canine rabies remains a serious threat for persons traveling to and living in developing countries. Largely because of the ubiquitous presence of dogs in these countries, rates of human rabies sometimes exceed 1 per 100,000 people per year, and more than 1,000 per 100,000 persons each year may receive rabies postexposure prophylaxis (PEP) (11). United States residents are at a much higher risk of exposure to rabies in developing countries than in the United States and occasionally have developed the disease when they failed to receive proper PEP (70). Four U.S. citizens traveling or living outside the United States have contracted the disease since 1980 (29, 38, 90, 104); five other individuals (U.S. citizens or residents) acquired the disease during visits to India, Haiti, Nepal, and the Philippines (19, 25, 30, 33, 94). Ten persons from countries where canine rabies is enzootic developed the disease while in the United States, and with

one possible exception, all are believed to have acquired the disease before coming to this country (18, 23, 24, 26, 36, 40, 41, 48, 49, 52, 92, 113). The epidemiology and strategies for preventing rabies within the United States are different from those observed and implemented in other areas of the world and are addressed separately.

EPIDEMIOLOGY OF RABIES IN THE UNITED STATES

Demographic changes resulting in ever-expanding suburban sprawl and changes in recreational land use, including the increased popularity of recreational activities such as hiking, camping, hunting, and visiting petting zoos and drive-through wildlife parks, as well as close contact with pets provide countless situations for human contact with a variety of animal species in the United States. Thus, rabies prevention strategies in this country focus on education and on a working knowledge of the epizootiology of the disease in animals, rather than relying solely on the prophylaxis of exposed individuals and on vaccination and control of dog populations, as is the case in much of the developing world.

Wildlife

In the United States, rabies is primarily a disease of wildlife. Reported rabies cases among wild animals have increased markedly since 1960, when their total first exceeded those reported among domestic animals, and exceeded 90% of all reported cases in 1991. Numbers of reported cases among wild animals have continued to exceed those among domestic animals, although the relative contributions of wildlife reservoir species most frequently reported as rabid have changed markedly. Historically, skunks have represented the reservoir species most reported to have rabies in the United States. However, in 1990, reported cases in raccoons first exceeded those in skunks, and in 2006, bats further supplanted skunks in the number of reported cases (7, 121). During 2007, cases in one or more wildlife species were reported in 49 of the 50 states and Puerto Rico (Table 1; Fig. 1 and 2) (9). Hawaii is currently the only state in the United States that is considered rabies free.

Compartmentalization of the disease by species and geographic area has led to the evolution of distinctive variants of rabies virus which can be identified by reaction with panels of monoclonal antibodies or by patterns of nucleotide substitution identified by genetic analysis (112, 114). Temporally dynamic boundaries can be identified in a given geographic area both for the principal animal species or reservoirs for rabies virus and for the variant of rabies virus associated with the reservoir species. Affected areas usually expand gradually and are bounded by natural barriers to animal movements, such as mountain ranges and bodies of water or unsuitable habitats; however, unusual animal dispersal patterns or human-mediated translocation of infected animals can result in more-rapid and unexpected introductions of rabies into new areas (60, 111). Spillover infection from reservoir species to other animal species occurs but rarely initiates sustained intraspecific transmission. Though rare, a recent case of spillover and adaptation occurred in Flagstaff, AZ, where sustained transmission of a big brown bat rabies virus variant was identified in a local skunk population. Rapid identification of this event led to intervention campaigns consisting of domestic animal vaccination, trapping, and parenteral vaccination of skunks, as well as oral rabies vaccination (ORV) campaigns. These activities appear to have contained and potentially eliminated the skunk-to-skunk transmission of this potential new terrestrial rabies virus variant (95). Once established, transmission within a species can persist at enzootic levels for decades and perhaps centuries.

Geographic separation currently allows recognition of eight distinct geographic areas in the continental United States, each with its respective reservoir species (Fig. 3). In each of

TABLE 1 Rabies in animals and humans in the United States (including Puerto Rico) from 2002 to 2007

Type(s) of animal	Avg no. of cases/yr, 2002–2006	Range, 2002–2006	No. of cases, 2007
Total	7,070	6,418–7,970	7,060
Wild animals	6,508	5,923–7,375	6,590
Raccoons	2,648	2,534–2,891	2,549
Skunks	1,875	1,478–2,433	1,476
Bats	1,410	1,212–1,692	1,935
Foxes	432	376–508	462
Mongooses[a]	58	47–66	32
Groundhogs	36	25–49	46
Coyotes	7	4–10	33
Other wildlife	42	29–47	53
Other rodents, lagomorphs	4	1–7	4
Domestic animals	559	494–614	469
Cats	298	269–321	262
Dogs	93	76–117	93
Cattle	101	82–116	57
Horses and mules	53	43–63	41
Goats and sheep	12	9–15	13
Other domestic animals	3	0–5	3
Humans	4	1–8	1

[a] Puerto Rico only.

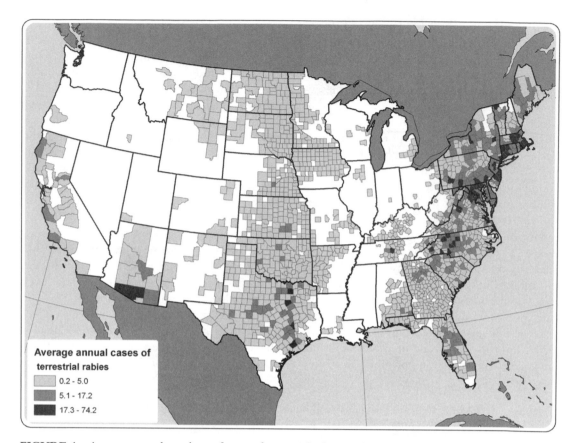

FIGURE 1 Average annual numbers of cases of terrestrial rabies in the United States, 2003 to 2007.

these areas, other rabid terrestrial animals (including domestic species) appear to acquire the disease as a result of spillover from a wildlife reservoir species (112). Multiple independent reservoirs for specific rabies virus variants circulating in several species of bats overlay the distribution of the disease in terrestrial animals (Fig. 2). Geographic boundaries for enzootic rabies in bats cannot be defined beyond the known ranges of individual species. Sporadic transmission of rabies from bats to terrestrial mammals (spillover) occurs but appears to be infrequent (101).

Raccoons *(Procyon lotor)* have been recognized as a reservoir for rabies virus in the southeastern states since the 1950s. An outbreak that began during the late 1970s in the Mid–Atlantic states was attributed to the probable translocation by humans of infected rac-

coons from the long-recognized epizootic in the Southeast (88). Although described as separate epizootics, these two outbreaks continued to expand, merging in North Carolina in 1995. Today, all of the eastern coastal states as well as Alabama, Pennsylvania, Vermont, West Virginia, eastern Ohio, and parts of Tennessee are affected. The spread of the raccoon rabies virus variant has significantly shifted the burden of disease in the United States due to the considerable amount of spillover into nonreservoir species. This variant now accounts for approximately 75% of reported cases of animal rabies in terrestrial species (9).

In response to the expansion of the raccoon rabies virus variant epizootic into areas previously free of the disease (Fig. 4), public health officials have been forced to allocate limited

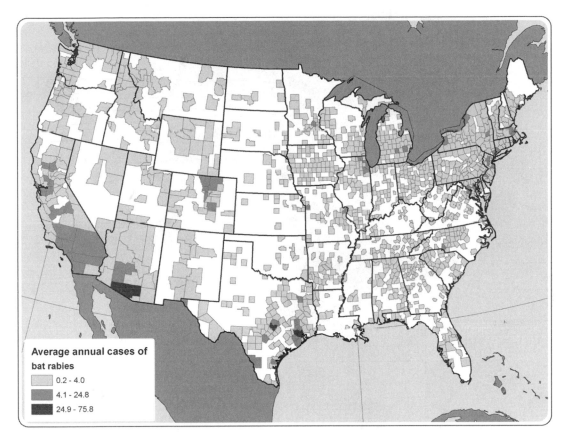

FIGURE 2 Average annual numbers of cases of bat rabies in the United States, 2003 to 2007.

resources for public education, vaccination programs for domestic animals, and PEP for humans (61, 62, 91, 108, 127). Despite the spread of the disease and the marked increase in the number of cases, no raccoon-associated human cases were reported in the United States until 2003, when a 25-year-old male from northern Virginia died from a rabies virus which was identified as the raccoon variant (16).

Bats are the most widely distributed wild animals in the United States. Rabies is present in at least 30 species of bats indigenous to the United States (with the exception of Hawaii) and the temperate parts of Canada (67). Although the vast majority of animal rabies cases are attributable to the dominant terrestrial species in the area, bats appear to be responsible for isolated cases of spillover infection. Of im-

portance in this regard is the fact that 40 of the 44 human rabies virus infections acquired in the United States between 1980 and 2008 were attributable to variants of the rabies virus associated with bats (four cases were due to organ transplantation of tissue from a donor infected with a bat rabies virus variant) (9, 93, 104). More remarkable is the fact that antigenic and genetic analyses revealed that over half of these infections (22 of 40) were caused by a variant associated with rabid silver-haired *(Lasionycteris noctivagans)* and eastern pipistrelle *(Pipistrellus subflavus)* bats. Although none of these cases were attributable to specific recreational pursuits, two spelunkers developed rabies in 1960 (66, 86).

It is unclear why exposure of humans in the United States to members of this order (Chiroptera [bats]) of mammals appears to

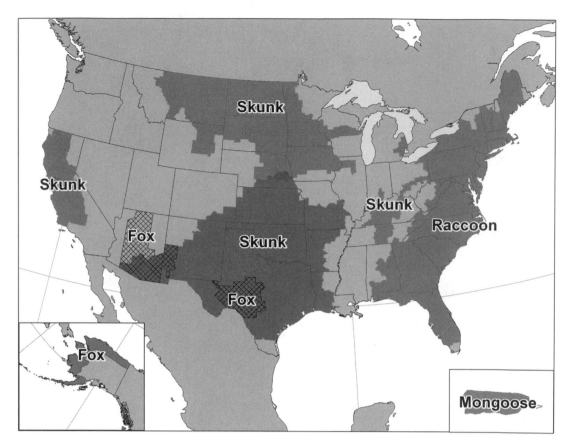

FIGURE 3 Distribution of terrestrial rabies virus variants and associated reservoirs in the United States, 2007.

pose a higher risk for acquiring rabies than exposure to other orders of mammals (Table 2).
The number of bats reported as rabid gradually
increased from the 1950s, when rabies was
first recognized in insectivorous bats in the
United States, to the 1970s; this increase was
likely due to factors associated with surveillance and awareness. Following this period,
the numbers of reported cases of rabies in bats
remained fairly constant, ranging between approximately 600 and 1,000 per year from 1976
through 1997 before the numbers again increased in 2006, when the bat became the
second-most-reported animal with rabies; a
record 1,935 cases were reported in 2007.
While not accurately known, the number of
humans bitten by bats is not particularly large,
and rabid *L. noctivagans* (silver-haired) and *P.*

subflavus (eastern pipistrelle) bats are not common among bats submitted to state health departments for testing (67). Although it is unknown why bat-associated rabies cases in
humans are reported more frequently than
cases associated with other mammals, it is clear
that even seemingly insignificant exposures to
bats must be carefully evaluated (50). The
small degree of injury inflicted by a bat (in
contrast to wounds inflicted by terrestrial carnivores) might cause it to remain undetected
and unreported, thereby limiting the ability of
health care providers to determine the rabies
risk resulting from an encounter with a bat.

Enzootic transmission of rabies in skunks
has been recognized in three major regions in
the United States since the late 1960s (63).
One region stretches from Alberta, Canada,

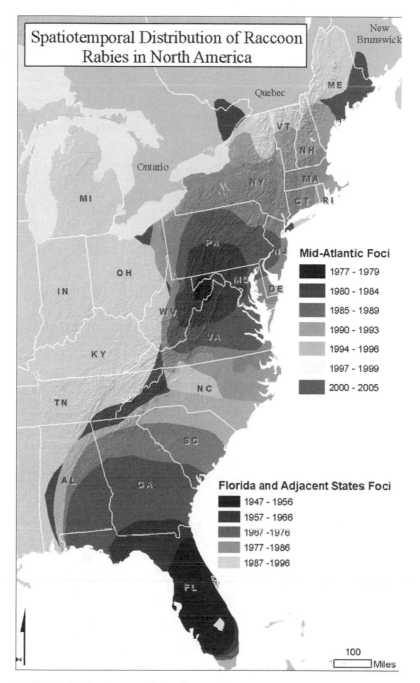

FIGURE 4 Spatiotemporal distribution of raccoon rabies in North America.

TABLE 2 Locations and presumed animal sources of human rabies in the United States from 1980 to 2008

Date of death (mo/day/yr) of patient	State of residence	Exposure history, location[a]	Rabies virus variant[b]
7/4/1981	Oklahoma	Unknown	Skunk, south-central United States
9/11/1981	Arizona	Dog bite, Mexico	Dog, Mexico
1/28/1983	Massachusetts	Dog bite, Nigeria	Dog, Nigeria
3/9/1983	Michigan	Unknown (interactions?)	Bat (Ln/Ps)
8/8/1984	Texas	Unknown, Laos	Dog, Laos
9/29/1984	Pennsylvania	Unknown	Bat (Msp)
10/1/1984	California	Dog bite, Guatemala	Dog, Guatemala
5/20/1985	Texas	Unknown, Mexico	Dog, Mexico
12/15/1987	California	Unknown, Philippines	Dog, Philippines
2/3/1989	Oregon	Unknown, Mexico	Dog, Mexico
6/5/1990	Texas	Bat bite, Texas	Bat (Tb)
8/20/1991	Texas	Unknown (interactions?)	Dog/coyote
8/25/1991	Arkansas	Unknown (interactions?)	Bat (Ln/Ps)
10/10/1991	Georgia	Unknown (interactions?)	Bat (Ln/Ps)
5/8/1992	California	Dog bite, India	Dog, India
7/11/1993	New York	Unknown (interactions?)	Bat (Ln/Ps)
11/9/1993	Texas	Unknown	Bat (Ln/Ps)
11/21/1993	California	Dog bite, Mexico	Dog, Mexico
1/18/1994	California	Unknown	Bat (Ln/Ps)
6/21/1994	Florida	Unknown, Haiti	Dog, Haiti
10/11/1994	Alabama	Unknown (interactions?)	Bat (Tb)
10/15/1994	West Virginia	Unknown (interactions?)	Bat (Ln/Ps)
11/23/1994	Tennessee	Unknown (interactions?)	Bat (Ln/Ps)
11/27/1994	Texas	Unknown (interactions?)	Dog/coyote
3/15/1995	Washington	Unknown (interactions?)	Bat (Msp)
9/21/1995	California	Unknown (interactions?)	Bat (Tb)
10/23/1995	Connecticut	Unknown (interactions?)	Bat (Ln/Ps)
11/9/1995	California	Unknown (interactions?)	Bat (Ln/Ps)
2/8/1996	Florida	Dog bite, Mexico	Dog, Mexico
8/20/1996	New Hampshire	Dog bite, Nepal	Dog, Southeast Asia
10/15/1996	Kentucky	Unknown	Bat (Ln/Ps)
12/19/1996	Montana	Unknown (interactions?)	Bat (Ln/Ps)
1/5/1997	Montana	Unknown (interactions?)	Bat (Ln/Ps)
1/18/1997	Washington	Unknown (interactions?)	Bat (Ef)
10/17/1997	Texas	Unknown (interactions?)	Bat (Ln/Ps)
10/23/1997	New Jersey	Unknown (interactions?)	Bat (Ln/Ps)
12/31/1998	Virginia	Unknown	Bat (Ln/Ps)
9/20/2000	California	Unknown (interactions?)	Bat (Tb)
10/9/2000	New York	Dog bite, Ghana	Dog, Africa
10/10/2000	Georgia	Unknown (interactions?)	Bat (Tb)
10/25/2000	Minnesota	Bat bite, Minnesota	Bat (Ln/Ps)
11/1/2000	Wisconsin	Unknown (interactions?)	Bat (Ln/Ps)
2/4/2001	California	Unknown	Dog, Philippines
3/31/2002	California	Unknown (interactions?)	Bat (Tb)
8/31/2002	Tennessee	Unknown (interactions?)	Bat (Ln/Ps)
9/28/2002	Iowa	Unknown (interactions?)	Bat (Ln/Ps)
3/10/2003	Virginia	Unknown	Eastern raccoon
6/5/2003	Puerto Rico	Dog bite, Puerto Rico	Mongoose/dog
9/14/2003	California	Bat bite, California	Bat (Ln/Ps)
2/15/2004	Florida	Dog bite, Haiti	Dog, Haiti
5/4/2004	Arkansas	Unknown (interactions?)	Bat (Tb)

(Table continues)

TABLE 2 *(continued)*

Date of death (mo/day/yr) of patient	State of residence	Exposure history, location[a]	Rabies virus variant[b]
5/31/2004	Texas	Organ transplant recipient	Bat (Tb)
6/9/2004	Texas	Organ transplant recipient	Bat (Tb)
6/21/2004	Texas	Organ transplant recipient	Bat (Tb)
6/10/2004	Texas	Tissue graft recipient	Bat (Tb)
Survived	Wisconsin	Bat bite, Wisconsin	None (no isolate)
10/26/2004	California	Unknown	Dog, El Salvador
9/11/2005	Mississippi	Unknown (interactions?)	None (no isolate)
5/12/2006	Texas	Unknown (interactions?)	Bat (Tb)
11/2/2006	Indiana	Unknown (interactions?)	Bat (Ln/Ps)
12/14/2006	California	Dog bite, Philippines	Dog, Philippines
10/20/2007	Minnesota	Bat bite, Minnesota	None (no isolate)
3/18/2008	California	Fox, Mexico	Bat (Tb?)

[a]Data for exposure history are reported only when the biting animal was available and tested positive for rabies, when plausible information was reported directly by the patient (if lucid or credible), or when a reliable account of an incident consistent with rabies exposure (e.g., a dog bite) was reported by an independent witness (usually a family member). In many instances where the exposure history is unknown, known or inferred interaction was elucidated from contact which, especially with bats, could have involved an unrecognized or unreported bite.

[b]Variants of the rabies virus associated with terrestrial animals in the United States are identified with the name of the animal reservoir, whereas variants of the rabies virus acquired outside the United States are identified with the names of the reservoir animal (dog, in all cases shown), followed by the name of the most definitive geographic entity (usually the country) from which the variant has been identified. Variants of the rabies virus associated with bats are identified with the names of the species of bat(s) in which they have been found to be circulating. Because information regarding the location of the exposure and the identity of the exposing animal is almost always gathered retrospectively and much information is frequently unavailable, the location of the exposure and the identity of the animal responsible for the infection are often limited to deduction. Ln/Ps, *L. noctivagans* or *P. subflavus,* the silver-haired bat or the eastern pipistrelle, respectively; Msp, *Myotis* species unknown; Tb, *Tadarida brasiliensis,* the Brazilian (Mexican) free-tailed bat; Ef, *Eptesicus fuscus,* the big brown bat.

south and east to portions of Tennessee and Virginia, and a second region extends from Nebraska and Missouri south to central Mexico (9, 122). The variant of the rabies virus circulating in skunks in a third region in northern California is similar to that found in skunks in the north-central states. Although the number of reported rabid skunks decreased throughout most of the 1980s, a subsequent increase was noted in the mid to late 1990s before again declining. Most increases are heavily augmented as a result of transmission of rabies from raccoons to skunks in the eastern United States. From 2000 to 2007, an overall decrease of 33.6% in skunks was reported; during the same time period, a 41.2% decrease in reported rabid skunks occurred in states where a skunk rabies virus variant is the predominant circulating variant (9, 93). The

last case of human rabies attributable to skunk rabies virus variant occurred in 1981 (35).

Long-standing reservoirs for rabies virus in Alaska are known to be red and Arctic foxes (*Vulpes vulpes* and *Alopex lagopus,* respectively). The disease spread during the 1950s to include foxes from the Northwest Territories, across Canada, and to adjoining areas of the New England states. Rabies remains a persistent problem in foxes in Alaska and Canada. However, ORV programs in Canada have been responsible for the elimination of this rabies virus variant in eastern Ontario (96). Two different variants of rabies virus are present in small but persistent numbers in gray foxes (*Urocyon cinereoargenteus*) in Arizona and Texas. A variant associated with coyotes (*Canis latrans*) and dogs in southern Texas, due to long-standing interactions between unvaccinated domestic dogs and coyotes at the Texas-Mexico border, was eliminated through ORV in 2004 (7).

The number of rabies cases in other wild animals is relatively small, although the number of such animals reported as rabid has increased markedly since 1990 because of the continuing spread of the raccoon rabies epizootic. The majority of the 462 foxes (26 states), 50 rodents and lagomorphs (14 states), and 118 other wild animals (20 states) reported as rabid in 2007 attest to the ability of rabies virus in terrestrial reservoir species to infect other species via spillover. In 2007, 46 cases of rabies among groundhogs *(Marmota monax)* and 4 cases among beavers *(Castor canadensis),* the largest species of rodents in the United States, accounted for all cases of rabies reported in rodents and lagomorphs. Smaller rodents (such as squirrels, hamsters, guinea pigs, gerbils, chipmunks, rats, and mice) and lagomorphs (rabbits and hares) are almost never found to be infected with the rabies virus, probably because they rarely survive the bite of the larger wild animals that expose them to rabies virus (50, 64). Another important wildlife species is the mongoose *(Herpestes javanicus),* which is a reservoir of rabies virus in Puerto Rico and other Caribbean islands (75).

Oral vaccines for wildlife have controlled and apparently eliminated fox rabies in much of western Europe as well as the variant associated with coyotes and dogs introduced into Texas from Mexico (65, 110, 123). A recombinant rabies virus vaccine for raccoons is now being used in ORV campaigns in the United States. The vaccine vector is the Copenhagen strain of vaccinia virus; the glycoprotein of rabies virus is inserted in the thymidine kinase region of the virus (109). Development of oral rabies vaccines continues as additional recombinant and attenuated viruses are developed (72, 73, 119). These novel vaccines under development may provide a better immune response, greater safety, and higher efficacy in a broader range of species than currently available oral rabies vaccines (8).

Domestic Animals

Only two cases of human rabies acquired in the United States since 1980 have been attributable to domestic animals; the exact circumstances of disease transmission were not elucidated (17, 44). Although most rabies cases occur in wild animals, the majority of humans who receive PEP are due to potential exposure from domestic animals (6, 68, 85, 91, 103, 105). This results in a tremendous cost for rabies prevention in domestic animals in the United States, ranging from approximately $500,000 per life saved to billions of dollars (71). While wild animals are more likely than domestic animals to be rabid in the United States, the amount of human contact with domestic animals greatly exceeds that with wild animals. This is especially true for companion species, which are therefore vaccinated to prevent them from acquiring rabies from wild animals and possibly transmitting it to humans. Hundreds of domestic animals acquire rabies from wild animals every year in the United States (469 [2007] to 1,082 [1981] cases reported annually since 1980), which seemingly justifies the recommendation for and cost of vaccinating all dogs and cats. The occurrence of only two indigenously acquired human rabies cases possibly attributable to indigenous pet domestic animals since 1979 as well as the elimination of the canine rabies virus variant responsible for dog-to-dog rabies transmission attests to the success of current prevention measures.

Rabid domestic animals accounted for only 6.6% of all rabies cases reported in 2007. Rabid cats that were reported represented approximately three times as many dogs reported and nearly five times as many cattle reported. The majority of cases in cats were reported from states where the raccoon rabies virus variant is enzootic. In fact, although the dog is probably the domestic animal most commonly associated with rabies in popular thought, reported cases of rabies in cats have outnumbered those in dogs during all but 1 of the past 27 years. During 2007, most of the reported

27

rabid cats were from states affected by the raccoon rabies epizootic, and a total of 29 states, Washington, DC, and Puerto Rico reported at least one rabid cat. Dogs were the second most commonly reported rabid domestic animal in 2007. Cattle were the third most commonly reported rabid domestic animal (57 cases), having lost their prior dominance in the 1980s, as skunk rabies has continued to decline in the north- and south central states. The 93 reported cases of rabies in dogs were presumably all due to spillover from the local terrestrial reservoir in the geographic region where the dog was exposed. Although Texas historically has reported higher numbers of rabid dogs, the successful elimination of the dog-coyote variant in south Texas through ORV has resulted in dramatic declines in numbers of reported rabid dogs. During earlier years, most cases of rabies in dogs were reported from south Texas and were the result of the epizootic of dog-coyote rabies that reemerged in the late 1970s and early 1980s. This had been the only area in the United States where dog-to-dog (enzootic) transmission of rabies was still reported. In 2007, cases of rabies in 57 other domestic animals, mainly horses, sheep, and goats, were reported (Table 1) (9). Monoclonal antibody and genetic analyses of rabies virus isolates from rabid domestic animals have demonstrated that these animals are almost always infected by the dominant terrestrial wildlife reservoir (101, 115).

RABIES OUTSIDE THE UNITED STATES

Dogs are the major reservoir of rabies in most developing countries of Asia, Africa, and Central and South America. In these countries, rabid dogs are responsible for tens of thousands of human rabies-related deaths each year (124). Rates of PEP in developing countries are about 10 times higher than those in the United States, and rates of human rabies are approximately 100 times higher (11). Due to underreporting and poor surveillance, especially in developing countries where rabies

has its highest burden, it is difficult to estimate accurately the number of cases globally. However, the World Health Organization (WHO) estimates that there are more than 55,000 human rabies cases each year worldwide, mostly in Asia and Africa, where infection is presumably due to exposure to circulating canine rabies virus variants (124).

In addition to dogs and the wild animal species discussed above, other important global rabies reservoirs include vampire bats *(Desmodus rotundus)* and mongooses *(H. javanicus)* (in much of Latin America and the Caribbean, respectively), red foxes *(V. vulpes)* and raccoon dogs *(Nyctereutes procyonoides)* (in Europe), black-backed jackals *(Canis mesomelas)* and yellow mongooses *(Cynictis penicillata)* (in southern Africa), and wolves *(Canis lupus)* (in Iran and Turkey). In addition to these reservoirs of *Rabies virus,* several species of bats outside the Western Hemisphere circulate additional lyssaviruses that cause rabies. Currently, seven species of lyssavirus and four putative species have been identified in Europe, Africa, Asia, and Australia. Most are maintained in chiropteran (bat) hosts. While *Rabies virus* remains the predominant species of lyssavirus responsible for human infection and commercially available rabies vaccines appear to be cross-reactive against several lyssaviruses, human cases attributable to some of these species have occurred (Australian bat virus, Duvenhage virus, European bat lyssaviruses 1 and 2, and Mokola virus), and the more divergent species have shown limited or no cross-reactivity to commercial rabies vaccines (i.e., Lagos bat virus, Mokola virus, and west Caucasian bat virus) (81, 99, 117).

PREVENTION OF HUMAN RABIES

The marked decrease in the number of human rabies cases in the United States since 1950 has been the direct result of the control of canine rabies. The introduction of potent, safe, and efficacious tissue culture-derived vaccines in the 1980s served to further supplement an already effective public health infrastructure.

Four human rabies cases that occurred between 1964 and 1970 were definitely attributable to exposure during recreational activities. All involved children sleeping (camping) or playing outdoors. Three were bitten by skunks, and the fourth was bitten by an unknown animal (4, 80, 82, 121). No human cases definitely known to be associated with recreational activities in the United States have been reported since 1970. Despite the lack of human rabies cases associated with leisure activities, reported mass exposure events in public spaces during recreational activities have increasingly been reported in the United States. The largest mass exposure event reported in the United States involved a rabid kitten sold in a pet store in New Hampshire in 1994. After potential contacts with the kitten were investigated, 665 persons received PEP (53). Additional recent mass exposure events have taken place in petting zoos, in public parks, at sporting tournaments, and at summer camps (54–56, 107). The adoption and importation of animals from abroad while traveling have also been responsible for the importation of canine variants of rabies virus into the United States, with a subsequent risk of reintroducing canine rabies (14, 57, 100). Also, the translocation of wild carnivores within the United States for the purpose of restocking hunting pens has been associated with the long-distance movement of isolated rabies virus variants and subsequent human and animal exposures (60).

In spite of repeated attempts, the remarkable success of the treatment and survival of a 15-year-old girl in 2004 following the clinical onset of rabies has not been repeated (59, 126). Additional evaluation of this potential treatment protocol is needed to determine its potential as a treatment for rabies after the onset of clinical disease. Regardless of future successes of this treatment protocol or of others which might be developed, the relative cost and level of medical sophistication required will continue to limit their use in countries with the highest burden of human rabies.

Routine public health activities consisting of animal rabies control, health communication and education, and preexposure prophylaxis and PEP will remain the most cost-effective methods for preventing human rabies.

Education and Pet Vaccinations

Although only 44 persons are known to have acquired rabies in the United States from 1980 through 2008, tens of thousands of people are exposed each year to animals capable of transmitting the disease. The most effective way to prevent exposure to rabies is to educate the public to avoid contact with all wild and unfamiliar domestic animals. In addition, all pet dogs, cats, and ferrets should be vaccinated against rabies in accordance with state regulations, and wild animals (many of which may be extremely susceptible to rabies) should not be kept as pets (15).

Travelers to countries where canine rabies is enzootic are at increased risk of exposure to rabies and have occasionally developed the disease when they failed to receive advice before departure about the risk of exposure or failed to heed recommendations regarding preexposure vaccination (10). A second opportunity to prevent rabies may be missed when PEP is either not administered or administered incorrectly or to immunocompromised patients (79, 118, 125). In addition, a lack of familiarity with rabies among physicians in developed countries can result in missed diagnoses, especially for patients with a concurrent recreational drug habit which might mask some symptoms, possibly leading to additional cases through organ donation (84, 116).

Because of the high incidence of human rabies and PEP among both residents and visitors in developing countries, travelers to these countries should be advised to avoid contact with dogs and other potential reservoirs of the disease. Persons at risk of possible unavoidable contact with such animals in areas where rabies is enzootic should carefully evaluate possible benefits of preexposure vaccination. In addition, when traveling abroad, especially in countries where rabies is enzootic, travelers should not adopt stray animals without a veterinarian's health assessment and assurance that appropriate vaccinations and precautions have been taken so that importation of an animal with rabies or other zoonotic diseases is prevented. Importation of rabid animals from countries where canine rabies is enzootic continues to challenge the elimination of canine rabies in the United States as well as the rabies status in other developed countries (13, 14, 57, 89, 100).

Evaluation of Possible Exposures of Humans to Rabies

Each year in the United States, as many as 40,000 persons receive rabies PEP (91) and perhaps as many as 20,000 receive preexposure vaccination. Although canine rabies has been eliminated in the United States, the close association and frequent contact between dogs and humans are still the primary reasons for most antirabies prophylaxis (6, 85, 105). Because of the fatal nature of the disease, medical personnel, public health officials, and the person exposed are almost always unwilling to accept even a minute risk of rabies developing in a person who has been bitten by a dog that cannot be observed or tested for rabies. Appropriate management of persons who may have been exposed to rabies requires reasonably rapid interpretation of the risk of infection. Each possible exposure to rabies virus should be evaluated by a physician and in consultation with local or state public health officials when exposure is not clear-cut. In the United States, factors to be considered include the identity of the species to which the patient was exposed, the type and circumstance of the exposure, the local epidemiology of rabies, and, when appropriate, the health and vaccination status of the exposed animal. Direct consultation with local and state health officials becomes even more important under situations in which the supply of rabies biologics is limited or inadequate, in order to prevent

unnecessary and/or inappropriate prophylaxis (9).

Rabies is transmitted only when the virus (present in saliva and nervous tissue) is introduced into open cuts or wounds in skin or mucous membranes. Thus, if the virus could not have been introduced or the material containing the virus was dry, PEP is not necessary. Contact such as petting a rabid animal or contact with the blood, urine, or feces of a rabid animal does not by itself constitute an exposure and is not an indication for prophylaxis.

Types of Exposure

It is useful to differentiate possible exposure into bite and nonbite types. Any penetration of the skin by teeth constitutes a bite exposure. Almost all rabies cases are the result of animal bites. Although bites to the face carry the highest risk, as opposed to bites to the lower extremities, all bites present a potential risk of rabies transmission, and the site of the bite should not influence the decision to administer prophylaxis (50). Once the decision to administer PEP has been made, however, the site of the bite often influences the urgency of such administration.

Contamination of scratches, abrasions, open wounds, or mucous membranes with saliva or other potentially infectious materials (such as nervous tissue) from a rabid animal constitutes nonbite exposures. Although occasional reports of transmission by nonbite exposure suggest that such an exposure is sufficient reason to begin PEP, nonbite exposures rarely cause rabies and are frequently unique and thus defy categorization (1). The limited risk of nonbite exposures (such as scratches and licks) to rabid animals is demonstrated in the unusual nature of human rabies cases that resulted from nonbite exposures. Two types of nonbite exposures have been implicated in the transmission of rabies in humans: those resulting from transplantation and those resulting from unusual aerosol scenarios. Eight cases of rabies in corneal transplant recipients (two each in Thailand, India, and Iran and one each in the United States and France) and seven cases of rabies in whole-organ transplantation (four patients from one donor in the United States and three patients from one donor in Germany) have been reported and represent the only instances of confirmed human-to-human transmission of rabies (50, 84, 87, 116). Retrospective investigations found that each of the cornea and tissue donors had died of an illness compatible with or proved to be rabies. Of the four cases of rabies attributable to aerosol exposures, two were due to infections acquired in rabies research laboratories and two were attributed to infections believed to have been acquired in a cave that was home to tens of millions of bats (58, 66). In addition, two possible cases (not laboratory confirmed) of human-to-human transmission of rabies (one via a bite and one via a kiss) in Ethiopia have been described (76).

Animals Involved in the Exposures

Information about the epidemiology of animal rabies in the geographic area where the exposure occurred is essential for the proper treatment of the patient and prevention of the disease. Exposures to specific domestic and wild animal species are extremely dangerous in some parts of the country and relatively free of risk in other parts. Carnivorous wild animals (especially raccoons, skunks, and foxes) and bats are the animals most often reported to be rabid and were the cause of most of the indigenously acquired cases of human rabies in the United States since 1960. These animals constitute the most important potential source of infection for humans in the United States. All bites by wild carnivores and bats must be evaluated as possible exposures to rabies. The signs of rabies and the period of rabies virus shedding in carnivorous wild animals and bats cannot be interpreted reliably (15); therefore, any such animal that bites or scratches a person should be killed at once (without unnecessary damage to the head), and the brain should be submitted for rabies testing (Fig. 5). If a person is bitten by such an animal, PEP should be initiated promptly but can be delayed if prompt diagnostic testing of the exposure animal is available.

The period of virus shedding in wild animals and the offspring of wild animals crossed with domestic animals is unknown. Such animals should not be kept as pets. When the biting animal is a particularly rare or valuable specimen (e.g., a zoo animal), public health authorities may choose to recommend PEP of the bite victim in lieu of killing the animal for

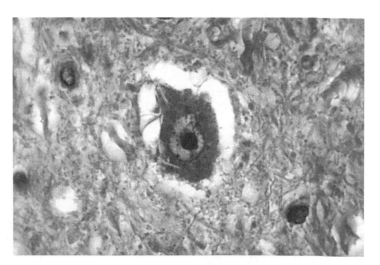

FIGURE 5 Brain biopsy showing Negri bodies, cellular inclusions found most frequently in the pyramidal cells of Ammon's horn and the Purkinje cells of the cerebellum. They are also found in the cells of the medulla and various other ganglia. In addition to the presence of these characteristic histopathologic changes, direct fluorescent antibody testing establishes a specific diagnosis of rabies. Source: CDC/Daniel P. Perl (http://phil.cdc.gov/phil/quicksearch.asp).

rabies testing (15). Since rodents rarely are found to be rabid, state or local health department officials should be consulted before a decision is made to initiate PEP for a person bitten by a rodent because PEP is rarely required.

The likelihood that a domestic animal is infected with rabies varies from region to region; hence, the need for PEP also varies. Because the canine rabies virus variant has been eliminated from the United States, no geographic region is at increased risk due to enzootic dog transmission. However, because of the proficient spillover of the raccoon rabies virus variant to nonreservoir species, a significant proportion of the rabies cases identified in domestic species are located in states where this variant is enzootic. However, overall in the United States, relatively small proportions of tested cats and dogs are found to be positive for rabies: 0.9% and 0.3%, respectively (9). As mentioned above, more cats are routinely reported to be rabid in the United States than dogs. This is possibly a result of less-consistent state vaccination and leash laws for cats, the roaming habits of cats, and the popularity of cats as pets.

A healthy domestic dog, cat, or ferret that bites a person should be confined and observed for 10 days. Any illness in the animal during confinement should be evaluated by a veterinarian and reported immediately to the local health department. If signs suggestive of rabies develop or if the animal is a stray or unwanted, the animal should be killed immediately and the head should be removed and shipped, under refrigeration, to a laboratory for rabies examination (15). If the dog, cat, or ferret is unavailable for observation, other epidemiological factors should be taken into account. An unprovoked attack by a domestic animal is more likely than a provoked attack to indicate that the animal is rabid. Bites inflicted on a person attempting to feed or handle an apparently healthy animal should generally be regarded as provoked. A fully vaccinated dog or cat is very unlikely to be-

come infected with rabies virus. However, rare vaccine failures have been reported for cats and dogs that received only one or two doses of vaccine (51, 74).

Exposures to dogs carry an extremely high risk of rabies in most developing countries (124). For dog and cat exposures that occur in these areas, PEP should be initiated immediately after exposure (PEP can be discontinued if the animal remains healthy during a 10-day observation period). All nine of the U.S. residents who acquired rabies while traveling or living outside the country since 1980 had exposures that were improperly managed. In each case, the victim either did not recognize the risk of rabies or obtained incorrect advice regarding treatment (19, 25, 29, 30, 33, 38, 90, 94, 104). Although dogs are the main reservoir of rabies throughout much of the world, the epizootiology of the disease in other animals differs sufficiently from one region or country to another to warrant the evaluation of all animal bites in these countries.

Rabies PEP

The two essential components of PEP are local treatment of wounds and immunization, including the administration of both rabies immunoglobulin (RIG) and vaccine. Extensive laboratory evidence and field experience in many areas of the world indicate that the combination of local wound treatment and vaccination, including the administration of passive immunization, is uniformly effective when appropriately administered (3, 50). However, rabies occasionally has developed in humans when key elements of PEP were omitted or incorrectly administered. Rabies PEP is a medical urgency, not an emergency; however, prophylaxis should be started as soon as possible after a bite has occurred, especially if there is a strong suspicion of rabies in the biting animal.

The importance of immediate and thorough washing of all bite wounds and scratches with soap and water cannot be overemphasized, since it may, in itself, be one of the most effective measures for preventing rabies; tetanus prophylaxis and measures to control bacterial infection should be given as necessary. In experimental animals, simple local wound cleansing has been shown to markedly reduce the likelihood of rabies (69). The decision to suture large wounds should take into account the potential for inoculating rabies virus more deeply into the wound, the possibility of bacterial infections, and cosmetic factors.

PEP, consisting of the local and systemic administration of RIG and vaccine, is recommended for both bite and nonbite exposures regardless of the interval between exposure and initiation of PEP. Despite an average incubation period of 1 to 3 months, there have been instances in which the decision to begin PEP was made many months after the exposure because of a delay in recognizing that an exposure had occurred and awareness that incubation periods of more than 1 year have been reported, albeit rarely (113).

A variety of cell substrates have been used to produce modern cell culture rabies vaccines (12). In addition, production standards and potency have been defined by the WHO to ensure the production of quality rabies vaccines. The human diploid-cell vaccine (HDCV) was the first modern cell culture-based rabies vaccine, first licensed in the United States in 1980. Purified chick embryo cell rabies vaccine (PCEC) and purified Vero cell rabies vaccine represent the next generation of cell culture-based rabies vaccines following the development of HDCV. In addition, purified duck embryo vaccine is another modern rabies vaccine which has recently been transferred for manufacture in India (97).

Rabies PEP should be administered by one of the routes and schedules evaluated by the WHO and approved by national authorities to ensure the high efficacy achievable with modern rabies biologics. The Essen regimen is considered the standard intramuscular PEP schedule in many countries, including the United States. The Essen (or five-dose sched-

ule) consists of five doses of rabies vaccine administered intramuscularly (i.m.) on days 0, 3, 7, 14, and 28 into the deltoid region in addition to RIG administered on day 0 (50). The Zagreb schedule is another i.m. schedule used in some parts of Europe. It calls for two i.m. doses of vaccine on day 0, followed by one dose on days 7 and 21. In addition to these i.m. schedules, two multisite intradermal regimens have been reviewed and are commonly used in countries with a high burden of human rabies exposure. The Thai Red Cross schedule is used primarily in Thailand, Sri Lanka, and the Philippines. It consists of two intradermal doses (0.1 ml) of vaccine on days 0, 3, 7, and 28, usually given in the right and left upper arms. The Oxford (or eight-site intradermal) regimen is another intradermal regimen which has not been as widely implemented. It consists of eight intradermal doses on day 0 (0.1-ml doses administered to the upper arms, lateral thighs, suprascapular region, and lower abdomen), followed by four doses on day 7 (upper arms and lateral thighs) and one dose on days 28 and 90 (upper arm) (12). Intradermal regimens are frequently used in developing countries with a high incidence of human rabies so that limited and costly supplies of vaccine can be more efficiently used and because of the more rapid immunological response of these schedules due to the often very limited supply of RIG (106).

Nervous tissue vaccines (NTVs) produced from brain tissue of rabies virus-infected sheep, goats, or mice are still in use in some developing countries but fortunately are being rapidly replaced by modern cell culture vaccines. A high rate of adverse reactions has been associated with NTVs, and all have been found to be reactogenic, as well as to have low immunogenicity. The use of NTVs has been discouraged by the WHO (124).

HDCV and PCEC represent the only two rabies vaccines currently licensed in the United States and are approved for i.m. administration by the Essen regimen (50). For adults, the vaccine should always be administered in the deltoid area. For children, the outer aspect of the thigh is also acceptable. The gluteal area should never be used for vaccine injections because administration in this area results in lower neutralizing-antibody titers. Also, vaccine should never be administered at the same site or in the same syringe as RIG.

Human RIG (HRIG) is the only form of RIG available in the United States (equine RIG is not licensed for use in the United States, though it may be the only available form internationally). RIG is administered only once, at the beginning of PEP, to provide immediate antibodies until the patient responds to the vaccine by active production of antibodies. If RIG was not given when vaccination was begun, it can be given through the 7th day of the PEP schedule. After the 7th day, RIG is not indicated, since an antibody response to cell culture vaccine is presumed to have occurred and administration of RIG could interfere with active antibody production. The recommended dose of HRIG is 20 IU/kg of body weight. This concentration is applicable for all age groups, including children. As much of the dose of RIG as is anatomically feasible should be thoroughly infiltrated in the area around the wound, and the remainder should be administered i.m. at a site distal to the site of vaccine administration. The gluteal area is no longer considered optimal for HRIG administration. HRIG should never be administered in the same syringe or in the same anatomical site as the vaccine. Because HRIG may partially suppress active production of antibody, no more than the recommended dose should be given (50).

PEP for persons who have been previously vaccinated should receive two i.m. doses (1.0 ml each) of vaccine; one dose should be administered as soon as possible after exposure and the second dose 3 days later. In such cases, "previously vaccinated" refers to persons who previously received one of the recommended preexposure or postexposure regimens of HDCV or PCEC or who received another regimen or biologic and have a recently documented rabies virus antibody titer. RIG is unnecessary and should not be given in these cases because an anamnestic antibody response will follow the administration of a booster regardless of the prebooster antibody titer (77).

Primary, or Preexposure, Vaccination

Preexposure vaccination should be offered to persons in high-risk groups, such as veterinarians, animal handlers, and certain laboratory workers. Other persons whose activities bring them into frequent contact with rabies virus or with potentially rabid carnivores or bats and persons visiting areas where canine rabies is enzootic should also be considered for preexposure vaccination (50). Persons whose hobbies or vocations regularly bring them into frequent contact with rabies virus-infected or potentially rabid dogs, cats, skunks, raccoons, bats, or other species should also be considered for preexposure vaccination. However, preexposure vaccination is not recommended for hunters and other outdoor enthusiasts who may occasionally be exposed to the disease. These persons should be able to recognize exposures and report them to medical authorities, and such exposures are rare enough that the cost of administering preexposure vaccination to the entire group at risk almost always exceeds that of administering PEP to those exposed (98). Administration of preexposure vaccination to persons traveling to areas where rabies is enzootic is not strictly cost beneficial (5) but may be considered for persons whose travel might involve contact with animals or where PEP may be unavailable or not easily accessed. Although preexposure vaccination does not preclude the need for additional therapy after a rabies exposure, it simplifies therapy by eliminating the need for RIG and decreasing the number of doses of vaccine required after an exposure. Moreover, in many areas where rabies is enzootic, products for immunizing against rabies may not be available or the available product may carry a high risk of adverse reactions; thus, preexposure vaccination might be prudent when traveling to such areas.

The regimen for preexposure vaccination consists of three 1.0-ml doses (0.5 ml for purified Vero cell rabies vaccine) given i.m. in the deltoid area on days 0, 7, and 21 or 28 (50). Serologic testing is not routinely necessary except for certain high-risk-occupation groups (rabies laboratory workers and veterinarians in areas where rabies is enzootic) and persons who are immunocompromised. Persons who work with live rabies virus in research laboratories or vaccine production facilities are at the highest risk of inapparent exposures and therefore should submit a serum sample for rabies antibody testing every 6 months. Booster doses of vaccine should be given as needed to maintain a serum titer corresponding to at least complete neutralization at a 1:5 serum dilution by the rapid-fluorescence focus inhibition test. Other laboratory workers (such as those doing rabies diagnostic testing), spelunkers, veterinarians and their staff, and animal control and wildlife officers in areas where terrestrial rabies is enzootic should have a serum sample tested for rabies antibody every 2 years. Veterinarians, animal control workers, and wildlife officers working in areas of low rabies enzooticity do not require routine testing and booster doses of vaccine following completion of primary preexposure vaccination (50).

SUMMARY

Although terrestrial rabies is enzootic across most of the United States, there have been few human infections involving variants of rabies virus associated with terrestrial reservoirs since 1980. No recreationally (or vocationally) associated human rabies cases are known to have occurred since 1977, when a laboratory worker developed rabies following an accident in a research facility (58). However, mass exposure to rabies during recreational activities at public event spaces has become more common over the past few decades. Insectivorous bats are now associated with the majority of human cases of rabies reported in the United States. Available information is sometimes conflicting because of missing details and subsequent interpretations. However, most of these cases appear to have been largely unpreventable, as no medical advice was sought by the persons exposed. Although wild animals have not been involved in most human rabies virus infections since 1980, the large number of wild animals reported rabid each year serves as a reminder of the potential threat that rabies in these animals poses to the naïve camper, hiker, or other outdoor enthusiast. Persons in the United States should be advised to avoid contact with wild animals, especially bats, and stray or unknown domestic animals.

In developing countries, enzootic canine rabies is the most serious threat to Americans. Travelers to such countries can substantially reduce the risk of rabies exposure by avoiding all dogs and wild animals. Americans planning to travel to or reside in countries where canine rabies is enzootic should be informed about the risk of rabies and consider the possible benefits of rabies preexposure vaccination.

PRACTICAL TIPS

- Appropriate behavior around unfamiliar animals reduces the risk of exposure to rabies. Avoid contact with wild animals, and vaccinate companion animals.
- Bats may represent a higher risk of rabies exposure to humans due to the minor wounds inflicted by their teeth compared to those of other carnivores. Direct contact with a bat should be evaluated by a physician or public health official if a person is uncertain if a bite could have occurred.
- The highest risk of rabies exposure remains in countries where canine rabies has not been controlled.
- Rabies is preventable if proper action is taken after a potential exposure; proper action consists of wound washing and timely and appropriate administration of RIG and vaccine according to an approved schedule.

REFERENCES
1. **Afshar, A.** 1979. A review of non-bite transmission of rabies virus infection. *Br. Vet. J.* **135:** 142–148.

2. **Anderson, L. J., K. G. Nicholson, R. V. Tauxe, and W. G. Winkler.** 1984. Human rabies in the United States, 1960 to 1979: epidemiology, diagnosis, and prevention. *Ann. Intern. Med.* **100:**728–735.

3. **Anderson, L. J., R. K. Sikes, C. W. Langkop, J. M. Mann, J. S. Smith, W. G. Winkler, and M. W. Deitch.** 1980. Postexposure trial of a human diploid cell strain rabies vaccine. *J. Infect. Dis.* **142:**133–138.

4. **Bell, G. R.** 1967. Death from rabies in a ten-year-old boy (one of two cases in United States in 1966). *S. D. J. Med.* **20:**28–29.

5. **Bernard, K. W., and D. B. Fishbein.** 1991. Pre-exposure rabies prophylaxis for travellers: are the benefits worth the cost? *Vaccine* **9:**833–836.

6. **Blanton, J. D., N. Y. Bowden, M. Eidson, J. D. Wyatt, and C. A. Hanlon.** 2005. Rabies postexposure prophylaxis, New York, 1995–2000. *Emerg. Infect. Dis.* **11:**1921–1927.

7. **Blanton, J. D., C. A. Hanlon, and C. E. Rupprecht.** 2007. Rabies surveillance in the United States during 2006. *J. Am. Vet. Med. Assoc.* **231:**540–556.

8. **Blanton, J. D., A. Meadows, S. M. Murphy, J. Manangan, C. A. Hanlon, M. L. Faber, B. Dietzschold, and C. E. Rupprecht.** 2006. Vaccination of small Asian mongoose (Herpestes javanicus) against rabies. *J. Wildl. Dis.* **42:**663–666.

9. **Blanton, J. D., D. Palmer, K. Christian, and C. E. Rupprecht.** 2008. Rabies surveillance in the United States during 2007. *J. Am. Vet. Med. Assoc.* **233:**884–897.

10. **Blanton, J. D., and C. E. Rupprecht.** 2008. Travel vaccination for rabies. *Expert. Rev. Vaccines* **7:**613–620.

11. **Bogel, K., and E. Motschwiller.** 1986. Incidence of rabies and post-exposure treatment in developing countries. *Bull. W. H. O.* **64:**883–887.

12. **Briggs, D. J.** 2007. Human rabies vaccines, p. 505–515. *In* A. C. Jackson and W. H. Wunner (ed.), *Rabies*, 2nd ed. Academic Press, London, United Kingdom.

13. **Briggs, D. J., and K. Schweitzer.** 2001. Importation of dogs and cats to rabies-free areas of the world. *Vet. Clin. N. Am. Small Anim. Pract.* **31:**573–583, viii.

14. **Castrodale, L., V. Walker, J. Baldwin, C. Hofmann, and C. Hanlon.** 2008. Rabies in a puppy imported from India to the USA, March 2007. *Zoonoses Public Health* **55:**427–430.

15. **CDC.** 2008. Compendium of animal rabies prevention and control, 2008: National Association of State Public Health Veterinarians, Inc. (NASPHV). *MMWR Recommend. Rep.* **57:**1–9.

16. **CDC.** 2003. First human death associated with raccoon rabies—Virginia, 2003. *MMWR Morb. Mortal. Wkly. Rep.* **52:**1102–1103.

17. **CDC.** 1995. Human rabies—Alabama, Tennessee, and Texas, 1994. *MMWR Morb. Mortal. Wkly. Rep.* **44:**269–272.

18. **CDC.** 1988. Human rabies—California, 1987. *MMWR Morb. Mortal. Wkly. Rep.* **37:**305–308.

19. **CDC.** 1992. Human rabies—California, 1992. *MMWR Morb. Mortal. Wkly. Rep.* **41:**461–463.

20. **CDC.** 1994. Human rabies—California, 1994. *MMWR Morb. Mortal. Wkly. Rep.* **43:**455–458.

21. **CDC.** 1996. Human rabies—California, 1995. *MMWR Morb. Mortal. Wkly. Rep.* **45:**353–356.

22. **CDC.** 2002. Human rabies—California, 2002. *MMWR Morb. Mortal. Wkly. Rep.* **51:**686–688.

23. **CDC.** 2000. Human rabies—California, Georgia, Minnesota, New York, and Wisconsin, 2000. *MMWR Morb. Mortal. Wkly. Rep.* **49:**1111–1115.

24. **CDC.** 1996. Human rabies—Florida, 1996. *MMWR Morb. Mortal. Wkly. Rep.* **45:**719–720, 727.

25. **CDC.** 2005. Human rabies—Florida, 2004. *MMWR Morb. Mortal. Wkly. Rep.* **54:**767–768.

26. **CDC.** 2007. Human rabies—Indiana and California, 2006. *MMWR Morb. Mortal. Wkly. Rep.* **56:**361–365.

27. **CDC.** 2003. Human rabies—Iowa, 2002. *MMWR Morb. Mortal. Wkly. Rep.* **52:**47–48.

28. **CDC.** 1997. Human rabies—Kentucky and Montana 1996. *MMWR Morb. Mortal. Wkly. Rep.* **46:**397–400.

29. **CDC.** 1983. Human rabies—Kenya. *MMWR Morb. Mortal. Wkly. Rep.* **32:**494–495.

30. **CDC.** 1994. Human rabies—Miami, 1994. *MMWR Morb. Mortal. Wkly. Rep.* **43:**773–775.

31. **CDC.** 1983. Human rabies—Michigan. *MMWR Morb. Mortal. Wkly. Rep.* **32:**159–160.

32. **CDC.** 1997. Human rabies—Montana and Washington, 1997. *MMWR Morb. Mortal. Wkly. Rep.* **46:**770–774.

33. **CDC.** 1997. Human rabies—New Hampshire, 1996. *MMWR Morb. Mortal. Wkly. Rep.* **46:**267–270.

34. **CDC.** 1993. Human rabies—New York, 1993. *MMWR Morb. Mortal. Wkly. Rep.* **42:**799, 806.

35. **CDC.** 1981. Human rabies—Oklahoma. *MMWR Morb. Mortal. Wkly. Rep.* **30:**343–344, 349.

36. **CDC.** 1989. Human rabies—Oregon, 1989. *MMWR Morb. Mortal. Wkly. Rep.* **38:**335–337.

37. **CDC.** 1984. Human rabies—Pennsylvania. *MMWR Morb. Mortal. Wkly. Rep.* **33:**633–635.

38. **CDC.** 1982. Human rabies—Rwanda. *MMWR Morb. Mortal. Wkly. Rep.* **31:**135.

39. **CDC.** 2002. Human rabies—Tennessee, 2002. *MMWR Morb. Mortal. Wkly. Rep.* **51:**828–829.

40. **CDC.** 1984. Human rabies—Texas. *MMWR Morb. Mortal. Wkly. Rep.* **33**:469–470.

41. **CDC.** 1994. Human rabies—Texas and California, 1993. *MMWR Morb. Mortal. Wkly. Rep.* **43**:93–96.

42. **CDC.** 1998. Human rabies—Texas and New Jersey, 1997. *MMWR Morb. Mortal. Wkly. Rep.* **47**:1–5.

43. **CDC.** 1991. Human rabies—Texas, 1990. *MMWR Morb. Mortal. Wkly. Rep.* **40**:132–133.

44. **CDC.** 1991. Human rabies—Texas, Arkansas, and Georgia, 1991. *MMWR Morb. Mortal. Wkly. Rep.* **40**:765–769.

45. **CDC.** 1999. Human rabies—Virginia, 1998. *MMWR Morb. Mortal. Wkly. Rep.* **48**:95–97.

46. **CDC.** 1995. Human rabies—Washington, 1995. *MMWR Morb. Mortal. Wkly. Rep.* **44**:625–627.

47. **CDC.** 1995. Human rabies—West Virginia, 1994. *MMWR Morb. Mortal. Wkly. Rep.* **44**:86–87, 93.

48. **CDC.** 1985. Human rabies acquired outside the United States. *MMWR Morb. Mortal. Wkly. Rep.* **34**:235–236.

49. **CDC.** 1985. Human rabies diagnosed 2 months postmortem—Texas. *MMWR Morb. Mortal. Wkly. Rep.* **34**:700, 705–707.

50. **CDC.** 2008. Human rabies prevention—United States, 2008: recommendations of the Advisory Committee on Immunization Practices. *MMWR Recommend. Rep.* **57**:1–28.

51. **CDC.** 1988. Imported dog and cat rabies—New Hampshire, California. *MMWR Morb. Mortal. Wkly. Rep.* **37**:559–560.

52. **CDC.** 1983. Imported human rabies. *MMWR Morb. Mortal. Wkly. Rep.* **32**:78–80, 85–86.

53. **CDC.** 1995. Mass treatment of humans exposed to rabies—New Hampshire, 1994. *MMWR Morb. Mortal. Wkly. Rep.* **44**:484–486.

54. **CDC.** 1999. Public health response to a potentially rabid bear cub—Iowa, 1999. *MMWR Morb. Mortal. Wkly. Rep.* **48**:971–973.

55. **CDC.** 2008. Public health response to a rabid kitten—four states, 2007. *MMWR Morb. Mortal. Wkly. Rep.* **56**:1337–1340.

56. **CDC.** 2002. Rabies in a beaver—Florida, 2001. *MMWR Morb. Mortal. Wkly. Rep.* **51**:481–482.

57. **CDC.** 2008. Rabies in a dog imported from Iraq—New Jersey, June 2008. *MMWR Morb. Mortal. Wkly. Rep.* **57**:1076–1078.

58. **CDC.** 1977. Rabies in a laboratory worker—New York. *MMWR Morb. Mortal. Wkly. Rep.* **26**:183–184.

59. **CDC.** 2004. Recovery of a patient from clinical rabies—Wisconsin, 2004. *MMWR Morb. Mortal. Wkly. Rep.* **53**:1171–1173.

60. **CDC.** 1995. Translocation of coyote rabies—Florida, 1994. *MMWR Morb. Mortal. Wkly. Rep.* **44**:580–581, 587.

61. **CDC.** 2000. Update: raccoon rabies epizootic—United States and Canada, 1999. *MMWR Morb. Mortal. Wkly. Rep.* **49**:31–35.

62. **Chang, H. G., M. Eidson, C. Noonan–Toly, C. V. Trimarchi, R. Rudd, B. J. Wallace, P. F. Smith, and D. L. Morse.** 2002. Public health impact of reemergence of rabies, New York. *Emerg. Infect. Dis.* **8**:909–913.

63. **Charlton, K. M., W. A. Webster, G. A. Casey, and C. E. Rupprecht.** 1988. Skunk rabies. *Rev. Infect. Dis.* **10**(Suppl. 4):S626–S628.

64. **Childs, J. E., L. Colby, J. W. Krebs, T. Strine, M. Feller, D. Noah, C. Drenzek, J. S. Smith, and C. E. Rupprecht.** 1997. Surveillance and spatiotemporal associations of rabies in rodents and lagomorphs in the United States, 1985–1994. *J. Wildl. Dis.* **33**:20–27.

65. **Cliquet, F., and M. Aubert.** 2004. Elimination of terrestrial rabies in Western European countries. *Dev. Biol.* (Basel) **119**:185–204.

66. **Constantine, D. G.** 1962. Rabies transmission by nonbite route. *Public Health Rep.* **77**:287–289.

67. **Constantine, D. G.** 1979. An updated list of rabies-infected bats in North America. *J. Wildl. Dis.* **15**:347–349.

68. **Conti, L., S. Wiersma, and R. Hopkins.** 2002. Evaluation of state-provided postexposure prophylaxis against rabies in Florida. *South. Med. J.* **95**:225–230.

69. **Dean, D., M. K. Abelseth, and P. Atanasiu.** 1996. The fluorescent antibody test, 4th ed. World Health Organization, Geneva, Switzerland.

70. **Devriendt, J., M. Staroukine, F. Costy, and J. J. Vanderhaeghen.** 1982. Fatal encephalitis apparently due to rabies. Occurrence after treatment with human diploid cell vaccine but not rabies immune globulin. *JAMA* **248**:2304–2306.

71. **Dhankhar, P., S. A. Vaidya, D. B. Fishbien, and M. I. Meltzer.** 2008. Cost effectiveness of rabies post exposure prophylaxis in the United States. *Vaccine* **26**:4251–4255.

72. **Dietzschold, B., and M. J. Schnell.** 2002. New approaches to the development of live attenuated rabies vaccines. *Hybrid. Hybridomics* **21**:129–134.

73. **Dietzschold, M. L., M. Faber, J. A. Mattis, K. Y. Pak, M. J. Schnell, and B. Dietzschold.** 2004. In vitro growth and stability of recombinant rabies viruses designed for vaccination of wildlife. *Vaccine* **23**:518–524.

74. **Eng, T. R., D. B. Fishbein, et al.** 1990. Epidemiologic factors, clinical findings, and vaccination status of rabies in cats and dogs in the United States in 1988. *J. Am. Vet. Med. Assoc.* **197**:201–209.

75. **Everard, C. O., and J. D. Everard.** 1992. Mongoose rabies in the Caribbean. *Ann. N. Y. Acad. Sci.* **653**:356–366.

76. **Fekadu, M., T. Endeshaw, W. Alemu, Y. Bogale, T. Teshager, and J. G. Olson.** 1996. Possible human-to-human transmission of rabies in Ethiopia. *Ethiop. Med. J.* **34:**123–127.

77. **Fishbein, D. B., K. W. Bernard, K. D. Miller, T. Van der Vlugt, C. E. Gains, J. T. Bell, J. W. Sumner, F. L. Reid, R. A. Parker, J. T. Horman, et al.** 1986. The early kinetics of the neutralizing antibody response after booster immunizations with human diploid cell rabies vaccine. *Am. J. Trop. Med. Hyg.* **35:** 663–670.

78. **Foroutan, P., M. I. Meltzer, and K. A. Smith.** 2002. Cost of distributing oral raccoon-variant rabies vaccine in Ohio: 1997–2000. *J. Am. Vet. Med. Assoc.* **220:**27–32.

79. **Gacouin, A., H. Bourhy, J. C. Renaud, C. Camus, E. Suprin, and R. Thomas.** 1999. Human rabies despite postexposure vaccination. *Eur. J. Clin. Microbiol. Infect. Dis.* **18:**233–235.

80. **Gomez, M. R., R. G. Siekert, and E. C. Herrmann.** 1965. A human case of skunk rabies. Case report with comment on virological studies and the prophylactic treatment. *JAMA* **194:**333–335.

81. **Hanlon, C. A., I. V. Kuzmin, J. D. Blanton, W. C. Weldon, J. S. Manangan, and C. E. Rupprecht.** 2005. Efficacy of rabies biologics against new lyssaviruses from Eurasia. *Virus Res.* **111:**44–54.

82. **Hattwick, M. A., F. H. Hochberg, P. J. Landrigan, and M. B. Gregg.** 1972. Skunk-associated human rabies. *JAMA* **222:**44–47.

83. **Held, J. R., E. S. Tierkel, and J. H. Steele.** 1967. Rabies in man and animals in the United States, 1946–65. *Public Health Rep.* **82:**1009–1018.

84. **Hellenbrand, W., C. Meyer, G. Rasch, I. Steffens, and A. Ammon.** 2005. Cases of rabies in Germany following organ transplantation. *Euro Surveill.* **10:**E0502246.

85. **Helmick, C. G.** 1983. The epidemiology of human rabies postexposure prophylaxis, 1980–1981. *JAMA* **250:**1990–1996.

86. **Humphrey, G. L., G. E. Kemp, and E. G. Wood.** 1960. A fatal case of rabies in a woman bitten by an insectivorous bat. *Public Health Rep.* **75:**317–326.

87. **Javadi, M. A., A. Fayaz, S. A. Mirdehghan, and B. Ainollahi.** 1996. Transmission of rabies by corneal graft. *Cornea* **15:**431–433.

88. **Jenkins, S. R., and W. G. Winkler.** 1987. Descriptive epidemiology from an epizootic of raccoon rabies in the Middle Atlantic states, 1982–1983. *Am. J. Epidemiol.* **126:**429–437.

89. **Jones, R. D., L. Kelly, A. R. Fooks, and M. Wooldridge.** 2005. Quantitative risk assessment of rabies entering Great Britain from North America via cats and dogs. *Risk Anal.* **25:**533–542.

90. **Krebs, J. W., R. C. Holman, U. Hines, T. W. Strine, E. J. Mandel, and J. E. Childs.** 1992. Rabies surveillance in the United States during 1991. *J. Am. Vet. Med. Assoc.* **201:** 1836–1848.

91. **Krebs, J. W., S. C. Long-Marin, and J. E. Childs.** 1998. Causes, costs, and estimates of rabies postexposure prophylaxis treatments in the United States. *J. Public Health Manag. Pract.* **4:** 56–62.

92. **Krebs, J. W., E. J. Mandel, D. L. Swerdlow, and C. E. Rupprecht.** 2005. Rabies surveillance in the United States during 2004. *J. Am. Vet. Med. Assoc.* **227:**1912–1925.

93. **Krebs, J. W., A. M. Mondul, C. E. Rupprecht, and J. E. Childs.** 2001. Rabies surveillance in the United States during 2000. *J. Am. Vet. Med. Assoc.* **219:**1687–1699.

94. **Krebs, J. W., H. R. Noll, C. E. Rupprecht, and J. E. Childs.** 2002. Rabies surveillance in the United States during 2001. *J. Am. Vet. Med. Assoc.* **221:**1690–1701.

95. **Leslie, M., S. L. Messenger, R. E. Rohde, J. S. Smith, R. Cheshier, C. A. Hanlon, and C. E. Rupprecht.** 2006. Bat-associated rabies virus in skunks. *Emerg. Infect. Dis.* **12:** 1274–1277.

96. **MacInnes, C. D., S. M. Smith, R. R. Tinline, N. R. Ayers, P. Bachmann, D. G. Ball, L. A. Calder, S. J. Crosgrey, C. Fielding, P. Hauschildt, J. M. Honig, D. H. Johnston, K. F. Lawson, C. P. Nunan, M. A. Pedde, B. Pond, R. B. Stewart, and D. R. Voigt.** 2001. Elimination of rabies from red foxes in eastern Ontario. *J. Wildl. Dis.* **37:** 119–132.

97. **Mahendra, B. J., S. N. Madhusudana, D. H. Ashwathnarayana, G. Sampath, S. S. Datta, M. K. Sudarshan, G. M. Venkatesh, K. Muhamuda, G. Bilagumba, and M. Shamanna.** 2007. A comparative study on the immunogenicity, safety and tolerance of purified duck embryo vaccine (PDEV) manufactured in India (Vaxirab) and Switzerland (Lyssavac-N): a randomized simulated post-exposure study in healthy volunteers. *Vaccine* **25:**8405–8409.

98. **Mann, J. M.** 1984. Routine pre-exposure rabies prophylaxis: a reassessment. *Am. J. Public Health* **74:**720–722.

99. **Markotter, W., C. Van Eeden, I. V. Kuzmin, C. E. Rupprecht, J. T. Paweska, R. Swanepoel, A. R. Fooks, C. T. Sabeta, F. Cliquet, and L. H. Nel.** 2008. Epidemiology and pathogenicity of African bat lyssaviruses. *Dev. Biol.* (Basel) **131:**317–325.

100. **McQuiston, J. H., T. Wilson, S. Harris, R. M. Bacon, S. Shapiro, I. Trevino, J. Sinclair, G. Galland, and N. Marano.** 2008.

Importation of dogs into the United States: risks from rabies and other zoonotic diseases. *Zoonoses Public Health* **55:**421–426.

101. **McQuiston, J. H., P. A. Yager, J. S. Smith, and C. E. Rupprecht.** 2001. Epidemiologic characteristics of rabies virus variants in dogs and cats in the United States, 1999. *J. Am. Vet. Med. Assoc.* **218:**1939–1942.

102. **Meltzer, M. I., and C. E. Rupprecht.** 1998. A review of the economics of the prevention and control of rabies. Part 2. Rabies in dogs, livestock and wildlife. *Pharmacoeconomics* **14:**481–498.

103. **Moore, D. A., W. M. Sischo, A. Hunter, and T. Miles.** 2000. Animal bite epidemiology and surveillance for rabies postexposure prophylaxis. *J. Am. Vet. Med. Assoc.* **217:**190–194.

104. **Noah, D. L., C. L. Drenzek, J. S. Smith, J. W. Krebs, L. Orciari, J. Shaddock, D. Sanderlin, S. Whitfield, M. Fekadu, J. G. Olson, C. E. Rupprecht, and J. E. Childs.** 1998. Epidemiology of human rabies in the United States, 1980 to 1996. *Ann. Intern. Med.* **128:**922–930.

105. **O'Bell, S. A., J. McQuiston, L. J. Bell, S. C. Ferguson, and L. A. Williams.** 2006. Human rabies exposures and postexposure prophylaxis in South Carolina, 1993–2002. *Public Health Rep.* **121:**197–202.

106. **Phanuphak, P., P. Khawplod, S. Sirivichayakul, W. Siriprasomsub, S. Ubol, and M. Thaweepathomwat.** 1987. Humoral and cell-mediated immune responses to various economical regimens of purified Vero cell rabies vaccine. *Asian Pac. J. Allergy Immunol.* **5:**33–37.

107. **Robbins, A., M. Eidson, M. Keegan, D. Sackett, and B. Laniewicz.** 2005. Bat incidents at children's camps, New York State, 1998–2002. *Emerg. Infect. Dis.* **11:**302–305.

108. **Rosatte, R., D. Donovan, M. Allan, L. A. Howes, A. Silver, K. Bennett, C. MacInnes, C. Davies, A. Wandeler, and B. Radford.** 2001. Emergency response to raccoon rabies introduction into Ontario. *J. Wildl. Dis.* **37:**265–279.

109. **Rupprecht, C. E., A. N. Hamir, D. H. Johnston, and H. Koprowski.** 1988. Efficacy of a vaccinia-rabies glycoprotein recombinant virus vaccine in raccoons (Procyon lotor). *Rev. Infect. Dis.* **10**(Suppl. 4):S803–S809.

110. **Sidwa, T. J., P. J. Wilson, G. M. Moore, E. H. Oertli, B. N. Hicks, R. E. Rohde, and D. H. Johnston.** 2005. Evaluation of oral rabies vaccination programs for control of rabies epizootics in coyotes and gray foxes: 1995–2003. *J. Am. Vet. Med. Assoc.* **227:**785–792.

111. **Slate, D., C. E. Rupprecht, J. A. Rooney, D. Donovan, D. H. Lein, and R. B. Chipman.** 2005. Status of oral rabies vaccination in wild carnivores in the United States. *Virus Res.* **111:**68–76.

112. **Smith, J. S.** 1989. Rabies virus epitopic variation: use in ecologic studies. *Adv. Virus Res.* **36:**215–253.

113. **Smith, J. S., D. B. Fishbein, C. E. Rupprecht, and K. Clark.** 1991. Unexplained rabies in three immigrants in the United States. A virologic investigation. *N. Engl. J. Med.* **324:**205–211.

114. **Smith, J. S., L. Orciari, and P. Yager.** 1995. Molecular epidemiology of rabies in the United States. *Semin. Virol.* **6:**387–400.

115. **Smith, J. S., L. A. Orciari, P. A. Yager, H. D. Seidel, and C. K. Warner.** 1992. Epidemiologic and historical relationships among 87 rabies virus isolates as determined by limited sequence analysis. *J. Infect. Dis.* **166:**296–307.

116. **Srinivasan, A., E. C. Burton, M. J. Kuehnert, C. Rupprecht, W. L. Sutker, T. G. Ksiazek, C. D. Paddock, J. Guarner, W. J. Shieh, C. Goldsmith, C. A. Hanlon, J. Zoretic, B. Fischbach, M. Niezgoda, W. H. El-Feky, L. Orciari, E. Q. Sanchez, A. Likos, G. B. Klintmalm, D. Cardo, J. LeDuc, M. E. Chamberland, D. B. Jernigan, and S. R. Zaki.** 2005. Transmission of rabies virus from an organ donor to four transplant recipients. *N. Engl. J. Med.* **352:**1103–1111.

117. **Stantic-Pavlinic, M.** 2005. Public health concerns in bat rabies across Europe. *Euro Surveill.* **10:**217–220.

118. **Tantawichien, T., W. Jaijaroensup, P. Khawplod, and V. Sitprija.** 2001. Failure of multiple-site intradermal postexposure rabies vaccination in patients with human immunodeficiency virus with low CD4+ T lymphocyte counts. *Clin. Infect. Dis.* **33:**E122–E124.

119. **Tordo, N., A. Foumier, C. Jallet, M. Szelechowski, B. Klonjkowski, and M. Eloit.** 2008. Canine adenovirus based rabies vaccines. *Dev. Biol.* (Basel) **131:**467–476.

120. **Uhaa, I. J., V. M. Dato, F. E. Sorhage, J. W. Beckley, D. E. Roscoe, R. D. Gorsky, and D. B. Fishbein.** 1992. Benefits and costs of using an orally absorbed vaccine to control rabies in raccoons. *J. Am. Vet. Med. Assoc.* **201:**1873–1882.

121. **Uhaa, I. J., E. J. Mandel, R. Whiteway, and D. B. Fishbein.** 1992. Rabies surveillance in the United States during 1990. *J. Am. Vet. Med. Assoc.* **200:**920–929.

122. **Velasco-Villa, A., L. A. Orciari, V. Souza, V. Juarez-Islas, M. Gomez-Sierra, A. Castillo, A. Flisser, and C. E. Rupprecht.** 2005. Molecular epizootiology of rabies associated

with terrestrial carnivores in Mexico. *Virus Res.* **111:**13–27.

123. **Wandeler, A. I., S. Capt, A. Kappeler, and R. Hauser.** 1988. Oral immunization of wildlife against rabies: concept and first field experiments. *Rev. Infect. Dis.* **10**(Suppl. 4)**:**S649–S653.

124. **WHO.** 2005. *WHO expert consultation on rabies. First report,* p. 121. WHO Tech. Rep. Ser. 931. WHO, Geneva, Switzerland.

125. **Wilde, H., S. Sirikawin, A. Sabcharoen, D. Kingnate, T. Tantawichien, P. A. Harischandra, N. Chaiyabutr, D. G. de Silva, L. Fernando, J. B. Liyanage, and V. Sitprija.** 1996. Failure of postexposure treatment of rabies in children. *Clin. Infect. Dis.* **22:**228–232.

126. **Willoughby, R. E., Jr., K. S. Tieves, G. M. Hoffman, N. S. Ghanayem, C. M. Amlie-Lefond, M. J. Schwabe, M. J. Chusid, and C. E. Rupprecht.** 2005. Survival after treatment of rabies with induction of coma. *N. Engl. J. Med.* **352:**2508–2514.

127. **Wyatt, J. D., W. H. Barker, N. M. Bennett, and C. A. Hanlon.** 1999. Human rabies postexposure prophylaxis during a raccoon rabies epizootic in New York, 1993 and 1994. *Emerg. Infect. Dis.* **5:**415–423.

SPORTS: THE INFECTIOUS HAZARDS

Arezou Minooee, Leland S. Rickman, and Geeta Gupta

11

Recreational sporting events and organized athletic competitions are popular pastimes of our generation. With a high level of spectator interest in, even reverence towards, national and international games such as the Super Bowl or World Cup, sporting events have become the focus of many societies. Not only is participation in fitness activities enjoyable and sometimes challenging, it is also beneficial to one's health. Still, there are hazards. In addition to risking physical injuries, athletes face the possibility of contracting infectious diseases (2, 15, 16, 22, 49, 49a, 57, 58, 64, 74, 86, 92, 100, 107, 110, 141, 143, 144).

There are several mechanisms by which infectious agents may be spread during sports. The main routes of transmission include direct- and indirect-contact, droplet, common-source, and airborne transmission. Direct-contact transmission involves person-to-person contact in which infectious agents are physically transferred to a susceptible host

from an infected player. Indirect-contact transmission occurs when a susceptible host comes into contact with contaminated objects or fomites, such as equipment, towels, or clothing. A type of indirect contact is droplet transmission, which occurs when large droplets containing infectious agents are generated through coughing, sneezing, or talking and are deposited on the host's conjunctivae, nasal mucosa, or mouth after being propelled in the air a short distance. Common-source transmission happens when infectious agents are transmitted by contaminated items, such as food, water, beverage containers, or other equipment with which multiple people may have had contact. Airborne transmission occurs when extremely small particles called droplet nuclei which contain infectious agents are suspended in the air for long periods and are subsequently inhaled by the susceptible host. Vector-borne diseases are spread by insects, mites, ticks, animals, or other carriers and may pose a risk to the host exposed in areas of endemicity. Table 1 summarizes potential sports-related infectious diseases.

BLOOD-BORNE PATHOGENS

Human Immunodeficiency Virus

The human retrovirus known as human immunodeficiency virus (HIV) is the etiologic agent which leads to the suppression of the

Arezou Minooee, Department of Internal Medicine, University of California Irvine Medical Center, Bldg. 200, Suite 720, 101 The City Dr. S., Orange, CA 92868. *Leland S. Rickman (deceased)*, Epidemiology Unit, Division of Infectious Diseases, University of California, San Diego, San Diego, CA 92103. *Geeta Gupta*, Division of Infectious Diseases, University of California Irvine Medical Center, Route 81, Bldg. 53, Rm. 215, 101 The City Dr. S., Orange, CA 92868.

Infections of Leisure, Fourth Edition, Edited by David Schlossberg,
© 2009 ASM Press, Washington, DC

TABLE 1 Common etiologies of
sports-related infections

Blood-borne infections
HIV infection, AIDS
Hepatitis B
Hepatitis C

Skin infections
Viral infections
   HSV infection
   Molluscum contagiosum
   HPV (warts)
Bacterial infections
   Staphylococcus aureus
   Streptococcus
   Corynebacterium minutissimum
   Pseudomonas aeruginosa
Fungal infections
   Tinea infections

Nonskin infectious syndromes
Conjunctivitis
IM
Meningitis
Upper respiratory tract infections
Vector-borne infections
Water sports-associated transmission[a]

[a]See Table 2 for a list of related infections.

immune system and the development of AIDS (acquired immunodeficiency syndrome). Modes of transmission include sexual contact, parenteral exposure to blood or blood components, contamination of open wounds or mucous membranes by infected blood or body fluids, needle sharing, and perinatal transmission from infected mother to fetus (82). The virus is distributed throughout a variety of bodily fluids but is found in high concentrations in blood (28).

Millions of people worldwide have been affected by HIV and AIDS. In the absence of a cure or vaccine, there is much concern regarding infection during athletic competitions in which bleeding and skin abrasions are common, such as in boxing and football (23, 27, 29, 50, 56, 59, 68, 81, 86a, 102a, 108, 131, 136, 163). Since the initial description of AIDS in 1981, there have been no definitive studies indicating transmission of the virus through sweat, tears, urine, sputum, vomitus, saliva, or respiratory droplets (171, 172).

American football is the one sport for which the potential risk of HIV transmission has been investigated. Based on the frequency of bleeding injuries and player contact observed in one study, the risk of infection was estimated to be less than 1 per 85 million game contacts (26). Athletes actually have a greater probability of becoming infected off the field through unsafe sexual practices and injection of drugs or anabolic steroids. For example, a bodybuilder who injected intramuscular steroids with a shared, unsterilized needle became infected with HIV (138a). Other risk factors were ruled out for this individual.

There has been only one documented case of HIV transmission during sports contact. The report concerned an Italian soccer player who allegedly seroconverted after a bloody head-to-head collision with an HIV-positive individual during a recreational soccer match (162). However, after careful review of the case, health officials were unable to rule out other risk factors to verify the actual mode of transmission (63).

At least two instances of HIV transmission have been reported to be due to fistfighting episodes involving bloody injuries (77a, 120a). Such reports reinforce the theoretical risks that face athletes and indicate the necessity of taking precautions during events in which blood exposure may occur. The following preventive strategies and recommendations adopted from the American Medical Society for Sports Medicine (9), American Academy of Sports Medicine (9), American Academy of Pediatrics (8), National Football League (25), National Collegiate Athletic Association (109), and World Health Organization (171) should be considered with regard to HIV in sports.

1. If a skin lesion is observed, it should be immediately cleansed with a suitable antiseptic and securely covered with an occlusive dressing that will withstand the demands of competition.
2. If a bleeding wound occurs, the individual's participation should be interrupted until the bleeding has been stopped and the

#30

wound has been both cleansed with antiseptics and securely covered or occluded. Any participant whose uniform is saturated with blood, regardless of the source, must have it changed before returning to competition.

3. Coaches and athletic trainers should receive training in first aid and emergency care; they should also be provided with the necessary supplies to treat open wounds, such as latex or vinyl gloves, disinfectant, bleach, antiseptic, designated receptacles for soiled equipment or uniforms, bandages or dressings, and a container for appropriate disposal of needles, syringes, or scalpels.

4. Athletic equipment that is visibly contaminated with blood should be wiped clean and disinfected with a bleach solution before being used

5. Gloves should be worn by persons attending to injuries when direct contact with blood or body fluids is anticipated. The gloves should be changed after individual participants have been treated, and hands should be washed after every glove removal. Emergency care, however, should never be delayed when protective equipment is not available.

6. Athletes should not be restricted from participating in sports merely on the basis of their HIV status unless substantial numbers of cases of transmission in sporting competitions occur.

7. The enforcement of mandatory HIV testing in athletic settings is unnecessary. Instead, voluntary testing and HIV education should be promoted to achieve public health benefits.

Viral Hepatitis

Hepatitis B virus (HBV) and hepatitis C virus (HCV) are transmitted via the same routes as HIV: sexual contact, parenteral blood exposure, and perinatally (57). Although the routes of transmission are similar to those of HIV, HBV transmission rates are 100-fold higher than those of HIV (73, 118, 171). A well-documented outbreak of HBV infection was reported among several members of a high school sumo wrestling club (87). It was suggested that HBV was transmitted percutane-

ously through the cuts and abrasions suffered during wrestling. In another report, horizontal transmission of HBV was documented among five players of an American-football team due to contact with open wounds during training (161).

Other sports-related outbreaks of HBV have occurred among Swedish orienteers (61, 129, 130). Orienteering is a sport in which runners are given the bearings of a number of checkpoints and, with the aid of a compass and map, choose their own route to the finish line. It was suggested that inoculation of HBV might have occurred when the runners scratched themselves on the same bushes or, after the competition, when the participants bathed in stagnant waters or shared the same plastic bathtubs. Immediately after preventive measures were applied, the incidence of HBV infection among the orienteers decreased.

The risk of HCV infection from percutaneous exposure to infected blood is estimated to be 10 times greater than that of HIV but lower than that of HBV (8). Although there are no confirmed cases of HCV transmission through sporting activities, there is some evidence of increased risk in athletes who play contact sports (85). Transmission resulting from nonathletic bloody fistfights has been reported (24). However, the greatest risk of HCV acquisition in athletes is not from the sport itself but rather from the injection use of anabolic steroids, vitamins, or other performance-enhancing agents (115, 121, 150). The risk of HIV, HBV, or HCV transmission to other athletes is generally very low; therefore, on the basis of risk of infection, infected athletes should be allowed to participate in sporting activities (8).

SKIN INFECTIONS

Viral Infections

HSV

Herpes simplex virus (HSV) is the cause of a contagious viral infection of the skin and mucous membranes. Herpes labialis (cold sores) and herpes progenitalis are two forms of the disease, so named because of their anatomical locations. Since HSV infection is so prevalent among rugby players and wrestlers, it is also referred to as herpes gladiatorum (140), herpes venatorum (106), herpes rugbeiorum (165a), and scrumpox (145). The virus may be transmitted directly through skin-to-skin contact or indirectly through the sharing of towels, clothes, or other equipment. Athletes participating in contact sports are at the greatest risk for infection. Several cases have been reported to occur among wrestlers and rugby players as a result of close person-to-person contact (17, 20, 52, 90, 106, 125, 133, 140, 145, 146, 155, 165a, 167, 169). Symptomatic athletes should refrain from participating in contact sports to avoid spreading the virus. Wearing protective clothing may also help prevent infection by eliminating contact with the lesions, although it has been suggested that abrasive shirts may actually contribute to infection (155).

Even though cutaneous HSV infections are rarely life threatening, herpetic lesions are unsightly and cause discomfort. Events such as trauma, exposure to sunlight, illness, surgery, stress, or menstruation may trigger recurrence of the lesions. For example, recurrent herpes labialis was reported among Alpine skiers exposed to increased UV irradiation at high altitudes (111). The prophylactic use of acyclovir has been shown to reduce the incidence of UV light-induced herpes labialis in skiers (126, 151).

MOLLUSCUM CONTAGIOSUM

Molluscum contagiosum is a benign viral skin infection caused by a poxvirus. The lesions present as 2- to 5-mm smooth papules that are often umbilicated. The incubation period ranges between 14 and 50 days. Minor skin injuries are thought to be the sites at which the virus is introduced. Athletes participating in close-contact sports where skin trauma is common are at risk of infection. Wrestlers and boxers, for example, are commonly infected in the areas of the hands, face, and upper body. The virus may also be spread in connection with bathing and washing. In one study, the infection was recognized among young children who used communal swimming pools (120). Infections may also arise if athletes come into direct skin contact with each other in the sauna or shower or on benches and also if they share their soap, brushes, and towels (111a).

Cutaneous transmission of molluscum contagiosum was reported in cross-country runners (111a) and in a 48-year-old woman during an orienteering competition (42a). The female orienteer had endured minor abrasions around her knees after running through a bush, and she developed lesions in the same area several weeks later. Because this individual had no other opportunity for contact with the virus, it was thought to have been spread by other athletes who had passed along the same track and brushed vigorously against the same plants.

Untreated infections usually resolve spontaneously within 6 to 9 months. Prolonged or severe infection can be seen in patients with untreated HIV infection or impaired cellular immunity (42a, 72). Some methods of treatment include curettage, skin abrasion with granules or an abrasive pad after bathing, topical tretinoin (Retin-A) gel or cream, liquid nitrogen, and chemical treatments with retinoic acid, phenol, salicylic acid, lactic acid, or cantharidin (21, 57). Protective clothing and good hygienic conditions are recommended to help prevent infection.

HPV

Warts, also called verrucae, are benign epithelial tumors caused by several human papillomaviruses (HPVs), with an average incubation period of approximately 6 months. Common warts seen on the hands appear as raised areas that are irregular and rough. Plantar warts, seen on weight-bearing surfaces such as the feet, appear as flat lesions extending deep into the skin with hyperkeratotic surfaces. Athletes are predisposed to infection due to the effects of perspiration, since moist environments create conditions favoring the spread of verrucae.

Although the infectivity rate is generally low, it is postulated that repetitive trauma to wet skin surfaces increases the risk of inoculation of HPV (132). Individuals competing in sports in which calluses are likely to develop, such as gymnastics, track, football, tennis, baseball, and wrestling, are more susceptible to acquiring warts.

In the athletic setting, it is likely that plantar warts are transmitted by contaminated floors, such as swimming pool decks or shower rooms, while hand warts are transmitted by contaminated gym equipment or weight apparatus (43). To prevent the transmission of HPV, warts should always be covered during contact sports. Athletes who are prone to warts should consider using drying powders on their feet and wearing rubber sandals in the locker room and shower (60).

Since warts may cause irritation in crucial locations, such as the fingers or hands, an athlete's performance in sports such as golf and bowling may be hampered. Effective treatment methods are available but may sometimes cause short-term disabilities. For example, athletic participation is likely to be interrupted when cryotherapy with liquid nitrogen is applied. Surgical removal and electrical desiccation techniques are also quite disabling. Less aggressive treatments include the application of salicylic acid plasters, tretinoin gel, and other topical preparations.

Bacterial Infections

STAPHYLOCOCCUS AUREUS

Bacterial skin infections are commonly caused by *Staphylococcus aureus*. *S. aureus* may cause abscesses, cellulitis, impetigo, folliculitis, furuncles, and carbuncles. In recent years, the incidence of community-acquired skin infections caused by methicillin-resistant *Staphylococcus aureus* (MRSA) has significantly risen.

MRSA. Although the clinical presentations of methicillin-sensitive *Staphylococcus aureus* and MRSA may be identical, community MRSA strains have a greater propensity to

lead to abscesses and give a more toxic presentation. The severity may be due to certain virulence factors unique to the community MRSA strain.

Community outbreaks of MRSA infections have been reported with increasing frequency over the past decade among young persons without health care exposures or associated risk factors, such as athletes. During the 2003 National Football League season, eight MRSA infections occurred among five St. Louis Rams players at turf abrasion sites. Some opposing team members also developed MRSA abscesses, which suggests that transmission occurred during game play (89). Other reported outbreaks involved direct-contact transmission or common-source transmission of MRSA resulting from the sharing of gym equipment or hygiene products, such as towels, soaps, razors, and other objects, among athletes involved in wrestling, rugby, baseball, basketball, fencing, canoeing, and other sporting activities (39, 42).

Staphylococcus aureus infections are usually treated with semisynthetic penicillins; however, MRSA is resistant to all semisynthetic penicillins, including cephalosporins. Therefore, commonly used antibiotics such as dicloxacillin and cephalexin are not effective. Obtaining cultures in suspected cases of infection and performing antimicrobial-susceptibility testing facilitate early identification of MRSA infection and appropriate treatment. Unlike hospital-acquired strains, community-acquired MRSA is often susceptible to tetracyclines, trimethoprim-sulfamethoxazole, or clindamycin. Abscesses should be drained and the wounds covered and contained with clean, dry dressings. Infected persons should receive guidance regarding enhanced hand and personal hygiene to prevent further transmission. Chlorhexidine-containing soap and nasal decolonization with mupirocin have been recommended to control outbreaks; however, data demonstrating the independent benefit of these agents in controlling MRSA in community clusters are lacking (89).

Folliculitis and Furunculosis. Folliculitis is an infection of hair follicles usually caused by *Staphylococcus aureus,* but it may also be caused by gram-negative organisms. Lesions usually emerge on areas of the skin that have been traumatized by maceration, such as under shoulder pads or sweaty garments, and on the legs, arms, and trunks of wrestlers. In one report, an outbreak of pustular follicular dermatitis among college students was the result of skin trauma endured during mud wrestling (5). Folliculitis often resolves spontaneously within a few days. Treatment is usually topical, with compresses, topical antibacterials, and/or astringent lotions or drying agents that remove the tops of pustules to prevent furuncles from developing.

Furunculosis is an infection involving the hair follicles, sebaceous glands, or skin compromised by abrasions, wounds, or burns. It is usually caused by *S. aureus* and can arise from preexisting folliculitis. Outbreaks of staphylococcal skin infections reported among high school football teams and river-rafting guides have been attributed to direct person-to-person contact, with an increased risk of infection in the presence of skin injuries (14, 46, 83a, 101, 149, 153). Wearing uniforms that cover all parts of the body may reduce the frequency of ecchymoses and microabrasions on the skin. To prevent the spread of infection, infected athletes should refrain from participation in contact sports until lesions have resolved. Also, ointments and powders should not be distributed by hand from common containers. Treatment consists of warm compresses and benzoyl peroxide along with oral antibiotics. Large deep lesions (carbuncles) may require surgical drainage.

Impetigo. Impetigo is a contagious bacterial skin infection caused by *S. aureus* or *Streptococcus pyogenes* and is most commonly seen among wrestlers, swimmers, gymnasts, football players, and soccer players. Lesions are superficial and vary from small vesicles to large bullae on the face and body. After the lesions become pustular and rupture, they become covered with a heavy, honey-colored serosanguineous crust. The infection spreads quickly to multiple areas of the body and may lead to deeper, invasive infections. A bacterial skin culture can confirm the microbiologic diagnosis. Treatment consists of local cleansing and debridement with hydrogen peroxide. Administration of oral or topical antibiotic treatments directed at the specific causative agent may also be helpful. As the infection is contagious, epidemics can occur if coaches and athletes pay little attention to the lesions. To prevent the spread of infection, athletic equipment and towels should not be shared and infected athletes should be discouraged from participation until their infections have healed.

STREPTOCOCCAL INFECTIONS

Skin infections caused by *Streptococcus pyogenes* are typically transmitted by close physical contact. A possible complication of *Streptococcus pyogenes* is acute glomerulonephritis. Epidemic pyoderma caused by nephritogenic streptococci has been documented among members of college athletic teams (62, 103). Strategies such as keeping players with cutaneous streptococcal infections from participating on the field and applying skin antiseptics to traumatized skin after competition may help prevent the spread of infection.

OTHER BACTERIAL INFECTIONS

Erythrasma. Erythrasma is an infection caused by *Corynebacterium minutissimum* that may clinically mimic a fungal infection in appearance. The typical rash develops as a reddish-brown patch with desquamation in the axillae and groin. The lesions are erythematous, with a fine scale, and are well demarcated at their borders. The infection may be pruritic and can be diagnosed with a Wood's light (black light), which reveals a coral red fluorescence. It is often confused with a fungal infection. Erythrasma may be treated with topical cleansing agents, topical germicidal agents, or oral antibiotics. Using antibacterial soaps and wearing loose clothing may help prevent or eliminate infection (48, 95).

Pitted Keratolysis. Pitted keratolysis, also known as "stinky foot" or "toxic-sock syndrome," is an asymptomatic skin infection associated with the growth of *Corynebacterium minutissimum*. Athletes participating in basketball, tennis, volleyball, and track often develop pitted keratolysis. The lesions are superficial pits up to 7 mm in diameter and are typically seen on weight-bearing areas of the body. The feet and toes are more frequently involved and are typically malodorous (157). Two cases of pitted keratolysis in non-weight-bearing areas involved a volleyball player and a field athlete (158). It was presumed that the non-weight-bearing areas of the body were infected with the organism following infection of the weight-bearing regions. Infections are precipitated by occlusive footwear and excessive sweating. The lesions can clear rapidly with the elimination of local moisture, which may be achieved by wearing absorbent cotton socks and with the application of drying agents to the foot. More-resistant infections may require treatment with oral erythromycin or with mupirocin ointment (141, 165).

"Hot Tub" Folliculitis. Hot tub folliculitis differs from typical folliculitis in that it is caused by *Pseudomonas aeruginosa* and is associated with water exposure. This infection has been associated with the use of hot tubs, whirlpools, and swimming pools. In one report, hot tub associated folliculitis was described to occur among individuals who had bathed in a tub that was shared by several people and had not been cleaned for 10 days (40). In another report, infection in a college football player following whirlpool use for the treatment of an ankle strain was described (65). To prevent infection, it is necessary to reduce the quantity of the bacterial organism in the water. This is achieved by appropriate monitoring of the temperature, pH, disinfectant level, and chlorine concentration. Hot tub folliculitis is a self-limiting condition lasting 7 to 10 days and therefore requires no specific treatment.

Fungal Infections

TINEA CORPORIS, CRURIS, PEDIS, AND VERSICOLOR

Tinea is the name applied to fungal infections in the keratin of the skin, hair, and nails. They are named according to the site of infection, such as tinea corporis (body), tinea cruris (groin), tinea pedis (feet), tinea capitis (scalp), and tinea onychomycosis (nail) (21). A definitive diagnosis may be made by fungal cultures or KOH preparations of skin scrapings. The treatments may vary according to the type of fungal organism involved and the site of infection. The factors contributing to most cases in athletes are the presence of increased moisture from sweat (worsened by occlusive footwear), shared towels, skin injuries, and contaminated floors in the locker room, gymnasium, or showering facilities (30, 60, 128).

Tinea pedis, also known as athlete's foot, is most commonly seen among marathon runners, swimmers, and professional ice hockey players, as well as persons active in basketball, judo, tennis, water polo, and football (84, 98, 112). *Trichophyton rubrum,* which generally causes an erythematous and scaling eruption on the plantar surface of the foot, and *Trichophyton mentagrophytes,* which may present as painful, pruritic blisters, are the most common organisms involved (11). One study suggests that fungal infections of the toenail (onychomycosis) are three times more prevalent among swimmers and athletes already infected with tinea pedis than among the general population (67). Keeping the feet dry by wearing appropriate shoes and socks, using drying powders, and wearing sandals in the locker room or shower may help prevent infection. Topical treatments with antifungal agents are effective and should be applied several times a day. Oral antifungal therapy is also available.

Tinea corporis, also known as tinea corporis gladiatorum or ringworm (154, 166a), is a fungal infection usually occurring on the face, trunk, and limbs. Athletes participating in close-contact sports such as football, rugby, and wrestling are at risk of becoming infected. Although *T. rubrum* is the most frequent causative organism, several outbreaks involving *Trichophyton tonsurans* have been reported among high school and college wrestlers (4, 19, 55, 75, 94, 124, 154, 166a). Athletes should either cover lesions or refrain from participating in sports to prevent the spread of infection. Other preventive strategies include inspecting the skin regularly and avoiding the use of shared equipment. Prophylactic treatment of tinea gladiatorum with intermittent doses of oral itraconazole (70) or 100 mg of fluconazole once weekly has been shown to be effective (93). Though antifungals are effective prophylactic agents, the cost, the increased risk of microbial resistance, and the potential adverse effects of the medications make general prophylaxis for all team members unattractive (3).

Tinea cruris, also known as "jock itch," is an infection involving the groin and upper thighs. The fungal organisms and treatment methods involved are similar to those of tinea pedis. The pruritic rash appears as red, scaly patches, usually with sharp margins, covering the moist areas. Symptoms include pain and pruritus with occasional production of a weeping discharge. Keeping the areas dry and maintaining good hygiene may help prevent infection.

Tinea versicolor, or "fungus of many colors," is caused by a yeast called *Malassezia furfur*. The diagnosis is confirmed by KOH staining of a skin scraping, and a characteristic yellow-orange color appears under inspection with a Wood's light. Typical lesions are asymptomatic, irregularly shaped, scaly, hyperpigmented, or hypopigmented patches which are located on the back, trunk, neck, arms, and upper extremities. After acne, tinea versicolor is the most common skin affliction observed in athletes participating in college football and basketball (108a). Topical anti-

fungal treatments and oral regimens are effective therapeutic measures.

OTHER INFECTIOUS SYNDROMES

Conjunctivitis

Several etiologic agents of conjunctivitis may be spread by direct contact, through contaminated swimming pools, or by fomites. The most common bacterial organisms involved are *S. aureus, Staphylococcus epidermidis,* and *Haemophilus* species (147). Direct contact with HSV lesions can also result in conjunctival infection. Athletes competing in contact sports such as rugby and wrestling are usually at greater risk.

In one case, follicular conjunctivitis was among the complications observed when two players of a rugby team contracted HSV infections while in competition (169). In another report, conjunctival erythema among seven members of a college wrestling team who had developed extensive cutaneous herpesvirus infections during a 2-week period in the wrestling season was described (125). The best preventive strategy is to carefully screen out symptomatic athletes before competition. Swimmers with conjunctivitis must also refrain from entering swimming pools to avoid spreading viral agents in the water.

Waterborne transmission of adenoviruses has also been shown to cause communitywide outbreaks of febrile disease with conjunctivitis. It can be prevented by proper chlorination of swimming pools (80, 164).

Infectious Mononucleosis

The most common cause of infectious mononucleosis (IM) is Epstein-Barr virus, which is a herpesvirus. Cytomegalovirus and *Toxoplasma gondii* are other causes of IM. Transmission may occur by direct contact but is more common through droplet transmission (i.e., through infected oral secretions, such as saliva). It has been demonstrated that repeated and prolonged exposure to the virus does not necessarily contribute to infection. In one study, it was concluded that college roommates of infected patients had no increased risk of infection (137). The incubation period for primary Epstein-Barr virus infection is generally 30 to 45 days. The illness may persist for 1 to several weeks, while the infectious state may last for up to a year in some cases. Even though life-threatening complications are remarkably infrequent, spontaneous rupture of the spleen and airway obstruction due to massive lymphoid hyperplasia during the acute phase of illness have accounted for a number of reported deaths (100, 135, 152).

Treatment consists of rest, fluids, and analgesics. Acetaminophen is recommended for fever, headache, and muscle pain, along with lozenges, saltwater gargles, or viscous lidocaine for sore throats. Although athletes may recover from IM more quickly than nonathletes, their athletic performance may be suboptimal for up to 3 months. It is important to restrict all kinds of strenuous activity for at least a month after the onset of clinical illness, since most splenic ruptures occur within the first 21 days (105, 152). Treatment for IM should be individualized, and athletes should return to activity only when they feel physically ready.

Meningitis

Meningitis may be caused by one of several microorganisms, including bacteria or viruses. *Neisseria meningitidis,* for example, can be transmitted by droplet transmission or direct contact of infectious fluid from the nose or throat of an infected person. The infection is normally spread in places where people live closely together, such as in school dormitories, on religious pilgrimages, or in military camps. Although there have been episodes of infections occurring in overcrowded environments, such as in dance clubs and bars, no cases pertaining to the crowded conditions of sporting events have been cited (44, 53, 77, 156).

Viral meningitis is commonly associated with enteroviral infections, such as echoviruses and coxsackie B viruses. Several outbreaks of viral meningitis have been reported among members of high school football teams (7, 12, 31, 113). Most of the reports indicate that infections were associated with the peak seasonal incidence of aseptic meningitis (summer and fall) and occurred through close physical contact among the athletes or by common-source transmission, such as the unhygienic sharing of water containers or the dipping of cups into a common water source.

Upper Respiratory Tract Infection

Upper respiratory tract infections (URI), which are caused by a number of viruses and bacteria, are some of the most common illnesses encountered in sports. Symptoms vary according to the type of agent and the individual's immune response. The most-common symptoms include runny nose, sneezing, congestion, sore throat, cough, myalgias, and a general feeling of weakness. There are over 200 viruses that may cause URI, but the most common ones include rhinoviruses, coronaviruses, respiratory syncytial viruses, parainfluenza viruses, and adenoviruses (57). Although viruses account for over 60 to 90% of URI, bacteria also cause respiratory infections. In one report, three cases of respiratory infection relating to deep-sea diving involved a penicillin-resistant strain of *Streptococcus pneumoniae* (127).

Transmission may occur by contact with respiratory secretions, such as virus-containing droplets produced by a cough or sneeze, or by contact with hands contaminated with secretions from mucous membranes or with shared athletic equipment (71, 138). Good personal hygiene and avoidance of close contact with infected individuals may help prevent infections. It has been suggested that there is a relationship between acute stress and susceptibility to infection. In one study, it was observed that faster marathon runners developed more URI symptoms than slower or more moderate runners, and the frequency of symptoms was inversely proportional to the time taken to complete a race (123).

WATER SPORTS-ASSOCIATED INFECTIONS

Water acts as a passive carrier for numerous infectious agents. Athletes participating in water sports may be at risk, depending on the type of activity and water quality (41, 47, 69, 91, 97, 102, 119, 142, 160, 166). Water-based infections known to have been acquired by athletes either by prolonged contact with water or by ingestion during a sporting event are listed in Table 2 and reference 51. Leptospirosis and otitis externa, two of the prominent water-based diseases faced by athletes, are discussed below.

TABLE 2 Potential infectious diseases associated with water sports

Disseminated infections
Leptospirosis

Enteric infections
Amoebic dysentery
Cryptosporidiosis (33)
Escherichia coli infections (1, 34)
Gastroenteritis
Giardiasis
Infectious hepatitis
Norwalk virus infection (13, 96)
Salmonellosis
Shigellosis (134, 148)
Typhoid fever

Eye infections
Acanthamoebic keratitis
Adenoviruses

Skin and soft tissue infections
Otitis externa
Schistosome dermatitis (swimmer's itch) (99)
Schistosomiasis

Respiratory infections
Legionnaires' disease (e.g., Pontiac fever) (104)
Pneumonia following near drowning

Wound infections
Aeromonas primary wound infection (83)

Leptospirosis

Small rodents and some domesticated animals act as the reservoir for leptospirosis. Humans can become infected by means of direct contact with infected tissue or urine or by exposure to contaminated water, such as lakes or streams. Usually the infection is asymptomatic or an acute self-limited illness with chills, fever, headache, and myalgias. In 10% of patients, the acute illness is followed by a severe illness, with fever, inflammation of the liver, kidney damage, and bleeding, which can be fatal. Enthusiasts participating in water sports in environmental waters are at greater risk of infection. Several leptospiral outbreaks involving white-water rafters, swimmers, kayakers, and other recreational water users have been documented (10, 35, 78, 79, 88, 122). Outbreaks involving athletes participating in triathlons (races consisting of swimming, biking, and running competitions) with exposure to contaminated waters have also been reported (36, 37, 38, 66, 114, 139, 159). Antimicrobial agents such as doxycycline, amoxicillin, or ceftriaxone should be administered to treat the disease, and preventive measures, such as wearing protective clothing to minimize contact with potentially contaminated water, should be implemented (170).

Otitis Externa

Acute otitis externa, also known as swimmer's ear, is an inflammation of the external auditory canal. It is typically seen among athletes participating in water sports who commonly experience mechanical trauma to the external ear. Swimmers, divers, surfers, sailboarders, and kayakers who are exposed to polluted bodies of water are at risk of infection. The infection is most commonly caused by *Pseudomonas aeruginosa* but may also be caused by organisms such as *S. aureus* or *Aspergillus* (6, 18). Prolonged exposure to water causes maceration of the epithelial tissue in the ear canal and removes the ear wax, which normally aids in repelling water and maintaining an acidic pH to prevent bacterial and fungal growth. Cleaning the external auditory canal and keeping it as dry as possible are important aspects of therapy, along with topical steroid and antimicrobial agents. Systemic therapy is recommended in severe cases of otitis externa.

COMMON-SOURCE TRANSMISSION

Common-source exposure to infectious diseases in athletic settings normally occurs in cases where water or food containers are contaminated and shared. Such outbreaks may involve a myriad of different infectious agents. For example, an outbreak of hepatitis A occurred among players and coaching staff of a college football team as a result of a contaminated water supply (116, 117). Enteroviral infections, such as aseptic meningitis and pleurodynia, have also been documented to occur by similar means in other studies involving athletic teams (7, 12, 31, 76, 113).

AIRBORNE TRANSMISSION

There is a potential risk of spreading infectious diseases by airborne transmission during indoor sporting events where large groups of people are gathered in a confined environment. A packed, humid gym or stadium provides the classic conditions for the spread of illnesses such as measles, chickenpox (which is caused by varicella–zoster virus), and influenza (107). Although usually not life threatening, such illnesses may keep an athlete from competing, postpone sporting events, or compromise a team's competitive edge. Airborne infections, however, are not confined to the athletes competing on the field. Spectators watching sporting events from afar are at risk of infection as well. For example, several outbreaks of measles have been reported in association with mass spectator sporting events (32, 45, 54). However, outdoor sports, such as track and field, baseball, and football, do not pose a high risk for airborne infections because of adequate ventilation (168). Immunizations

are recommended to help prevent the spread of infections.

VECTOR-BORNE PATHOGENS

Vector-borne pathogens are spread by carriers such as ticks, insects, or animals. Extreme-sport athletes competing in marathons or triathlons in exotic or foreign locations such as jungles, mountains, and deserts may be susceptible to unusual diseases endemic in the environment (173). For example, in the correct geographic scenario, mosquito bites may transmit the agents of malaria, dengue, chikungunya, or yellow fever. Even the more ordinary sports enthusiast may be exposed to vector-borne diseases while golfing, running, or hiking. Examples of vector-borne diseases include tick-borne infections such as Lyme disease, caused by the spirochete *Borrelia burgdorferi,* Rocky Mountain spotted fever, caused by *Rickettsia rickettsii,* human monocytic ehrlichiosis, caused by *Ehrlichia chaffeensis,* and babesiosis. While there have been no specific reports of outbreaks of vector-borne diseases among athletes, their risks are similar to those of others, such as travelers and campers, while participating in outdoor activities in areas of endemicity. Physicians caring for such athletes must take a careful exposure history and maintain a high level of suspicion for such diseases. For a more detailed discussion of vector-borne infectious diseases, please see chapter 3.

CONCLUSION

Individual athletes, team members, persons who come into contact with the participants, and spectators who merely watch the events from afar are at risk of infection at sporting events. Often, these infections can be avoided with proper hygiene, appropriate immunizations, early recognition, or subsequent exclusion of infected participants during the game. Physicians caring for athletes must play an active role in educating them about effective preventive strategies and in providing advice on appropriate treatment methods based on consideration of their individual situations. Fortunately, being a healthy population in general, athletes tend to respond well to treatments provided.

PRACTICAL TIPS

- Blood-borne infections such as HIV, HBV, and HCV are very difficult to acquire through sports contacts; these infections are more likely to be acquired via off-the-field risk behaviors.
- Athletes should refrain from sharing or borrowing personal items such as towels and razors and should clean common gym or locker room equipment with a disinfectant before use to prevent the spread of infections such as MRSA.
- To avoid the spread of fungal infections of the feet, athletes should wear proper footwear, keep the feet and socks dry during sporting activities, and avoid going barefoot in shared areas, such as the locker room and shower.
- Physicians caring for athletes must take a careful exposure history and have a high index of suspicion for diseases transmittable during sporting activities.

REFERENCES

1. **Ackman, D., S. Marks, P. Mack, M. Caldwell, T. Root, and G. Birkhead.** 1997. Swimming-associated haemorrhagic colitis due to Escherichia coli O157:H7 infection: evidence of prolonged contamination of a fresh water lake. *Epidemiol. Infect.* **119:**1–8.
2. **Adams, B. B.** 2002. Dermatologic disorders of the athlete. *Sports Med.* **32:**309–321.
3. **Adams, B. B.** 2002. Tinea corporis gladiatorum. *J. Am. Acad. Dermatol.* **47:**286–290.
4. **Adams, B. B.** 2000. Tinea corporis gladiatorum: a cross-sectional study. *J. Am. Acad. Dermatol.* **43:**1039–1041.
5. **Adler, A. I., and J. Altman.** 1993. An outbreak of mud-wrestling-induced pustular dermatitis in college students. Dermatitis palaestrae limosae. *JAMA* **269:**502–504.
6. **Agius, A. M., J. M. Pickles, and K. L. Burch.** 1992. A prospective study of otitis externa. *Clin. Otolaryngol.* **17:**150–154.
7. **Alexander, J. P., Jr., L. E. Chapman, M. A. Pallansch, W. T. Stephenson, T. J. Török, and L. J. Anderson.** 1993. Coxsackievirus B2 infection and aseptic meningitis: a focal outbreak among members of a high school football team. *J. Infect. Dis.* **167:**1201–1205.
8. **American Academy of Pediatrics Committee on Sports Medicine and Fitness.** 1999. Human immunodeficiency virus and other blood-borne viral pathogens in the athletic setting. *Pediatrics* **104:**1400–1403.
9. **American Medical Society for Sports Medicine and American Academy of Sports Medicine.** 1995. Human immunodeficiency virus (HIV) and other blood-borne pathogens in sports (joint position statement): the American Medical Society for Sports Medicine (AMSSM) and the American Academy of Sports Medicine (AASM). *Am. J. Sports Med.* **23:**510–514.
10. **Anderson, D. C., D. S. Folland, M. D. Fox, C. M. Patton, and A. F. Kaufmann.** 1978. Leptospirosis: a common-source outbreak due to leptospires of the grippotyphosa serogroup. *Am. J. Epidemiol.* **107:**538–544.
11. **Auger, P., G. Marquis, J. Joly, and A. Attye.** 1993. Epidemiology of tinea pedis in marathon runners: prevalence of occult athlete's foot. *Mycoses* **36:**35–41.
12. **Baron, R. C., M. H. Hatch, K. Kleeman, and J. N. MacCormack.** 1982. Aseptic meningitis among members of a high school football team: an outbreak associated with echovirus 16 infection. *JAMA* **248:**1724–1727.
13. **Baron, R. C., F. D. Murphy, H. B. Greenberg, C. E. Davis, D. J. Bregman, G. W. Gary, J. M. Hughes, and L. B. Schonberger.** 1982. Norwalk gastrointestinal illness: an outbreak associated with swimming in a recreational lake and secondary person-to-person transmission. *Am. J. Epidemiol.* **115:**163–172.
14. **Bartlett, P. C., R. J. Martin, and B. R. Cahill.** 1982. Furunculosis in a high school football team. *Am. J. Sports Med.* **10:**371–374.
15. **Basler, R. S. W.** 1983. Skin lesions related to sports activity. *Prim. Care* **10:**479–494.
16. **Basler, R. S. W.** 1989. Sports-related skin injuries. *Adv. Dermatol.* **4:**29–50.
17. **Becker, T. M., R. Kodsi, P. Bailey, F. Lee, R. Levandowski, and A. J. Nahmias.** 1988. Grappling with herpes: herpes gladiatorum. *Am. J. Sports Med.* **16:**665–669.
18. **Bell, D. N.** 1985. Otitis externa: a common, often self-inflicted condition. *Postgrad. Med.* **78:**101–104, 106.
19. **Beller, M., and B. D. Gessner.** 1994. An outbreak of tinea corporis gladiatorum on a high

school wrestling team. *J. Am. Acad. Dermatol.* **31:** 197–201.

20. **Belongia, E. A., J. L. Goodman, E. J. Holland, C. W. Andres, S. R. Homann, R. L. Mahanti, M. W. Mizener, A. Erice, and M. T. Osterholm.** 1991. An outbreak of herpes gladiatorum at a high-school wrestling camp. *N. Engl. J. Med.* **325:**906–910.

21. **Bergfeld, W. F.** 1984. Dermatologic problems in athletes. *Prim. Care* **11:**151–160.

22. **Bergfeld, W. F., and J. S. Taylor.** 1985. Trauma, sports, and the skin. *Am. J. Ind. Med.* **8:** 403–413.

23. **Bitting, L. A., C. A. Trowbridge, and L. E. Costello.** 1996. A model for a policy on HIV-AIDS and athletics. *J. Athl. Train.* **31:**356–357.

24. **Bourlière, M., P. Halfon, Y. Quentin, P. David, C. Mengotti, I. Portal, H. Khiri, S. Benali, H. Perrier, C. Boustière, M. Jullien, and G. Lambot.** 2000. Covert transmission of hepatitis C virus during bloody fisticuffs. *Gastroenterology* **119:**507–511.

25. **Brown, L. S., Jr., D. P. Drotman, A. Chu, C. L. Brown, Jr., and D. Knowlan.** 1995. Bleeding injuries in professional football: estimating the risk of HIV transmission. *Ann. Intern. Med.* **122:**271–274.

26. **Brown, L. S., Jr., R. Y. Phillips, C. L. Brown, Jr., D. Knowlan, L. Castle, and J. Moyer.** 1994. HIV-AIDS policies and sports: the National Football League. *Med. Sci. Sports Exerc.* **26:**403–407.

27. **Calabrese, L. H., H. A. Haupt, L. Hartman, and R. H. Strauss.** 1993. HIV and sports: what is the risk? *Phys. Sportsmed.* **21:**173–180.

28. **Calabrese, L. H., and D. Kelley.** 1989. AIDS and athletes. *Phys. Sportsmed.* **17:**126.

29. **Calabrese, L. H., and A. LaPerriere.** 1993. Human immunodeficiency virus infection, exercise and athletics. *Sports Med.* **15:**6–13.

30. **Caputo, R., K. De Boulle, J. Del Rosso, and R. Nowicki.** 2001. Prevalence of superficial fungal infections among sports-active individuals: results from the Achilles survey, a review of the literature. *J. Eur. Acad. Dermatol. Venereol.* **15:** 312–316.

31. **Centers for Disease Control.** 1981. Aseptic meningitis in a high school football team—Ohio. *MMWR Morb. Mortal. Wkly. Rep.* **29:**631–637.

32. **Centers for Disease Control.** 1992. Measles at an international gymnastics competition—Indiana, 1991. *MMWR Morb. Mortal. Wkly. Rep.* **41:**109–111.

33. **Centers for Disease Control and Prevention.** 1994. Cryptosporidium infections associated with swimming pools—Dane County, Wisconsin, 1993. *MMWR Morb. Mortal. Wkly. Rep.* **43:**561–563.

34. **Centers for Disease Control and Prevention.** 1996. Lake-associated outbreak of Escherichia coli O157:H7—Illinois, 1995. *MMWR Morb. Mortal. Wkly. Rep.* **45:**437–439.

35. **Centers for Disease Control and Prevention.** 1997. Outbreak of leptospirosis among whitewater rafters—Costa Rica, 1996. *JAMA* **278:**808.

36. **Centers for Disease Control and Prevention.** 1998. Update: leptospirosis and unexplained acute febrile illness among athletes participating in triathlons—Illinois and Wisconsin, 1998. *MMWR Morb. Mortal. Wkly. Rep.* **47:**673–676.

37. **Centers for Disease Control and Prevention.** 2001. Update on emerging infections: news from the Centers for Disease Control and Prevention. *Ann. Emerg. Med.* **38:**83–86.

38. **Centers for Disease Control and Prevention.** 2001. Update: outbreak of acute febrile illness among athletes participating in Eco-Challenge-Sabah 2000—Borneo, Malaysia, 2000. *MMWR Morb. Mortal. Wkly. Rep.* **50:**21–24.

39. **Centers for Disease Control and Prevention.** 2003. Methicillin-resistant *Staphylococcus aureus* infections among competitive sports participants—Colorado, Indiana, Pennsylvania, and Los Angeles County, 2000–2003. *MMWR Morb. Mortal. Wkly. Rep.* **52:**793–795.

40. **Chandrasekar, P. H., K. V. I. Rolston, D. W. Kannangara, J. L. Le Frock, and S. A. Binnick.** 1984. Hot tub-associated dermatitis due to Pseudomonas aeruginosa. *Arch. Dermatol.* **120:**1337–1340.

41. **Chang, W. J., and F. D. Pien.** 1986. Marine-acquired infections. Hazards of the ocean environment. *Postgrad. Med.* **80:**30–32, 37, 41.

42. **Cohen, P. R.** 2008. The skin in the gym: a comprehensive review of the cutaneous manifestations of community-acquired methicillin-resistant *Staphylococcus aureus* infection in athletes. *Clin. Dermatol.* **26:**16–26.

42a.**Commens, C. A.** 1987. Letter. *Med. J. Aust.* **146:**117.

43. **Conklin, R. J.** 1990. Common cutaneous disorders in athletes. *Sports Med.* **9:**100–119.

44. **Cookson, S. T.** 1998. Disco fever: epidemic meningococcal disease in northeastern Argentina associated with disco patronage. *J. Infect. Dis.* **178:**266–269.

45. **Davis, R. M., E. D. Whitman, W. A. Orenstein, S. R. Preblud, L. E. Markowitz, and A. R. Hinman.** 1987. A persistent outbreak of measles despite appropriate prevention and control measures. *Am. J. Epidemiol.* **126:**438–449.

46. **Decker, M. D., J. A. Lybarger, W. K. Vaughn, R. H. Hutcheson, Jr., and W. Schaffner.** 1986. An outbreak of staphylococcal skin infections among river rafting guides. *Am. J. Epidemiol.* **124:**969–976.

47. **Dewailly, E., C. Poirier, and F. M. Meyer.** 1986. Health hazards associated with windsurfing on polluted water. *Am. J. Public Health* **76:**690–691.

48. **Dodge, B. G., W. R. Knowles, M. E. McBride, W. C. Duncan, and J. M. Knox.** 1968. Treatment of erythrasma with an antibacterial soap. *Arch. Dermatol.* **97:**548–552.

49. **Dorman, J. M.** 2000. Contagious diseases in competitive sport: what are the risks? *J. Am. Coll. Health* **49:**105–109.

49a. **Dorman, M.** 1994. Letter. *JAMA* **272:**436.

50. **Drotman, D. P.** 1996. Professional boxing, bleeding, and HIV testing. *JAMA* **276:**193.

51. **Dufour, A. P.** 1986. Diseases caused by water contact, p. 23–41. *In* G. F. Craun (ed.), *Waterborne Diseases in the United States.* CRC Press, Boca Raton, FL.

52. **Dyke, L. M., U. R. Merikangas, O. C. Bruton, S. G. Trask, and F. M. Hetrick.** 1965. Skin infection in wrestlers due to herpes simplex virus. *JAMA* **194:**1001–1002.

53. **Edmond, M. B., R. J. Hollis, A. K. Houston, and R. P. Wenzel.** 1995. Molecular epidemiology of an outbreak of meningococcal disease in a university community. *J. Clin. Microbiol.* **33:**2209–2211.

54. **Ehresmann, K., C. Hedberg, and M. Grimm.** 1995. An outbreak of measles at an international sporting event with airborne transmission in a domed stadium. *J. Infect. Dis.* **171:**679–683.

55. **El-Fari, M., Y. Gräser, W. Presber, and H.-J. Tietz.** 2000. An epidemic of tinea corporis caused by Trichophyton tonsurans among children (wrestlers) in Germany. *Mycoses* **43:**191–196.

56. **Feller, A., and T. P. Flanigan.** 1997. HIV-infected competitive athletes. What are the risks? What precautions should be taken? *J. Gen. Intern. Med.* **12:**243–246.

57. **Fields, K. B., and P. A. Fricker (ed.).** 1997. *Medical Problems in Athletes.* Blackwell Science, Inc., Malden, MA.

58. **Freeman, M. J., and W. F. Bergfeld.** 1977. Skin diseases of football and wrestling participants. *Cutis* **20:**333–341.

59. **Gauthier, M. M.** 1987. Sports health workers respond to AIDS. *Phys. Sportsmed.* **15:**51–54.

60. **Gentles, J. C., E. G. V. Evans, and G. R. Jones.** 1974. Control of tinea pedis in a swimming bath. *Br. Med. J.* **1:**577–580.

61. **Gille, G., O. Ringertz, and B. Zetterberg.** 1967. Serum hepatitis among Swedish track-finders. II. A clinical study. *Acta Med. Scand.* **182:**129–135.

62. **Glezen, P. W., J. L. DeWalt, R. L. Lindsay, and H. C. Dillon.** 1972. Epidemic pyoderma caused by nephritogenic streptococci in college athletes. *Lancet* **i:**301–303.

63. **Goldsmith, M. F.** 1992. When sports and HIV share the bill, smart money goes on common sense. *JAMA* **267:**1311–1314.

64. **Goodman, R. A., S. B. Thacker, S. L. Solomon, M. T. Osterholm, and J. M. Hughes.** 1994. Infectious diseases in competitive sports. *JAMA* **271:**862–867.

65. **Green, J. J.** 2000. Localized whirlpool folliculitis in a football player. *Cutis* **65:**359–362.

66. **Guarner, J., W.-J. Shieh, J. Morgan, S. L. Bragg, M. D. Bajani, J. W. Tappero, and S. R. Zaki.** 2001. Leptospirosis mimicking acute cholecystitis among athletes participating in a triathlon. *Hum. Pathol.* **32:**750–752.

67. **Gudnadóttir, G., I. Hilmarsdóttir, and B. Sigurgeirsson.** 1999. Onychomycosis in Icelandic swimmers. *Acta Dermato-Venereol.* **79:**376–377.

68. **Gunby, P.** 1988. Boxing: AIDS? *JAMA* **259:**1613–1614.

69. **Harris, J. R., M. L. Cohen, and E. C. Lippy.** 1983. Water-related disease outbreaks in the United States, 1981. *J. Infect. Dis.* **148:**759–762.

70. **Hazen, P. G., and M. L. Weil.** 1997. Itraconazole in the prevention and management of dermatophytosis in competitive wrestlers. *J. Am. Acad. Dermatol.* **36:**481–482.

71. **Heath, G. W., C. A. Macera, and D. C. Nieman.** 1992. Exercise and upper respiratory tract infections. Is there a relationship? *Sports Med.* **14:**353–365.

72. **Highet, A. S.** 1992. Molluscum contagiosum. *Arch. Dis. Child.* **67:**1248–1249.

73. **Ho, D. D., T. Moudgil, and M. Alam.** 1989. Quantitation of human immunodeficiency virus type 1 in the blood of infected persons. *N. Engl. J. Med.* **321:**1621–1625.

74. **Houston, S. D., and J. M. Knox.** 1977. Skin problems related to sports and recreational activities. *Cutis* **19:**487–491.

75. **Hradil, E., K. Hersle, P. Nordin, and J. Faergemann.** 1995. An epidemic of tinea corporis caused by Trichophyton tonsurans among wrestlers in Sweden. *Acta Dermato-Venereol.* **75:**305–306.

76. **Ikeda, R. M., S. F. Kondracki, P. D. Drabkin, G. S. Birkhead, and D. L. Morse.** 1993. Pleurodynia among football players at a high school. An outbreak associated with coxsackievirus B1. *JAMA* **270:**2205–2206.

77. **Imrey, P. B., L. A. Jackson, P. H. Ludwinski, A. C. England III, G. A. Fella, B. C. Fox, L. B. Isdale, M. W. Reeves, and J. D. Wenger.** 1996. Outbreak of serogroup C meningococcal disease associated with campus bar patronage. *Am. J. Epidemiol.* **143:**624–630.

77a.Ippolito, G., P. Del Poggio, C. Arici, G. P. Gregis, G. Antonelli, E. Riva, and F. Dianzani. 1994. Letter. *JAMA* **272:**433–434.

78. Jackson, L. A., A. F. Kaufmann, W. G. Adams, M. B. Phelps, C. Andreasen, C. W. Langkop, B. J. Francis, and J. D. Wenger. 1993. Outbreak of leptospirosis associated with swimming. *Pediatr. Infect. Dis. J.* **12:**48–54.

79. Jevon, T. R., M. P. Knudson, P. A. Smith, P. S. Whitecar, and R. L. Blake, Jr. 1986. A point-source epidemic of leptospirosis. Description of cases, cause, and prevention. *Postgrad. Med.* **80:**121–122, 127–129.

80. Jiang, S. C. 2006. Human adenovirus in water: occurrence and health implications: a critical review. *Environ. Sci. Technol.* **40:**7132–7140.

81. Johnson, R. J. 1992. HIV infection in athletes. What arc the risks? Who can compete? *Postgrad. Med.* **92:**73–75, 79–80.

82. Jones, W. K., and J. W. Curran. 1994. Epidemiology of AIDS and HIV infection in industrialized countries, p. 91–108. In J. J. Pine (ed.), *Textbook of AIDS Medicine*. Williams & Wilkins, Baltimore, MD.

83. Joseph, S. W., O. P. Daily, W. S. Hunt, R. J. Seidler, D. A. Allen, and R. R. Colwell. 1979. Aeromonas primary wound infection of a diver in polluted waters. *J. Clin. Microbiol.* **10:**46–49.

83a.Joyce, D. 1990. Letter. *Am. J. Sports Med.* **18:**219–220.

84. Kamihama, T., T. Kimura, J.-I. Hosokawa, M. Ueji, T. Takase, and K. Tagami. 1997. Tinea pedis outbreak in swimming pools in Japan. *Public Health* **111:**249–253.

85. Kamochkine, M., F. Carrat, O. Dos Santos, P. Cacoub, and G. Ragum. 2006. A case-control study of risk factors for hepatitis C infection in patients with unexplained routes of infection. *J. Viral Hepat.* **13:**775–782.

86. Kantor, G. R., and W. F. Bergfeld. 1988. Common and uncommon dermatologic diseases related to sports activities. *Exerc. Sport Sci. Rev.* **16:**215–253.

86a.Karjalainen, J., and G. Friman. 1995. Letter. *Ann. Intern. Med.* **123:**635–636.

87. Kashiwagi, S., J. Hayashi, H. Ikematsu, S. Nishigori, K. Ishihara, and M. Kaji. 1982. An outbreak of hepatitis B in members of a high school sumo wrestling club. *JAMA* **248:**213–214.

88. Katz, A. R., S. J. Manea, and D. M. Sasaki. 1991. Leptospirosis on Kauai: investigation of a common source waterborne outbreak. *Am. J. Public Health* **81:**1310–1312.

89. Kazakova, S. V., J. C. Hageman, M. Matava, A. Srinivasan, L. Phelan, B. Garfinkel, T. Boo, S. McAllister, J. Anderson, B. Jensen, D. Dodson, D. Lonsway, L. M. McDougal, M. Arduino, V. J. Fraser, G. Killgore, F. C. Tenover, S. Cody, and D. B. Jernigan. 2005. A clone of methicillin-resistant *Staphylococcus aureus* among professional football players. *N. Engl. J. Med.* **352:**468–475.

90. Keilhofner, M., and D. S. McKinsey. 1988. Herpes gladiatorum in a high school wrestler. *Mo. Med.* **85:**723–725.

91. Kincaid, C. K. 1967. Lake pollution and human disease. *Wis. Med. J.* **66:**371–372.

92. Klein, A. W., and D. C. Rish. 1992. Sports related skin problems. *Compr. Ther.* **18:**2–4.

93. Kohl, T. D., D. C. Martin, R. Nemeth, T. Hill, and D. Evans. 2000. Fluconazole for the prevention and treatment of tinea gladiatorum. *Pediatr. Infect. Dis. J.* **19:**717–722.

94. Kohl, T. D., D. P. Giesen, J. Moyer, and M. Lisney. 2002. Tinea gladiatorum: Pennsylvania's experience. *Clin. J. Sport Med.* **12:**165–171.

95. Kooistra, J. A. 1965. Prophylaxis and control of erythrasma of the toe webs. *J. Investig. Dermatol.* **45:**399–400.

96. Koopman, J. S., E. A. Eckert, H. B. Greenberg, B. C. Strohm, R. E. Isaacson, and A. S. Monto. 1982. Norwalk virus enteric illness acquired by swimming exposure. *Am. J. Epidemiol.* **115:**173–177.

97. Krishnaswami, S. K. 1971. Health aspects of water quality. *Am. J. Public Health* **61:**2259–2268.

98. Lacroix, C., M. Baspeyras, P. de-La-Salmonière, M. Benderdouche, B. Couprie, I. Accoceberry, F. Weill, and F. Derouin. 2002. Tinea pedis in European marathon runners. *J. Eur. Acad. Dermatol. Venereol.* **16:**139–142.

99. Lévesque, S., P. Giovenazzo, P. Guerrier, D. Laverdière, and H. Prud'Homme. 2002. Investigation of an outbreak of cercarial dermatitis. *Epidemiol. Infect.* **129:**379–386.

100. Levine, N. 1980. Dermatologic aspects of sports medicine. *J. Am. Acad. Dermatol.* **3:**415–424.

101. Lindenmayer, J. M., S. Schoenfeld, R. O'Grady, and J. K. Carney. 1998. Methicillin-resistant Staphylococcus aureus in a high school wrestling team and the surrounding community. *Arch. Intern. Med.* **158:**895–899.

102. Losonsky, G. 1991. Infections associated with swimming and diving. *Undersea Biomed. Res.* **18:**181–185.

102a.Loveday, C. 1990. Letter. *Lancet* **335:**1532.

103. Ludlam, H., and B. Cookson. 1986. Scrum kidney: epidemic pyoderma caused by a nephritogenic Streptococcus pyogenes in a rugby team. *Lancet* **ii:**331–333.

104. Lüttichau, H. R., C. Vinther, S. A. Uldum, J. Møller, M. Faber, and J. S. Jensen. 1998. An outbreak of Pontiac fever among children following use of a whirlpool. Clin. Infect. Dis. 26:1374–1378.

105. Maki, D. G., and R. M. Reich. 1982. Infectious mononucleosis in the athlete. Diagnosis, complications, and management. Am. J. Sports Med. 10:162–173.

106. Maré, J. B., C. M. J. Keyzer, and W. B. Becker. 1978. Traumatic Herpesvirus hominis infection during rugby (herpes venatorum): a discussion of four cases. S. Afr. Med. J. 54:752–754.

107. Mast, E. E., and R. A. Goodman. 1997. Prevention of infectious disease transmission in sports. Sports Med. 24:1–7.

108. Mast, E. E., R. A. Goodman, W. W. Bond, M. S. Favero, and D. P. Drotman. 1995. Transmission of blood-borne pathogens during sports: risk and prevention. Ann. Intern. Med. 122:283–285.

108a. McDaniel, W. E. 1997. Letter. Arch. Dermatol. 113:519–520.

109. McGrew, C. A., R. W. Dick, K. Schniedwind, and P. Gikas. 1993. Survey of NCAA institutions concerning HIV/AIDS policies and universal precautions. Med. Sci. Sports Exerc. 25:917–921.

110. Midtvedt, T., and K. Midtvedt. 1982. Sport and infection. Scand. J. Soc. Med. Suppl. 29:241–244.

111. Mills, J., L. Hauer, A. Gottlieb, S. Dromgoole, and S. Spruance. 1987. Recurrent herpes labialis in skiers. Clinical observations and effect of sunscreen. Am. J. Sports Med. 15:76–78.

111a. Mobacken, H., and P. Nordin. 1987. Letter. J. Am. Acad. Dermatol. 17:519–520.

112. Möhrenschlager, M., H. P. Seidl, C. Schnopp, J. Ring, and D. Abeck. 2001. Professional ice hockey players: a high-risk group for fungal infection of the foot? Dermatology 203:271.

113. Moore, M., R. C. Baron, M. R. Filstein, J. P. Lofgren, D. L. Rowley, L. B. Schonberger, and M. H. Hatch. 1983. Aseptic meningitis and high school football players: 1978 and 1980. JAMA 249:2039–2042.

114. Morgan, J., S. L. Bornstein, A. M. Karpati, M. Bruce, C. A. Bolin, C. C. Austin, C. W. Woods, J. Lingappa, C. Langkop, B. Davis, D. R. Graham, M. Proctor, D. A. Ashford, M. Bajani, S. L. Bragg, K. Shutt, B. A. Perkins, and J. W. Tappero. 2002. Outbreak of leptospirosis among triathlon participants and community residents in Springfield, Illinois, 1998. Clin. Infect. Dis. 34:1593–1599.

115. Morrison, C. L. 1994. Anabolic steroid users identified by needles and syringe exchange program. Drug Alcohol Depend. 36:153–155.

116. Morse, L. J., J. A. Bryan, L. W. Chang, J. P. Hurley, J. F. Murphy, and T. F. O'Brien. 1970. Holy Cross football team hepatitis outbreak. Antimicrob. Agents Chemother. 10:30–32.

117. Morse, L. J., J. A. Bryan, J. P. Hurley, J. F. Murphy, T. F. O'Brien, and W. E. C. Wacker. 1972. The Holy Cross college football team hepatitis outbreak. JAMA 219:706–708.

118. Mullan, R. J., E. L. Baker, D. M. Bell, W. W. Bond, M. C. Chamberland, M. S. Favero, J. S. Garner, S. C. Hadler, J. M. Hughes, H. W. Jaffe, M. A. Kane, R. Marcus, W. J. Martone, M. J. Scally, and P. W. Strine. 1989. Guidelines for prevention of transmission of human immunodeficiency virus and hepatitis B virus to health-care and public safety workers. MMWR Morb. Mortal. Wkly. Rep. 38:1–37.

119. Mumford, C. J. 1989. Leptospirosis and water sports. Br. J. Hosp. Med. 41:519.

120. Niizeki, K., O. Kano, and Y. Kondo. 1984. An epidemic study of molluscum contagiosum: relationship to swimming. Dermatologica 169:197–198.

120a. O'Farrell, N., S. J. Tovey, and P. Morgan-Capner. 1992. Letter. Lancet 339:246.

121. Parana, A., Lyra, L., and C. Trepo. 1999. Intravenous vitamin complexes used in sporting activities and transmission of HCV in Brazil. Am. J. Gastroenterol. 94:857–858.

122. Perra, A., V. Servas, G. Terrier, D. Postic, G. Baranton, G. André-Fontaine, V. Vaillant, and I. Capek. 2002. Clustered cases of leptospirosis in Rochefort, France, June 2001. Euro Surveill. 7:131–136.

123. Peters, E. M., and E. D. Bateman. 1983. Ultramarathon running and upper respiratory tract infections: an epidemiological survey. S. Afr. Med. J. 64:582–584.

124. Piqu, E., R. Copado, A. Cabrera, M. Olivares, M. C. Farina, P. Escalonilla, M. L. Soriano, and L. Requena. 1999. An outbreak of tinea gladiatorum in Lanzarote. Clin. Exp. Dermatol. 24:7–9.

125. Porter, P. S., and R. D. Baughman. 1965. Epidemiology of herpes simplex among wrestlers. JAMA 194:998–1000.

126. Raborn, G. W., A. Y. Martel, M. G. A. Grace, and W. T. McGaw. 1997. Herpes labialis in skiers: randomized clinical trial of acyclovir cream versus placebo. Oral Surg. Oral Med. Oral Pathol. Oral Radiol. Endod. 84:641–645.

127. **Raymond, L. W., D. T. Kingsbury, and J. F. Duncan.** 1971. Penicillin resistance of D. pneumoniae in upper respiratory infections associated with diving. *Aerosp. Med.* **42:**196–198.

128. **Resnik, S. S., L. A. Lewis, and B. H. Cohen.** 1977. The athlete's foot. *Cutis* **20:**351–353, 355.

129. **Ringertz, O.** 1971. Some aspects of the epidemiology of hepatitis in Sweden. *Postgrad. Med. J.* **47:**465–472.

130. **Ringertz, O., and B. Zetterberg.** 1967. Serum hepatitis among Swedish track finders. An epidemiologic study. *N. Engl. J. Med.* **276:**540–546.

131. **Risser, W. L.** 1992. HIV makes caution necessary in sports settings. *Phys. Sportsmed.* **20:**190.

132. **Roach, M. C., and J. H. Chretien.** 1995. Common hand warts in athletes: association with trauma to the hand. *J. Am. Coll. Health* **44:**125–126.

133. **Rosenbaum, G. S., M. J. Strampfer, and B. A. Cunha.** 1990. Herpes gladiatorum in a male wrestler. *Int. J. Dermatol.* **29:**141–142.

134. **Rosenberg, M. L., K. K. Hazlet, J. Schaefer, J. G. Wells, and R. C. Pruneda.** 1976. Shigellosis from swimming. *JAMA* **236:**1849–1852.

135. **Rutkow, I. M.** 1978. Rupture of the spleen in infectious mononucleosis. *Arch. Surg.* **113:**718–720.

136. **Sadovsky, R.** 1995. Transmission of bloodborne pathogens during sports contact. *Am. Fam. Physician* **51:**2011.

137. **Sawyer, R. N., A. S. Evans, J. C. Niederman, and R. W. McCollum.** 1971. Prospective studies of a group of Yale University freshmen. I. Occurrence of infectious mononucleosis. *J. Infect. Dis.* **123:**263–270.

138. **Schouten, W. J., R. Verschuur, and H. C. G. Kemper.** 1988. Physical activity and upper respiratory tract infections in a normal population of young men and women: the Amsterdam growth and health study. *Int. J. Sports Med.* **9:**451–455.

138a. **Scott, M. J., and M. J. Scott, Jr.** 1989. Letter. *JAMA* **262:**207–208.

139. **Sejvar, J., E. Bancroft, K. Winthrop, J. Bettinger, M. Bajani, S. Bragg, K. Shutt, R. Kaiser, N. Marano, T. Popovic, J. Tappero, D. Ashford, L. Mascola, D. Vugia, B. Perkins, N. Rosenstein, and the Eco-Challenge Investigation Team.** 2003. Leptospirosis in "Eco-Challenge" athletes, Malaysian Borneo, 2000. *Emerg. Infect. Dis.* **9:**702–707.

140. **Selling, B., and S. Kibrick.** 1964. An outbreak of herpes simplex among wrestlers (herpes gladiatorum). *N. Engl. J. Med.* **270:**979–982.

141. **Sevier, T. L.** 1994. Infectious disease in athletes. *Med. Clin. N. Am.* **78:**389–412.

142. **Seyfried, P. L., R. S. Tobin, N. E. Brown, and P. F. Ness.** 1985. A prospective study of swimming-related illness. *Am. J. Public Health* **75:**1068–1070.

143. **Sharp, J. C.** 1994. ABC of sports medicine: infections in sport. *Br. Med. J.* **308:**1702–1706.

144. **Sharp, J. C.** 1989. Viruses and the athlete. *Br. J. Sports Med.* **23:**47–48.

145. **Shute, P., D. J. Jeffries, and A. C. Maddocks.** 1979. Scrum-pox caused by herpes simplex virus. *Br. Med. J.* **2:**1629.

146. **Skinner, G. R. B., J. Davies, A. Ahmad, P. McLeish, and A. Buchan.** 1996. An outbreak of herpes rugbiorum managed by vaccination of players and sociosexual contacts. *J. Infect.* **33:**163–167.

147. **Snyder, R. W., and D. B. Glasser.** 1994. Antibiotic therapy for ocular infection. *West. J. Med.* **161:**579–584.

148. **Sorvillo, F. J., S. H. Waterman, J. K. Vogt, and B. England.** 1988. Shigellosis associated with recreational water contact in Los Angeles county. *Am. J. Trop. Med. Hyg.* **38:**613–617.

149. **Sosin, D. M., R. A. Gunn, W. L. Ford, and J. W. Skaggs.** 1989. An outbreak of furunculosis among high school athletes. *Am. J. Sports Med.* **17:**828–832.

150. **Souto, F. J., A. G. Silva, and F. Yonamine.** 2003. Risk of hepatitis C among Brazilian ex-soccer players. *Mem. Inst. Oswaldo Cruz* **98:**1025–1026.

151. **Spruance, S. L., M. L. Hamill, W. S. Hoge, L. G. Davis, and J. Mills.** 1988. Acyclovir prevents reactivation of herpes simplex labialis in skiers. *JAMA* **260:**1597–1599.

152. **Srivastava, K. P., E. C. Quinlan, and T. V. Casey.** 1972. Spontaneous rupture of the spleen secondary to infectious mononucleosis. *Int. Surg.* **57:**171–173.

153. **Stacey, A. R., K. E. Endersby, P. C. Chan, and R. R. Marples.** 1998. An outbreak of methicillin resistant Staphylococcus aureus infection in a rugby football team. *Br. J. Sports Med.* **32:**153–154.

154. **Stiller, M. J., W. P. Klein, R. I. Dorman, and S. Rosenthal.** 1992. Tinea corporis gladiatorum: an epidemic of Trichophyton tonsurans in student wrestlers. *J. Am. Acad. Dermatol.* **27:**632–633.

155. **Strauss, R. H., D. J. Leizman, R. R. Lanese, and M. F. Para.** 1989. Abrasive shirts may contribute to herpes gladiatorum among wrestlers. *N. Engl. J. Med.* **320:**598–599.

156. **Stuart, J. M., K. A. Cartwright, J. A. Dawson, J. Rickard, and N. D. Noah.** 1988. Risk

factors for meningococcal disease: a case control study in south west England. *Community Med.* **10**:139–146.

157. **Takama, H., Y. Tamada, K. Yano, Y. Nitta, and T. Ikeya.** 1997. Pitted keratolysis: clinical manifestations in 53 cases. *Br. J. Dermatol.* **137**:282–285.

158. **Takama, H., Y. Tamada, K. Yokochi, and T. Ikeya.** 1998. Pitted keratolysis: a discussion of two cases in non-weight-bearing areas. *Acta Dermato-Venereol.* **78**:225–226.

159. **Teichmann, D., K. Göbels, J. Simons, M. P. Grobusch, and N. Suttorp.** 2001. A severe case of leptospirosis acquired during an iron man contest. *Eur. J. Clin. Microbiol. Infect. Dis.* **20**:137–138.

160. **Tillett, H. E., J. de Louvois, and P. G. Wall.** 1998. Surveillance of outbreaks of waterborne infectious disease: categorizing levels of evidence. *Epidemiol. Infect.* **120**:37–42.

161. **Tobe, K., K. Matsuura, T. Ogura, Y. Tsuo, Y. Iwasaki, M. Mizuno, K. Yamamoto, T. Higashi, and T. Tsuji.** 2000. Horizontal transmission of hepatitis B virus among players of an American football team. *Arch. Intern. Med.* **160**:2541–2545.

162. **Torre, D., C. Sampietro, G. Ferraro, C. Zeroli, and F. Speranza.** 1990. Transmission of HIV-1 infection via sports injury. *Lancet* **335**:1105.

163. **Tranquilli, C., O. Armignacco, and M. Ilardi.** 1994. Sport activity and HIV infection. *Med. Sport* (Turin) **47**:47–52.

164. **Turner, M., G. R. Istre, H. Beauchamp, M. Baum, and S. Arnold.** 1987. Community outbreak of adenovirus type 7a infection associated with a swimming pool. *South. Med. J.* **80**:712–715.

165. **Vazquez-Lopez, F., and N. Perez-Oliva.** 1996. Mupirocin ointment for symptomatic pitted keratolysis. *Infection* **24**:55.

165a. **Verbov, J., and N. J. Lowe.** 1974. Letter, *Lancet* **ii**:1523–1524.

166. **Walker, A.** 1992. Swimming—the hazards of taking a dip. *Br. Med. J.* **304**:242–245.

166a. **Werninghaus, K.** 1993. Letter. *J. Am. Acad. Dermatol.* **28**:1022–1023.

167. **Wheeler, C. E., Jr., and W. H. Cabaniss, Jr.** 1965. Epidemic cutaneous herpes simplex in wrestlers (herpes gladiatorum). *JAMA* **194**:993–997.

168. **White, J.** 1991. Measles: a hazard of indoor sports. *Phys. Sportsmed.* **19**:21.

169. **White, W. B., and J. M. Grant-Kels.** 1984. Transmission of herpes simplex virus type 1 infection in rugby players. *JAMA* **252**:533–535.

170. **World Health Organization.** 1982. Guidelines for the control of leptospirosis. *WHO Offset Publ.* **67**:1–171.

171. **World Health Organization.** 1992. World Health Organization consensus statement: consultation on AIDS and sports. *JAMA* **267**:1312.

172. **Wormser, G. P., S. Bittker, G. Forseter, I. K. Hewlett, I. Argani, B. Joshi, J. S. Epstein, and D. Bucher.** 1992. Absence of infectious human immunodeficiency virus type 1 in "natural" eccrine sweat. *J. Infect. Dis.* **165**:155–158.

173. **Young, C. C., M. W. Niedfeldt, L. M. Gottschlich, C. S. Peterson, and M. R. Gammons.** 2007. Infectious disease and the extreme sport athlete. *Clin. Sports Med.* **26**:473–487.

TRAVELING ABROAD

Martin S. Wolfe

12

Approximately 15 million Americans travel abroad each year, and about half of this number go to the developing world. Tourists usually visit these remoter parts of the world for a period of weeks, where they may be exposed to diseases that are not present, or are at most rare, in the United States. Other individuals may be longer-term travelers or residents in the developing world.

In response to the hazards posed to travelers, the medical specialty of travel medicine has evolved, and numerous travel clinics are in operation. Travel medicine involves both the prevention of travel-related diseases and the diagnosis and treatment of exotic, primarily tropical, diseases upon the traveler's return (34, 38).

PRETRAVEL ADVICE
The main areas involved in prevention include pretravel advice, preparation of an individualized medical kit, immunizations, malaria prophylactic measures, and prophylaxis and self-treatment of traveler's diarrhea.

A pretravel physical examination, best performed by a personal physician, is indicated for travelers with serious medical problems and for those planning a long or physically demanding trip. A medical summary, including recent chest X-rays and electrocardiogram, should be carried. A serious medical condition can be summarized on a health card or an engraved bracelet. The names of recognized, preferably English-speaking, physicians or specialists in the countries to be visited should be known by the traveler.

In addition, adequate medical insurance should be obtained to cover conditions acquired abroad, as well as hospitalization and medical evacuation if required. Those with chronic illness should carry a needed supply of required drugs.

Individualized Medical Kits
Items to be included in an individualized medical kit depend on preexisting and other potential needs. General items could include a thermometer, bandages, gauze, tape, a germicidal soap solution, aspirin, antacids, anti-motion-sickness medication, and a mild laxative. Particular antibiotic, antifungal, and anti-inflammatory ointments should be included. A sunscreen is indicated for tropical areas. Antibiotics can be carried by travelers to

Martin S. Wolfe, Traveler's Medical Service of Washington, DC, and George Washington University Medical School, Washington, DC 20037.

Infections of Leisure, Fourth Edition, Edited by David Schlossberg,
© 2009 ASM Press, Washington, DC

remote areas where medical assistance may not be readily available. Suggested specific items for a medical kit and information on their use can be found in a publication of the American Society of Tropical Medicine, *Health Hints for the Tropics* (71). Specific items are discussed below.

Immunizations

Vaccine requirements by country are published annually by the Centers for Disease Control and Prevention (CDC) (*Health Information for International Travel* [21]) and by the World Health Organization (*International Travel and Health: Vaccination Requirements and Health Advice* [75]). A number of commercial computer programs are also available (29).

YELLOW FEVER

Yellow fever is currently the only disease for which vaccination is required for international travel. Yellow fever occurs in tropical Africa and South America, and vaccination can be required for entry into countries in these regions or for travelers entering certain other countries if they have come from a country with regions where infections occur (21). Vaccination must be validated in an International Certificate of Vaccination. Yellow fever vaccine requires continuous cold storage and must be used within 60 min following reconstitution. Because of this, yellow fever vaccine is given only in approved state-licensed official vaccination centers. A single dose is valid for 10 years, and side effects are minimal. The vaccine is contraindicated for those with an altered immune status or known hypersensitivity to eggs, children below the age of 9 months, pregnant women, and those with a history of thymus disease. These individuals must be advised not to enter any area with active yellow fever infection and should be given a letter of contraindication to satisfy any entrance requirement. Persons older than 60 years of age may be at increased risk for systemic adverse events following vaccination compared with younger persons. Travelers

older than 60 years should discuss with their physicians the risks and benefits of vaccination in the context of their destination-specific risk for yellow fever exposure (21).

CHOLERA

At present, no countries officially require a cholera certificate, and the vaccine is not recommended, even for travel to areas with epidemic cholera. The manufacture and sale of the only cholera vaccine licensed in the United States have been discontinued. New and improved oral cholera vaccines are available abroad but are not yet licensed in the United States (49).

SMALLPOX

Smallpox is considered to be eradicated worldwide, and vaccination is no longer required or recommended for travelers.

HEPATITIS A

Hepatitis A is the most common type of hepatitis contracted by unprotected travelers to areas of endemicity (70). Two hepatitis A vaccines are available in the United States. Havrix (GlaxoSmithKline) was approved in 1995, and Vaqta (Merck) became available in 1996. Adults receive an adult dose, and children and adolescents aged 1 to 17 years receive a reduced dose. An initial dose of either vaccine will induce protective immunity within 4 weeks. A booster dose given 6 to 12 months after the first dose is expected to lead to long-term protection (estimated as possibly >20 years) (56). A combined hepatitis A and B vaccine (Twinrix) is also available (4).

HEPATITIS B

Vaccination against hepatitis B is recommended for travelers who anticipate direct contact with blood or sexual contact with residents of high-risk areas and for resident expatriates (21). Three doses are required, and the vaccine is expensive. At this time, there is no recommendation for booster doses, as the primary series leads to long-term protection.

#39

IMMUNOGLOBULIN
Immunoglobulin is an alternative method for short-term protection from hepatitis A. Persons undertaking travel for less than 3 months will be protected by a single intramuscular dose (0.02 ml/kg of body weight). Those traveling for longer periods, as well as expatriate residents, should receive an intramuscular dose of 0.06 ml/kg at 4-month to no more than 6-month intervals. Immunoglobulin offers no protection against hepatitis types B, C, and E.

INFLUENZA AND PNEUMOCOCCAL VACCINES
Travelers at high risk for contracting influenza and its complications and travelers to the tropics should receive influenza vaccine. Travelers who are young children or elderly and those of all ages with chronic medical conditions should receive pneumococcal vaccine.

JAPANESE ENCEPHALITIS VACCINE
Japanese encephalitis is endemic in much of the Far East, Southeast Asia, and southern Asia. Occasional cases have occurred in expatriates, usually in those in long-term residence. Persons who plan to live in rural-agricultural locations of infected areas should consider receiving this vaccine (18). The currently used mouse brain-derived vaccine is no longer being produced and will soon be replaced by an inactivated cell culture-derived vaccine (21).

MENINGOCOCCAL MENINGITIS
Epidemic meningococcal meningitis occurs annually in the meningitis belt in sub-Saharan Africa during the dry season (December through June). Immunization with quadrivalent meningitis type A/C/Y/W 135 vaccine is recommended for travelers to this area during the epidemic season. A single dose offers protection for 3 years. Pilgrims and some visa applicants to Saudi Arabia are required to have evidence of this vaccination for entry (44).

PLAGUE
Plague occurs sporadically, usually in remote locations. Vaccination is particularly indicated for field workers who could have direct contact with potentially plague-infected wild rodents in rural areas where plague is endemic. A case of plague imported into the United States by an American rodent collector infected in rural Bolivia emphasizes the importance of vaccination for such workers (66). A primary series requires three doses, and periodic boosters are required when exposure risk continues. In the absence of vaccine, when there is a potential exposure, a 7-day course of doxycycline or trimethoprim-sulfamethoxazole may be taken as postexposure prophylaxis.

POLIO
Because of polio eradication efforts, the number of countries in which polio is endemic has decreased to four. The western hemisphere, the western Pacific region (including China), and the European region are now considered free of polio. Most of the remaining cases of poliovirus transmission occur in Afghanistan, India, Pakistan, and Nigeria. Most travelers have had a basic polio immunization series during childhood, but not all have had a necessary subsequent booster. A single inactivated polio vaccine booster dose is recommended for travelers who have received a primary polio vaccine series and are going to countries where polio is still endemic or epidemic. Those who travel to areas where polio occurs but who have not been vaccinated adequately against polio should receive a primary inactivated polio vaccine series (21).

RABIES
Rabies is endemic in practically all of the developing world. The usual traveler is at minimal risk, and the expensive three-dose human diploid cell or purified chicken embryo cell vaccine preexposure series is rarely indicated for this group. This series can be recommended for higher-risk groups, such as young

children, joggers, animal handlers, and field workers (63). The preexposure series offers added protection but does not eliminate the need for additional therapy following rabies exposure. All travelers in areas where rabies is endemic should not approach stray dogs or cats, primates, or other wild animals (see chapter 10).

TUBERCULOSIS (*MYCOBACTERIUM TUBERCULOSIS* BCG)

Although tuberculosis is a potential hazard to visitors to the developing world, the use of the BCG vaccine is not usually recommended by American travel medicine specialists because of troublesome side effects and questionable efficacy of available vaccines (19). Pre- and posttravel tuberculin skin test screening is considered preferable.

TYPHOID

Typhoid and paratyphoid fevers are endemic in much of the developing world. There are no available vaccines for paratyphoid, but there are oral and injectable typhoid vaccines which are recommended for travelers to developing countries where typhoid is endemic. The oral live-attenuated Ty21a strain vaccine is administered in capsule form, with one capsule taken every other day for four doses. A booster dose is required every 5 years (11). A single-dose parenteral vaccine offers similar (approximately 70%) protection for 2 years (69).

TYPHUS

No American traveler has contracted epidemic typhus in the last 40 years. Typhus vaccine is no longer recommended and is not available in the United States.

ROUTINE AND CHILDHOOD VACCINATIONS

All Americans should be up to date on routine immunizations regardless of travel plans, and indicated boosters must be given before travel. Boosters of adult tetanus and diphtheria are necessary every 10 years. *Haemophilus influen-*zae type b vaccine should be given to all children older than 2 months. Measles/mumps/rubella vaccine is usually given as a single dose at age 15 months. However, the age of vaccination should be lowered to age 6 to 11 months for children traveling to areas where they are at increased risk of endemic or epidemic measles (21). Adult travelers may also be at increased risk of measles infection. Persons born in or after 1957 should be vaccinated with a single-dose measles vaccine if they have not previously received two doses of measles vaccine or have no history of measles (34). Varicella vaccine should be considered for travelers who do not have immunity to varicella-zoster virus, especially if close personal contact with local populations is expected (77).

Malaria Prophylaxis

Malaria infection is a very serious risk for travelers to areas where malaria is endemic. The emergence and continued spread of chloroquine-resistant and other drug-resistant *Plasmodium falciparum* malaria and the complexities involved with contraindications and toxic effects of available malaria prophylactic drugs make it difficult to offer appropriate advice to travelers. Expert opinion is required to determine the areas of drug resistance and to make decisions on the best drug and antimosquito measures for particular situations (24).

Chloroquine is the drug of choice for the relatively few malarious areas where *P. falciparum* parasites remain sensitive to it (Central America, Haiti, and parts of the Middle East). In all other malarious areas, chloroquine-resistant *P. falciparum* malaria occurs, and other drugs must be used (38). Drugs should be started before travel and should be taken while in and for 4 weeks after leaving the malarious area. Atovaquone-proguanil need be taken for only 7 days after leaving. Chloroquine tablets are available in the United States, and liquid preparations are available abroad. The adult dose is 500 mg of salt (300 mg of base) once weekly for adults and 5 mg/kg weekly for children. Chloroquine is considered safe for young children and pregnant women (65). Minor side effects are common, but marked intolerance is rare. In recent years, chloroquine-resistant *Plasmodium vivax* malaria has occurred in parts of Southeast Asia and South America (73).

In the United States, there are currently three main drugs recommended for prophylaxis. Mefloquine (Lariam) has the advantage of being taken weekly. The adult dose is 250 mg, and the drug is administered in reduced doses by weight for children. There is a high degree of mefloquine resistance in *P. falciparum* along the Thai-Burmese and Thai-Cambodian borders and in western Cambodia; rare cases of confirmed resistance have been reported in tropical Africa. Reported side effects of mefloquine include insomnia, bad dreams, dizziness, headache, irritability, and gastrointestinal symptoms. More serious reactions, such as toxic psychosis, depression, suicidal thoughts, and hallucinations, occur in approximately 1 in 10,000 users. Since many of these adverse reactions occur within the first 3 weeks of initial usage, first-time users should ideally begin taking mefloquine 3 weeks before travel to allow potential adverse events to occur before travel. Contraindications to mefloquine use include a history of epilepsy, serious psychiatric disorders, and cardiac conduction abnormalities. Mefloquine is considered safe for infants and young children as well as for pregnant women when there is a significant risk of contracting malaria (21, 24).

Malarone, a fixed combination of atovaquone and proguanil, is an alternative to mefloquine. Dosage is on a daily basis, beginning 1 day before entering a malarious area, while in the area, and for 7 days after leaving the area. This drug is therefore particularly useful and cost-effective for trips of 14 days or less. The adult dose is one adult tablet daily. Pediatric dose tablets are available, and doses vary by weight. The available data on safety and efficacy of atovaquone-proguanil for prevention of malaria in children weighing less than 11 kg and in pregnant women are insufficient;

the drug is contraindicated for these groups. Severe renal impairment is another contraindication. Atovaquone-proguanil should not be used together with tetracyclines, rifampin, or metoclopromide. The most common adverse effects with this drug are abdominal pain, nausea, vomiting, and headache (14).

The third commonly recommended prophylactic drug is daily doxycycline. It is particularly indicated for travelers to the mefloquine-resistant areas mentioned above. The daily dose for adults is 100 mg. This is begun 1 day before arrival in and continued for 4 weeks after leaving the malarious area. Doxycycline is contraindicated for pregnant women and children younger than 8 years of age. Potential adverse effects include photosensitivity, gastrointestinal effects, and candidiasis (21).

Particularly for short trips, primaquine at a daily dose of 30 mg can be taken the day before entering, while in, and for 7 days after leaving the malarious area (9). Primaquine is also used to prevent potential relapsing malaria due to persisting liver forms of *P. vivax* and *Plasmodium ovale,* which are not eliminated by other antimalaria prophylactic drugs. This is particularly important for persons who have had intense or prolonged exposure in malarious areas. Primaquine is taken in a daily dose for 14 days, after completing the terminal suppressive doses of one of the above-mentioned drugs. The usual adult dose is 15 mg of base daily. However, in some malarious areas, including the southwest Pacific, Southeast Asia, and Central and South America, *P. vivax* parasites have acquired resistance to this standard dose of primaquine. Travelers returning from these areas for whom terminal primaquine is indicated should take a dose of 30 mg of base daily for 14 days (9, 24). Primaquine may cause severe hemolysis in persons with glucose-6-phosphate dehydrogenase deficiency, and this condition must be ruled out before primaquine is used. Primaquine is contraindicated during pregnancy.

Some drugs are no longer recommended for prophylaxis by American experts because of potentially serious side effects; these include pyrimethamine-sulfadoxine (Fansidar), amodiaquine, and pyrimethamine-sulfone (Maloprim).

Travelers who are in very remote areas without access to medical care may take along a dose of antimalarial medication for emergency self-treatment. This should be taken promptly if fever, chills, or other influenza-like illness develops. This self-treatment is only a temporary measure, and prompt medical evaluation is imperative. The drug of choice for presumptive self-treatment is atovaquone-proguanil for those not taking this drug for prophylaxis. The adult dose is four adult tablets in a single dose daily for 3 days (21).

In addition to drug prophylaxis, mosquito avoidance measures should be practiced. Malaria transmission by mosquitoes occurs primarily between dusk and dawn. Measures to prevent mosquito bites during these hours include the following:

1. Remaining in well-screened areas
2. Use of permethrin-impregnated mosquito nets (3)
3. Wearing clothes that cover most of the body
4. Application of permethrin repellent to clothing
5. Use of repellents containing DEET (*N*,*N*-diethyl-*m*-toluamide) on exposed parts of the body (28)
6. Use of pyrethrum-containing flying-insect spray in living areas

Traveler's Diarrhea

Up to 50% of travelers to the developing world are affected by traveler's diarrhea. This can be caused by bacteria (particularly toxigenic *Escherichia coli*), viruses, and less commonly, parasites. Infection is usually contracted from contaminated water or food (67).

To prevent traveler's diarrhea, water should be boiled for 3 min or disinfected with iodine tablets or a portable iodine resin filter prior to ingestion (8). Foods should be well cooked, and hot salads and cold foods should be avoided. Raw or poorly cooked shellfish, unwashed vegetables and fruits, and suspect dairy products should not be eaten.

Prophylactic antibiotics are generally not recommended by experts because of the potential for side effects and widespread bacterial resistance (30). Bismuth subsalicylate (Pepto-Bismol), taken as two tablets four times a day for up to 3 weeks, has proven to be a safe means of reducing the occurrence of traveler's diarrhea by about 65% (26).

Should diarrhea occur during travel, lost fluids should be replaced by drinking water, tea, broth, or carbonated beverages. Oral rehydration electrolyte mixtures are even better (27). Cramps or moderate diarrhea can be relieved by such antimotility agents as loperamide (Imodium) (27). Bismuth subsalicylate liquid, taken at 1 oz every half hour for eight doses, is useful, particularly for diarrhea due to toxigenic *E. coli* (27). If these measures are not adequate or if fever, chills, or blood or mucus in the stool occurs, a physician should be contacted for appropriate diagnosis and treatment. In an emergency, self-treatment, preferably with a quinolone antibiotic or azithromycin, can be administered (1).

POSTTRAVEL MANAGEMENT

The most common problems in returning travelers are diarrhea or other gastrointestinal difficulties, fever, unexplained eosinophilia, and skin rashes. Drugs for parasitic infections are summarized in reference 7.

Diarrhea or Other Gastrointestinal Difficulties

Diarrhea and gastrointestinal complaints are the most common problems for travelers, both during and after a trip. The most common cause of acute diarrhea during or just after return is toxigenic *E. coli,* but infection may also be due to a variety of viral, bacterial, fungal, and protozoal organisms or toxic marine organisms (i.e., fish or shellfish poisoning). Symptoms developing sometime following travel are most commonly due to pathogenic intestinal protozoa. Less likely causes are tropical sprue (39) or enteropathy, celiac disease, postinfectious lactose intolerance, intestinal helminths, or postinfectious irritable bowel.

VIRAL INTESTINAL INFECTIONS

Rotavirus spread by the fecal-oral route is a cause of enteric disease worldwide (13). After an incubation period of less than 48 h, there is the onset of frequent watery diarrhea, nausea, and malaise. Symptoms usually last for 5 to 7 days. The viral etiology is usually suspected from the clinical picture and the absence of other organisms. Specific diagnosis can be made from a variety of available assays which detect rotavirus in stool.

Norwalk virus also occurs worldwide, has an incubation period of 18 to 48 h, and causes a 24- to 48-h illness with diarrhea and vomiting (13). There is currently no available routine diagnostic assay. Treatment of both these viral infections is supportive, with particular emphasis on fluid replacement.

BACTERIAL INTESTINAL INFECTIONS

Toxigenic *E. coli* causes approximately 50 to 70% of traveler's diarrhea cases. Other relatively common bacterial etiological agents include *Shigella* and *Salmonella* species, *Campylobacter jejuni,* and *Vibrio parahaemolyticus.* Less common etiologies include other *Vibrio* species (*Vibrio cholerae* is distinctly uncommon), *Clostridium, Staphylococcus aureus,* and *Yersinia enterocolitica* (27, 67).

Most severe infections leading to dysentery with fever, chills, and blood and mucus in the stool are caused by large-bowel-invasive *C. jejuni, Shigella* species, and certain invasive *Salmonella* species. Other organisms, such as toxigenic *E. coli,* are noninvasive and usually cause symptoms by producing an enterotoxin, leading to watery diarrhea and a relatively short, self-limiting illness. A wet mount of stool stained with methylene blue usually reveals sheets of polymorphonuclear leukocytes and red blood cells with the former, more invasive organisms, while these cells are gener-

ally absent with noninvasive bacteria colonizing the small bowel (67).

Definitive diagnosis is made with stool culture using various media, including those for *Salmonella* and *Shigella,* and special selective media for *C. jejuni* and *Vibrio* species. Symptoms caused by noninvasive *Vibrio* and *Salmonella* species are generally self-limiting and usually do not require treatment. The other invasive organisms can be treated with a quinolone antibiotic or azithromycin (1).

In a traveler who has recently taken antibiotics, diarrhea may be due to *Clostridium difficile* infection. This is diagnosed by detecting *C. difficile* toxin in the stool. If the toxin is present, treatment is carried out with metronidazole or vancomycin.

FUNGAL ENTERITIS

Recent use of broad-spectrum antibiotics or metronidazole can eliminate normal intestinal bacteria and allow candidal overgrowth. In some cases, this can lead to diarrhea and other gastrointestinal symptoms. Intestinal candidiasis should be considered the etiology when budding yeast and mycelial forms are found in large numbers on direct fecal examinations after antimicrobial treatment. Rapid improvement is seen with oral nystatin (41).

FISH AND SHELLFISH TOXINS

Fish and shellfish toxins may initially cause acute diarrhea, which can then be followed by prolonged neurological symptoms. Ciguatera poisoning from ingestion of large marine reef fish (including grouper, snapper, and barracuda) containing ciguatoxin is the most common form of fish poisoning (25).

INTESTINAL PARASITES

Pathogenic intestinal protozoa commonly affecting travelers include *Giardia lamblia* (most frequently recognized), *Entamoeba histolytica,* and *Dientamoeba fragilis.* Less common are *Cryptosporidium parvum, Cyclospora cayetanensis,* and *Isospora belli.* Since the incubation period of these organisms is generally considerably longer than that of viruses and bacteria, initial symptoms frequently do not develop until late in a trip or following return. Symptoms can also be more prolonged or recurrent (64).

G. lamblia is a worldwide threat to travelers. Infection is usually acquired from contaminated water, and the incubation period is approximately 9 to 15 days. Typical symptoms include recurrent or persistent soft, foul-smelling stools and flatus, intestinal bloating and gurgling, belching, indigestion, weight loss, and fatigue. Diagnosis is usually from a series of stool specimens, best collected in a preservative. However, up to 30% of those infected can be "low excretors" of the parasite and can be difficult to diagnose by stool examination. Enzyme-linked immunosorbent assays to detect Giardia antigen in stool are available (2), but it remains to be proven that these tests are consistently positive for low excretors with negative stool samples. Other methods which can be used to confirm infection include examination of upper intestinal fluid obtained with a nasogastric tube or with an Enterotest duodenal string test (10), examination of a biopsy impression smear, or histological examination of a small-bowel biopsy specimen. In some cases with typical travel and exposure history and typical Giardia-like symptoms, it is not possible to confirm infections. In this situation, empiric treatment is advocated. Available drugs in the United States include metronidazole (Flagyl) and furazolidone (Furoxone) (68). Quinacrine (Atabrine), a very effective treatment, is not currently commercially available but can be put into capsules by certain pharmaceutical compounders. Nitazoxanide (Alinia) is available as a liquid preparation for children 1 to 11 years old, and a tablet formulation of nitazoxanide for use in adults is given in a 3-day course. This drug is generally well tolerated and effective (5). Tinidazole (Tindamax), which can be administered in a single dose, is now available in the United States (6). Lactase deficiency is common with giardiasis and may persist after successful treatment, causing symptoms mimicking persistent giardiasis (68).

E. histolytica is also contracted worldwide by travelers. Many of those infected with En-tamoeba are asymptomatic cyst passers who harbor the nonpathogenic species Entamoeba dispar. E. histolytica and E. dispar are morphologically identical but can be differentiated with a two-stage rapid stool antigen detection kit (55). At the other clinical extreme, amebic dysentery is uncommon. Intermediate non-dysenteric symptoms include alternating constipation and diarrhea, lower abdominal cramps, bloating and flatus (not foul smelling), and fatigue. Diagnosis is made by finding typical cysts or trophozoites in the stool and confirming E. histolytica identification by stool antigen detection. In cases of dysentery, proctoscopic examination reveals typical ulcers; scrapings or biopsy of these ulcers can reveal E. histolytica trophozoites. Amebic serology is usually positive with invasive amebic bowel disease. In mild cases, a nonabsorbed luminal drug such as paromomycin or iodoquinol is usually curative. Moderate to severe (dysenteric) symptoms require initial metronidazole, followed by a luminal drug (64).

D. fragilis is an amoeba-like noninvasive flagellate of the large bowel found worldwide. This protozoan has no cyst form and occurs only in the very labile trophozoite form. To confirm infection with this parasite, stools must be collected in preservative and permanently stained slides must be examined. Not all those infected have symptoms, but diarrhea, abdominal bloating, flatulence, and fatigue may occur (31). Treatment is carried out with paromomycin, with iodoquinol as an alternative (64).

Cryptosporidium is usually associated with AIDS patients, but infection can occur in travelers with healthy immune systems (51). The incubation period can be as little as 4 days, and symptoms can mimic those of giardiasis. Diagnosis may require special stool concentration tests and staining. Nitazoxanide is effective for treatment, although infection in nonimmunosuppressed persons is usually self-limited within 7 to 30 days (5).

Cyclospora is present throughout the world and has been identified in travelers from various regions. The incubation period varies from 2 to 11 days. Symptoms include watery

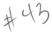

diarrhea, indigestion, cramps, weight loss, and marked fatigue. Left untreated, infection is self-limiting in immunocompetent persons, usually after 4 to 6 weeks. Diagnosis is based on finding oocysts on fecal examinations. Trimethoprim-sulfamethoxazole is an effective treatment (52).

I. belli is a rarely diagnosed parasite which can give symptoms similar to those of giardiasis (50). *Blastocystis hominis* is a ubiquitous parasite whose pathogenicity is debated. It is frequently present in asymptomatic travelers. In one careful study of symptomatic individuals with only *B. hominis* parasites, most were later found to have another difficult-to-recognize pathogenic protozoan (43).

A number of nonpathogenic intestinal protozoa must be differentiated from pathogenic parasites. This requires fecal smears permanently stained with iron hematoxylin or trichrome. Intestinal helminths seldom cause chronic diarrhea; a major exception is *Strongyloides stercoralis*.

Travelers with chronic diarrhea who have had relatively prolonged residence in southern Asia, Southeast Asia, or parts of the Caribbean may have tropical sprue (39). This malabsorption syndrome is rare in short-term travelers. It should be considered for those with a history of geographic exposure who have persistent diarrhea, indigestion, flatulence, and weight loss when no pathogenic organism can be found.

Fever in the Returned Traveler

Many febrile illnesses in the traveler have a cosmopolitan rather than exotic etiology, and they are frequently self-limiting. The major exotic tropical fevers occurring in travelers include malaria, enteric fever, hepatitis, bacterial dysentery, and rickettsial and arboviral infections (42).

MALARIA

A febrile traveler returning from an area where malaria is endemic must first and foremost be considered to have possible malaria. Most malaria infections occur in those travelers who have had no, irregular, or inappropriate che-

moprophylaxis. However, all febrile travelers from a malarious area must be examined for malaria, since no chemoprophylaxis regimen can be considered fully protective. Potentially lethal falciparum malaria usually occurs within 4 weeks after leaving a malarious area. *P. vivax* and *P. ovale* malaria may occur up to 3 years after exposure if primaquine has not been taken to eliminate persistent latent parasites in the liver. *Plasmodium malariae* does not have a latent liver phase and is the least common species seen in travelers. Typical malaria symptoms are high fever, shaking chills, sweats, headache, and myalgias. Symptoms may be modified or masked depending on the malaria immune status (as in an immune native of an area of endemicity) or by the use of prophylactic antimalarial drugs. Severe *P. falciparum* infections can rapidly lead to such lethal complications as cerebral malaria, renal failure, severe hemolysis, and adult respiratory distress syndrome (74).

Diagnosis is made by appropriately prepared and carefully examined Giemsa-stained thin and thick malaria smears (Fig. 1). A single negative set of smears cannot rule out malaria, and smears should be repeated at 6-h intervals for a 24- to 48-h period. A malaria rapid diagnostic test is now available in the United States; it can allow rapid diagnosis of malaria and result in prompt treatment (22). Blood smears, however, are considered the gold standard for malaria diagnosis and should be carried out to confirm results of the rapid test.

Falciparum malaria contracted in one of the relatively few areas with chloroquine-sensitive malaria can be treated with chloroquine alone. Initially, 1 g of chloroquine phosphate salt (600 mg of base) is given orally. Six hours later, 500 mg of salt (300 mg of base) is taken, and this dose is repeated 24 and 48 h later. For falciparum malaria contracted in chloroquine-resistant malarial areas, with a low level of parasitemia (<1%) and no complications, oral treatment can be given. Atovaquone-proguanil can be taken in an adult course of four adult tablets as a single dose on three consecutive days. Mefloquine in a single adult dose of 1,250 mg can be used for those with-

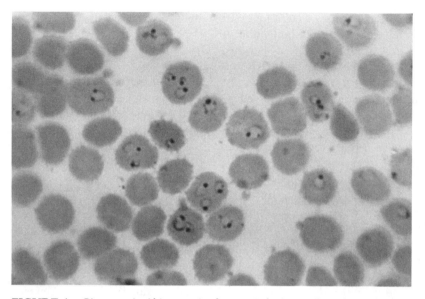

FIGURE 1   Giemsa stain (thin smear) of severe infection with *P. falciparum*. Numerous ring forms are visible. Source: Steven Glenn, Laboratory and Consultation Division, CDC (http://phil.cdc.gov/phil/quicksearch.asp).

out a contraindication for this drug. Vomiting and neuropsychiatric side effects can occur in a small percentage of those taking mefloquine. Alternatively, oral quinine, given as 650 mg of salt three times a day for 3 days, can be used, to be followed by oral tetracycline at 250 mg four times a day for 7 days (60). Patients with severe or complicated falciparum malaria must be hospitalized and managed with intensive care, immediate intravenous antimalarial drug treatment, and necessary supportive management (74). In the United States, intravenous quinine is not available, and treatment must be carried out with intravenous quinidine (47). A continuous infusion of quinidine gluconate is recommended. A loading dose of 10 mg of quinidine gluconate salt (equal to 6.2 mg of quinidine base) per kg of body weight is given over 1 to 2 h, followed by constant infusion of 0.02 mg of quinidine gluconate salt (0.0125 mg of base) per kg per min. This regimen is highly effective and well tolerated in monitored patients. Quinidine is given for 3 days and is then followed by tetracycline, as described above. In patients with a malaria parasitemia level of >10% or with

marked clinical deterioration, exchange transfusion along with constant quinidine infusion can be lifesaving (45). Intravenous artesunate is now available in the United States as an investigational new drug application and can be obtained for use in severe malaria infections. It can be obtained from the CDC Drug Service or from one of the CDC Quarantine Stations. A follow-on antimalarial drug should be given after the artesunate course (23, 48).

P. malariae, P. vivax, and *P. ovale* can be treated with chloroquine alone, like chloroquine-sensitive *P. falciparum*. Chloroquine-resistant *P. vivax* should be treated with atovaquone-proguanil or mefloquine. With *P. vivax* or *P. ovale,* this should be followed by primaquine, given as 15 mg of base daily for 14 days (30 mg of base in areas where primaquine-resistant *P. vivax* is found), after a normal glucose-6-phosphate dehydrogenase status is established.

ENTERIC FEVER

Typhoid and paratyphoid fevers (enteric fever) can be contracted from contaminated food or water in the developing world, where the prevalence of the causative bacteria is high. Currently available typhoid vaccines offer protection from *Salmonella enterica* serovar Typhi to no more than 70% of recipients (11). Enteric fever should be suspected in travelers returning from an area of endemicity with fever, headache, abdominal pain, diarrhea, or cough. Symptoms may not develop until several weeks after return. Diagnosis is confirmed by positive blood, stool, or urine cultures. Febrile agglutinin (Widal) tests or *Salmonella* antibodies may be useful. *Salmonella* serovar Typhi organisms worldwide have developed multiple antibiotic resistance, and a quinolone is the usual drug of choice for most areas. However, *Salmonella* serovar Typhi in southern Asia is frequently resistant to quinolones, and infections contracted in this region should be treated with azithromycin. Similar resistance can be seen with *S. enterica* serovar Paratyphi A infection (32).

HEPATITIS

Travelers to the developing world who have not received immunoglobulin or hepatitis A vaccine run a significant risk of contracting hepatitis A from contaminated water or food. Rare cases of hepatitis E have been contracted in southern Asia and elsewhere. There is no available vaccine, and immunoglobulin does not protect against hepatitis E (17). Hepatitis B is usually contracted through sexual contact and is uncommon in travelers. In the preicteric phase of acute hepatitis, fever, chills, myalgias, and fatigue may occur, and this syndrome can mimic malaria and other acute tropical fevers. Hepatitis serologic testing can confirm infection, but when these tests are negative for a patient with apparent hepatitis, cytomegalovirus or Epstein-Barr virus (mononucleosis) infection should be considered.

AMEBIC LIVER ABSCESS

A period of acute diarrhea frequently precedes development of an amebic liver abscess. A returned traveler with fever and right upper quadrant pain should be suspected of this disorder. Sonography or scanning of the liver shows a filling defect, and an amebic serology test confirms infection. Needle aspiration is not usually required for diagnosis or treatment. There is usually a very rapid clinical response to oral or intravenous metronidazole. Follow-up treatment should be given with paromomycin or iodoquinol (as for intestinal amebiasis) to eliminate any bowel cysts and prevent relapse. Abscess cavities may take some months to fill in (55).

RICKETTSIAL INFECTIONS

Tick typhus can be contracted in West, East, and southern Africa and in the Mediterranean littoral. Infection typically begins with a skin eschar at the tick bite site, fever, chills, and headache; in a few days, a diffuse papular rash may develop. Epidemic typhus, scrub typhus, and murine typhus are much less commonly contracted by travelers. The Weil-Felix agglutination battery can be used for initial screening, and confirmation can be obtained from indirect fluorescent-antibody tests for specific rickettsial organisms. Tetracycline is a highly effective and rapid treatment (37).

VIRAL FEVERS

Dengue fever is endemic in most parts of the tropical world and is the most commonly imported arbovirus infection. Symptoms include fever, headache, body aches, and eye pain (54). Typically, a diffuse rash appears on the third to fifth day as other symptoms abate. Japanese B encephalitis is a rare infection of travelers to rural areas of the Far East (18). A number of other rarer acute viral illnesses have been imported from areas of endemicity, including those caused by lethal Lassa, Ebola, and Marburg fever viruses from West and Central Africa (36). Diagnosis is usually confirmed serologically. Treatment is generally supportive; ribavirin has been found useful in Lassa fever cases. In recent years, a major outbreak of chikungunya virus infection occurred on islands of the Indian Ocean, in Africa, and in India, and imported cases have been seen in North America and Europe (56).

LESS COMMON FEBRILE ILLNESSES

African trypanosomiasis was contracted by 15 American travelers from 1967 through 1987 (15). Although the actual risk is low, even short-term travelers to game parks in East and Central Africa should take precautions against tsetse fly bites. Travelers should inform their physicians of exposure history if symptoms such as trypanosomal chancre at a bite site, fever, evanescent rash, headache, and lethargy develop up to 4 weeks following return.

Tuberculosis. Tuberculosis remains a threat worldwide. Although infection in travelers is uncommon, any returnee with fever, cough, and chest radiographic evidence of pulmonary disease should be evaluated for tuberculosis. Pre- and posttravel tuberculin skin testing is recommended for long-term travelers. A newly available tuberculosis blood test is considered more accurate than the tuberculin skin test (20).

Brucellosis. Brucellosis is contracted from contaminated raw goat's or cow's milk or soft cheese. Those infected can present with fever, chills, sweats, body aches, headache, monarticular arthritis, weight loss, fatigue, or depression. Generalized lymphadenopathy and splenomegaly are common. Diagnosis is by blood culture and specific agglutination tests (76).

Leptospirosis. Leptospirosis is common in the tropics but is rarely contracted by travelers. Infection is acquired through direct or indirect contact with infected animals or through contaminated water exposure. Most infections are anicteric and mild. Initial symptoms can include high remittent fever, chills, headache, myalgias, nausea, and vomiting. No more than 10% of patients develop jaundice. Diagnosis is usually made with serologic techniques. Early therapy with penicillin or doxycycline is usually beneficial (57).

Anthrax. Anthrax is very rarely contracted from contact with contaminated animal by-products, such as hides and wool. Most infections occur on the face or arms after a minor abrasion, presenting as an initial painless papule which vesiculates and becomes hemorrhagic, necrotic, and covered with an eschar. Treatment is carried out with penicillin or tetracycline.

Melioidosis. Melioidosis is an uncommon infection in travelers to Southeast Asia. Presentation resembles that of acute pulmonary tuberculosis. Less commonly, chronic infection may develop (61).

Histoplasmosis. Histoplasmosis is a cosmopolitan disease and has rarely infected travelers to Latin America. Visitors to caves contaminated with bat droppings are at particular risk (59). Consideration should be given to possible histoplasmosis in a returned traveler with pulmonary or, less likely, disseminated disease.

Visceral Leishmaniasis. Visceral leishmaniasis (kala-azar) is extremely rare in American tourists, though European travelers have been infected around the Mediterranean littoral. Symptoms include fever, hepatosplenomegaly, and wasting. Diagnosis is confirmed by demonstrating leishmanial organisms in a biopsy specimen of liver, spleen, or bone marrow (12).

American Trypanosomiasis. American trypanosomiasis (Chagas' disease) is very common in Latin America, and travelers engaged there in hiking, camping, and archaeological projects can be exposed. However, naturally acquired, documented infection is extremely rare in travelers.

Lyme Disease. Lyme disease occurs in Europe and may also be present in other parts of the world. Hikers, in particular, should take precaution against tick bites in any recognized area of endemicity.

HIV. Human immunodeficiency virus (HIV) infection is a particular hazard from sexual contact, blood transfusion, or contact with contaminated needles or syringes in areas of high-level endemicity in the tropics. A number of disposable syringes and needles can be carried by travelers who might need injections while traveling in areas where only non-disposable products are used. HIV serology screening should be done on any traveler with the above-mentioned exposure (16).

Eosinophilia in the Returned Traveler

A returned traveler with eosinophilia of >5% who has been in the developing world should be considered to have possible helminthic infection. With some exceptions, protozoal infections do not cause eosinophilia. Allergic problems usually cause an eosinophilia of <15%, but some drug reactions can cause a much higher eosinophilia (72).

HELMINTH INFECTIONS

High eosinophilia of up to 80% can occur during the acute stage of certain helminth infections, particularly those with a tissue larval migration.

Adult intestinal helminths can cause mild to moderate (6% to 30%) eosinophilia. Patients are usually asymptomatic with *Ascaris lumbricoides,* hookworms, *Trichuris trichiura, Enterobius vermicularis* (pinworms), and various tapeworms. Diagnosis is made by finding typical eggs or tapeworm segments in the stool. Pinworm eggs are best diagnosed by applying sticky paddles or cellophane tape to the perianal area. Treatment of all these infections is carried out with mebendazole (Vermox) or albendazole (Albenza). Tapeworms are treated with praziquantel (7). *Ascaris* and hookworms have an early larval migration through the lungs which can cause pulmonary symptoms and infiltrates and quite high eosinophilia.

S. STERCORALIS

S. stercoralis and the much less commonly acquired *Trichostrongylus* species infect through the skin. *S. stercoralis,* however, can complete its life cycle without leaving the host, and infections persisting for more than 40 years have been recognized. Eosinophilia is particularly high during the early years of infection, but in long-established infections eosinophil counts can be normal. Many infections are asymptomatic, but some individuals may have epigastric pain, diarrhea, cough, and urticarial rashes occurring on the buttocks and thighs (related to larval migration from the anus). Unsuspected asymptomatic infections can become disseminated throughout the body in the presence of immunosuppression, with steroid treatment, or with cancer therapy. Definitive diagnosis is done by finding larvae in the stool, but larvae are not present in all cases. Special stool concentration tests or examination of duodenal fluid may be required to find larvae. An enzyme-linked immunosorbent serologic test (available from the CDC) is very useful in making a presumptive diagnosis. Treatment is performed with ivermectin (Stromectol).

SCHISTOSOMIASIS

Schistosomiasis is acquired through contact with fresh water containing snails, which are intermediate hosts. *Schistosoma mansoni* occurs in northeastern South America, certain Caribbean islands, Africa, and the Middle East. *Schistosoma hematobium* occurs in Africa and the Middle East. *Schistosoma japonicum* and *Schistosoma mekongi* are present in the Far East. *Schistosoma intercalatum* infection is an uncommon intestinal infection in West and Central Africa. Acute schistosomiasis (Katayama syndrome) is more often associated with *S. mansoni* and *S. japonicum* infections, and symptoms may occur 6 to 8 weeks after exposure, when adult worms begin producing eggs. Symptoms include hypereosinophilia, fever, chills, pulmonary complaints, headache, abdominal pain, and urticaria. The majority of established schistosome infections are asymptomatic, and eosinophilia seldom exceeds 3,000 eosinophils/mm^3. Intestinal infections with *S. mansoni, S. japonicum, S. mekongi,* and *S. intercalatum* can cause abdominal pain, diarrhea, and fatigue. *S. hematobium* can give hematuria and other urinary tract symptoms. Diagnosis is done by finding eggs in the stool or urine, depending on the geographic area of exposure, symptoms, and species. Infection in travelers is often light, and eggs can be absent on routine stool and urine examinations. Special concentration tests of stool and urine and rectal or bladder biopsy may be required to confirm infection. Serologic tests (available at the CDC) may be used to screen travelers with an exposure history. Treatment is performed with praziquantel (Biltricide) (7, 62).

LIVER FLUKES

Liver flukes in the early acute phase can cause hypereosinophilia, painful liver, and fever. *Fasciola hepatica* occurs almost worldwide and is contracted from eating watercress containing infective-stage metacercariae. *Clonorchis sinensis* and *Opisthorchis viverrini* occur in Southeast and East Asia and are contracted from eating raw fish containing metacercariae. In early *F. hepatica* infections, eggs may not occur in the stool, and diagnosis is made by suggested filling defects in the liver and hypereosinophilia; confirmation of *F. hepatica* infection is made on the basis of a positive serologic test. Ultrasonography or cholangiography can demonstrate *C. sinensis* or *O. viverrini* flukes in the bile ducts and gallbladder. In chronic infections, which are frequently asymptomatic, eggs may be found in the stool and mild eosinophilia may be present. *F. hepatica* infection is best treated with bithionol, and *Clonorchis* and *Opisthorchis* infections are treated with praziquantel (7).

FILARIAE

A number of filariae infect humans and can cause quite high eosinophilia. *Wuchereria bancrofti* and *Brugia malayi* are rare in travelers; long-term residence in an area of high-level endemicity seems necessary for infection. *Mansonella perstans* is a common parasite in tropical Africa and is the most commonly diagnosed filarial infection in the United Kingdom. *Loa loa* and *Onchocerca volvulus* are the two most commonly diagnosed causes of filarial infections in the United States, usually in longer-term residents of tropical Africa. The incubation period can be 6 months to 1 year, and symptoms may develop some time after return from an area of endemicity. The classic presentation of *L. loa* infection is the migra-

tion of the adult worm across the eye and/or subcutaneous evanescent swellings (Calabar swellings) on the arms or legs, associated with hypereosinophilia. Onchocerciasis usually presents with a very pruritic maculopapular eruption on the hips, back, buttocks, and thighs in the presence of hypereosinophilia. Filariasis should be suspected in travelers from areas of endemicity with hypereosinophilia and suggestive signs and symptoms. Microfilariae should be searched for in the blood or, in the case of onchocerciasis, in skin snips or biopsy samples. Filariasis serology can be useful. If infection is confirmed or strongly suspected, diethylcarbamazine is the treatment of choice for all species except *Onchocerca* and *M. perstans*. Onchocerciasis is treated with ivermectin, and *M. perstans* infection is treated with mebendazole or albendazole (46).

INTESTINAL PROTOZOA

Eosinophilia is distinctly uncommon in pure infections with *E. histolytica* and *G. lamblia*. Eosinophilia has been associated with other pathogenic intestinal protozoa, i.e., *D. fragilis* and *I. belli*.

Skin Disorders in the Returned Traveler

Common skin disorders acquired by travelers are cutaneous mycoses. Tinea versicolor is frequently contracted in the tropics, and depigmentation of the lesions may persist for some months after effective treatment. Tinea pedis ("athlete's foot") is particularly common in moist climates, as is tinea cruris ("jock itch"). The former can be prevented by regular use of foot powder and dry socks, while the latter can be prevented by use of a drying powder and frequent change of clothing. Superficial mycoses are diagnosed from skin scrapings in potassium hydroxide or by culture. Treatment is performed with a broad-spectrum cutaneous antimycotic preparation.

CUTANEOUS MYIASIS

Cutaneous myiasis is contracted by travelers to Latin America *(Dermatobia hominis)* and by travelers to Africa *(Cordylobia anthropophaga,* the tumbu fly). Infection with *C. anthropophaga* results from eggs deposited on clothes which are air dried and unironed. Larvae hatch in a few days and penetrate the skin, causing persistent, pruritic, and sometimes painful furuncular lesions with central necrosis. These lesions can often be confused with bacterial infections. A larva, which can be extracted, is seen in the center of the lesion, and healing is generally rapid after removal.

The sand flea, *Tunga penetrans,* invades the skin (often around the toes) when a person is walking barefoot. These fleas are easily removed with fine forceps.

Scabies and louse infestations are cosmopolitan conditions and are contracted when hygiene is poor. There is usually severe pruritus. Infection is confirmed by observing moving lice or, in the case of scabies, by examination of scrapings of scabetic burrows or papules. Scabies are treated with topical 5% permethrin or 10% crotamiton. Lice can be treated similarly. Oral ivermectin can also be used for both of these conditions.

Dog and cat hookworm larvae deposited in sandy soil can penetrate exposed skin and lead to cutaneous larva migrans (creeping eruption). This leaves migrating pruritic serpiginous tunnels in the epidermis. *S. stercoralis* can cause a particular form of hive-like cutaneous lesions (larva currens), usually on the buttocks or thighs. These lesions can be treated with oral ivermectin (35).

A number of cutaneous ulcers are contracted in the tropics. Most common is cutaneous leishmaniasis, transmitted by sandflies in the Middle East, the Mediterranean littoral, and parts of Asia, Africa, and Latin America. The incubation period can be 1 to 3 months or, rarely, longer. Typically, a papule develops which gradually enlarges and ulcerates into a painless sore with rolled edges. The causal *Leishmania* parasites can be identified in Giemsa-stained preparations, cultures of aspirate, or biopsy specimens from the edge of the ulcer. Treatment is carried out with pentavalent antimonial compounds (12). Similar but rare ulcers caused by *Corynebacterium diphtheriae* may occur in hot, dry, tropical areas.

A generalized maculopapular eruption can be seen with various typhus infections. Most common is tick typhus contracted in Africa, which often presents with an eschar at a tick bite site associated with rash, fever, chills, and headache. It is very responsive to tetracycline (37).

ROUTINE POSTTRAVEL SCREENING
Posttravel evaluation is usually not necessary for the short-term traveler who remains well while traveling and after return. However, ill travelers and their physicians must be aware of the long latency periods of some infections. Prior travel must then be considered in the presence of symptoms beginning some months or even a few years after travel or residence in the developing world. Longer-term travelers or residents from the tropics should have certain routine screening tests following return. These can include complete blood count, urinalysis, liver function tests, hepatitis B virus and HIV tests, tuberculin skin test, stool examinations for ova and parasites, and serologic tests for schistosomiasis if possible exposure has occurred (42).

PRACTICAL TIPS
- Main areas in prevention include general pretravel advice, use of an individualized medical kit, immunizations, malaria prophylaxis and prevention, and self-treatment of traveler's diarrhea.
- For malaria drug prophylaxis, expert opinion is required to determine areas of drug resistance and to decide on the best drug and antimosquito measures for particular situations.
- Traveler's diarrhea is usually contracted from contaminated food or water and can be caused by viruses, bacteria, and less commonly, parasites.
- Emergency self-treatment for presumed malaria is best carried out with atovaquone-proguanil for those not taking this drug for prophylaxis.
- Routine screening tests for returned travelers might include routine blood tests, urinalysis, hepatitis B virus and HIV tests, tu-

berculin skin test, stool examinations for ova and parasites, and serologic tests for schistosomiasis.

REFERENCES

1. **Adachi, J. A., L. Ostrosky-Zeichner, H. L. Du Pont, and C. D. Ericsson.** 2000. Empirical antimicrobial therapy for travelers' diarrhea. *Clin. Infect. Dis.* **31:**1079–1083.

2. **Aldeen, W. E. K., K. Carroll, A. Robison, M. Morrison, and D. Hale.** 1998. Comparison of nine commercially available enzyme-linked assays for detection of *Giardia lamblia* in fecal specimens. *J. Clin. Microbiol.* **36:**1338–1340.

3. **Anonymous.** 1991. Editorial. *Lancet* **337:**1515–1516.

4. **Anonymous.** 2001. Twinrix: a combination hepatitis A and B vaccine. *Med. Lett. Drugs Ther.* **43:**67–68.

5. **Anonymous.** 2003. Nitazoxanide (Alinia)—a new antiprotozoal agent. *Med. Lett. Drugs Ther.* **45:**29–31.

6. **Anonymous.** 2004. Tinidazole (Tindamax)—a new anti-protozoal drug. *Med. Lett. Drugs Ther.* **46:**70–72.

7. **Anonymous.** 2007. Drugs for parasitic infections. Treatment guidelines. *Med. Lett.* **5**(Suppl.): e1–e15. http://www.medletter.com.

8. **Backer, H.** 2002. Water disinfection for international and wilderness travelers. *Clin. Infect. Dis.* **34:**355–364.

9. **Baird, J. K., D. J. Fryauff, and S. L. Hoffman.** 2003. Primaquine for prevention of malaria in travelers. *Clin. Infect. Dis.* **37:**659–667.

10. **Beal, C. B., P. Viens, R. G. L. Grant, and J. M. Hughes.** 1970. A new technique for sampling duodenal contents—demonstration of upper small bowel pathogens. *Am. J. Trop. Med. Hyg.* **19:**349–352.

11. **Bennish, M. L.** 1995. Immunization against *Salmonella typhi. Infect. Dis. Clin. Pract.* **4:**114–122.

12. **Berman, J.** 1997. Human leishmaniasis: clinical, diagnostic, and chemotherapeutic developments in the last 10 years. *Clin. Infect. Dis.* **24:**684–703.

13. **Blacklow, N. R., and H. B. Greenberg.** 1991. Viral gastroenteritis. *N. Engl. J. Med.* **325:**252–264.

14. **Boggild, A. K., M. E. Parise, L. S. Lewis, and K. C. Kain.** 2007. Atovaquone-proguanil: report from the CDC Expert Meeting on Malaria Chemoprophylaxis (II). *Am. J. Trop. Med. Hyg.* **76:**208–223.

15. **Bryan, R. T., H. A. Waskin, F. O. Richards, T. M. Bailey, and D. D. Juranek.** 1988. African trypanosomiasis in American travelers: a 20 year review, p. 384–388. *In* R. Steffen, H. O. Lobel, J. Haworth, and D. J. Bradley (ed.), *Travel Medicine.* Springer-Verlag, Berlin, Germany.

16. **Castelli, F., and A. Patroni.** 2000. The human immunodeficiency virus infected traveler. *Clin. Infect. Dis.* **31:**1403–1408.

17. **Centers for Disease Control and Prevention.** 1993. Hepatitis E among US travelers, 1989–1992. *MMWR Morb. Mortal. Wkly. Rep.* **42:**1–4.

18. **Centers for Disease Control and Prevention.** 1993. Inactivated Japanese encephalitis vaccine. Recommendations of the ACIP. *MMWR Morb. Mortal. Wkly. Rep.* **42**(RR-1):1–15.

19. **Centers for Disease Control and Prevention.** 1996. The role of BCG vaccine in the prevention and control of tuberculosis in the United States. *MMWR Recomm. Rep.* **45**(RR-4):1–18.

20. **Centers for Disease Control and Prevention.** 2005. Guidelines for using the Quantiferon-TB Gold test for detecting *Mycobacterium tuberculosis* infection, United States. *MMWR Morb. Mortal. Wkly. Rep.* **54**(RR-15):49–55.

21. **Centers for Disease Control and Prevention.** 2007. *Health Information for International Travel 2008.* U.S. Department of Health and Human Services, Public Health Service, Atlanta, GA.

22. **Centers for Disease Control and Prevention.** 2007. Notice to readers: malaria rapid diagnostic test. *MMWR Morb. Mortal. Wkly. Rep.* **56:**286.

23. **Centers for Disease Control and Prevention.** 2007. Notice to readers: new medication for severe malaria available under an investigational new drug protocol. *MMWR Morb. Mortal. Wkly. Rep.* **56:**769–770.

24. **Chen, L. H., M. E. Wilson, and P. Schlagenhauf.** 2007. Controversies and misconceptions in malaria chemoprophylaxis for travelers. *JAMA* **20:**2251–2263.

25. **Dembert, M. L., K. F. Strosahl, and R. L. Baumgarner.** 1981. Diseases from fish and shellfish ingestion. *Am. Fam. Physician* **24:**103–108.

26. **DuPont, H. L., C. D. Ericsson, P. C. Johnson, J. M. Bitsura, M. W. DuPont, and F. J. de la Cabada.** 1987. Prevention of travelers' diarrhea by the tablet formulation of bismuth subsalicylate. *JAMA* **257:**1347–1350.

27. **Ericsson, C. D.** 1998. Travelers' diarrhea: epidemiology, prevention, and self-treatment. *Infect. Dis. Clin. N. Am.* **83:**285–304.

28. **Fradin, M. S., and J. F. Day.** 2002. Comparative efficacy of insect repellants against mosquito bites. *N. Engl. J. Med.* **347:**13–18.

29. **Freedman, D. O.** 2008. Sources of travel medicine information, p. 29–34. *In* J. S. Keystone, P. E. Kozarsky, D. O. Freedman, H. D. Northdurft, and B. A. Connor (ed.), *Travel Medicine,* 2nd ed. Mosby Elsevier, Philadelphia, PA.

30. Gorbach, S. L., and R. Edelman (ed.). 1986. Travelers' diarrhea: National Institutes of Health Consensus Development Conference. *Rev. Infect. Dis.* **8:**S109–S227.

31. Grendon, J. H., R. F. Di Giacomo, and F. J. Frost. 1995. Descriptive features of *Dientamoeba fragilis* infections. *J. Trop. Med. Hyg.* **98:**309–315.

32. Gupta, S. K., F. Medalla, M. W. Omondi, J. M. Whichard, P. I. Fields, P. Gerner-Smidt, N. J. Patel, K. L. F. Cooper, T. M. Chiller, and E. D. Mintz. 2008. Laboratory-based surveillance of paratyphoid fever in the United States: travel and antimicrobial resistance. *Clin. Infect. Dis.* **46:**1656–1663.

33. Hill, D. R., and F. J. Bia. 2005. Coming of age in travel medicine and tropical diseases: a need for continued advocacy and mentorship. *Infect. Dis. Clin. N. Am.* **19:**XV–XXI.

34. Hill, D. R., and R. D. Pearson. 1989. Editorial. *Ann. Intern. Med.* **111:**699–701.

35. Hochedez, P., and E. Caumes. 2008. Common skin infections in travelers. *J. Travel Med.* **15:**252–262.

36. Isaacson, M. 2001. Viral hemorrhagic fever hazards for travelers in Africa. *Clin. Infect. Dis.* **33:**1707–1712.

37. Jensenius, M., P. E. Fournier, and D. Raoult. 2004. Rickettsioses and the international traveler. *Clin. Infect. Dis.* **39:**1493–1499.

38. Jong, E. C., and H. D. Nothdurft. 2001. Current drugs for antimalarial chemoprophylaxis: a review of safety and efficacy. *J. Travel Med.* **8**(Suppl. 3):548–556.

39. Klipstein, F. A. 1981. Tropical sprue in travelers and expatriates living abroad. *Gastroenterology* **80:**590–600.

40. Kozarsky, P. E., and J. S. Keystone. 2002. Body of knowledge for the practice of travel medicine. *J. Travel Med.* **9:**112–115.

41. Levine, J., R. K. Dykoski, and E. N. Janoff. 1995. Candida-associated diarrhea: a syndrome in search of credibility. *Clin. Infect. Dis.* **21:**881–886.

42. MacLean, J. D., and M. Libman. 1998. Screening returning travelers. *Infect. Dis. Clin. N. Am.* **12:**431–443.

43. Markell, L. K., and M. P. Udkow. 1986. *Blastocystis hominis*: pathogen or fellow traveler? *Am. J. Trop. Med. Hyg.* **35:**1023–1026.

44. Memish, Z. 2002. Meningococcal disease and travel. *Clin. Infect. Dis.* **34:**84–90.

45. Miller, K. D., A. E. Greenberg, and C. C. Campbell. 1989. Treatment of severe malaria in the United States with a continuous infusion of quinidine gluconate and exchange transfusion. *N. Engl. J. Med.* **321:**65–70.

46. Ottesen, E. 1993. Filarial infections. *Infect. Dis. Clin. N. Am.* **7:**619–633.

47. Rosenthal, P. J., C. Peterson, F. R. Geertsma, and S. Kohl. 1996. Availability of intravenous quinidine for falciparum malaria. *N. Engl. J. Med.* **348:**621.

48. Rosenthal, P. J. 2008. Artesunate for the treatment of severe falciparum malaria. *N. Engl. J. Med.* **358:**1829–1836.

49. Ryan, E. T., and S. B. Calderwood. 2000. Cholera vaccines. *Clin. Infect. Dis.* **31:**561–565.

50. Shaffer, N., and L. Moore. 1989. Chronic travelers' diarrhea in normal host due to *Isospora belli*. *J. Infect. Dis.* **159:**596–597.

51. Soave, R., and P. Ma. 1985. Cryptosporidiosis. Travelers' diarrhea in two families. *Arch. Intern. Med.* **145:**70–72.

52. Soave, R. 1996. Cyclospora. An overview. *Clin. Infect. Dis.* **23:**429–437.

53. Suh, K. N., P. E. Kozarsky, and J. S. Keystone. 1999. Evaluation of fever in the returned traveler. *Med. Clin. N. Am.* **83:**997–1017.

54. Sung, V., D. P. O'Brien, E. Matchett, G. V. Brown, and J. Torresi. 2003. Dengue fever in travelers returning from Southeast Asia. *J. Travel Med.* **10:**208–213.

55. Tanyuksel, M., and W. A. Petri. 2003. Laboratory diagnosis of amebiasis. *Clin. Microbiol. Rev.* **16:**713–729.

56. Taubitz, W., J. P. Cramer, A. Kapaun, M. Pfeffer, C. Drosten, G. Dobles, G. D. Burchard, and T. Löscher. 2007. Chikungunya fever in travelers: clinical presentation and course. *Clin. Infect. Dis.* **45:**e1–e4.

57. Van Creval, R., P. Speelman, and C. Gravekamp. 1994. Leptospirosis in travelers. *Clin. Infect. Dis.* **19:**132–134.

58. Van Damme, P., J. Banatvala, O. Fay, O. Iwarson, B. McMahon, K. Van Herck, P. Shouval, P. Bonanni, B. Connor, G. Cooksley, G. Leroux-Roels, and F. Von Sonnenburg. 2003. Hepatitis A booster vaccination: is there a need? *Lancet* **362:**1065–1071.

59. Weinberg, M., J. Weeks, S. Lance-Parker, M. Traeger, S. Wiersma, Q. Phan, D. Dennison, P. MacDonald, M. Lindsley, J. Guarner, P. Connolly, M. Cetron, and R. Hajjeh. 2003. Severe histoplasmosis in travelers to Nicaragua. *Emerg. Infect. Dis.* **9:**1322–1325.

60. White, N. 1996. The treatment of malaria. *N. Engl. J. Med.* **335:**800–806.

61. White, N. 2003. Melioidosis. *Lancet* **361:**1715–1722.

62. Whitty, C. J. M., D. C. Mabey, M. Armstrong, S. G. Wright, and P. Chiodini. 2000. Presentation and outcome of 1107 cases of schistosomiasis from Africa diagnosed in a nonendemic country. *Trans. R. Soc. Trop. Med. Hyg.* **94:**531–534.

63. **Wilde, H., D. J. Briggs, F.-X. Meslin, T. Hemachudha, and V. Sitprija.** 2003. Rabies update for travel medicine advisors. *Clin. Infect. Dis.* **37:**96–100.

64. **Wolfe, M. S.** 1982. The treatment of intestinal protozoa. *Med. Clin. N. Am.* **66:**707–720.

65. **Wolfe, M. S., and J. F. Cordero.** 1985. Safety of chloroquine in chemosuppression of malaria. *Br. Med. J.* **290:**1466–1467.

66. **Wolfe, M. S., C. Tuazon, and R. Schultz.** 1990. Imported bubonic plague—District of Columbia. *MMWR Morb. Mortal. Wkly. Rep.* **39:** 895–901.

67. **Wolfe, M. S.** 1990. Acute diarrhea associated with travel. *Am. J. Med.* **88**(Suppl. 6A)**:**34S–37S.

68. **Wolfe, M. S.** 1992. Giardiasis. *Clin. Microbiol. Rev.* **5:**93–100.

69. **Wolfe, M. S.** 1995. Typhim Vi: a new typhoid vaccine. *Infect. Dis. Clin. Pract.* **4:**186–188.

70. **Wolfe, M. S.** 1995. Hepatitis A and the American traveler. *J. Infect. Dis.* **171**(Suppl. 1)**:**S29–S32.

71. **Wolfe, M. S. (ed.).** 2005. *Health Hints for the Tropics,* 13th ed. American Society of Tropical Medicine and Hygiene, Northbrook, IL.

72. **Wolfe, M. S.** 2008. The eosinophilia patient with suspected parasitic infection, p. 637–649. *In* E. G. Jong and C. Stanford (ed.), *The Travel and Tropical Medicine Manual,* 4th ed. Elsevier, Philadelphia, PA.

73. **Wongsrichanalai, C., A. L. Pickard, W. H. Wernsdorfer, and S. R. Meshnick.** 2002. Epidemiology of drug-resistant malaria. *Lancet Infect. Dis.* **2:**209–218.

74. **World Health Organization.** 2000. Severe falciparum malaria. *Trans. R. Soc. Trop. Med. Hyg.* **94**(Suppl. 1)**:**S1–S74.

75. **World Health Organization.** 2008. *International Travel and Health: Vaccination Requirements and Health Advice.* World Health Organization, Geneva, Switzerland.

76. **Young, E. J.** 1983. Human brucellosis. *Rev. Infect. Dis.* **5:**821–842.

77. **Zimmerman, R. K.** 1996. Varicella vaccine: rationale and indications for use. *Am. Fam. Physician* **53:**647–652.

FROM BOUDOIR TO BORDELLO: SEXUALLY TRANSMITTED DISEASES AND TRAVEL

Jonathan M. Zenilman

13

Travel has historically been an important risk factor for acquisition of sexually transmitted infections (STIs) (1, 16). Travel is often associated with a sense of adventure, periods of loneliness, and exploration away from one's home environment—which often form a milieu in which sexual activity can occur with new partners. Survey data clearly demonstrate that out-of-country travel is associated with recruitment of new sex partners and increased STI risk. Pretravel counseling to prevent STI risk is variable, and there is controversy about the efficacy impact of counseling. Some travel occurs specifically for sexual purposes, such as the sexual tourism junkets to Southeast Asian destinations which became popular during the 1980s. Some travel situations pose particularly high risk. For example, military deployments and assignments to work camps such as those for oil extraction occur in the context of large groups of individuals of reproductive age, often predominantly males, exposed to high levels of stress in unfamiliar environments. Over the past decade, travel has also been associated with a resurgence of genital ulcer diseases, es-

pecially syphilis and lymphogranuloma venereum (LGV), in homosexual men.

The types of diseases acquired during travel are dependent on the types of sexual activity, the types of sexual partners, and the reasons/type of travel that occurred. For example, the diseases and social situation of a military base are different from those of a refugee camp, which in turn are much different from the situations encountered by casual travelers. Travel is an important factor in the spread of new types of infections, such as antimicrobial-resistant *Neisseria gonorrhoeae* and human immunodeficiency virus (HIV) infection. In areas where STI incidence is low, travelers are often implicated in the reestablishment of new epidemic foci (reintroductions), as occurred in the reintroduction of syphilis and LGV to disease-free areas in Europe and North America. In this chapter, I review the clinical syndromes and epidemiology of the most commonly encountered STIs, as well as the clinical and behavioral aspects of travel and sexually transmitted disease (STD) epidemiology.

STIs have a major public health impact. In the United States, over 18 million cases of STIs (89) occur annually, with the highest incidence in adolescents and young adults. The different types of common STIs are described in Table 1.

Jonathan M. Zenilman, Division of Infectious Diseases, Johns Hopkins Bayview Medical Center, 4940 Eastern Ave., Baltimore, MD 21224.

Infections of Leisure, Fourth Edition, Edited by David Schlossberg,
© 2009 ASM Press, Washington, DC

TABLE 1 Major STDs

Genital ulcer diseases
Syphilis *(Treponema pallidum)*
Granuloma inguinale *(Calymmatobacterium granulomatis)*
LGV *(Chlamydia trachomatis* LGV serovars)
Chancroid *(Haemophilus ducreyi)*
Genital herpes (HSV-1 and HSV-2)
HPV infection

Exudative diseases
Gonorrhea *(Neisseria gonorrhoeae)*
Chlamydia *(Chlamydia trachomatis)*
Trichomoniasis *(Trichomonas vaginalis)*
BV (vaginal flora ecological disturbance)

Systemic diseases
HIV
Hepatitis B virus infection
Human T-lymphotropic virus type 1 (HTLV-1)
  infection
Cytomegalovirus infection
Human herpesvirus 8 (Kaposi's sarcoma-associated
  herpes virus) infection

Infestations
Scabies
Pediculosis

TRANSMISSION MODE: DEFINITION OF AN STD

STIs are transmitted through sexual intercourse. Sexual intercourse is clinically and epidemiologically defined as sexual contact, including vaginal intercourse, oral intercourse (either type of receptive oral intercourse, i.e., fellatio or cunnilingus), and rectal intercourse. STDs can be transmitted between heterosexual or homosexual partners. Different types of sexual activity may result in increased risks. Receptive rectal intercourse and vaginal intercourse carry the highest risks of STI transmission (73).

STIs are completely dependent on behavioral factors for transmission. Abstinent individuals will not contract an STI (37). Acquisition of STIs is also dependent on the probability that one will come into contact with an STI-infected partner, the susceptibility of the host, and the efficiency of transmission of the organism through sexual intercourse. Not only is the absolute number of sexual partners important, but the type of sexual partner contributes to potential infection risk. Individuals with partners who are more likely to be infected with STIs (for example, those involved in commercial sex work or drug use or those from an environment where diseases are highly prevalent) are much more likely to contract an STI than are other individuals who do not have high-risk sexual partners. Similarly, persons with serial partners (but only one sexual partner at a time) are less likely to spread STIs than are persons with multiple concurrent sex partners (2, 60). In parts of the world such as Western Europe and North America, travelers to areas where STIs are highly endemic account for a disproportionate share of new bacterial STIs (28, 34).

STD COVARIATES

Socioeconomic factors have been associated with an increased incidence of bacterial STIs (55). Decreased availability of health services, especially preventive health services, has also been associated with an increased incidence of STDs. For example, in Eastern Europe since the dissolution of the Soviet Union, there has been social and economic disruption, disintegration of the health system, increased levels of intravenous drug use, and loosening of travel restrictions. Economic upheaval in parts of Asia and Africa and in Eastern European countries such as the Ukraine and Moldova, coupled with a demand for commercial sex workers (CSWs) in other areas of the world, resulted in these becoming "source countries" for trafficked CSWs (81). The combination of economic disparity, commercial sex work, and travel has the potential for developing large STI and HIV epidemics.

Urbanization in developing countries is strongly associated with an increased incidence of STIs (67). In the United States, illicit drug use and its associated sexual behaviors are associated with the incidence of STIs, especially syphilis and HIV infection (29, 54). This is related in part to direct pharmacologic activities of the drugs themselves (cocaine and methamphetamine may stimulate increased sexual activity) but is more often due to the behaviors associated with drug use and the marketing of drugs, including prostitution.

Alcohol and other drug use is particularly associated with high-risk sexual activity. Similarly, studies of travelers find consistent relationships between alcohol use and, in some studies (where it was assessed), marijuana use and having sex with a new partner (9, 45, 46). Alcohol use is a frequent accompaniment of travel, and CSW establishments often are bars. Strategies for disease prevention in these settings should focus on identifying triggers or high-risk situations before they occur. If sexual activity is a possibility, then the individual should prepare beforehand (i.e., by having condoms available). Furthermore, individuals should take care not to overindulge, because the technical capacity to use a condom correctly may become impaired with high levels of alcohol or drug use.

EPIDEMIOLOGY OF TRAVEL AND STIs

Most studies of travelers' sexual behavior have been performed in Western Europe. In an early survey, 27% of women queried in a Swedish family planning setting reported a history of casual sex while traveling, mostly to destinations in Western Europe (5). Casual sex was associated with more frequent alcohol and marijuana use, a past history of STDs, and paradoxically, a higher education level (although this may be correlated with income and ability to travel). In Britain, a survey conducted in the early 1990s at the largest STI clinic in London (45) found that 18% of participants had traveled abroad within the previous 6 months, mostly to Western Europe. Of this subgroup, 25% reported a new sex partner while abroad, of whom 19% were from developing countries. Twenty-two percent of heterosexual men with new sex partners while abroad paid for these services, and two-thirds did not practice consistent condom use. A 2002 study in Australia suggested that up to one-quarter of new HIV infections may be acquired overseas, especially in Vietnam, where intravenous drug use and sexually trans-

mitted transmission have increased rapidly (31).

More recent surveys (published since 2004) are summarized in Table 2. Mercer et al. (65) estimated that residents of the United Kingdom made 66.4 million trips abroad in 2005. A survey embedded in the population-based and methodologically rigorous British National Survey of Sexual Attitudes and Lifestyles assessed travel-related sexual behaviors in persons aged 16 to 44 years. Within the previous 5 years, 13.9% of men and 7.1% of women reported a new sexual partner while overseas. Half of these partners were nationals of the United Kingdom, one-third were from other European Union countries, and 11% were from North America. Fewer than 5% reported partners from sub-Saharan Africa, the Caribbean, or South America. Bellis et al. (9) surveyed British vacationers who went to Ibiza, Spain, and found that of those surveyed, more than half had sex with a new partner, and 26% of men and 14% of women had multiple partners, nearly all of whom were residents of the United Kingdom. Alcohol and illicit drugs were very common. This may, however, reflect the destination, as Ibiza was marketed specifically to younger vacationers. Cabada et al. (14) studied vacationers who went to Cuzco, Peru, and found that 5.6% of travelers to Cuzco were sexually active with a new partner. Besides the demographic data, the study reported that 39% of travelers had received prior pretravel advice—but paradoxically this group had higher rates of sexual activity. A novel part of the reported Cuzco experience was the description of a specific indigenous group, the *bricheros,* who interact with foreigners, especially in bars and discos. Cabada et al. also studied tour guides (13) in Peru and found that 11% had had sex with a foreigner, but 46% of male and 4% of female guides would have sex with a traveler if the opportunity arose. Croughs et al. (20) studied travel clinic attendees in Holland and Belgium. This study was different from the others because it was a mailed questionnaire (response rate, 55%) but also because the travel-

TABLE 2 Recent papers on travel STDs

Study population	n	Sample frame	Yr(s) of survey	Findings	Comment(s)	Authors and reference
UK National Survey of Sexual Attitudes and Lifestyles (NATSAL)	12,100	Age of 16–44 yr; probability sample	1999–2001	13.9% of men and 7.1% of women had a new partner within previous 5 years	Nearly all partners were from United Kingdom, European Union, or North America; population-based weighted sample	Mercer et al. (65)
Travelers to Cuzco, Peru	2,540	Age of 15–50 yr; convenience sample at bus station	2001	5.6% of travelers had a new partner during their stay	54% of partners were other travelers, 41% were local partners, and 2% were CSWs; consistent condom use was practiced by 69%	Cabada et al. (14)
Travelers to Ibiza	1,241	Age of 16–35 yr; airport surveys, convenience sample	2000–2002	Of those who arrived without a sexual partner, 21% had one partner and 26% had two or more partners; one-third had unprotected sex acts; 20% of men had a non-UK sexual partner	Difficult to identify within study those who came with partners and those who did not	Bellis et al. (9)
Travel clinic attendees	1,907	Age of 16–50 yr; mailed questionnaires	2005	61% traveled with a steady partner; 5% of all travelers had a new partner; 31% did not consistently use condoms	Response rate was 55%; most travel was to Africa, Asia, and Turkey	Croughs et al. (20)
MSM visiting Key West, FL	247	Convenience samples at venues	2004	34% had anal sex with new a partner; avg no. of partners was 1.95; 77% did not disclose HIV status; 60% of sexually active men had unprotected sex	94% were gay, and 6% were bisexual; 8% were known to be HIV positive	Benotsch et al. (10)
HIV-infected travelers	290	Patients at Toronto HIV clinic; 93% were male	2001	46% traveled outside Canada and the United States; 90% were on antiretroviral therapy; 23% had casual sex while traveling; 35% of these encounters were with another traveler, and 87% were with local residents	Small study, but demonstrates increasing importance of HIV-infected travelers; few sought pretravel advice; only 58% reported consistent condom use.	Salit et al. (74)

ers' destinations were high-risk areas—24% of travel was to sub-Saharan Africa. Sixty-one percent of respondents were traveling with a regular sex partner. Overall, 5% had a new sex partner abroad, and 31% were not consistent condom users.

The themes which are evident in these studies are as follows:

1. Sexual activity can occur within a large variety of settings.

2. Only a minority of travelers receive pretravel sexual counseling.

3. With the exception of sexual tourists, the vast majority of exposures are "assortative"—i.e., new partners are usually other travelers from the same host country.

4. Condom use is relatively high but is affected by alcohol and other drug use.

SPECIFIC STUDIES OF MSM AND HIV-POSITIVE INDIVIDUALS

Few studies have specifically addressed these issues in the era of effective antiretroviral therapy. Salit et al. (74) studied travel and sexual behaviors in HIV-infected patients in a large Toronto HIV clinic. Disturbingly, they found that of those traveling outside North America, 23% had a casual sexual exposure, mostly with local residents. Only 58% of these exposures were condom protected 100% of the time, and 13% of sexually active respondents reported not using a condom at all when traveling. Pinkerton and colleagues (10) studied men who have sex with men (MSM) by use of venue-based surveys in Key West and found that almost one-third of participants had a new partner while traveling to the island and that 60% had at least one unprotected exposure. HIV status disclosure was rare. They also concluded through a modeling exercise that travel-related exposures may be an important contributor to HIV incidence among gay men. Besides these studies, there is a substantial literature which has documented the spread of bacterial STIs, such as syphilis, LGV, and antimicrobial-resistant gonococcal infections, in MSM travelers (48, 75, 82).

Most of the reported literature on travel describes persons from developed countries visiting developing countries and ignores the risks associated with indigenous travel. STI risk in developing countries is often associated with personal mobility as well as with geographic proximity to trading centers in rural areas. Travel has affected HIV epidemiology in developed countries, especially those in Europe, where ties to Africa and Asia are often close. Increasingly, travel-associated infections are being diagnosed in émigrés living in a developed country who return home to visit friends and relatives. For example, among Londoners of sub-Saharan ancestry, 40% of men and 21% of women reported a new sex partner when traveling home (33). Specific recommendations have been developed for these groups (7).

MILITARY POPULATIONS

Military personnel and the merchant marine are at high risk of STIs. Studies from the 1960s and 1970s suggest that the annual incidence rate of STIs in merchant seamen was 17 to 23% per year (19). Military campaigns where there has been interaction with the local population have been associated with very high rates of STI acquisition. For example, in the Boer War, British STD rates were >50% (3), and attack rates of 37% among Dutch soldiers in the East Indies in 1913, 16% among Dutch East Indies troops in the late 1940s, 27% among Australian troops in Vietnam (44), and 10% among U.S. naval personnel and marines deployed to Mediterranean staging areas, South America, and Africa between 1989 and 1991 (61) were observed. Similar problems were observed in military personnel deployed for noncombat roles. For example, of 1,885 Dutch marines deployed to Cambodia in 1992 to 1993, all received intensive STD education before deployment, and condoms were available. Eight hundred forty two (45%) reported sexual contact during deployment; 301 (36%) had one to three contacts, and 541 (64%) had four or more contacts (52). The overall unadjusted attack rate (including non-sexually active soldiers in the denominator) was 3.5%, and no cases were reported among consistent condom users. More recent studies of U.S. Navy personnel based in the Western Pacific found that the prevalence of asymptomatic urethritis ranged from 3.4 to 6.9% (76).

EXPATRIATES

Long-term travelers such as expatriates are at increased risk for HIV and STIs. Because of increasing numbers of HIV/AIDS cases in Belgian expatriates, a case-control study of 33 expatriate HIV patients and 119 seronegative controls in 1985 to 1987 found that HIV patients were more likely to have had an increased number of local sex partners (odds ratio [OR], >34) and CSW contact (OR, >10) (12). A study of U.S. Peace Corps volunteers ($n = 1,602$) found that 60% of respondents had sex while overseas, and 29% of these persons had sex with a local country partner (66). Only 32% of volunteers reported consistent condom use; alcohol use and low perceived HIV risk were the most important predictors of condom nonuse. A study of 847 Dutch expatriates found that 22% of men and 19% of women had a local steady sexual partner and that 29% of men and 17% of women had local casual partners (24). Condom use rates were 17 to 21% for the steady partners and 64 to 69% for the casual partners. Of the men with casual partners, 19% had CSW exposure.

OCCUPATIONAL TRAVEL AND EXPOSURE

Sudden economic development can also impact STI risk behaviors, especially in isolated areas where workers or travelers have rapid access to large amounts of funds and little activity. Goldenberg et al. (41, 42) performed qualitative work in the oil and gas boom towns of northern Canada. The work environment typically involved interim stays of 20 to 28 days and was located several hours from the nearest urban center. Important factors in high STI risk were mobility, high rates of partner turnover, binge partying, and a lack of community, which in turn impedes communication of disease status with sex partners.

Another factor described was that the workers often had steady partners or spouses at home, which in turn makes this situation very much like that in Africa. Also identified were local barriers to STI testing for youth among the workers, including the logistics related to work schedule and deployments, waits at the clinics, lack of public transportation, geographic inaccessibility of the clinics and the limited time that the workers have, stigma and labeling which would result from being tested, and prior poor interactions with health care workers. The authors suggest that active outreach efforts for both service delivery and patient education should take place in settings where there are large numbers of persons at risk.

CSWs

Sexual intercourse with CSWs is very common among travelers, expatriates, and military personnel and is one of the major risk factors for HIV and other STDs. In most parts of the world, CSWs are economically stratified. The lowest strata include brothel-based workers and CSWs who recruit customers on the street ("streetwalkers"). The next level are workers who recruit customers in bars (often karaoke bars in Asia) and have intercourse in hourly hotels. At the highest stratum are workers who have preset appointments and have one partner per day. The prices for services vary accordingly. Since STD rates are intrinsically tied to partner turnover rates and socioeconomic class, the lowest strata have the highest STD rates (22, 85).

Besides unprotected sexual intercourse, several practices of CSWs may increase STI risk even higher. This can include use of preexposure antibiotics, use of vaginal products and disinfectants (56), and the presence of other communicable diseases, such as tuberculosis (40). Condom use with CSWs may vary by locale, which may be attributed to socioeconomic disparity (between CSW and client), social or local norms, and enforcement. Most studies in this area were performed in Hong Kong and Singapore. A study of Hong Kong residents found that condom use was higher when they used CSWs in Hong Kong (91%) than when they used CSWs from mainland China (66%) and that self-reported STD rates were four times higher in those who had traveled to the mainland (58), 33% of travelers to the mainland had used services of CSWs, and 11% had used these services on the most recent trip (59).

In Singapore, a study of STD clinic attendees ($n = 372$) found that half of the clients had visited sex workers in Singapore and outside the country. Interestingly, 87.5% of the Singapore CSW contacts were condom protected, whereas outside the country, the rate was 41 to 77%, with the lowest rates in China and Indonesia (91, 92). The important finding here is that the most important variable which predicted condom use was initiation by the CSW, and it was not associated with demographic or other factors, including perceived risk of HIV/STI. This demonstrates that among risky clients, there are still tremendous education needs, even in areas where STI education is prioritized. It also highlights the need for local structural interventions which target CSWs.

From a human rights standpoint, CSWs present important issues (81). Many are engaged in commercial sex work because of poverty or oppression, especially in developing countries. The work environments are oppressive because the activity is illegal in most settings and therefore prone to corruption and organized criminal syndicates. Trafficking is increasingly recognized as an international problem. Health services, including sexual health services and contraception, are often nonexistent. In the developed world, commercial sex work is associated with drug use and a lack of effective income and drug treatment options. In addition to the objective disease risks, travelers should also consider the social context of commercial sex work and its associated issues.

TRAVEL FOR HEALTH PROFESSIONALS

Few data are available on travel-associated STD and HIV risk for health professionals. One small study of British medical students found that 18 of 23 medical schools surveyed provided starter packs for postexposure prophylaxis (all for bloodborne exposure) for students traveling to developing countries (80). Large proportions of fluid exposure and invasive procedures were reported by students, which reflects a combination of setting, health care system supply shortages, and local practices.

CLINICAL ASPECTS OF COMMON STDs

Gonorrhea and Chlamydia

Gonorrhea is caused by *Neisseria gonorrhoeae,* a fastidious gram-negative coccus (50). In men, urethritis is the most common syndrome. Discharge or dysuria usually appears within 1 week of exposure, although as many as 5 to 10% of patients never have signs or symptoms. Asymptomatic disease can exist in men for up to several weeks after infection. In women, gonorrhea typically causes cervical disease (cervicitis). Women with untreated gonococcal cervicitis develop upper tract infection-pelvic inflammatory disease (PID) (69). Symptomatic anorectal gonococcal disease occurs in men with a history of receptive rectal intercourse. Approximately 50% have symptoms which include rectal pain, discharge, constipation, and tenesmus. Because rectal gonorrhea in men implies a history of unprotected rectal intercourse, surveillance of rectal gonorrhea has been useful as a surrogate marker for HIV risk in gay men. Gonococcal pharyngitis occurs in men or women after oral sexual exposure and is clinically indistinguishable from any other bacterial pharyngitis. Disseminated gonococcal infection (gonococcal septicemia) occurs in approximately 0.1 to 0.5% of total gonococcal cases.

The syndromes for chlamydia are similar to those seen for gonorrhea, but they tend to be less aggressive in the acute context yet cause significant numbers of complications, especially PID and adverse perinatal outcomes (68). In men, *Chlamydia* urethritis accounts for approximately 40% of all cases of nongonococcal urethritis. Urethritis in men typically

#47

49

48

presents as a mucoid discharge, often associated with dysuria. Asymptomatic infection occurs in over 30% of cases seen in clinical settings but >90% of cases diagnosed in population-based prevalence studies. The time from infection to development of symptoms is longer than that for gonorrhea, usually about 7 to 14 days.

In women, cervical infection is the most commonly reported syndrome. Over one-half of women with cervical infection are asymptomatic. When symptoms occur, they may manifest as vaginal discharge or poorly differentiated abdominal or lower abdominal pain. At clinical examination, there are often no clinical signs present. When they are present, they include mucopurulent cervical discharge, cervical friability, and cervical edema. Left untreated, approximately 30% of women with chlamydial infection will develop PID. Rectal chlamydia infection occurs predominantly in homosexual men who have had receptive rectal intercourse, although there are cases in heterosexual women where similar exposures are reported. Oropharyngeal chlamydial infection appears not to be a clinically important entity.

DIAGNOSIS

Current approaches to diagnosis largely use nucleic acid amplification tests (38), which have largely replaced culture.

ANTIMICROBIAL RESISTANCE

Antimicrobial resistance is not a clinical issue in chlamydia treatment. Antimicrobial-resistant gonorrhea has been an ongoing problem since the development of plasmid-mediated β-lactam resistance (by penicillinase-producing *N. gonorrhoeae* in 1976 [84]), first diagnosed in returning travelers from Southeast Asia. Since 1989, quinolones and cephalosporins have been the drugs of choice, since they were effective against the known β-lactam and tetracycline resistance determinants. However, since the mid-1990s, resistance has developed rapidly, initiating from foci in Southeast Asia and widely disseminated by travelers with sexual contact in

that region (6, 39). Quinolone resistance has become widespread, and these drugs are no longer recommended as therapy. Treatment (15) for mucosal gonorrhea infections is based on providing single-dose regimens, preferably oral, that are effective against most or all of the known resistance determinants. Current single-dose oral regimens include cefixime (400 mg) and ceftriaxone (125 mg intramuscularly). All patients treated for gonorrhea should also be treated for chlamydia. The base chlamydia regimen is either azithromycin (1-g single dose) or doxycycline (100 mg twice daily for 1 week).

Pelvic Inflammatory Disease

PID encompasses soft tissue upper tract inflammation, including endometritis, oophoritis, and pelvic peritonitis (43, 70). PID usually follows an untreated lower genital tract infection, such as gonorrhea or chlamydia. Organisms that are isolated from the upper tract, for example, at laparoscopy or surgery, include *N. gonorrhoeae*, *Chlamydia trachomatis*, organisms associated with the vaginal flora, such as *Streptococcus* (group B), *Gardnerella*, *Escherichia coli*, and *Veillonella*, and intra-abdominal colonic organisms such as *Bacteroides* and other anaerobes. The inflammation caused by PID often results in tubal scarring, which may cause later tubal infertility and increased risk of ectopic pregnancy. Accurate clinical diagnosis is difficult because up to one-fourth of PID patients may manifest no symptoms, especially for disease associated with chlamydia. Therefore, many practitioners currently will treat women with mild cervical motion tenderness with treatment regimens effective against PID under the assumption that the benefit of preventing PID or curing early PID outweighs the costs in terms of increased cost of treatment and potential side effects. Treatment strategies for PID are based on the underlying microbiology, including antimicrobial coverage for *N. gonorrhoeae*, *C. trachomatis*, streptococci, gram-negative rods, and anaerobes. Treatment regimens are therefore complex and beyond the scope of this chapter. Despite the efforts toward developing effective antimicrobial regimens, treatment efficacy has been difficult to assess because of the need to evaluate long-term impact.

Vaginal Infections

When individuals with vaginal infections or vaginal discharge (Fig. 1) are evaluated, it is imperative to differentiate primary vaginal infections from cervical infections presenting as vaginitis. Vaginitis has a number of causes, including trichomoniasis, bacterial vaginosis (BV), and candidiasis (77). Since *Candida* infection is not an STI and has very few long-term health effects, it is not considered here for the sake of brevity. However, the clinician should recognize that patients often confuse any vaginal discharge disorder with a yeast infection and treat it with over-the-counter drugs before seeking medical attention.

TRICHOMONAS

Trichomonas infection occurs in approximately 3 million women annually and is caused by *Trichomonas vaginalis,* a flagellated protozoan (78). Signs and symptoms include a watery vaginal discharge, punctate hemorrhagic lesions on the cervix, and occasionally a frank cervicitis occurring in response to the vaginal infection. The prevalence of trichomoniasis in women is high—some studies report rate ranges of 5 to 40%. In men, *Trichomonas* can present as a nonchlamydial, nongonococcal urethritis, and the prevalence in men in developing country settings ranges from 6 to 12%. Wet mount is the most inexpensive and widely used method for diagnosis. Treatment

#50

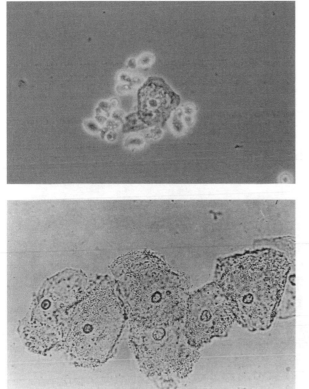

FIGURE 1 (Top) Vaginal discharge syndrome. *T. vaginalis* organisms on a wet mount are shown. (Bottom) BV. Clue cells with a ground-glass appearance are shown.

for trichomoniasis is metronidazole (2 g as a single dose).

BACTERIAL VAGINOSIS

BV is a disorder which occurs as a result of ecological disturbances in the vaginal flora (36, 63). The normal vaginal flora overwhelmingly consists of lactobacilli. As a result, the vaginal host environment is acidic, with a pH of <4.5. In BV, alteration of the microflora occurs, with the population of lactobacilli being replaced by gram-negative rods and anaerobes.

BV occurs most commonly as a secondary disorder due to cervical infection and inflammation (such as gonorrhea or chlamydia), alteration of the vaginal microflora as a result of antibiotic use, or use of vaginal douches. Clinical recommendations include specific recommendations not to douche. BV is a risk for premature rupture of membranes and premature delivery in pregnant women. Diagnosis of BV is made on either evaluation of a vaginal smear Gram stain demonstrating the characteristic alteration of the vaginal flora or clinical criteria. The clinical criteria are three of the following: homogenous vaginal discharge, pH of >4.5, presence of an amine odor, and presence of "clue cells" (vaginal epithelial cells which have large amounts of adherent bacteria, causing a ground-glass-type appearance). Treatment of BV uses antimicrobials effective against anaerobes, such as metronidazole or clindamycin, which results in reestablishment of the normal vaginal microflora.

Genital Ulcer Diseases

SYPHILIS

Syphilis (51) is a multistage disease caused by *Treponema pallidum*. Syphilis is typically seen in situations where there are multiple opportunities for large numbers of anonymous sex partners.

Initial infection occurs through sexual contact at a mucosal membrane. The incubation period ranges from 10 to 30 days until a chancre develops (Fig. 2). The chancre is a painless lesion with an indurated border and has as-

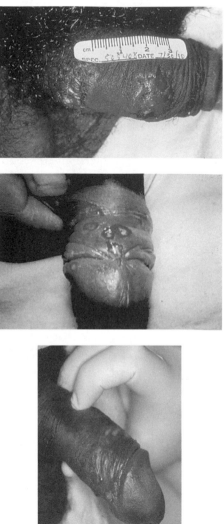

FIGURE 2 Classical and nonclassical examples of genital ulcers. These lesions could not be differentiated solely on the basis of physical examination. (Top) Primary syphilis chancre. Note that the edges are ragged and the lesion is hemorrhagic, in contrast to the classical description. (Middle) Chancroid. This multicentric ulcer was painful and had an undermined border. (Bottom) Primary herpes. These lesions were extremely painful and presented after the vesicle phase. There was large associated lymphadenopathy.

sociated painless lymphadenopathy. Left untreated, the chancre will heal spontaneously within 2 to 3 weeks. Four to eight weeks later, the secondary syphilis syndrome will develop. Secondary syphilis is a systemic vasculitis caused by high levels of *T. pallidum* in the blood and associated immunologic responses. The most characteristic findings are dermatological, including the classic palmar plantar rash, but other manifestations include alopecia (hair loss), mucosal lesions, and visceral involvement, which can include granulomatous hepatitis, nephrotic syndrome, optic neuritis, and rarely, meningovascular syphilis. Left untreated, the secondary syphilis syndrome will spontaneously resolve, usually within 1 to 2 months of onset.

The late complications of syphilis, such as neurosyphilis, cardiovascular syphilis, and gummatous syphilis, do not develop until 10 to 20 years after the resolution of early syphilis. For HIV patients, case reports have suggested that late complications may occur earlier and ulcers may be more severe (32, 72).

Early latent syphilis is a serologic diagnosis in which a fourfold increase in titer (i.e., 2 dilutions [see below]) is seen within 1 year, with previous documentation of the earlier serology. Late latent syphilis is a serologic diagnosis of syphilis occurring more than 1 year after baseline diagnosis.

Diagnosis of Primary Syphilis. Darkfield examination of the ulcer exudate establishes the diagnosis. Realistically, dark-field microscopy is not available in most settings. False-negative results may occur if patients apply bactericidal creams to the lesions. Therefore, diagnosis is most often established clinically as the presence of a lesion in association with serological findings.

Serological Diagnosis. Serological diagnosis of syphilis is a two-step procedure. Initially, a nontreponemal screening test is performed. The most widely used tests are the Venereal Disease Research Laboratory and rapid plasma reagin tests. Results for these tests are reported as titers, i.e., the dilutions required to achieve a negative reaction with standard reagents. Patients with a positive nontreponemal test should have a confirmatory test such as the fluorescent treponemal antibody-absorbed test or microhemagglutination test. Up to 20% of patients with positive nontreponemal tests will have negative confirmatory tests. These are termed benign false-positive results. Most frequently, these are seen for patients with past series of intravenous drug abuse, pregnancy, systemic disorders such as lupus, and other infectious processes such as Lyme disease.

All stages of syphilis are seen more commonly in HIV-infected patients. HIV prevalence in patients with syphilis is up to three times higher than that in nonsyphilis patients in these settings (32, 72).

Treatment. Treatment (15) of primary, secondary, and early latent syphilis with benzathine penicillin is recommended. For patients who are allergic to penicillin, doxycycline may be used. Treatment for patients with late latent syphilis, late syphilis, or syphilis of unknown duration (serological syphilis in which an initial benchmark cannot be defined) should be treated with benzathine penicillin at 2.4 million units intramuscularly for 3 weeks. Treatment is not different for persons with HIV coinfection, although more careful serological follow-up is recommended.

CHANCROID AND LGV

Chancroid. Chancroid is a genital ulcer disease caused by the organism *Haemophilus ducreyi*. Chancroid is predominantly seen in developing countries and in subtropical areas of the developing world. Occasional outbreaks are seen in the United States, usually associated with prostitution and drug use (26, 27). The incubation period of chancroid is 4 to 7 days. The ulcer develops initially as a tender papule with erythema. The ulcer typically is undermined, and in contrast to the case with syphilis, it is often painful, is not indurated, and has a purulent exudate. Painful large adenopathy is seen in up to 50% of patients. These can develop into large purulent nodes that can develop spontaneously in sinus tracts and rupture (buboes). Chancroid does not disseminate and has not been associated with major perinatal or neonatal complications. Diagnosis of chancroid is difficult because culture requires special growing conditions and is not widely available. Nucleic acid amplification tests are available only in research settings.

LGV. LGV is a genital ulcer disease caused by the L1, L2, and L3 serovars of *C. trachomatis.* This infection is found most frequently in tropical and subtropical areas of the world (8, 82). Since 2003, large outbreaks have been reported in Western Europe and North America, primarily in MSM. The majority of these cases have presented as proctitis. In these outbreaks, over two-thirds of patients are also HIV positive. Primary infection is characterized by a genital ulcer or a mucosal inflammatory reaction at the site of inoculation. The incubation period is 3 to 12 days. The lesions heal spontaneously within a few days. The secondary stage appears 2 to 6 weeks later and is related to local direct extension of the infection to regional lymph nodes. Most commonly, in persons who have had receptive rectal intercourse, an anorectal syndrome can also occur, which results in an inflammatory mass present in the rectum and retroperitoneum. Patients may present with rectal discharge, anal pain, constipation, fever, and/or tenesmus. There may be hemorrhagic proctocolitis and hyperplasia of intestinal and perirectal lymphatic tissue. This can be mistaken for inflammatory bowel disease or surgical disease. Complications include chronic colorectal fistulas and strictures. Diagnosis is difficult because the genital ulcer phase, during which *Chlamydia* can be identified, is relatively short and is often missed by clinicians. Serology is most commonly used to establish the diagnosis. Treatment regimens include either macrolides, such as azithromycin, or quinolones (15).

GENITAL HERPES INFECTION

Herpes simplex virus (HSV) infections are characterized by lifelong infection, latency, and recurrences. Genital herpes is almost exclusively sexually transmitted and can be caused by either HSV type 1 (HSV-1) or HSV-2 (17, 18). Primary infection is often asymptomatic. Genital herpes can occur at any exposed mucosal site (genitalia, rectum, and mouth). In primary disease, the ulceration develops 5 to 10 days after exposure; there may also be associated systemic signs, such as fever, myalgias, headache, and occasionally meningeal irritation. Recurrent herpes can develop at any time after the primary infection. In many settings, patients report a prodrome, which may consist of low-grade fever, pruritus, and tingling at the site of recurrence. Patients often report that they are able to feel the recurrence developing with nonspecific signs and symptoms, which is most likely related to irritation of the peripheral nerve roots.

Since many patients have asymptomatic primary infection, differentiation of a clinical first episode into primary disease or recurrence (in patients who have had an asymptomatic primary episode) requires serological testing (17, 84). Symptomatic recurrences are less symptomatic and heal faster than the primary episode. Recurrences occur most frequently within the first year after primary infection, and frequency decreases thereafter. Asymptomatic shedding plays a major role in transmission of HSV. Asymptomatic shedding occurs between clinical outbreaks, especially in the first few years after diagnosis. Initial culture studies of women with a recent diagnosis of primary herpes found that asymptomatic shedding occurred approximately 1% of the time (79, 83). Asymptomatic culture-diagnosed shedding definitely represents a potential infectious inoculum (about 10^4 viral particles).

Diagnosis of active genital herpes is made by either culture or other direct virus-specific tests, using specimens obtained from the lesions. In persons without active disease, serological testing with HSV-1/HSV-2-specific tests can define serological status, but results need to be interpreted in the context of the clinical history. Treatment is effective in managing symptoms but is not curative. The nucleoside analogue drugs—acyclovir, famciclovir, and valacyclovir—all reduce symptom severity and shorten the time to healing of lesions. For individuals who have more than six recurrences per year or who are profoundly immunosuppressed and have recurrent disease (such as those with advanced HIV disease, transplant recipients, and patients undergoing chemotherapy), suppressive therapy is indicated. Suppressive regimens are over 90% protective in preventing recurrences.

HPV INFECTION

Human papillomaviruses (HPVs) are small RNA viruses which have the unique capacity of causing chronic infection and malignant transformation, resulting in vulvar, anal, cervical, and penile squamous cell carcinomas, but they also cannot be cultured in vitro (97). There are over 80 subtypes of HPV. The HPV types that most commonly infect the genital tract are HPV-6, -11, -16, and -18. HPV-6 and -11 cause genital warts. HPV-16 and -18 are implicated in cervical infection, resulting in cellular changes and Pap smear abnormalities, and can cause eventual malignant transformation and cervical cancer.

HPV infections are very common (21, 62). One carefully performed study of college students found that one-third of college students became infected within a year of initiating sexual intercourse (90). Estimates indicate that approximately 1% of the sexually active population in the United States has clinically apparent genital warts, and in STD clinic populations the percentage is much higher. Estimates of infection range from 20 to above 90%, depending on the specific populations studied, with college students, adolescents, and CSWs demonstrating the highest rates.

The vast majority of HPV infections are asymptomatic. The incubation period is esti-

mated to be 3 months (range of 3 weeks to 8 months). Lesions may occur anywhere on the external genitalia, anus, rectum, and cervix and, in men, inside the urethra. In women, cervical warts are occasionally observed; in men, lesions may be present inside the urethra.

Treatment for condylomata is based on surgical excision of the lesions, tissue-destructive therapy such as liquid nitrogen cryotherapy, chemical destruction with trichloroacetic acid or podophyllin, or local immunotherapy with imiquamod or interferons. An eradication of HPV-containing tissue is impossible because grossly and histologically appearing tissues may be infected with HPV and cannot be detected unless specifically probed for by DNA analysis. Therefore, the treatment of genital wart lesions due to HPV by traditional destructive methods, such as liquid nitrogen or surgery, leads to substantial recurrence rates because HPV infection is often present in the histologically normal surgical margins.

The availability of a quadrivalent HPV vaccine has revolutionized the approach to HPV prevention (57). The currently approved HPV vaccine prevents genital wart types 6 and 11 and cervical cancer types 16 and 18. Vaccination is recommended for women aged 9 to 26, and vaccination recommendations for men are currently being considered.

RELATIONSHIPS BETWEEN STDs AND HIV

Sexually transmitted HIV is prevalent in many parts of the world, especially South Asia and Africa. Cross-sectional and prospective studies in the developed and developing world have firmly established that bacterial and viral STIs are biological cofactors in facilitating HIV transmission (87, 88). As noted above, since the late 1990s, there has been a resurgence of both STDs and HIV infection, especially syphilis and gonorrhea, in gay men, often associated with high-risk sexual behavior at popular travel venues.

Studies of HIV transmission consistently demonstrate that the presence of STDs increases HIV transmission risk three- to five-fold. Travelers to areas where there are high rates of HIV-STI coinfection should be especially careful to practice safer sex and consistent condom use.

INTERVENTIONS TO REDUCE THE RISK OF SEXUAL EXPOSURE

Promoting condom use has been one of the central tenets of HIV and STD risk reduction strategies, both in the United States and abroad. Condoms are effective when used correctly and consistently and are highly effective against transmitting HIV, genital herpes, and bacterial STIs (4, 49, 86). The most dramatic studies were performed early in the HIV epidemic, using HIV-discordant heterosexual couples in California and Italy, and conclusively demonstrated that consistent use in controlled settings results in an approximately sevenfold decrease in HIV seroconversions.

Probably the most intensive and successful effort has been implemented in Thailand, where the "100% Condom" program (35, 47, 71) has been implemented since 1991 and includes intensive advertising, an infrastructure to purchase and distribute condoms, and linkages in promoting condoms with stakeholders, including the army, provincial and municipality governments, and CSWs. The Thai program provides a useful model for the development of an effective condom promotion and sexual risk reduction campaign, was adopted by the World Health Organization as a model program, and has been implemented in other countries, especially in Asia. The program includes open discussion of HIV prevention and condom promotion, mass media campaigns, and the active participation of a large variety of stakeholders, including the military, government, medical community, and even brothels. In other words, this effective program's major accomplishment was to change the social norms across a broad spectrum of society to encourage condom use.

In developing countries, condom promotion and safer sex education campaigns have often been innovative in responding to local situations. For example, a highly successful Kenyan campaign to increase condom use focused on truck drivers and their assistants and was delivered at truck and rest stops, which resulted in decreasing STDs by >30% (53). In Nicaragua, the health ministry successfully implemented a condom promotion campaign in a CSW district by providing condoms on the beds of local motels (30). Both of these efforts utilize a harm reduction and nonjudgmental approach.

PREVENTION ISSUES SPECIFIC TO WOMEN

If a woman regularly takes hormonal contraceptives, she should continue her regimen if there is even the remote possibility of sexual activity while traveling abroad. Under most circumstances, the risk of unintended pregnancy from unprotected intercourse is as high as or higher than that of STD. Hormonal contraceptives should be used in addition to condom use, i.e., the "dual method" approach.

There has been much interest in developing vaginal microbicides as a female-controlled method of STD prevention (25). The ideal vaginal microbicides should demonstrate physical and chemical stability in the vaginal environment, allowing insertion some time before intercourse, should not interfere with sexual intercourse, and should also be inexpensive. The ideal compound would be cidal to bacterial and viral pathogens while being nontoxic to the host epithelium. Unfortunately, despite tremendous efforts, effective microbicides have yet to be developed.

HIV-INFECTED TRAVELERS

The advent of effective antiretroviral therapy has made prolonged overseas travel possible for persons infected with HIV. Several review papers have addressed special problems facing

HIV-infected travelers (11, 64). Risky sexual behavior was described for Toronto HIV clinic patients and for MSM visiting Key West. Relatively high rates of risky sexual behavior while traveling were described, and about 10% of patients discontinued their medications while traveling. These data clearly demonstrate the need for more intensive and frank counseling pretravel. A major concern for all HIV-infected travelers is the risk for opportunistic infections. HIV patients under treatment and immune reconstitution are still at increased risk for opportunists. Therefore, water and food precautions are particularly important because of the risk of cryptosporidiosis, salmonellosis, and campylobacter infection in HIV-infected persons. Traveler's diarrhea prophylaxis should strongly be considered. HIV-infected persons should also ensure that all of their vaccinations are up to date, especially those for hepatitis A and B. Live typhoid vaccine is contraindicated. Yellow fever vaccine is contraindicated for persons with CD4 counts of <200 but is considered safe for persons with CD4 counts of >200. Malaria prophylaxis in HIV-infected persons is a major clinical problem because of the myriad interactions between antimalarials and antiretrovirals. Doxycycline has the least number of interactions, but generally, this issue should be addressed with the health care provider prior to travel.

CLASSIFICATION OF SEXUAL RISK AND THE TRAVELER

Travelers who are at risk for unprotected sexual activity while abroad have been categorized into the following five major categories (23):

1. Persons who travel with a regular partner and who anticipate being sexually active while abroad, but within a monogamous relationship. These persons do not need any additional counseling, especially for short trips. Additional counseling may be indicated if there are signs or anticipation that either partner may be interested in additional partners while abroad. Furthermore, persons on long-term travel assignments may benefit from additional counseling.

2. The "unprepared." These are persons who are traveling and not anticipating being sexually active but have an unexpected sexual relationship while abroad. Since this is unexpected, by definition, all persons traveling should have pretravel sexual counseling and be aware especially of local triggers or customs. For example, travelers to countries where there is a large commercial sex industry based in alcohol establishments may have unexpected sexual exposures in these settings.

3. The "fanatical" (who must have sex to have a successful vacation). These individuals fall into two categories. The data clearly show that especially for young singles, recruiting an associative (from the same background and country) sex partner is quite common. The second group are the sex tourists, who are at extraordinarily high risk for STI-HIV infection unless condoms are used consistently.

4. The "unaffected" (who feel that sex abroad is the same as sex at home). These individuals should be counseled on the specific risks posed by local environments.

5. The "slightly accessible" (who feel that sex abroad is different and come prepared). These are the individuals who require informational counseling but have already understood the message.

AN STI PREVENTION STRATEGY

The epidemiological data consistently show that travelers are sexually active. From the standpoint of primary prevention, abstinence would be an impractical approach, although this would clearly reduce the risk to zero! Preventing sexual infection in travelers therefore emphasizes reducing risk (Table 3). In developing countries, such as in Africa, Southeast Asia, and Eastern Europe, STI rates are extraordinarily high and heterosexual transmission of HIV is extremely common. Therefore, unprotected sexual contacts in these areas

TABLE 3 STD prevention strategy

Reduce number of sex partners
Recognize trigger situations for intercourse with new partners (alcohol use, drug use)
Eliminate or reduce contact with CSWs
100% condom use and use of hormonal contraceptives
Periodic screening for STDs and HIV at home and abroad
Postexposure
    Emergency contraception
    Syndromic treatment (postexposure prophylaxis)

carry substantial risk. The context of sexual activity is clearly related to risk—for example, CSW contacts are more risky (in most situations) than expatriates. However, the reader should note with caution that these conclusions are based on population-based statistics and that an individual's risk may vary substantially.

Travelers and those counseling travelers should emphasize that if there is even a remote possibility of sexual relations, the traveler should ensure that condoms are available and easily accessible. Counseling needs to be non-judgmental and should also ascertain "triggers" or "risk situations" which put the traveler at risk. The best example of the above is the expatriate who does not anticipate being sexually active but does so because of an unforeseen opportunity, often associated with alcohol use. Counseling in prior recognition of these settings is critical.

Persons who are sexually active with multiple partners should have periodic screening for STDs, especially gonorrhea, chlamydia, syphilis, and HIV, at least on an annual basis. Herpes serology, using new, type-specific serological tests, should also be considered to identify asymptomatic HSV infection.

MANAGEMENT STRATEGY AFTER EXPOSURE

Anyone who may have been exposed to an STD and develops either a vaginal or urethral discharge, an unexplained rash or genital lesion, or genital or pelvic pain should cease sexual activity and promptly seek competent medical care. Because STDs are often asymptomatic, especially in women, anyone who believes that they may have been exposed to an STD should consult their health care provider for the advisability of screening for STDs.

When available, diagnostic services should include a physical examination, including a pelvic examination for women, and diagnostic tests for *N. gonorrhoeae*, *C. trachomatis*, and syphilis. Women should have a vaginal wet mount to evaluate for *Trichomonas* infection and BV. HSV testing should be performed in appropriate situations. All persons evaluated for a travel-related unprotected sexual exposure should also receive HIV counseling and testing. If the initial test is negative, the person should be retested a second time, >3 months after the last unprotected sexual exposure, to ensure that the individual is not in the "seroconversion window." Treatment for STDs should follow the current Centers for Disease Control and Prevention guidelines. Persons should not have unprotected sex until the diagnostic and therapeutic process is completed and HIV testing is confirmed to be negative. If possible, partners should also be notified of the potential exposure.

In many settings, however, diagnostic facilities and testing services are not available. In these situations, syndromic management strategies for STDs should be utilized, and HIV counseling and testing should still be offered.

The Centers for Disease Control and Prevention's Travelers' Health Service and the Canadian Department of Public Health have both published extensive recommendations on travel and STI prevention. In particular, the Canadian document provides extensive guidelines and resources and can be viewed at http://www.phac-aspc.gc.ca/publicat/ccdr-rmtc/06vol32/acs-05/index.html.

In summary, health care providers should consider travel a potential risk factor for unprotected intercourse and STD exposure, in both pretravel counseling settings and post-travel evaluations.

PRACTICAL TIPS
- Sexual health counseling should be an integral part of travel advice.
- Travelers should be advised to recognize potentially risky situations, for example, alcohol establishments where there is an integral link with prostitution.
- Structural interventions, such as 100% condom regulations or increasing access to preventive methods, are usually the most effective.
- Health care providers should be cognizant that the allure of traveling for many people includes the possiblity of new sexual partners. Barrier protection should be used for all sexual encounters unless they are with a monogamous partner.
- STI and HIV rates in countries can vary substantially.
- Most new sexual partners are other travelers, usually from the same country and background. Travelers should not assume that their counterparts are free of STI risk!
- Expatriates and persons on long-term overseas detail should receive sexual health counseling.

REFERENCES
1. **Abdullah, A. S., S. H. Ebrahim, R. Fielding, and D. E. Morisky.** 2004. Sexually transmitted infections in travelers: implications for prevention and control. *Clin. Infect. Dis.* **39:**533–538.
2. **Adimora, A. A., V. J. Schoenbach, and I. A. Doherty.** 2006. HIV and African Americans in the southern United States: sexual networks and social context. *Sex. Transm. Dis.* **33:**S39–S45.
3. **Adler, M. W.** 1980. The terrible peril: a historical perspective on the venereal diseases. *Br. Med. J.* **281:**206–211.
4. **Anonymous.** 2003. *Workshop Summary: Scientific Evidence on Condom Effectiveness for STD Prevention.* National Institutes of Health, Bethesda, MD.
5. **Arvidson, M., I. Kallings, S. Nilsson, D. Hellberg, and P. A. Mardh.** 1997. Risky behavior in women with history of casual travel sex. *Sex. Transm. Dis.* **24:**418–421.
6. **Australian Gonococcal Surveillance Programme.** 2005. Annual report of the Australian Gonococcal Surveillance Programme, 2004. *Commun. Dis. Intell.* **29:**137–142.
7. **Bacaner, N., B. Stauffer, D. R. Boulware, P. F. Walker, and J. S. Keystone.** 2004. Travel medicine considerations for North American immigrants visiting friends and relatives. *JAMA* **291:**2856–2864.
8. **Bauwens, J. E., H. Orlander, M. P. Gomez, M. Lampe, S. Morse, W. E. Stamm, R Cone, R. Ashley, P. Swenson, and K. K. Holmes.** 2002. Epidemic lymphogranuloma venereum during epidemics of crack cocaine use and HIV infection in the Bahamas. *Sex. Transm. Dis.* **29:**253–259.
9. **Bellis, M. A., K. Hughes, R. Thomson, and A. Bennett.** 2004. Sexual behaviour of young people in international tourist resorts. *Sex. Transm. Infect.* **80:**43–47.
10. **Benotsch, E. G., J. J. Mikytuck, K. Ragsdale, and S. D. Pinkerton.** 2006. Sexual risk and HIV acquisition among men who have sex with men travelers to Key West, Florida: a mathematical modeling analysis. *AIDS Patient Care STDS* **20:**549–556.
11. **Bhadelia, N., M. Klotman, and D. Caplivski.** 2007. The HIV-positive traveler. *Am. J. Med.* **120:**574–580.
12. **Bonneux, L., P. Van der Stuyft, H. Taelman, P. Cornet, C. Goilav, G. van der Groen, and P. Piot.** 1988. Risk factors for infection with human immunodeficiency virus among European expatriates in Africa. *BMJ* **297:**581–584.
13. **Cabada, M. M., F. Maldonado, I. Bauer, K. Verdonck, C. Seas, and E. Gotuzzo.** 2007. Sexual behavior, knowledge of STI prevention, and prevalence of serum markers for STI among tour guides in Cuzco/Peru. *J. Travel Med.* **14:**151–157.
14. **Cabada, M. M., M. Montoya, J. I. Echevarria, K. Verdonck, C. Seas, and E. Gotuzzo.** 2003. Sexual behavior in travelers visiting Cuzco. *J. Travel Med.* **10:**214–218.
15. **Centers for Disease Control and Prevention, K. A. Workowski, and S. M. Berman.** 2006. Sexually transmitted diseases treatment guidelines, 2006. *MMWR Recomm. Rep.* **55:**1–94.
16. **Committee to Advise on Tropical Medicine and Travel (CATMAT).** 2006. Statement on travellers and sexually transmitted infections. An Advisory Committee statement (ACS). *Can. Commun. Dis. Rep.* **32:**1–24.
17. **Corey, L., and H. H. Handsfield.** 2000. Genital herpes and public health: addressing a global problem. *JAMA* **283:**791–794.
18. **Corey, L., and P. G. Spear.** 1986. Infections with herpes simplex viruses (2). *N. Engl. J. Med.* **314:**749–757.

19. **Cross, A. B., and J. R. Harris.** 1976. Reappraisal of the problem of British mariners and sexually transmitted infection. *Br. J. Vener. Dis.* **52:** 71–77.

20. **Croughs, M., A. Van Gompel, E. de Boer, and J. Van Den Ende.** 2008. Sexual risk behavior of travelers who consulted a pretravel clinic. *J. Travel Med.* **15:**6–12.

21. **Datta, S. D., L. A. Koutsky, S. Ratelle, E. R. Unger, J. Shlay, T. McClain, B. Weaver, P. Kerndt, J. Zenilman, M. Hagensee, C. J. Suhr, and H. Weinstock.** 2008. Human papillomavirus infection and cervical cytology in women screened for cervical cancer in the United States, 2003–2005. *Ann. Intern. Med.* **148:**493–500.

22. **Day, S., and H. Ward.** 1997. Sex workers and the control of sexually transmitted disease. *Genitourin. Med.* **73:**161–168.

23. **de Graaf, R., G. van Zessen, and H. Houweling.** 1998. Underlying reasons for sexual conduct and condom use among expatriates posted in AIDS endemic areas. *AIDS Care* **10:** 651–665.

24. **de Graaf, R., G. van Zessen, H. Houweling, R. J. Ligthelm, and R. van den Akker.** 1997. Sexual risk of HIV infection among expatriates posted in AIDS endemic areas. *AIDS* **11:**1173–1181.

25. **Dhawan, D., and K. H. Mayer.** 2006. Microbicides to prevent HIV transmission: overcoming obstacles to chemical barrier protection. *J. Infect. Dis.* **193:**36–44.

26. **DiCarlo, R. P., B. S. Armentor, and D. H. Martin.** 1995. Chancroid epidemiology in New Orleans men. *J. Infect. Dis.* **172:**446–452.

27. **Dillon, S. M., M. Cummings, S. Rajagopalan, and W. C. McCormack.** 1997. Prospective analysis of genital ulcer disease in Brooklyn, New York. *Clin. Infect. Dis.* **24:**945–950.

28. **Dupin, N., R. Jdid, Y. T. N'Guyen, I. Gorin, N. Franck, and J. P. Escande.** 2001. Syphilis and gonorrhoea in Paris: the return. *AIDS* **15:**814–815.

29. **Edlin, B. R., K. L. Irwin, S. Faruque, C. B. McCoy, C. Word, Y. Serrano, J. A. Inciardi, B. P. Bowser, R. F. Schilling, S. D. Holmberg, et al.** 1994. Intersecting epidemics—crack cocaine use and HIV infection among inner-city young adults. *N. Engl. J. Med.* **331:**1422–1427.

30. **Egger, M., J. Pauw, A. Lopatatzidis, D. Medrano, F. Paccaud, and G. D. Smith.** 2000. Promotion of condom use in a high-risk setting in Nicaragua: a randomised controlled trial. *Lancet* **355:**2101–2105.

31. **Elliott, J. H., A. M. Mijch, A. C. Street, and N. Crofts.** 2003. HIV, ethnicity and travel: HIV infection in Vietnamese Australians associated with injecting drug use. *J. Clin. Virol.* **26:**133–142.

32. **Erbelding, E. J., D. Vlahov, K. E. Nelson, A. M. Rompalo, S. Cohn, P. Sanchez, T. C. Quinn, W. Brathwaite, and D. L. Thomas.** 1997. Syphilis serology in human immunodeficiency virus infection: evidence for false-negative fluorescent treponemal testing. *J. Infect. Dis.* **176:** 1397–1400.

33. **Fenton, K. A., M. Chinouya, O. Davidson, and A. Copas.** 2001. HIV transmission risk among sub-Saharan Africans in London travelling to their countries of origin. *AIDS* **15:**1442–1445.

34. **Fenton, K. A., C. Ison, A. P. Johnson, E. Rudd, M. Soltani, I. Martin, T. Nichols, and D. M. Livermore.** 2003. Ciprofloxacin resistance in Neisseria gonorrhoeae in England and Wales in 2002. *Lancet* **361:**1867–1869.

35. **Fontanet, A. L., J. Saba, V. Chandelying, C. Sakondhavat, P. Bhiraleus, S. Rugpao, C. Chongsomchai, O. Kiriwat, S. Tovanabutra, L. Dally, J. M. Lange, and W. Rojanapithayakorn.** 1998. Protection against sexually transmitted diseases by granting sex workers in Thailand the choice of using the male or female condom: results from a randomized controlled trial. *AIDS* **12:**1851–1859.

36. **Fredricks, D. N., T. L. Fiedler, K. K. Thomas, B. B. Oakley, and J. M. Marrazzo.** 2007. Targeted PCR for detection of vaginal bacteria associated with bacterial vaginosis. *J. Clin. Microbiol.* **45:**3270–3276.

37. **Garnett, G. P.** 1998. The basic reproductive rate of infection and the course of HIV epidemics. *AIDS Patient Care STDs* **12:**435–449.

38. **Gaydos, C. A., and T. C. Quinn.** 2005. Urine nucleic acid amplification tests for the diagnosis of sexually transmitted infections in clinical practice. *Curr. Opin. Infect. Dis.* **18:**55–66.

39. **Ghanem, K. G., J. A. Giles, and J. M. Zenilman.** 2005. Fluoroquinolone-resistant Neisseria gonorrhoeae: the inevitable epidemic. *Infect. Dis. Clin. N. Am.* **19:**351–365.

40. **Gilks, C. F., P. Godfrey-Faussett, B. I. Batchelor, J. C. Ojoo, S. J. Ojoo, R. J. Brindle, J. Paul, J. Kimari, M. C. Bruce, J. Bwayo, F. A. Plummer, and D. A. Warrell.** 1997. Recent transmission of tuberculosis in a cohort of HIV-1-infected female sex workers in Nairobi, Kenya. *AIDS* **11:**911–918.

41. **Goldenberg, S., J. Shoveller, M. Koehoorn, and A. Ostry.** 2008. Barriers to STI testing among youth in a Canadian oil and gas community. *Health Place* **14:**718–729.

42. **Goldenberg, S., J. Shoveller, A. Ostry, and M. Koehoorn.** 2008. Youth sexual behaviour in a boomtown: implications for the control of sex-

ually transmitted infections. *Sex. Transm. Infect.* **84:**220–223.

43. **Gray-Swain, M. R., and J. F. Peipert.** 2006. Pelvic inflammatory disease in adolescents. *Curr. Opin. Obstet. Gynecol.* **18:**503–510.

44. **Hart, G.** 1974. Factors influencing venereal infection in a war environment. *Br. J. Vener. Dis.* **50:**68–72.

45. **Hawkes, S., G. J. Hart, E. Bletsoe, C. Shergold, and A. M. Johnson.** 1995. Risk behaviour and STD acquisition in genitourinary clinic attenders who have travelled. *Genitourin. Med.* **71:**351–354.

46. **Hawkes, S., G. J. Hart, A. M. Johnson, C. Shergold, E. Ross, K. M. Herbert, P. Mortimer, J. V. Parry, and D. Mabey.** 1994. Risk behaviour and HIV prevalence in international travellers. *AIDS* **8:**247–252.

47. **Hearst, N., and S. Chen.** 2004. Condom promotion for AIDS prevention in the developing world: is it working? *Stud. Fam. Plann.* **35:**39–47.

48. **Hiltunen-Back, E., O. Haikala, P. Koskela, A. Vaalasti, and T. Reunala.** 2002. Epidemics due to imported syphilis in Finland. *Sex. Transm. Dis.* **29:**746–751.

49. **Holmes, K. K., R. Levine, and M. Weaver.** 2004. Effectiveness of condoms in preventing sexually transmitted infections. *Bull. W. H. O.* **82:**454–461.

50. **Hook, E. W., III, and K. K. Holmes.** 1985. Gonococcal infections. *Ann. Intern. Med.* **102:**229–243.

51. **Hook, E. W., III, and C. M. Marra.** 1992. Acquired syphilis in adults. *N. Engl. J. Med.* **326:**1060–1069.

52. **Hopperus Buma, A. P., R. L. Veltink, E. J. van Ameijden, C. H. Tendeloo, and R. A. Coutinho.** 1995. Sexual behaviour and sexually transmitted diseases in Dutch marines and naval personnel on a United Nations mission in Cambodia. *Genitourin. Med.* **71:**172–175.

53. **Jackson, D. J., J. P. Rakwar, B. Chohan, K. Mandaliya, J. J. Bwayo, J. O. Ndinya-Achola, N. J. Nagelkerke, J. K. Kreiss, and S. Moses.** 1997. Urethral infection in a workplace population of East African men: evaluation of strategies for screening and management. *J. Infect. Dis.* **175:**833–838.

54. **Jones, D. L., K. L. Irwin, J. Inciardi, B. Bowser, R. Schilling, C. Word, P. Evans, S. Faruque, H. V. McCoy, B. R. Edlin, et al.** 1998. The high-risk sexual practices of crack-smoking sex workers recruited from the streets of three American cities. *Sex. Transm. Dis.* **25:**187–193.

55. **Karpati, A., S. Galea, T. Awerbuch, and R. Levins.** 2002. Variability and vulnerability at the ecological level: implications for understanding the social determinants of health. *Am. J. Public Health* **92:**1768–1772.

56. **Kilmarx, P. H., K. Limpakarnjanarat, S. Supawitkul, S. Korattana, N. L. Young, B. S. Parekh, R. A. Respess, T. D. Mastro, and M. E. St Louis.** 1998. Mucosal disruption due to use of a widely-distributed commercial vaginal product: potential to facilitate HIV transmission. *AIDS* **12:**767–773.

57. **Koutsky, L. A., K. A. Ault, C. M. Wheeler, D. R. Brown, E. Barr, F. B. Alvarez, L. M. Chiacchierini, and K. U. Jansen.** 2002. A controlled trial of a human papillomavirus type 16 vaccine. *N. Engl. J. Med.* **347:**1645–1651.

58. **Lau, J. T., A. S. Tang, and H. Y. Tsui.** 2003. The relationship between condom use, sexually transmitted diseases, and location of commercial sex transaction among male Hong Kong clients. *AIDS* **17:**105–112.

59. **Lau, J. T., and J. Thomas.** 2001. Risk behaviours of Hong Kong male residents travelling to mainland China: a potential bridge population for HIV infection. *AIDS Care* **13:**71–81.

60. **Lenoir, C. D., N. E. Adler, D. L. Borzekowski, J. M. Tschann, and J. M. Ellen.** 2006. What you don't know can hurt you: perceptions of sex-partner concurrency and partner-reported behavior. *J. Adolesc. Health* **38:**179–185.

61. **Malone, J. D., K. C. Hyams, R. E. Hawkins, T. W. Sharp, and F. D. Daniell.** 1993. Risk factors for sexually-transmitted diseases among deployed U.S. military personnel. *Sex. Transm. Dis.* **20:**294–298.

62. **Manhart, L. E., K. K. Holmes, L. A. Koutsky, T. R. Wood, D. L. Kenney, Q. Feng, and N. B. Kiviat.** 2006. Human papillomavirus infection among sexually active young women in the United States: implications for developing a vaccination strategy. *Sex. Transm. Dis.* **33:**502–508.

63. **Marrazzo, J. M., H. C. Wiesenfeld, P. J. Murray, B. Busse, L. Meyn, M. Krohn, and S. L. Hillier.** 2006. Risk factors for cervicitis among women with bacterial vaginosis. *J. Infect. Dis.* **193:**617–624.

64. **McCarthy, A. E., and M. D. Mileno.** 2006. Prevention and treatment of travel-related infections in compromised hosts. *Curr. Opin. Infect. Dis.* **19:**450–455.

65. **Mercer, C. H., K. A. Fenton, K. Wellings, A. J. Copas, B. Erens, and A. M. Johnson.** 2007. Sex partner acquisition while overseas: results from a British national probability survey. *Sex. Transm. Infect.* **83:**517–522.

66. **Moore, J., C. Beeker, J. S. Harrison, T. R. Eng, and L. S. Doll.** 1995. HIV risk behavior

among Peace Corps volunteers. *AIDS* **9:**795–799.

67. **Moses, S., E. Muia, J. E. Bradley, N. J. Nagelkerke, E. N. Ngugi, E. K. Njeru, G. Eldridge, J. Olenja, K. Wotton, and F. A. Plummer.** 1994. Sexual behaviour in Kenya: implications for sexually transmitted disease transmission and control. *Soc. Sci. Med.* **39:**1649–1656.

68. **Peipert, J. F.** 2003. Clinical practice. Genital chlamydial infections. *N. Engl. J. Med.* **349:**2424–2430.

69. **Peipert, J. F., R. B. Ness, J. Blume, D. E. Soper, R. Holley, H. Randall, R. L. Sweet, S. J. Sondheimer, S. L. Hendrix, A. Amortegui, G. Trucco, and D. C. Bass.** 2001. Clinical predictors of endometritis in women with symptoms and signs of pelvic inflammatory disease. *Am. J. Obstet. Gynecol.* **184:**856–863.

70. **Peipert, J. F., R. B. Ness, D. E. Soper, and D. Bass.** 2000. Association of lower genital tract inflammation with objective evidence of endometritis. *Infect. Dis. Obstet. Gynecol.* **8:**83–87.

71. **Rojanapithayakorn, W., and R. Hanenberg.** 1996. The 100% condom program in Thailand. *AIDS* **10:**1–7.

72. **Rompalo, A. M., J. Lawlor, P. Seaman, T. C. Quinn, J. M. Zenilman, and E. W. Hook III.** 2001. Modification of syphilitic genital ulcer manifestations by coexistent HIV infection. *Sex. Transm. Dis.* **28:**448–454.

73. **Royce, R. A., A. Sena, W. Cates, Jr., and M. S. Cohen.** 1997. Sexual transmission of HIV. *N. Engl. J. Med.* **336:**1072–1078.

74. **Salit, I. E., M. Sano, A. K. Boggild, and K. C. Kain.** 2005. Travel patterns and risk behaviour of HIV-positive people travelling internationally. *CMAJ* **172:**884–888.

75. **Sarwal, S., T. Wong, C. Sevigny, and L. K. Ng.** 2003. Increasing incidence of ciprofloxacin-resistant Neisseria gonorrhoeae infection in Canada. *CMAJ* **168:**872–873.

76. **Shafer, M. A., C. B. Boyer, R. A. Shaffer, J. Schachter, S. I. Ito, and S. K. Brodine.** 2002. Correlates of sexually transmitted diseases in a young male deployed military population. *Mil. Med.* **167:**496–500.

77. **Sobel, J. D.** 1997. Vaginitis. *N. Engl. J. Med.* **337:**1896–1903.

78. **Soper, D.** 2004. Trichomoniasis: under control or undercontrolled? *Am. J. Obstet. Gynecol.* **190:**281–290.

79. **Sucato, G., A. Wald, E. Wakabayashi, J. Vieira, and L. Corey.** 1998. Evidence of latency and reactivation of both herpes simplex virus (HSV)-1 and HSV-2 in the genital region. *J. Infect. Dis.* **177:**1069–1072.

80. **Tilzey, A. J., and J. E. Banatvala.** 2002. Protection from HIV on electives: questionnaire survey of UK medical schools. *BMJ* **325:**1010–1011.

81. **United States Department of State.** 2002. *Trafficking in Persons Report—2002.* Government Printing Office, Washington, DC.

82. **Van der Bij, A. K., J. Spaargaren, S. A. Morre, H. S. Fennema, A. Mindel, R. A. Coutinho, and H. J. de Vries.** 2006. Diagnostic and clinical implications of anorectal lymphogranuloma venereum in men who have sex with men: a retrospective case-control study. *Clin. Infect. Dis.* **42:**186–194.

83. **Wald, A., M. L. Huang, D. Carrell, S. Selke, and L. Corey.** 2003. Polymerase chain reaction for detection of herpes simplex virus (HSV) DNA on mucosal surfaces: comparison with HSV isolation in cell culture. *J. Infect. Dis.* **188:**1345–1351.

84. **Wald, A., J. Zeh, S. Selke, T. Warren, A. J. Ryncarz, R. Ashley, J. N. Krieger, and L. Corey.** 2000. Reactivation of genital herpes simplex virus type 2 infection in asymptomatic seropositive persons. *N. Engl. J. Med.* **342:**844–850.

85. **Ward, H., S. Day, A. Green, K. Cooper, and J. Weber.** 2004. Declining prevalence of STI in the London sex industry, 1985 to 2002. *Sex. Transm. Infect.* **80:**374–376.

86. **Warner, L., M. Macaluso, D. Newman, H. Austin, D. Kleinbaum, M. Kamb, J. Douglas, C. K. Malotte, and J. M. Zenilman.** 2006. Condom effectiveness for prevention of C trachomatis infection. *Sex. Transm. Infect.* **82:**265.

87. **Wasserheit, J. N.** 1992. Epidemiological synergy. Interrelationships between human immunodeficiency virus infection and other sexually transmitted diseases. *Sex. Transm. Dis.* **19:**61–77.

88. **Wasserheit, J. N., and S. O. Aral.** 1996. The dynamic topology of sexually transmitted disease epidemics: implications for prevention strategies. *J. Infect. Dis.* **174**(Suppl. 2)**:**S201–S213.

89. **Weinstock, H., S. Berman, and W. Cates, Jr.** 2004. Sexually transmitted diseases among American youth: incidence and prevalence estimates, 2000. *Perspect. Sex Reprod. Health* **36:**6–10.

90. **Winer, R. L., S. K. Lee, J. P. Hughes, D. E. Adam, N. B. Kiviat, and L. A. Koutsky.** 2003. Genital human papillomavirus infection: incidence and risk factors in a cohort of female university students. *Am. J. Epidemiol.* **157:**218–226.

91. **Wong, M. L., R. K. Chan, and D. Koh.** 2007. HIV prevention among travelers: why do men not use condoms when they engage in commercial sex overseas? *Sex. Transm. Dis.* **34:**237–244.

92. **Wong, M. L., R. K. Chan, D. Koh, M. E. Barrett, S. K. Chew, and S. S. Wee.** 2005. A comparative study of condom use and self-reported sexually transmitted infections between foreign Asian and local clients of sex workers in Singapore. *Sex. Transm. Dis.* **32:**439–445.

INFECTIONS FROM BODY PIERCING AND TATTOOS

Mukesh Patel and C. Glenn Cobbs

14

Tattoos and body piercing have received increased attention in recent years. The increasing acceptance of tattoo and body piercing culture by society is evidenced by the popularity of reality television shows such as "LA Ink," "Miami Ink," and "Inked." Temporary tattoos and body jewelry (without actual piercing) are popular decorative items for children as well. The term "body modification" or "body art" has been used to describe procedures that "enhance" appearance, whether permanent or temporary. These procedures include tattooing, body piercing, scarification, branding, and surgical modifications. For many people, body modification represents a form of artistic or creative expression that provides long-term enjoyment and thus can be considered a recreational pursuit. A positive effect of the increased interest in tattoos and body piercing has been the development of standardized protocols of infection control to protect the health and safety of both the client and the tattooist or piercer. Though the incidence of serious postprocedure complications appears to be low, a significant number of tattoos and body piercings are still performed by personnel who often do not follow appropriate precautions, thus increasing the possibility of infectious and noninfectious complications.

PREVALENCE OF TATTOOS AND BODY PIERCINGS

The prevalence of tattoos and body piercing has most certainly increased in recent decades, though previous studies may have been affected by underreporting of tattoos, as many older persons still consider their own tattoos and piercings a sensitive topic. A visit to almost any high school or university in North America will provide proof that body art is especially popular among adolescents and college students, with estimates of prevalence ranging from 13 to 23% (17, 69). The prevalence of body piercing has been noted to range from 8 to 32%, with the highest prevalence noted in college students and young adults (8, 9, 59, 66).

Though the arms, legs, and back are most commonly decorated, virtually any part of the body may be tattooed, including the palms and soles, eyelids, face, genitals, and tongue. The most common locations for tattoos differ between gender but generally are the arms, upper back, shoulders, and legs, with men

Mukesh Patel and C. Glenn Cobbs, Division of Infectious Diseases, University of Alabama at Birmingham, Birmingham, AL 35294-0006.

Infections of Leisure, Fourth Edition, Edited by David Schlossberg,
© 2009 ASM Press, Washington, DC

more likely than women to have an exposed tattoo (89% versus 48%) (59). In addition to the earlobe, common piercing sites include nonearlobe portions of the ear, the navel, oral sites, and the eyebrow (59).

TATTOOING

History

Tattooing has been performed since antiquity by numerous cultures. The word "tattoo" may have been derived from a Polynesian word, *tatau,* meaning to "strike twice" and referring to the tattoo techniques used by the Polynesians. Captain James Cook was reported to refer to tatau after visiting the South Pacific. The modern word was subsequently derived and spread throughout Western cultures. Individual expression, decoration, storytelling, identification within a specific social group, and rites of passage are common reasons people have sought tattoos. More recently, tattooing has become a technique for application of permanent forms of makeup or as a permanent cosmetic camouflage of skin blemishes or scars (26). An apparent increase in the popularity of tattoos in Western cultures has been described since the 18th century, with members of the military and prison inmates commonly decorated with tattoos (64). However, tattoos were also fashionable among high-society circles; Lady Randolph Churchill, Winston Churchill's mother, started a trend for tattooing among her peers in the late 19th century (109). It is estimated that more than 20 million people presently have tattoos in the United States alone (8).

Though we generally consider tattoos to be decorative, tattooing has had a legitimate role in medical practice, including the use of injected dye to mark areas of the colon during colonoscopy for later reidentification. An interesting and short-lived practice utilizing tattoos in the United States was Operation Tat-Type during 1951 and 1952. Fearing major blood shortages for transfusion during the Korean War, various government and medical groups considered the use of community-wide blood typing and the application of blood type tattoos on volunteers in order to allow for rapid identification of blood donor types. While only two communities adopted these proposals, nevertheless thousands of adults and children received blood type tattoos. Ultimately, the program fell out of favor, though individuals from these communities may still bear these faded tattoos today (115).

Techniques

The tools of tattooing have changed over time, though the basic application techniques remain very similar. Pigment is deposited to a depth of 1 to 2 mm into the dermis by the use of various instruments. Traditional techniques involve using a sharp instrument to cut the surface of the skin, with the pigment pressed into the wound. Burning the skin followed by rubbing of pigment into the wound is a less commonly used technique. Traditional Samoan tattooing remains an important cultural rite of passage and is performed with a sharpened, serrated bone or shark's tooth attached to the end of a long stick. The cutting edge or skin is saturated in ink, and the stick is tapped to create a shallow incision in the skin, into which the ink is deposited (72). Tattoo dye or ink may be made from any number of pigmented substances, including ashes, oils, and synthetic dyes. Modern techniques of tattooing accomplish the same goal, but with the aid of a motorized tattoo machine, which is less painful and allows for a more controlled application of ink, and thus more intricate designs. As skin is punctured, minor bleeding commonly accompanies application of the tattoo. Generally, the fresh tattoo should remain covered with a bandage until bleeding resolves. "Homemade" or "prison" tattoo techniques using any available needle and ink are still commonly practiced by individuals unable to access modern tattooing equipment or resources or by "scratchers"—a term used to describe persons who have little training in tattoo application techniques.

#57

Infectious Complications

The skin is an important physical barrier and immune mechanism. Disruption of the normal skin anatomy may predispose individuals to infectious complications. Numerous bacterial and fungal microorganisms colonize the surface of the skin. Coagulase-negative staphylococci and diphtheroids are common skin colonizers, though a recent study suggests that *Pseudomonas* species may also be important colonizing bacteria in some people (43). Infectious disorders occurring after tattooing may be classified by the source of the infectious agent and may be separated into those due to endogenous and exogenous agents. Those due to endogenous agents represent diseases caused by normal flora following disruption of the skin's normal barriers. Infections associated with endogenous microorganisms are not completely preventable, although the use of appropriate sterile techniques during tattoo application and proper aftercare of the new tattoo may serve to minimize the risk. Infections due to exogenous agents are due to inoculation of a microbe not present on the host initially and should typically be preventable if hygienic techniques are followed. Reuse of tattoo ink or needles, contamination of equipment between tattoo recipients, and use of contaminated body fluids during the tattoo process (e.g., saliva used to wet the needle) have all been implicated in transmission of pathogenic microbes. Viral hepatitis, tuberculosis, syphilis, and human immunodeficiency virus (HIV) disease are examples of infections following inoculation from an exogenous source. Both endogenously and exogenously acquired infections have the potential to widely disseminate in the body via the bloodstream.

Infectious Disorders Due to Endogenous Flora

Streptococci and staphylococci are the most common bacterial causes of local infection at the tattoo site and may cause cellulitis, impetigo, erysipelas, or furunculosis (63). More in-vasive syndromes, including bacteremic illness, may follow these disorders.

Disseminated endogenous infection following tattooing has occurred, caused by both bacteria and fungi. Bacteremia typically complicates cellulitis and may result in metastatic infection. Polymicrobial sepsis with *Pseudomonas aeruginosa* and *Streptococcus pyogenes* (56), *Staphylococcus aureus* epidural abscess (23), and necrotizing fasciitis (84) following traditional Samoan tattooing have been reported. *S. aureus* aortic valve endocarditis following repeated tattooing occurred in a patient with a bicuspid aortic valve (93). *Candida albicans* endophthalmitis has been described for an asplenic individual with a recent tattoo application that required surgical drainage of the infected eye and long-term antifungal therapy with amphotericin B and fluconazole (3). There was no apparent local wound disease. Finally, tetanus, a disease due to toxins produced by *Clostridium tetani,* has followed tattooing in Maori individuals in New Zealand (103) as well as in persons in the United States (18, 19). Of course, the risk of tetanus is inversely proportional to the level of protective antibody associated with prior immunization.

Infectious Disorders Due to Exogenous Infections

VIRAL HEPATITIS

Among the exogenously acquired diseases associated with tattoos, viral hepatitis has probably been reported most commonly. The earliest reported outbreaks of acute hepatitis following tattooing occurred in military personnel who had received their tattoos at the same parlor (in which hygienic techniques were not employed) (102). Both hepatitis B virus (HBV) and HCV are transmitted by transfusion of contaminated blood products, intravenous drug use (IVDU), and occupational needlestick injuries. The risk of HBV transmission following needlestick with a hollow-bore needle is estimated to be between 2 and 40%, and the risk of HCV trans-

#58

mission is estimated to be between 3 and 10% (39). There are no precise data on specific risks for transmission of viral hepatitis during tattoo application.

During the last 50 years, numerous common-source outbreaks of acute hepatitis have been associated with recent tattooing (cited in reference 63). In some instances, the person applying the tattoo had an illness with jaundice in the months preceding the outbreaks. Patients developed acute hepatitis when contaminated needles were reused, inadequate techniques were employed to sterilize needles or dye, or an infected tattoo artist tested the needle on himself before using it on a client. Earlier cases of hepatitis were mostly likely due to HBV, though HCV could have been implicated in some.

Nishioka and Gyorkos (76) have summarized a number of studies that evaluated the association between tattooing and seropositivity for viral hepatitides. Despite accounting for confounding variables in these studies, there was no consensus on the association between receiving a tattoo and chronic HBV or HCV infection. One study from the United States did not find tattoos to be a statistically significant risk factor for chronic viral hepatitis (HBV and HCV), comparing tattooed emergency room patients to matched controls (99). Other risk factors for acquisition of viral hepatitis were noted for almost all of the individuals who had chronic viral hepatitis (e.g., body piercing, multiple sexual partners, and IVDU). However, the association between tattooing and viral hepatitis transmission is more strongly suggested among populations with a history of incarceration than among the general tattooed population. Receipt of a tattoo in prison has been associated strongly with HBV and HCV infection in several studies (47, 77, 92). Clearly, the risk of transmitting viral hepatitis appears to be vastly increased for tattooing under nonsterile conditions and in populations with a high prevalence of chronic viral hepatitis.

HIV

Concern about tattoo-associated HIV transmission is related to the known risks of transmitting HIV by needlestick injury. Though the risk of transmitting HIV is relatively low for a single needle puncture (approximately 0.1%) (39), repeated punctures, as utilized during application of a tattoo, may increase the risk. Epidemiological studies suggest that tattoo application is a risk factor for acquiring HIV in some prison populations (16, 34) and in military personnel who travel to high-prevalence countries (79). In contrast, a study of HIV infection of prisoners in Canada did not find tattooing to be a risk factor for HIV infection (31). Only one report of HIV transmission following tattooing has been published. In that instance, possible HIV transmission was reported for two prisoners who denied other risk factors (IVDU, sex with other men, or prior blood transfusions) but who had extensive tattooing with a needle used to apply tattoos on other prisoners (29). Both were found to be positive for HIV during incarceration, presumably with prior documented negative HIV tests. Of course, the potential risk of HIV transmission via tattooing may be much higher in regions of the world where HIV prevalence is itself significantly greater. Genital tattooing is practiced by some cultural groups in central and western Africa and has been considered a possible mode of HIV transmission through reuse of tattoo needles (50). Clearly, a theoretical risk for transmitting HIV exists and should be considered by those who wish to have tattoos applied outside a "professional" setting.

TUBERCULOSIS AND ATYPICAL MYCOBACTERIA

Tuberculous cellulitis following cutaneous inoculation of *Mycobacterium tuberculosis* has been well described for more than a century. Historically, morticians and physicians who performed postmortem examinations on patients who died with active tuberculosis were prone to "prosector's wart"—cutaneous tuberculosis at the site of a skin injury with instruments contaminated by *M. tuberculosis* (4, 58). Similarly, inoculation tuberculosis following application of a tattoo has been documented since the late 19th century. In one instance, a child with pulmonary tuberculosis used ink mixed with his saliva and tattooed three friends who subsequently developed pustules, local adenopathy, and giant cells, as determined by skin biopsy at the site of the tattoos (24). Another report describes the development of presumed tuberculosis in a fresh tattoo contaminated by cow's milk that may have come from an infected cow. The use of techniques considered nonhygienic by modern standards was apparently commonplace at the time of the reported infections of inoculation tuberculosis (48, 63). Papular eruptions within a tattoo appear to be a commonly described manifestation of inoculation tuberculosis (40, 41, 116).

Inoculation leprosy, presumably from the use of contaminated needles, has been well described (42, 65, 85, 94–97, 101). *Mycobacterium leprae,* the agent of leprosy, is an important cause of infection in some parts of the world, particularly sub-Saharan Africa and Asia. Many of these cases describe the development of lepromatous skin lesions confined to a tattoo and developing years after the initial tattoo application. Presumably, a person with unrecognized leprosy was tattooed and the needle was reused on subsequent individuals. The long latency period frequently described makes determining the exact source of the infection difficult in most cases, though descriptions of inoculation leprosy in American servicemen who received tattoos in countries with endemic leprosy and no other risk factors support the hypothesis that tattooing transmitted the infection.

SYPHILIS (LUES)

Both primary syphilis and secondary syphilis have been reported to occur following tattoo application. Syphilis is a sexually transmitted infection caused by the spirochete *Treponema pallidum.* It is spread from person to person by infected body fluids, including semen, vaginal secretions, saliva, and blood. Less commonly, kissing or other close contact with an active syphilitic lesion or direct inoculation may transmit infection. Primary syphilis is the first stage of infection, with the development of a painless papule at the site of inoculation occurring approximately 3 weeks after exposure. This lesion erodes and becomes indurated, forming the classic chancre. Chancres are usually encountered on or near the genitals, but they may appear almost anywhere depending on the site of inoculation. The chancre contains spirochetes and is infectious. Two to eight weeks after the appearance of a chancre, secondary syphilis may occur. This is a generalized illness with diffuse skin lesions and systemic symptoms and signs. The rash may be macular, papular, pustular, or a combination of lesions. Any organ system may be involved, leading to the protean manifestations of secondary syphilis. If untreated, the rash will resolve over days to weeks, with potential for relapses. Chronic inflammation in an affected organ may lead to symptoms of tertiary syphilis (cardiovascular, neurological, and gumma late disease), usually occurring years after initial infection.

Primary syphilis at the site of a recently applied tattoo was described in the medical literature as early as 1853 (51) and subsequently reported by others (cited in reference 63). In the described cases, the tattoo artist had oral mucous patches thought to be chancres and used saliva to rewet the needle or ink, or saliva was applied directly to the tattoo site. Chancres formed within the newly applied tattoo. Lesions of secondary syphilis may localize within recently applied tattoos and may be due to chronic inflammation and decreased immune responses within the tattoo (90). Interestingly, rashes of secondary syphilis have been noted to preferentially affect portions of some tattoos, with higher concentrations of skin lesions in areas with blue ink and the absence of lesions in areas with red pigment. This preference for blue-pigmented tattoos is due to the use of red cinnabar, or mercuric sulfide, in older formulations of red inks. Mercury compounds have been recognized to possess antiluetic activity for centuries and appear to prevent localization of disseminated treponemal disease in the red-pigmented areas, while the blue-pigmented areas are susceptible to the appearance of the rash of secondary syphilis.

OTHER INFECTIONS

Staphylococcus aureus is usually considered an endogenous pathogen of tattoos. However, outbreaks of tattoo site infections where *S. aureus* appeared to be transmitted exogenously have occurred. Methicillin-resistant *S. aureus* (MRSA) was traditionally considered an important cause of infection in patients with significant health care exposures, such as hospitalization, residence in long-term care facilities, recent surgery, and dialysis, and in patients with the presence of indwelling devices. In recent years, MRSA infections have been recognized in persons without any of the previously identified risk factors. These community-associated MRSA (CA-MRSA) infections commonly present as skin or skin structure infections and are due to unique MRSA strains that may have recently evolved. Outbreaks of CA-MRSA skin infections following tattooing were noted to occur in 34 individuals from three states in the United States (20). None of the tattoos were applied in prison, but many were done in a nonprofessional setting without appropriate infection control practices. Some of the tattooists were noted to have skin infections on their hands at the time of the tattoo application, and homemade tattooing equipment was used in some cases. Manifestations of CA-MRSA infection included pustules, cellulitis, and abscesses in or adjacent to the recently applied tattoo, and some lesions required surgical drainage. All of the bacteria available for testing from patients were noted to be the USA300 genotype, the most common strain of CA-MRSA associated with skin infections.

Transmission of papillomavirus from contaminated ink or needles has resulted in the appearance of warts at the site of recently applied tattoos (63). Vaccinia has also been reported to occur near a recently applied tattoo and may have represented inoculation of virus (113). Tattoo-related fungal infections have also been reported. Sporotrichosis, typically a lymphocutaneous infection caused by the fungus *Sporothrix schenckii,* was described to occur starting at the site of a tattoo recently applied using traditional Samoan techniques (22). The infection was likely due to inoculation of the skin with *S. schenckii* at the time of tattooing, and cutaneous nodules persisted for 6 years until definitively treated with itraconazole. Invasive mold disease with members of the zygomycete family usually occurs in immunocompromised individuals but also may occur in others. A subcutaneous infection with *Saksenaea vasiformis* at the site of a tattoo applied 7 years previously has been described to occur in an immunocompetent individual (83), though it is unclear whether the mold infection was inoculated at the time of tattoo application or acquired more recently.

BODY PIERCING

Body piercing has gained popularity recently in developed countries but has been performed in primitive cultures for thousands of years, often as a rite of passage or associated with religious ceremonies. Piercing of the male genitals was described in the 4th-century Indian text the *Kama Sutra* as follows: "In southern countries, the penis is pierced during childhood, just as one pierces the ears" (111). "Purists" of body piercing often do not consider earlobe piercings true body piercings and prefer to consider piercings of the face, navel, nipples, and genitals to be true body piercings. More recently, "surface piercings," where jewelry is embedded in almost any surface of the body (especially the chest, neck, or arms), and implanting of jewelry or other foreign material (e.g., plastic beads, metal, and even natural pearls) into the subcutaneous tissue has become popular. Jewelry has even been inserted into the conjunctiva of the eye in The Netherlands, a controversial procedure that appears to risk serious complications (http://www.niioc.nl/cei-eng.htm). However, we were unable to find reports of infectious complications from these procedures. Since any body piercing may result in various complications, for purposes of this discussion we define body piercing as Samantha et al. (91) do, as "the use of needles, rings, steel posts, or other adornments that penetrate the skin and other structures of the human body." We include earlobe piercings in this definition.

Body Piercing Techniques

Specific techniques of body piercing vary depending on the site of the piercing but are generally similar. Most piercings are accomplished using a sharp, hollow needle designed for this purpose. The site to be pierced is usually held in place by a surgical clamp (Pennington or Foerster clamp), through which the needle is pushed by hand into a cork or rubber stopper. The needle is typically 14 or 16 gauge (though larger sizes are available) and is made of stainless steel. An open end of the jewelry is introduced into the rear blunt end of the piercing needle and pulled through the opening made by the needle, and the needle and stopper are removed.

Modern body jewelry implanted during piercing is fabricated of stainless steel, titanium, gold, niobium, or acrylic. Nickel-containing alloys are not recommended due to the risk of hypersensitivity. Frequently, a barbell-shaped device with two threaded beads at the ends or an open loop closed with a bead is used as the initial choice of jewelry. However, many styles of jewelry exist, with unique shapes being used with increasing frequency. Traditional jewelry used by cultures in developing countries where body piercing is common includes items made of bone, wood, metal, shells, or feather quills.

General Infectious Complications

The risk of infection itself and the precise types of infectious disorders that follow body piercing depend upon the site of the piercing,

extent of hygienic techniques utilized during the procedure, experience of the person performing the piercing, general host defenses of the individual receiving the piercing, and aftercare of the pierced site. Healing time, generally a function of blood supply and tissue integrity, varies greatly with body location and is an important factor in the risk of infection. As with tattooing, infections associated with body piercing may be generally classified as either endogenous or exogenous depending on the suspected source of infection. Local inflammatory reactions must be distinguished from early local infections and may be due to direct mechanical irritation, allergic reactions to the metal, or granulomatous foreign-body reactions. Local cellulitis at the site of new piercings is the most common infectious complication, with an overall estimated prevalence ranging from 10 to 30% (44, 104). The most common sites where local infections have been described to occur include the navel, ear, nose, and nipple. Less commonly, piercings of the tongue, genitals, and other sites appear to be complicated by infectious disorders. Cellulitis, characterized by redness, swelling, pain, and purulent drainage from the piercing site, is most commonly caused by *S. aureus,* group A streptococci, and aerobic gram-negative bacilli, particularly *Pseudomonas* species. Table 1 summarizes the infectious disorders associated with body piercing.

Endogenously Acquired Infectious Complications by Site of Piercing

EARS

The ear remains the most commonly pierced site; as many as 80 to 90% of women in North America have at least one ear piercing (15, 100), and a growing number of men report having had their ears pierced. In addition to the earlobe, the cartilaginous portions of the ear, including the tragus, antitragus, helix, and antihelix, may be pierced. In addition, "flesh tunnels," stretched earlobe piercings, are common in many indigenous cultures and have become quite popular in contemporary pierc-

TABLE 1 Overview of infectious complications of body piercing[a]

Site	Infectious complication	Associated pathogen(s)
General	Local infections, cellulitis, hepatitis, HIV	Staphylococci, streptococci, HBV, HCV
Ear	Chondritis, bacteremia, hepatic abscess, meningitis, osteomyelitis, toxic shock syndrome, glomerulonephritis, infective endocarditis, tetanus, tuberculosis	*Staphylococcus aureus,* group A streptococci, *Pseudomonas* species
Oral	Glossitis, abscess, Ludwig's angina, Lemierre's syndrome, cerebellar abscess, IE, tetanus, warts	Oral flora, *Haemophilus aphrophilus, Neisseria mucosa, Staphylococcus aureus,* papillomavirus
Nose	IE	*Staphylococcus aureus*
Nipple	Mastitis, IE, infected prosthetic breast implants	Staphylococci, streptococci, *Mycobacterium abscessus, Mycobacterium fortuitum, Prevotella melaninogenica, Gordonia terrae*
Navel	Cellulitis, IE, tetanus	*Staphylococcus aureus,* viridans group streptococci
Genital	Warts, sexually transmitted infections	Papillomavirus

[a]See text for references.

ing practices. Techniques of ear piercing include the use of a piercing "gun," which uses pressure to push the earring post through the earlobe, and use of a needle in the earlobe or cartilage to create a hole through which jewelry is placed. Piercing guns are apparently difficult to thoroughly disinfect. Local infections of the earlobe are most commonly caused by *S. aureus* and group A streptococci (73). A history of poorly controlled diabetes mellitus was noted in a woman who developed local inflammation and local infection of the ears, suggesting that conditions that compromise the immune system or wound healing may lead to complications following even typical ear lobe piercings (7). Cellulitis and erysipelas at ear piercing sites have been well recognized since the 19th century (105). Chondritis following piercing of the cartilaginous portions of the ear is most commonly due to *Pseudomonas* species (36, 38, 54, 73, 108, 110). The decreased vascularity of ear cartilage compared to that of the soft tissue of the earlobe increases the risk of bacterial infection at that location (73, 108).

As in other situations, cellulitis may occasionally be complicated by bacteremia. Lovejoy and Smith described the occurrence of severe disseminated *S. aureus* infection in children with recent earlobe piercings (two patients) or subacutely infected earlobe piercing sites (one patient). Hepatic abscesses complicated one case of bacteremia, another was complicated by osteomyelitis, and a third was complicated by meningitis (64). In addition, spondylitis has also been associated with infection following ear piercing (98). Immune-mediated disease following ear piercing was described by Ahmed-Jushuf et al. (1), who reported poststreptococcal glomerulonephritis occurring in a boy who had recently pierced his own ear and developed group A streptococcal infection of the earlobe, and by McCarthy and Peoples (70), who reported toxic shock syndrome following earlobe piercing. In addition, tetanus has been noted following ear piercing (67; see references in reference 105). Infective endocarditis (IE) has followed ear piercing in several patients, including viridans group streptococcal aortic valve endocarditis complicated by a Gerbode ventricular septal defect in an otherwise healthy 15-year-old boy (13, 49, 60, 82).

ORAL PIERCINGS
Reports of infections following oral soft tissue piercings have a broad variety of microbiological etiologies reflecting the many commensal

#61

organisms in the oral cavity. Oral piercing sites include the tongue, lip, cheek, and rarely, the uvula. Metastatic infectious complications have been described most frequently for tongue piercings. This discussion focuses on tongue piercings, as the vast majority of reported infections involve complications of this procedure. However, Lemierre's disease with external jugular vein thrombosis and septic pulmonary emboli was tenuously associated with a lip piercing, occurring 6 weeks after the piercing (75). Lemierre's disease is a severe oropharyngeal infection, caused by *Fusobacterium necrophorum,* which may lead to jugular vein thrombosis and metastatic spread of infection to the lung, liver, joints, and other sites.

Tongue. Tongue piercings may be horizontal or vertical through the tongue or through the frenulum beneath the tongue. Despite the rich microbiological environment of the mouth, infections of tongue piercings remain uncommon, probably due to the rich vascularity of the tongue and the related rapid healing time for tongue injuries. Local inflammation following piercing is expected, with significant swelling and tenderness of the tongue, but this usually resolves in a few days to several weeks. Most tongue infections can be prevented with appropriate aftercare, usually involving regular use of antiseptic mouthwash during the initial healing period. Persistent swelling, tenderness, and pain may indicate glossitis, a local soft tissue infection of the tongue. If severe, glossitis justifies removal of the jewelry and systemic antimicrobial therapy.

Development of a lingual abscess requiring surgical drainage has been reported to occur in an adolescent who attempted to pierce his tongue (80). Ludwig's angina, a rapidly spreading cellulitis involving the submandibular and sublingual spaces, has also been reported to occur 4 days after placement of a tongue piercing (84). Bacteremia complicating tongue piercing may result in metastatic disease as well. A cerebellar abscess in a previously healthy woman who had a tongue piercing 4 weeks earlier has been reported (68). It seems that after the piercing, the patient had a self-limiting infection at the site, with purulent discharge. Headache, nausea, vomiting, and vertigo characterized the patient's illness, and the abscess required surgical drainage and long-term antimicrobial therapy. Cultures of the abscess revealed a polymicrobial infection with viridans group streptococci, *Peptostreptococcus micros, Actinomyces* species, and *Eikenella corrodens.* The bacteria cultured were consistent with an oral source of infection. No other infectious sources or predispositions could be found in this patient.

IE associated with tongue piercing has been reported for at least seven individuals (Table 2). Only one of the patients who developed IE after tongue piercing had a known predisposing cardiac valve defect. The microbiology of these infections was diverse, likely representing the flora of the oral cavity, and included streptococci, *S. aureus, Neisseria mucosa,* and *Haemophilus aphrophilus* (2, 12, 30, 45, 55, 62, 106). One individual developed mitral valve IE 3 days after replacing her tongue jewelry with (apparently) contaminated jewelry from a friend, highlighting the importance of not sharing body jewelry, especially immediately after a piercing has been placed (45).

A single case of cephalic tetanus associated with tongue piercing has been described, manifesting as jaw pain, trismus, dysarthria, and flu-like symptoms (33).

OTHER FACIAL PIERCINGS

Eyebrow, "antieyebrow" (piercings lateral to the eye or on the upper cheek below the eye), bridge, and nasal piercings are also common. Nasal piercing sites include the nostril or septum. In one reported complication of nasal piercing, *S. aureus* mitral valve IE occurred in a 14-year-old girl without known prior cardiac abnormalities (89). *Staphylococcus aureus* was cultured from the nose and was the possible source of infection.

TABLE 2 Endocarditis associated with tattooing and body piercing

Reference	Procedure	Organism	Valve affected	Predisposition
93	Tattooing	*Staphylococcus aureus*	Aortic	Bicuspid valve
13	Ear piercing	Viridans group streptococci	Aortic	None
60	Ear piercing	*Staphylococcus aureus*	Mitral	None
57	Ear piercing	*Staphylococcus aureus*	Tricuspid	None
82	Ear piercing	*Staphylococcus aureus*	Mitral	None
49	Ear piercing	*Staphylococcus aureus*	Homograft conduit	Tetralogy of Fallot
89	Nasal piercing	*Staphylococcus aureus*	Mitral	None
37	Lip piercing	*Haemophilus parainfluenzae*	Mitral	None
2	Tongue piercing	*Haemophilus aphrophilus*	Aortic	Bicuspid valve, repaired aortic stenosis (valvuloplasty)
106	Tongue piercing	*Neisseria mucosa*	Mitral	None
45	Tongue piercing	*Staphylococcus aureus*	Mitral	None
62	Tongue piercing	Viridans group streptococci	Aortic	None
55	Tongue piercing	Alpha-hemolytic streptococci	Mitral	None
30	Tongue piercing	*Staphylococcus aureus*	Mitral	None
12	Tongue piercing	*Streptococcus constellatus*	Aortic	None
78	Nipple piercing	*Staphylococcus epidermidis*	Aortic	Bicuspid valve, repaired aortic coarctation
112	Navel piercing	*Staphylococcus aureus*	Pulmonary	Corrected transposition of the great arteries
11	Navel piercing	Viridans group streptococci	Myocardial septum	Ventricular septal defect
88	Navel piercing	*Staphylococcus aureus*	Mitral	None
32	Navel piercing	*Staphylococcus aureus*	Tricuspid	None
35	Navel piercing	Culture negative	Mitral	Atrial septal defect

NIPPLES

In addition to cellulitis alone, infection may extend more deeply and has been noted to cause mastitis in both men and women after nipple piercing. Mastitis cases due to coagulase-negative staphylococci, group B streptococci, and microaerophilic staphylococci following nipple piercing have been described (52). Other reported bacteria causing mastitis, abscess, or granulomatous infection include *Mycobacterium abscessus* (107), *Mycobacterium fortuitum* (14, 61), *Prevotella melaninogenica* (14), and *Gordonia terrae* (117). Serious complications following nipple piercing include the development of *Staphylococcus epidermidis* aortic valve IE in a 24-year-old man with a bicuspid aortic valve and corrected aortic coarctation (78) and fatal toxic shock syndrome in a healthy 17-year-old girl (10). An unusual complication of nipple piercing is breast implant infection complicating cellulitis at the piercing site. Implant infection has been reported for both a female patient with silicone breast implants (53) and a male patient with solid pectoral implants who developed group A beta-hemolytic streptococcus infection after nipple piercing (27). Even more intriguing may be an association between nipple piercing, subsequent infection of the piercing site, and the development of hyperprolactinemia. Hyperprolactinemia was exacerbated following nipple piercing and local infection in a man who had previously well-controlled hyperprolactinemia (28) and was seen in a woman with no prior endocrine disorders following nipple piercing and local infection (71). It is possible that nipple stimulation by either infection, nipple jewelry, or both may lead to excessive prolactin secretion and could lead to galactorrhea, a disorder of inappropriate lactation.

NAVEL

The navel is probably the most common site of body piercing, after the ear. It is also the most likely body piercing site to experience a prolonged healing time (several months) and to be associated with infectious complications (104). Navel piercings may be performed through the subcutaneous tissue on any side of the navel. It should never include the umbilical remnant, which is more exposed in people with extroverted navels, as infection in this tissue may lead to intra-abdominal infection. Prolonged healing at the navel may be due to the presence of tight clothing irritating the pierced tissue and the presence of a persistent moist environment. There are few reports describing the precise bacterial etiology of cellulitis complicating navel piercing, but one may assume that staphylococci and streptococci are frequently implicated. A serious complication of navel piercing occurred in a 13-year-old girl with corrected D-transposition of the great arteries who developed *S. aureus* IE after she pierced her own navel (112). The patient did not take prophylactic antibiotics before the piercing, and a self-limiting local infection reportedly developed 2 days after the piercing, followed in 1 month by symptoms of IE. Several other cases of IE after navel piercing have also been reported (Table 2). Tetanus has been reported to occur in a 27-year-old woman with a remote history of tetanus vaccination who performed a navel piercing on herself and developed facial pain and trismus 10 days later (81).

GENITAL PIERCINGS

Anatomical sites for male and female genital piercings are extremely diverse, and no part of the genitalia has been spared (6). "Traditional" male genital piercings include the Prince Albert piercing (a ring passes through the urethra and ventral surface of the penis), dydoe (piercing the coronal ridge of the glans), ampallang (horizontal bar through the glans), apadravya (vertical piercing through the glans), hafada (piercing of the lateral scrotal tissue), guiche (piercing the perineal tissue between the scrotum and anus), frenulum piercing, and foreskin piercing. "Traditional" female genital piercings include piercings of the labia majora or minora, clitoris, and clitoral hood as well as the fourchette (a female version of the

guiche piercing). As with other piercings, the popularity of body piercings has spawned numerous other variations on the traditional piercings.

Serious infectious complications of genital piercings do not appear to be common. Infectious complications appear to usually reflect the local flora of the perineum or acquisition of disease through sexual activity. Aerobic gram-negative bacilli, such as *Escherichia coli,* and other enteric bacteria that are common causes of genitourinary infections are also likely causes of genital piercing infections, in addition to skin flora bacteria.

Recurrent genital warts have been noted at the site of a new penile frenulum piercing (5). The recent piercing caused local tissue damage that may have predisposed the patient to the recurrent papillomavirus infection.

Exogenously Acquired Diseases Associated with Body Piercing

Studies have attempted to define an association between body piercing and viral hepatitis, with the general consensus that body piercing is a risk factor for the spread of hepatitis B and C if aseptic techniques are not followed (46) and if the equipment used is contaminated by blood from prior infected clients. Sharing of contaminated body jewelry has also been implicated in the transmission of viral hepatitis (25).

Infection of the piercing recipient by HIV has been postulated but not well documented. A single case is described of a male with multiple documented seronegative tests for HIV antibody who subsequently seroconverted (87). During the year prior to seroconversion, he had multiple body piercings performed in several different countries. He also had three male sexual partners. Certainly, it is possible that the patient acquired HIV during a body piercing procedure, though it is difficult to prove. Regardless, the possibility of HIV transmission exists if contaminated needles are reused.

Inoculation of infectious agents at the time of piercing or during the healing period has also been reported to cause disease. Primary tuberculosis of the earlobe has been reported for an infant following ear piercing by her mother, who had active pulmonary tuberculosis and may have moistened the piercing needle with her saliva (74). Growth of warts due to human papillomavirus at the site of a new tongue piercing has been described, particularly following unprotected oral sex with a partner with genital warts (http://www.bmezine.com/risks/index.html). Piercing-associated warts usually do not resolve spontaneously and may require excision.

Sexually transmitted diseases are of particular concern for individuals with genital piercings. Unprotected sex with an unhealed piercing poses increased risk of transmission of many sexually transmitted diseases, including HIV, herpes simplex, syphilis, and gonorrhea. Even after a piercing is healed, it may cause mechanical irritation to mucous membranes and decrease the local barriers to transmission of viruses or bacteria.

PREVENTION OF INFECTIONS

Prevention of infectious complications following tattooing or body piercing begins with the person performing the procedure. In recent years, most states in the United States, as well as many Western countries, have developed specific legislation that requires tattoo and piercing parlors to follow strict hygiene and infection control policies. Usually, local public health departments (county and state) are responsible for ensuring that safe and sanitary practices are followed. In addition, professional piercing and tattooing associations have had some self-regulated infection control practices within their own industry. Generally, state laws mandate the use of single-use needles, sterilization of nondisposable equipment, needles, and jewelry prior to use, and appropriate environmental disinfection guidelines. Piercing guns are not recommended, nor are home piercing kits. Persons not experienced in appropriate tattooing or body piercing techniques, as well as those with equipment and jewelry that have not been properly sterilized, should not perform tattooing or body piercing. Professional establishments should provide appropriate aftercare instructions depending on the site of the piercing. For persons with genital piercings, sexual activity should be avoided during the healing period. The Association of Professional Piercers (http://www.safepiercing.org) provides general aftercare recommendations and precautions for different body piercings.

TREATMENT OF INFECTIONS ASSOCIATED WITH TATTOOING AND BODY PIERCING

Most cases of local infection following body piercing may be managed with local care (mild antiseptics or irrigation with saline solution). Removal of jewelry is not advocated if a local infection occurs, as it may result in a loculated infection in the pierced tract. Rather, the jewelry maintains a patent drainage site, aiding in healing of the infection. If the infection progresses, however, removal of the jewelry may be necessary, especially if a loculated abscess is already present, which would require irrigation and debridement. Systemic antibiotics may be indicated for local infections that do not resolve or in the case of associated signs and symptoms of systemic infectious disease, such as fever or chills. Antibiotic choices should take into account the role of the local flora at a specific piercing site. Infected oral piercings should be treated with antimicrobials with broad aerobic and anaerobic coverage. Genital piercings are predisposed to infections caused by aerobic gram-negative bacilli, especially the *Enterobacteriaceae,* as well as anaerobes, staphylococci, and streptococci. Antipseudomonal antimicrobials should be considered for treatment of auricular chondritis. All body piercing-associated infections should have adequate antimicrobial coverage for staphylococci and streptococci. For complicated infections (metastatic infection, bacteremia, and deep abscesses), blood cultures should be performed, and in the case of abscesses, operative cultures at the time of drainage should be performed to guide antimicrobial therapy.

An experienced tattoo artist should generally evaluate local infection of a recently applied tattoo. Topical antibiotic preparations are discouraged. If cellulitis or metastatic or systemic infection is suspected, evaluation by a physician and systemic antibiotics are warranted.

PRECAUTIONS FOR SPECIAL POPULATIONS

Certain medical conditions may increase the risk of infectious complications of body piercing, especially for those patients with congenital cardiac abnormalities, cardiac valvular disease, and immunologic disorders that predispose them to bacterial infections. The incidence of bacteremia following tattooing or body piercing is unknown. Bacteremia would be expected to place individuals with valvular or congenital heart disease at risk for IE. Of the 21 reported cases of IE that have been associated with body piercing or tattooing, seven occurred in persons with cardiac predispositions (Table 2). Patients with predisposing cardiac abnormalities should be made aware of the risk of serious infection, especially IE, and some authors recommend avoidance of tattoos and body piercing altogether or the use of prophylactic antibiotics (21). Though there are no specific guidelines for the prevention of IE in the setting of tattooing or body piercings, guidelines for the prevention of IE published by the American Heart Association may be useful, particularly in reference to oral piercings. Since perforation of the oral mucosa is considered a dental procedure, it may be reasonable to extrapolate the recommendations for prevention of IE in persons undergoing dental procedures. The cardiac conditions with the highest risk of endocarditis, for which antibiotic prophylaxis is recommended, include the presence of a prosthetic heart valve, previous IE, cardiac transplantation with development of cardiac valvulopathy, and specific congenital heart disease (unrepaired cyanotic congenital heart disease, completely repaired congenital heart defect with prosthetic material or device dur-

ing the first 6 months after the procedure, and repaired congenital heart disease with residual defects at or adjacent to the site of prosthesis that prevent endothelialization) (114). Similarly, patients who are predisposed to infections due to immunosuppression, immunocompromising disorders, or poorly controlled diabetes mellitus or those with chronic skin disorders should be aware of the risk of serious infection and should consider avoidance of these procedures.

SUMMARY

Medical practitioners and the general public should be aware of the potential risks of infection associated with tattooing and body piercing. Early recognition of infection following tattooing or body piercing is important to prevent potential complications, but such infections can be difficult to appreciate because most health care professionals are unfamiliar with the clinical characteristics of infections associated with these procedures. More recently, the popularity of these procedures has led to greater awareness and application of hygienic techniques and to use of sterile equipment, hopefully reducing the risk of transmitting blood-borne infections. In addition, public health departments have helped to regulate safe practices and procedures. Most infections seen today are due to endogenously acquired microorganisms, which may contaminate the healing tissue. Persons interested in getting a tattoo or body piercing should seek professional artists who follow established hygienic techniques. The Association for Professional Piercers (http://www.safepiercing.org) and the American Tattooing Institute (http://www.tatsmart.com) are resources that provide information on reputable tattooists and piercers. Certain populations, especially those with significant immunocompromise, skin disorders, or predisposing cardiac disease, should consider the infectious risks of tattooing and body piercing and take the appropriate precautions, discuss the procedure with their health care providers, or avoid these procedures altogether.

PRACTICAL TIPS

- Tattooing and body piercing should be performed only by professional practitioners who are licensed by state or local health departments.
- Persons with chronic skin conditions, congenital or valvular heart disease, diabetes mellitus, or other immunocompromising conditions should thoroughly discuss the risks of tattooing or body piercing with a medical professional.
- Persons undergoing these procedures should follow the aftercare instructions for a new tattoo or body piercing provided by a professional tattooist or piercer.
- If you suspect an infection is present, have the site evaluated by the tattooist or piercer.
- A medical professional should immediately evaluate systemic symptoms of infection, such as fevers or chills, or infections that are not responding to local wound care.

REFERENCES

1. **Ahmed-Jushuf, I. H., P. L. Selby, and A. M. Brownjohn.** 1984. Acute post-streptococcal glomerulonephritis following ear piercing. *Postgrad. Med. J.* **60:**73–74.
2. **Akhondi, H., and A. R. Rahimi.** 2002. *Haemophilus aphrophilus* endocarditis after tongue piercing. *Emerg. Infect. Dis.* **8:**850–851.
3. **Alexandridou, A.** 2002. Candida endophthalmitis after tattooing in an asplenic patient. *Arch. Ophthalmol.* **120:**518–519.
4. **Allen, R. K., D. L. Pierson, and O. G. Rodman.** 1979. Cutaneous inoculation tuberculosis, prosectors wart occurring in a physician. *Cutis* **23:**815–818.
5. **Altman, J. S., and K. S. Manglani.** 1997. Recurrent condyloma acuminatum due to piercing of the penis. *Cutis* **60:**237–238.
6. **Anderson, W. R., D. J. Summerton, D. M. Sharma, and S. A. Holmes.** 2003. The urologist's guide to genital piercing. *BJU Int.* **91:**245–251.
7. **Antoszewski, B., M. Jedrzejczak, and J. Kruk-Jeromin.** 2007. Complications after body piercing in a patient suffering from type 1 diabetes mellitus. *Int. J. Dermatol.* **46:**1250–1252.
8. **Armstrong, M. L.** 1994. Adolescents and tattoos: marks of identity or deviancy? *Dermatol. Nurs.* **6:**119–124.
9. **Armstrong, M. L., A. E. Roberts, D. C. Owen, and J. R. Koch.** 2004. Contemporary college students and body piercing. *J. Adolesc. Health* **35:**58–61.
10. **Bader, M. S., M. Hamodat, and J. Hutchinson.** 2007. A fatal case of *Staphylococcus aureus:* associated toxic shock syndrome following nipple piercing. *Scand. J. Infect. Dis.* **39:**741–743.
11. **Barkan, D., R. A. Fanne, A. Elazari-Scheiman, S. Maayan, and R. Beeri.** 2007. Naval piercing as a cause for Streptococcus viridans endocarditis: case report, review of the literature and implications for antibiotic prophylaxis. *Cardiology* **108:**159–160.
12. **Batiste, C., R. C. Bansal, and A. J. Razzouk.** 2004. Echocardiographic features of an unruptured mycotic aneurysm of the right aortic sinus of valsalva. *J. Am. Soc. Echocardiogr.* **17:**474–477.
13. **Battin, M., L. V. Fong, and J. L. Monro.** 1991. Gerbode ventricular septal defect following endocarditis. *Eur. J. Cardio-Thorac. Surg.* **5:**613–614.
14. **Bengualid, V., V. Singh, H. Singh, and J. Berger.** 2008. *Mycobacterium fortuitum* and anaerobic breast abscess following nipple piercing: case presentation and review of the literature. *J. Adolesc. Health* **42:**530–532.
15. **Biggar, R. J., and G. E. Haughie.** 1975. Medical problems of ear piercing. *N. Y. State J. Med.* **75:**1460–1462.
16. **Buavirat, A., K. Page-Shafer, G. J. van Griensven, J. S. Mandel, J. Evans, J. Chuaratanaphong, S. Chiamwongpat, R. Sacks, and A. Moss.** 2003. Risk of prevalent HIV infection associated with incarceration among injecting drug users in Bangkok, Thailand: case-control study. *BMJ* **326:**308–312.
17. **Carroll, S. T., R. H. Riffenburgh, T. A. Roberts, and E. B. Myhre.** 2002. Tattoos and body piercings as indicators of adolescent risk-taking behaviors. *Pediatrics* **109:**1021–1027.
18. **Centers for Disease Control and Prevention.** 1998. Tetanus surveillance—United States, 1995–1997. *MMWR Morb. Mortal. Wkly. Rep.* **47**(SS-02):1–13.
19. **Centers for Disease Control and Prevention.** 2003. Tetanus surveillance—United States, 1998–2000. *MMWR Morb. Mortal. Wkly. Rep.* **52**(SS-03):1–8.
20. **Centers for Disease Control and Prevention.** 2006. Methicillin-resistant *Staphylococcus aureus* skin infections among tattoo recipients—Ohio, Kentucky, and Vermont, 2004–2005. *MMWR Morb. Mortal. Wkly. Rep.* **55:**677–679.
21. **Cetta, F., L. C. Graham, R. C. Lichtenberg, and C. A. Warnes.** 1999. Piercing and tattooing

in patients with congenital heart disease: patient and physician perspectives. *J. Adolesc. Health* **24:** 160–162.

22. **Choong, K. Y., and L. J. Roberts.** 1996. Ritual Samoan body tattooing and associated sporotrichosis. *Australas. J. Dermatol.* **37:**50–53.

23. **Chowfin, A., A. Pott, A. Paul, and P. Carson.** 1999. Spinal epidural abscess after tattooing. *Clin. Infect. Dis.* **29:**225–226.

24. **Collings, D. W., and W. Murray.** 1895. Three cases of inoculation of tuberculosis from tattooing. *Br. Med. J.* **1:**1200–1201.

25. **Daniel, A. R., and T. Shehab.** 2005. Transmission of hepatitis C through swapping of body jewelry. *Pediatrics* **116:**1264–1265.

26. **De Cuyper, C.** 2008. Permanent makeup: indications and complications. *Clin. Dermatol.* **26:** 30–34.

27. **de Kleer, N., M. Cohen, J. Semple, A. Simor, and O. Antonyshyn.** 2001. Nipple piercing may be contraindicated in male patients with chest implants. *Ann. Plast. Surg.* **47:**188–190.

28. **Demirtas, Y., Y. Sariguney, O. Cukurluoglu, S. Ayhan, and C. Celebi.** 2004. Nipple piercing: it is wiser to avoid in patients with hyperprolactinemia. *Dermatol. Surg.* **30:**1184.

29. **Doll, A. C.** 1988. Tattooing in prison and HIV infection. *Lancet* **i:**66–67.

30. **Dubose, J., and J. W. Pratt.** 2004. Victim of fashion: endocarditis after oral piercing. *Curr. Surg.* **61:**474–477.

31. **Dufour, A., M. Alary, C. Poulin, F. Allard, L. Noel, G. Trottier, D. Lepine, and C. Hankins.** 1996. Prevalence and risk behaviours for HIV infection among inmates of a provincial prison in Quebec City. *AIDS* **10:**1009–1015.

32. **Dupont, P., P. Maragnes, G. de la Gastine, M. Jokic, and M. Morin.** 2006. Tricuspid valve endocarditis after umbilical piercing. *Arch. Mal. Coeur Vaiss.* **99:**629–631.

33. **Dyce, O., J. R. Bruno, D. Hong, K. Silverstein, M. J. Brown, and N. Mirza.** 2000. Tongue piercing . . . the new "rusty nail"? *Head Neck* **22:**728–732.

34. **Estebanez-Estebanez, P., C. Colomo-Gomez, M. V. Zunzunegui-Pastor, M. Rua Figueroa, M. Perez, C. Ortiz, P. Heras, and F. Babin.** 1990. Jails and AIDS. Risk factors for HIV infection in the prisons of Madrid. *Gac. Sanit.* **4:**100–105. (In Spanish.)

35. **Ferguson, A. W., A. Jollands, M. Kirkpatrick, S. D. Pringle, and N. D. George.** 2006. Infective endocarditis presenting with Parinaud's dorsal midbrain syndrome. *J. Pediatr. Ophthalmol. Strabismus* **43:**41–43.

36. **Fisher, C. G., M. A. Kacica, and N. M. Bennett.** 2005. Risk factors for cartilage infections of the ear. *Am. J. Prev. Med.* **29:**204–209.

37. **Friedel, J. M., J. Stehlik, M. Desai, and J. E. Granato.** 2003. Infective endocarditis after oral body piercing. *Cardiol. Rev.* **11:**252–255.

38. **George, J., and M. White.** 1989. Infection as a consequence of ear piercing. *Practitioner* **23:** 404–406.

39. **Gerberding, J. L.** 1995. Management of occupational exposures to blood-borne viruses. *N. Engl. J. Med.* **332:**444–451.

40. **Ghorpade, A.** 2003. Lupus vulgaris over a tattoo mark—inoculation tuberculosis. *J. Eur. Acad. Dermatol. Venereol.* **17:**569–571.

41. **Ghorpade, A.** 2006. Tattoo inoculation lupus vulgaris in two Indian ladies. *J. Eur. Acad. Dermatol. Venereol.* **20:**476–477.

42. **Ghorpade, A.** 2002. Inoculation (tattoo) leprosy: a report of 31 cases. *J. Eur. Acad. Dermatol. Venereol.* **16:**494–499.

43. **Grice, E. A., H. H. Kong, G. Renaud, A. C. Young, NISC Comparative Sequencing Program, G. G. Bouffard, R. W. Blakesley, T. G. Wolfsberg, M. L. Turner, and J. A. Segre.** 2008. A diversity profile of the human skin microbiota. *Genome Res.* **18:**1043–1050.

44. **Guiard-Schmid, J. B., H. Picard, L. Slama, C. Maslo, C. Amiel, G. Pialoux, M. G. Lebrette, and W. Rozenbaum.** 2000. Piercing and its infectious complications: a public health issue in France. *Presse Med.* **29:**1948–1956.

45. **Harding, P. R., M. W. Yerkey, G. Deye, and D. Storey.** 2002. Methicillin-resistant *Staphylococcus aureus* (MRSA) endocarditis secondary to tongue piercing. *J. Miss. State Med. Assoc.* **43:**109.

46. **Hayes, M. O., and G. A. Harkness.** 2001. Body piercing as a risk factor for viral hepatitis: an integrative research review. *Am. J. Infect. Control* **29:**271–274.

47. **Hellard, M. E., C. K. Aitken, and J. S. Hocking.** 2007. Tattooing in prisons—not such a pretty picture. *Am. J. Infect. Control* **35:**477–480.

48. **Horney, D. A., J. M. Gaither, R. Lauer, A. L. Norins, and P. N. Mathur.** 1985. Cutaneous inoculation tuberculosis secondary to "jailhouse tattooing." *Arch. Dermatol.* **121:**648–650.

49. **Hoyer, A., and M. Silberbach.** 2005. Infective endocarditis. *Pediatr. Rev.* **26:**394–400.

50. **Hrdy, D. B.** 1987. Cultural practices contributing to the transmission of human immunodeficiency virus in Africa. *Rev. Infect. Dis.* **9:**1109–1119.

51. **Hutin, J. M. F.** 1853. *Recherches sur les Tatouages.* J. B. Baillier, Paris, France.

52. **Jacobs, V. R., K. Golombeck, W. Jonat, and M. Kiechle.** 2002. Three case reports of breast

abscess after nipple piercing: underestimated health problems of a fashion phenomenon. *Zentbl. Gynaekol.* **124:**378–385. (In German.)

53. **Javaid, M., and M. Shibu.** 1999. Breast implant infection following nipple piercing. *Br. J. Plast. Surg.* **52:**676–677.

54. **Keen, W. E., A. C. Markum, and M. Samadpour.** 2004. Outbreak of *Pseudomonas aeruginosa* infections caused by commercial piercing of the upper ear cartilage. *JAMA* **291:**981–985.

55. **Kloppenburg, G., and J. G. Maessen.** 2007. Streptococcus endocarditis after tongue piercing. *J. Heart Valve Dis.* **16:**328–330.

56. **Korman, T. M., M. L. Grayson, and J. D. Turnidge.** 1997. Polymicrobial septicaemia with *Pseudomonas aeruginosa* and *Streptococcus pyogenes* following traditional tattooing. *J. Infect.* **35:**203.

57. **Kovarik, A., M. Setina, M. Sulda, P. Pazderkova, and A. Mokracek.** 2007. Infective endocarditis of the tricuspid valve caused by *Staphylococcus aureus* after ear piercing. *Scand. J. Infect. Dis.* **39:**266–268.

58. **Kramer, F., S. A. Sasse, J. C. Simms, and J. M. Leedom.** 1993. Primary cutaneous tuberculosis after a needlestick injury from a patient with AIDS and undiagnosed tuberculosis. *Ann. Intern. Med.* **119:**594–595.

59. **Laumann, A. E., and A. J. Derick.** 2006. Tattoos and body piercings in the United States: a national data set. *J. Am. Acad. Dermatol.* **55:**413–421.

60. **Lee, S., M. Chung, J. Lee, E. S. Kim, and J. Suh.** 2006. A case of *Staphylococcus aureus* endocarditis after ear piercing in a patient with normal cardiac valve and a questionnaire survey on adverse events of body piercing in college students of Korea. *Scand. J. Infect. Dis.* **38:**130–132.

61. **Lewis, C. G., M. K. Wells, and W. C. Jennings.** 2004. *Mycobacterium fortuitum* breast infection following nipple-piercing mimicking carcinoma. *Breast J.* **10:**363–365.

62. **Lick, S. D., S. N. Edozie, K. J. Woodside, and V. R. Conti.** 2005. Streptococcus viridans endocarditis from tongue piercing. *J. Emerg. Med.* **29:**57–59.

63. **Long, G. E., and L. S. Rickman.** 1994. Infectious complications of tattoos. *Clin. Infect. Dis.* **18:**610–619.

64. **Lovejoy, F. H., Jr., and D. H. Smith.** 1970. Life-threatening staphylococcal disease following ear piercing. *Pediatrics* **46:**301–303.

65. **Lowe, J., and S. N. Chatterjee.** 1939. Scarification, tattooing etc. in relation to leprous lesions of the skin. *Lepr. India* **11:**14–18.

66. **Makkai, T., and I. McAllister.** 2001. Prevalence of tattooing and body piercing in the Australian community. *Commun. Dis. Intell.* **25:**67–72.

67. **Mamtani, R., P. Malhotra, P. S. Gupta, and B. K. Jain.** 1978. A comparative study of urban and rural tetanus in adults. *Int. J. Epidemiol.* **7:**185–188.

68. **Martinello, R. A., and E. L. Cooney.** 2003. Cerebellar brain abscess associated with tongue piercing. *Clin. Infect. Dis.* **36:**e32–e34.

69. **Mayers, L. B., D. A. Judelson, B. W. Moriarty, and K. W. Rundell.** 2002. Prevalence of body art (body piercing and tattooing) in university undergraduates and incidence of medical complications. *Mayo Clin. Proc.* **77:**29–34.

70. **McCarthy, V. P., and W. M. Peoples.** 1988. Toxic shock syndrome after ear piercing. *Pediatr. Infect. Dis. J.* **7:**741–742.

71. **Modest, G. A., and J. J. W. Fangman.** 2002. Nipple piercing and hyperprolactinemia. *N. Engl. J. Med.* **347:**1626–1627.

72. **Moe, I.** 1989. Samoan navel tattoo, p. 117–119. *In* V. Vale and A. Juno (ed.), *Modern Primitives.* Re-Search, San Francisco, CA.

73. **More, D. R., J. S. Seidel, and P. A. Bryan.** 1999. Ear-piercing techniques as a cause of auricular chondritis. *Pediatr. Emerg. Care* **15:**189–192.

74. **Morgan, L. G.** 1952. Primary tuberculosis inoculation of an ear lobe: report of an unusual case and review of the literature. *J. Pediatr.* **40:**482–485.

75. **Morris, P., E. O'Sullivan, M. Choo, C. Barry, and C. J. Thompson.** 2006. A rare cause of sepsis in an 18 year old. Lemierre's syndrome with external jugular vein thrombosis. *Ir. Med. J.* **99:**24.

76. **Nishioka, S. A., and T. W. Gyorkos.** 2001. Tattoos as risk factors for transfusion-transmitted diseases. *Int. J. Infect. Dis.* **5:**27–34.

77. **Nishioka Sde, A., T. W. Gyorkos, L. Joseph, J.-P. Collet, and J. D. Maclean.** 2002. Tattooing and risk for transfusion-transmitted diseases: the role of the type, number and design of the tattoos, and the conditions in which they were performed. *Epidemiol. Infect.* **128:**63–71.

78. **Ochsenfahrt, C., R. Friedl, A. Hannekum, and B. A. Schumacher.** 2001. Endocarditis after nipple piercing in a patient with a bicuspid aortic valve. *Ann. Thorac. Surg.* **71:**365–366.

79. **Ollero, M., E. Pujol, A. Gimeno, A. Gea, P. Marquez, and J. M. Iturriaga.** 1991. Risky practices associated with HIV infection in seamen who travel in sub-Saharan West Africa. *Rev. Clin. Esp.* **189:**416–421. (In Spanish.)

80. **Olsen, J. C.** 2001. Lingual abscess secondary to body piercing. *J. Emerg. Med.* **20:**409.

81. **O'Malley, C. D., N. Smith, R. Braun, and D. R. Prevots.** 1998. Tetanus associated with body piercing. *Clin. Infect. Dis.* **27:**1343–1344.

82. **Papapanagioutou, V. A., M. G. Foukarakis, J. N. Fotiadis, E. P. Matsakas, and A. A. Zacharoulis.** 1998. Native tricuspid valve endocarditis in a young woman. *Postgrad. Med. J.* **74:**637–638.

83. **Parker, C., G. Kaminski, and D. Hill.** 1986. Zygomycosis in a tattoo, caused by *Saksenaea vasiformis*. *Aust. J. Dermatol.* **27:**107–111.

84. **Perkins, C. S., J. Meisner, and J. M. Harrison.** 1997. A complication of tongue piercing. *Br. Dent. J.* **182:**147–148.

85. **Poritt, R. J., and R. E. Olsen.** 1947. Two simultaneous cases of leprosy developing in tattoos. *Am. J. Pathol.* **23:**805–807.

86. **Porter, C. J. W., J. W. Simcock, and C. A. MacKinnon.** 2005. Necrotising fasciitis and cellulitis after traditional Samoan tattooing: case reports. *J. Infect.* **50:**149–152.

87. **Pugatch, D., M. Mileno, and J. D. Rich.** 1998. Possible transmission of human immunodeficiency virus type 1 from body piercing. *Clin. Infect. Dis.* **26:**767–768.

88. **Raja, S. G., S. K. Shad, and G. D. Dreyfus.** 2004. Body piercing: a rare cause of mitral valve endocarditis. *J. Heart Valve Dis.* **5:**854–856.

89. **Ramage, I. J., N. Wilson, and R. B. Thomson.** 1997. Fashion victim: infective endocarditis after nasal piercing. *Arch. Dis. Child.* **77:**187.

90. **Rukstinat, G. J.** 1941. Tattoos. A survey, with special reference to tattoos and scars as indicators of syphilis. *Arch. Pathol.* **31:**640–655.

91. **Samantha, S., M. Tweeten, and L. S. Rickman.** 1998. Infectious complications of body piercing. *Clin. Infect. Dis.* **26:**735–740.

92. **Samuel, M. C., P. M. Doherty, M. Bulterys, and S. A. Jenison.** 2001. Association between heroin use, needle sharing and tattoos received in prison with hepatitis B and C positivity among street-recruited injecting drug users in New Mexico, USA. *Epidemiol. Infect.* **127:**475–484.

93. **Satchitnananda, D. K., J. Walsh, and P. M. Schofield.** 2001. Bacterial endocarditis following repeated tattooing. *Heart* **85:**11–12.

94. **Sehgal, V. N.** 1971. Inoculation leprosy appearing after seven years of tattooing. *Dermatologica* **142:**58–61.

95. **Sehgal, V. N.** 1987. Upgrading borderline tuberculoid developing in tattoos. *Int. J. Dermatol.* **26:**332–333.

96. **Sehgal, V. N., and Joginder.** 1989. Tuberculoid (TT) leprosy: localization on a tattoo. *Lepr. Rev.* **60:**241–242.

97. **Sehgal, V. N., S. Jain, S. N. Bhattacharya, and S. Chouhan.** 1991. Borderline tuberculoid (BT) leprosy confined to a tattoo. *Int. J. Lepr.* **59:**323–325.

98. **Sewnath, M., T. Faber, and R. Castelein.** 2007. Pyogenic spondylitis as a complication of ear piercing: differentiating between spondylitis and discitis. *Acta Orthop. Belg.* **73:**128–132.

99. **Silverman, A. L., J. S. Sekhon, S. J. Saginaw, D. Wiedbrauk, M. Balasubramaniam, and S. C. Gordon.** 2000. Tattoo application is not associated with an increased risk for chronic viral hepatitis. *Am. J. Gastroenterol.* **95:**1312–1315.

100. **Simplot, T. C., and H. T. Hoffman.** 1998. Comparison between cartilage and soft tissue ear piercing complications. *Am. J. Otolaryngol.* **4:**305–310.

101. **Singh, G., M. A. Tutakne, V. D. Tiwari, and R. K. Dutta.** 1985. Inoculation leprosy developing after tattooing—a case report. *Indian J. Lepr.* **57:**887–888.

102. **Smith, B. F.** 1950. Occurrence of hepatitis in recently tattooed service personnel. *JAMA* **144:**1074–1076.

103. **Sow, P. S., B. M. Diop, H. L. Barry, S. Badiane, and A. M. Coll-Seck.** 1993. Tetanus and traditional practices in Dakar (report of 141 cases). *Dakar Med.* **38:**55–59.

104. **Stirn, A.** 2003. Body piercing: medical consequences and psychological motivations. *Lancet* **361:**1205–1215.

105. **Thorner, M.** 1894. Pathological conditions following piercing of the lobules of the ear. *JAMA* **22:**110–112.

106. **Tronel, H., H. Chaudemanche, N. Pechier, L. Doutrelant, and B. Hoen.** 2001. Endocarditis due to *Neisseria mucosa* after tongue piercing. *Clin. Microbiol. Infect.* **7:**275–276.

107. **Trupiano, J. K., B. A. Sebek, J. Goldfarb, L. R. Levy, G. S. Hall, and G. W. Procop.** 2001. Mastitis due to *Mycobacterium abscessus* after body piercing. *Clin. Infect. Dis.* **33:**131–134.

108. **Turkeltaub, S. H., and M. B. Habal.** 1990. Acute Pseudomonas chondritis as a sequel to ear piercing. *Ann. Plast. Surg.* **24:**279–282.

109. **Vale, V., and A. Juno.** 1989. Lyle Tuttle, p. 114–117. *In* V. Vale and A. Juno (ed.), *Modern Primitives.* Re-Search, San Francisco, CA.

110. **Vargas, J., M. Carballo, M. Hernandez, N. Rojas, O. Jimenez, J. Ricra, L. Romero, A. J. Rodriguez-Morales, and M. Silva.** 2005. Rapid development of auricular infection due to imipenem-resistant *Pseudomonas aeruginosa* following self-administered piercing of the high ear. *Clin. Infect. Dis.* **41:**1823–1824.

111. **Vatsyanyana.** 1994. *The Complete Kama Sutra: the First Unabridged Modern Translation of the Classic Indian Text.* Translated by Alain Danielou. Park Street Press, Rochester, NY.

112. **Weinberg, J. B., and R. A. Blackwood.** 2003. Case report of *Staphylococcus aureus* endocarditis after navel piercing. *Pediatr. Infect. Dis. J.* **22:**94–95.

113. **Wilde, A. G.** 1929–1930. Vaccinia infected tattoo: case report. *New Orleans Med. Surg. J.* **82:** 385–386.

114. **Wilson, W., K. A. Taubert, M. Gewitz, P. B. Lockhart, L. M. Baddour, M. Levison, A. Bolger, C. H. Cabell, M. Takahashi, R. S. Baltimore, J. W. Newburger, B. L. Strom, L. Y. Tani, M. Gerber, R. O. Bonow, T. Pallasch, S. T. Shulman, A. H. Rowley, J. C. Burns, P. Ferrieri, T. Gardner, D. Goff, and D. T. Durack.** 2007. Prevention of infective endocarditis: guidelines from the American Heart Association: a guideline from the American Heart Association Rheumatic Fever, Endocarditis and Kawasaki Disease Committee, Council on Cardiovascular Disease in the Young, and the Council on Clinical Cardiology, Council on Cardiovascular Surgery and Anesthesia, and the Quality of Care and Outcomes and Research Interdisciplinary Working Group. *J. Am. Dent. Assoc.* **138:**739–760.

115. **Wolf, E. K., and A. E. Laumann.** 2008. The use of blood-type tattoos during the Cold War. *J. Am. Acad. Dermatol.* **58:**472–476.

116. **Wong, H.-W., Y.-K. Tay, and C.-S. Sim.** 2005. Papular eruption on a tattoo: a case of primary inoculation tuberculosis. *Australas. J. Dermatol.* **46:**84–87.

117. **Zardawi, I. M., F. Jones, D. A. Clark, and J. Holland.** 2004. *Gordonia terrae*-induced suppurative granulomatous mastitis following nipple piercing. *Pathology* **36:**275–278.

INFECTIOUS DISEASES
AT HIGH ALTITUDE

*Buddha Basnyat, Thomas A. Cumbo,
and Robert Edelman*

15

EPIDEMIOLOGIC AND PHYSIOLOGIC FACTORS MODULATING INFECTIONS AT ALTITUDE

Travel to areas at high altitude (>2,500 m) is a popular activity enjoyed by many persons with various levels of experience and physical fitness. Activities range from relatively low-impact trekking at moderate altitude to extreme technical climbing. High mountain ranges are distributed in diverse ecosystems, cover approximately one-fifth of the earth's surface, are home to 150 million people, and are visited annually by millions who normally reside at low elevations (4). Many of these mountains exist in the developing world and require the sojourner to visit lowland areas for days to weeks before ascent, where they are exposed to infectious agents common in developing countries. Other mountains exist in more developed countries, where communi-

cable and arthropod-borne infections are less common. High altitude, however, still stresses the upper limits of human physiological reserve. Many host and environmental factors enhance susceptibility to infectious diseases, such as altered immune responses, hypoxia, physiological adaptation or lack of such adaptation, environmental stressors, increased UV radiation, cramped quarters, inability to maintain personal hygiene, and isolation from adequate medical care. The risk of contracting an infection varies depending on location, length of exposure, and nature of the high-altitude activity. There are few published data on this topic, and as a result, portions of this chapter are anecdotal and based on personal medical experience (B. Basnyat and T. A. Cumbo, unpublished data). The majority of our experience was gained in the Himalayas (Fig. 1). The Himalayas are among the world's tallest peaks and exist among some of the most impoverished areas of the globe. Therefore, this range provides an example of the complexities associated with high-altitude medicine and infectious diseases (Table 1).

Uniquely adapted flora and fauna exist in the low-barometric-pressure, hypoxic environment and harsh conditions of the higher altitudes. This ecosystem is one of gradual transformation from a nurturing lowland to

Buddha Basnyat, Nepal International Clinic, Himalayan Rescue Association, and Patan Hospital, Lal Durbar, GPO Box 3596, Kathmandu, Nepal. *Thomas A. Cumbo,* Private practice in infectious disease medicine, 17 Limestone Ct., Suite 3, Williamsville, NY 14221. *Robert Edelman,* Center for Vaccine Development, Division of Geographic Medicine, Department of Medicine, and Division of Infectious Diseases and Tropical Pediatrics, Department of Pediatrics, University of Maryland School of Medicine, 685 West Baltimore St., Room 480, Baltimore, MD 21201.

Infections of Leisure, Fourth Edition, Edited by David Schlossberg,
© 2009 ASM Press, Washington, DC

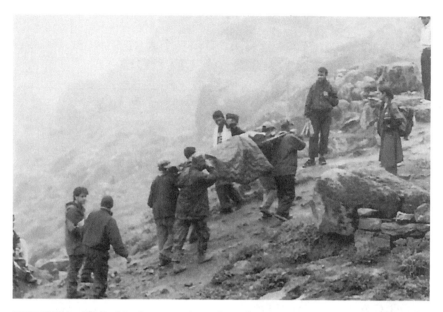

FIGURE 1 High-altitude evacuation of an ill Nepalese woman in the Himalayas during the Hindu festival of Janai Purnima in August 2000 near Lake Gosainkunda, Lang-Tang Region, Nepal. Photo by Paul Joseph Cumbo.

the inhospitable boundaries of space. Although the presence of microorganisms such as bacteria and fungi in the outer stratosphere has been recorded (40), there are no data linking such organisms with infections of trekkers. Moreover, the impact of high altitude on insect vector competence and microbial biology and virulence is largely unknown.

More is known about the changes in mammalian adaptive physiological capacity and im-munologic responses at high altitude. For example, in vitro studies using a hypobaric chamber revealed that T-lymphocyte function is compromised at high altitude, while B-cell function and mucosal immunity are not (29). T-cell-independent, B-cell antibody responses to various antigens seem to be preserved (12). Some hypothesize that adrenocorticotropic hormone, cortisol, and endorphins may partially mediate the impaired T-lymphocyte

TABLE 1 Infectious risks at high altitude[a]

Type of infection	Infection(s)
Gastrointestinal	Enteropathogenic bacteria *(Escherichia coli, Salmonella, Shigella, Campylobacter)*, viruses, protozoa *(Giardia, Cryptosporidium, Entamoeba, Cyclospora)*, typhoid fever, hepatitis, abdominal tuberculosis in local persons
Neurological	Rabies, JE, bacterial meningitis
Respiratory	Sinusitis, upper respiratory tract infection, bronchitis, pneumonia, influenza, tuberculosis
Dermatological	Pyoderma, furuncle, carbuncle, persistent wound infections, cellulitis, lymphangitis, herpes simplex, trauma and frostbite infections, scabies, lice, varicella
Urological and gynecological	Sexually transmitted diseases, genital candidiasis, urinary tract infections
Miscellaneous	Malaria, dengue, typhus, leptospirosis, dental caries, bone infections

[a]Adapted from reference 6 with permission from the publisher.

function noted at low atmospheric pressures and under hypoxic conditions (18). Murine studies have demonstrated an increased susceptibility to *Klebsiella pneumoniae, Salmonella enterica* serovar *Typhimurium, Escherichia coli, Chlamydia trachomatis,* and *Streptococcus* (30). Other work has shown an increased incidence of infectious symptoms, such as coryza, cough, pharyngitis, and diarrhea, especially in those subjects also suffering from acute mountain sickness (31). Murine studies have shown a decreased susceptibility to influenza A virus under hypoxic conditions (30), although other studies have demonstrated increased pulmonary vascular edema and permeability in rats with a laboratory-induced viral upper respiratory infection who were later exposed to a simulated high altitude (14). Respiratory infection may increase hypoxemia secondary to impaired diffusion capacity at high altitude. UV radiation exposure increases at high altitude because of the thin atmosphere. Although this energy results in the production of various immunomodulatory compounds (22), it is unclear if such compounds are clinically important. Other investigators have demonstrated increased amounts of systemic inflammatory markers, such as interleukin-6, interleukin-1 receptor agonist, and C-reactive protein, at high altitude (19). It is also postulated that free-radical-mediated changes in the peripheral metabolism of amino acids such as glutamine, known to influence immune function, may enhance susceptibility to or delay recovery from opportunistic infections at high altitude (3). Possible impaired immunity effected by high altitude needs to be anticipated in patients with trauma, burns, or systemic illnesses in that environment. In addition, the possibility that training at high altitude to enhance physical performance may cause some defect in the immune system also needs to be kept in mind (40).

The physician or other health care worker caring for patients at high altitude needs to recognize endogenous illness. Diagnosis in this environment is difficult because many diseases do not present in their typical fashion. For example, it can be difficult to differentiate bacterial pneumonia from high-altitude pulmonary edema (HAPE) or a pulmonary thromboembolism.

The local population in the developing world is at greater risk for diseases such as tuberculosis or parasitic infections than are travelers from developed countries. For example, hemoptysis at high altitude is more likely to represent tuberculosis in a local resident than in a trekker from North America, Europe, Australia, or other industrialized regions.

One must differentiate high-altitude travel in the developing world from such travel in more developed regions, such as the Rocky Mountains or the Alps. The hypoxic and hypobaric stresses are essentially the same, but the surrounding lowlands of the nonindustrialized world contain a higher prevalence and variety of infectious agents, which colors the differential diagnosis. In contrast, medical problems at high altitude in the developed world are more often noninfectious by nature.

GASTROINTESTINAL INFECTIONS

Enteric infections are the leading cause of illness in travelers, regardless of altitude (38). One study performed in the Himalayas found that 14% of a cohort of foreign outdoor trekkers developed gastroenteritis (7). This is approximately one-half of the incidence found at lower altitudes in the same region. Nevertheless, risk factors for gastrointestinal illness do exist; they include cramped sleeping arrangements, poor hygiene, concurrent illness, and medications that increase gastric pH (23).

No systematic surveys have examined the prevalence and epidemiology of enteric pathogens encountered at high altitude. The enteropathogenic bacteria are presumably the most common cause of diarrhea (1). Bacteria, *Giardia lamblia,* and amoebic dysentery are common causes in the Indian subcontinent (38), with *Cyclospora cayetanensis* infections occurring seasonally. *Campylobacter* spp. may cause a sizable number of diarrhea cases. Typhoid fever is one of the most common causes of fever within the Indian subcontinent (9). We have mistakenly diagnosed patients with high-altitude cerebral edema while they exhibited headache and fatigue found subsequently to be typhoid fever (unpublished data).

Local residents commonly develop large infestations with *Ascaris* worms, hookworms (21), or tapeworms. Travelers rarely develop symptomatic disease if they acquire low parasite inocula. If abdominal pain or unusual manifestations of diarrheal disease develop, however, stool screening examinations should be performed. Amoebic liver abscesses present with hepatomegaly and right upper quadrant abdominal pain. Abdominal tuberculosis manifests with ascites, wasting, and nonspecific signs and symptoms (24).

A fluoroquinolone effective against most aerobic bacterial pathogens and an antimotility drug are appropriate treatment for most cases of gastroenteritis in tourists at high altitude (1). Fluoroquinolone resistance is increasing in *Campylobacter* isolates from South and Southeast Asia, and for this reason a macrolide is preferred. Fluid intake should be encouraged, and attention should be directed towards potential electrolyte loss.

HEPATITIS VIRUS INFECTIONS
Hepatitis A, B, and E virus infections occur commonly in developing countries. Before the introduction of the hepatitis A vaccine, many outdoor trekkers in the Himalayas acquired this infection. Hepatitis E is one of the most common causes of jaundice in the adult population of the Indian subcontinent (37). Appropriate immunization with hepatitis A, hepatitis B, and typhoid vaccines helps to prevent liver and gastrointestinal disease. Women of childbearing age should be counseled about the high hepatitis E mortality rates that occur in pregnant women, and measures for avoidance need to be emphasized (39).

NEUROLOGICAL INFECTIONS
Those going into high-altitude regions in Latin America, Africa, and Asia are at risk of rabies infection. It is very difficult to arrange expedient postexposure rabies prophylaxis far from medical care. South Asia, including the Himalayas, accounts for 90% of the world's human rabies cases. Only Kathmandu, Bangkok, and Singapore have rabies immunoglobulin reliably available. Preventive measures include preexposure rabies vaccination and counseling trekkers to descend for postexposure immunoglobulin in the event of a dog or monkey bite.

Japanese encephalitis (JE) exists in rural areas of Southeast Asia and parts of the Indian subcontinent. No tourists to high-altitude regions have been diagnosed with JE, probably due to the rarity of the *Culex* mosquito vector at high altitudes. On the Indian subcontinent, JE must be differentiated from tuberculosis meningitis, bacterial meningitis, and typhoid encephalopathy seen in the local population in areas of endemicity. Treatment of JE is symptomatic. Prevention involves mosquito avoidance and vaccination.

Tick-borne encephalitis is endemic to central and eastern Europe and the former Soviet states and is seen sporadically throughout the eastern Mediterranean. Because areas of endemicity include deciduous forest below the altitude of 1,200 m, tick-borne encephalitis and perhaps its *Ixodes* tick vector may be uncommon in sojourners to the Alps and Ural Mountains, unless the disease was acquired at lower altitude.

Bacterial meningitis, although endemic in many developing countries, is uncommon in the traveler to high-altitude regions. However, it is important to consider in cases of acute confusion or severe headache and as a potential danger to the outdoor trekker.

Cysticercosis of the brain is one of the most common causes of epilepsy in Nepal (20). Cysticercosis should be considered if a local inhabitant presents with neurological findings or has a seizure at high altitude. Hypoxia may lower one's seizure threshold and promote clinical manifestation of a previously asymptomatic disease.

RESPIRATORY INFECTIONS
Respiratory problems are common at high altitudes (7, 10, 31). Pulmonary defense mechanisms are lessened by bronchospasm, congestion, and decreased mucociliary clearance (16).

Symptoms are exacerbated by hypoxic conditions, crowding, and cold dry air (41). Sinusitis, pharyngitis, bronchitis, and pneumonia may manifest in such an environment. While this is not firmly established, respiratory infections may predispose individuals to the development of acute mountain sickness (7, 10, 31).

Cough is ubiquitous in the mountains, and severe spasms of coughing leading to rib fracture are not uncommon. The specific etiology of cough at high altitude remains obscure because although cold air inhalation itself may cause coughing, study subjects exposed to controlled temperatures in hypobaric chambers also developed cough (26). Preventive measures such as keeping the head warm, adequate hydration, use of nasal decongestants, and breathing through a silk scarf to keep the air humidified are important (17). Influenza vaccination of all adults and pneumococcal vaccination of persons over 50 years of age should strongly be considered, especially for those trekking and climbing in developing countries. Pneumococcal vaccine may be indicated for those younger than 50 years if comorbid conditions are present. A booster dose of pertussis vaccine also needs to be considered, as vaccine-induced immunity wanes in adults. Anecdotally, bothersome cough in the mountains has been diagnosed as active pertussis infection.

The role of antibiotics is unclear, even with purulent sputum production (28). Respiratory infection can mimic HAPE. With prompt descent and oxygen, however, HAPE can improve rapidly, with a remarkable improvement in auscultative signs and disappearance of opacities from the chest X ray within a day or two, unlike lung opacities caused by bacterial pneumonia (43). We maintain a low threshold for descent for HAPE patients. Antibiotics may be used empirically in some patients. Pharyngitis accompanied by exudates and/or lymphadenopathy may represent a group A *Streptococcus* infection.

It is important to consider active pulmonary tuberculosis for local inhabitants who present with cough. Recent work has demonstrated a lower incidence of *Mycobacterium* *tuberculosis* infection at higher altitudes. However, an increased household clustering of tuberculosis occurs, hypothesized to be caused by crowded, poorly ventilated dwellings combined with increased UV light, hypoxia, and decreased humidity (33). An increased incidence of chronic obstructive pulmonary disease and cor pulmonale occurs in the mountain population of the Indian subcontinent. This is likely due to chronic smoke inhalation in poorly ventilated dwellings (34).

DERMATOLOGIC INFECTIONS

Pyoderma, carbuncles, furuncles, and wound infections are common problems encountered by those entering the mountains (8). Poor hygiene, prolonged exposure to moisture, local trauma from hiking boots, and frostbite are common in the mountain wilderness and can predispose individuals to skin infections. Wounds heal slowly at high altitude despite therapy with antibiotics. Superficial infections are often accompanied by cellulitis and lymphangitis (35). Descent to lower altitude may be required for cure. Scabies and lice are common in shared living quarters. Cold and sun exposure increases the likelihood of a herpesvirus reactivation.

Local inhabitants commonly present with advanced cases of skin infections. Septicemia and osteomyelitis can develop as a result of such uncontrolled skin infections. Suppurative otitis media can predispose patients to facial infection, bone infection, hearing loss, and meningitis. Varicella is common in children. Visitors unsure of their varicella immune status should consider antibody testing if time permits or varicella vaccination prior to travel (6).

Prevention of skin conditions and infections at high altitude includes the use of sunscreen on skin and lips, adequate hydration, avoidance of even minor trauma (including insect bites), good hygiene, and antibiotic therapy when warranted. Booster doses of tetanus vaccine should be administered before travel to prevent tetanus in the event that *Clostridium tetani* spores contaminate traumatized skin.

#65

INSECT-BORNE INFECTIONS

Arthropod-borne infections are extremely common in travel to developing countries, but arthropod vectors are less common at higher altitudes. Although malaria is an ever-present risk in most of the tropical world, *Plasmodium* species usually are not transmitted in high-altitude areas (32). Exceptions have been reported (15). Delayed febrile illness after initial plasmodial infection acquired at lower elevations may occur at higher elevations weeks or months later (13). Diagnosis is presumptive and must be followed by supervised evacuation to a lower altitude. Mosquito avoidance and malaria chemoprophylaxis in lowland areas of endemicity before ascent to high altitude offer a high degree of protection.

Dengue fever is endemic and epidemic in the tropics and subtropics (36). Similar to the case with malaria, travelers can become ill at high altitude with infections acquired in the lowlands. Dengue virus transmission usually occurs within 7 days before traveling to high altitude. As with malaria, mosquito avoidance and insect repellents can reduce the chance of acquiring dengue. Diagnosis is presumptive, and descent is imperative.

Typhus may be an underdiagnosed cause of fever in mountain travelers, although the evidence of its prevalence is anecdotal. Typhus as well as other rickettsial diseases should be considered for patients coming from areas of endemicity, since a delay in diagnosis can be lethal. For example, an individual treated with ciprofloxacin for diarrhea while trekking did not improve and was subsequently diagnosed in Bangkok, Thailand, as having typhus. Fortunately, treatment with doxycycline resulted in a rapid improvement (unpublished data).

Bartonella bacilliformis is transmitted by the *Phlebotomus* sand fly and occurs in the Andes Mountains between 600 and 2,500 m. Diagnosis is made by clinical presentation in the presence of anemia and by visualization of the pathogen in erythrocyte smears. Treatment options include tetracycline and chloramphenicol (27). Infrastructure in areas such as Peru allows one to reach areas of endemicity within a few hours of automobile travel.

OTHER INFECTIONS

Leptospirosis is spread by direct contact of abraded skin or mucous membranes with contaminated water or soil. Floods, heavy rains, and landslides common to the mountains can increase the concentration of spirochetes in water by washing hillside urinary waste contaminated with leptospires into lakes and streams. Trek and climb routes usually pass through such areas. Treatment involves the use of doxycycline (25) or azithromycin.

Sexually transmitted diseases, fungal vaginitis, and urinary tract infections usually present in typical fashion at high altitude. Increased frequency of sexual intercourse, new sexual partners, antibiotic use, and poor hygiene can predispose individuals variably to gonorrhea, chlamydia, trichomoniasis, candidiasis, genital herpes, and acute human immunodeficiency virus infection. An increased index of suspicion is usually required to recognize sexually transmitted diseases in this uncommon setting. Urinary tract infections can usually be diagnosed in the field with an adequate history and urine dipsticks to document the presence of white cells, leukocyte esterase, and nitrite in urine specimens. Treatment can often be instituted in the field if symptoms are mild and there is no indication of pyelonephritis. Finally, painful teeth and gum infections have caused climbers to abandon expeditions. A prior visit to the dentist may help.

SPECIAL CONSIDERATIONS

Immunocompromised travelers are at risk of contracting serious infections. Physicians counseling patients who travel with cancer, human immunodeficiency virus, chronic steroid or other immunosuppressive medication use, functional or anatomic asplenia, and renal insufficiency should familiarize themselves and their patients with the travel risks associated with these conditions. Older patients may be at increased risk for infectious disease because of comorbid conditions. Physicians and other health care professionals providing pretravel care should counsel such patients before they travel (2).

OTHER DISEASES AT HIGH ALTITUDE

The differential diagnosis of illness at high altitude includes other conditions that may be misdiagnosed as an infection. Documented examples include high-altitude cerebral edema, HAPE, subarachnoid hemorrhage, transient ischemic attack, seizures, cerebral neoplasm, migraine, syncope, Guillain-Barré syndrome, pulmonary embolism, chemical or plant toxin exposure, hypothermia, dehydration, carbon monoxide poisoning (from poorly ventilated indoor fires), acute psychiatric problems, asthma, and myocardial infarction (5).

Physicians who may treat infectious diseases at high altitude should carry appropriate chemotherapy and supportive equipment. Suggestions include a macrolide, a cephalosporin, trimethoprim-sulfamethoxazole, metronidazole, a fluoroquinolone, a tetracycline, hydrocortisone cream, a glucocorticoid, protective medical gloves, and water purification tablets or a reliable water filter. It is useful to carry both oral and intramuscular forms of steroid and antibiotics if possible. We also find it helpful to carry urine pregnancy test kits and urine dipsticks to help us to modify therapy in the field. It should be emphasized that the ultimate treatment of many medical problems will require descent.

In essence, infections and infectious diseases at high altitude often parallel those in adjacent lowland environments. Hypoxemia, hypobaria, physiological adaptation, harsh environmental stressors, exposure to foreign agents, and reckless behavior can enhance susceptibility to pathogens. The ultimate treatment may require descent. Prevention is crucial (see "Practical Tips" below). Counseling and immunization are essential. Clearly, more research needs to be done on high-altitude infections to better understand their pathogenic mechanisms and epidemiology and to improve treatment and prevention.

PRACTICAL TIPS

- Descend to a lower altitude, especially if infections do not improve with antibiotics alone.
- Wash hands with soap and/or liquid cleanser.
- Use insect repellents with DEET to help avoid mosquito and tick bites. Cover exposed skin, especially when trekking.
- Use pyrethrin-treated clothes and bed nets if necessary.
- Sterilize water.
- Avoid salads, ice, and other foods that can easily become contaminated.
- Breathe through a silk scarf at high altitude to help humidify the cold air.
- Use sunscreen on all exposed skin, including lips and ears.
- Maintain adequate hydration.
- Obtain appropriate immunizations.
- Review medical history, medication use, allergies, and pregnancy status prior to ascent.
- Visit a dentist before the trip.
- Purchase evacuation insurance, register at the local embassy, and become familiar with evacuation procedures.

REFERENCES

1. **Abramowicz, M.** 2006. Advice to travelers 2006, p. 25–34. *In Treatment Guidelines,* vol. 4. Medical Letter Inc., New York, NY.
2. **Albrecht, C., T. A. Cumbo, and S. Gambert.** 2003. Health issues, travel, and the elderly. *Clin. Geriatr.* **11:**24–33.
3. **Bailey, D. M., B. Davies, L. M. Castell, D. J. Collier, J. S. Milledge, D. A. Hullin, P. S. Seddon, and I. S. Young.** 2003. Symptoms of infection and acute mountain sickness; associated metabolic sequelae and problems in differential diagnosis. *High Alt. Med. Biol.* **4:**319–331.
4. **Basnyat, B., and D. Murdoch.** 2003. High altitude illness: an update of pathophysiology, prevention, and treatment. *Lancet* **361:**1967–1974.
5. **Basnyat, B., T. A. Cumbo, and R. Edelman.** 2000. Acute medical problems in the Himalayas outside the setting of altitude illness. *High Alt. Med. Biol.* **1:**167–174.
6. **Basnyat, B., T. A. Cumbo, and R. Edelman.** 2001. Infections at high altitude. *Clin. Infect. Dis.* **33:**1887–1891.
7. **Basnyat, B., J. Lemaster, and J. A. Litch.** 1999. Everest or bust: a cross sectional epidemiological study in the Himalayas at 4300 meters. *Aviat. Space Environ. Med.* **70:**867–873.
8. **Basnyat, B., and J. A. Litch.** 1997. Medical problems of porters and trekkers in the Nepal Himalaya. *Wilderness Environ. Med.* **8:**78–81.

9. **Basnyat, B., A. P. Maskey, M. D. Zimmerman, and D. R. Murdoch.** 2005. Enteric (typhoid) fever in travellers. *Clin. Infect. Dis.* **41:** 1467–1472.

10. **Basnyat, B., D. Subedi, J. Sleggs, G. Bhasyal, B. Aryal, and N. Subedi.** 2000. Disoriented and ataxic pilgrims: an epidemiological study of acute mountain sickness and high-altitude cerebral edema at a sacred lake at 4300 meters in the Nepal Himalayas. *Wilderness Environ. Med.* **11:** 89–93.

11. Reference deleted.

12. **Biselli, R., S. Le Moli, P. M. Matricardi, S. Farrace, A. Fattorossi, R. Nisini, and R. D'Amelio.** 1991. The effects of hypobaric hypoxia on specific B cell responses following immunization in mice and humans. *Aviat. Space Environ. Med.* **62:** 870–874.

13. **Bishop, R. A., and J. A. Litch.** 2000. Malaria at high altitude. *J. Travel Med.* **7:** 157–158.

14. **Carpenter, R. C., J. T. Reeves, and A. G. Durmowicz.** 1998. Viral respiratory infection increases susceptibility of young rats to hypoxia-induced pulmonary edema. *J. Appl. Physiol.* **84:** 1048–1054.

15. **Epstein, P. R., H. F. Diaz, S. Elias, G. Grabherr, N. E. Graham, W. J. M. Martens, E. Mosley-Thompson, and E. J. Susskind.** 1998. Biological and physical signs of climate change: focus on mosquito-borne disease. *Bull. Am. Meteorol. Soc.* **78:** 409–417.

16. **Giesbrecht, G. G.** 1995. The respiratory system in a cold environment. *Aviat. Space Environ. Med.* **66:** 890–902.

17. **Hackett, P. H., and R. C. Roach.** 2007. High-altitude medicine, p. 2–36. *In* P. S. Auerbach (ed.), *Wilderness Medicine.* C. V. Mosby, St. Louis, MO.

18. **Harris, M. D., J. Terrio, W. F. Miser, and J. F. Yetter III.** 1998. High-altitude medicine. *Am. Fam. Physician* **57:** 1907–1914, 1924–1926.

19. **Hartmann, G., M. Tschop, R. Fischer, C. Bidlingmaier, R. Riepl, K. Tschop, H. Hautmann, S. Endres, and M. Toepfer.** 2000. High altitude increases circulating interleukin-6, interleukin-1 receptor antagonist and C-reactive protein. *Cytokine* **12:** 246–252.

20. **Heap, B. J.** 1990. Cerebral cysticercosis as a common cause of epilepsy in Gurkhas in Hong Kong. *J. R. Army Med. Corps* **136:** 146–149.

21. **Houston, R., and E. Schwartz.** 1990. Helminthic infections among Peace Corps volunteers in Nepal. *JAMA* **263:** 373–374.

22. **Hug, D. H., J. K. Hunter, and D. D. Dunkerson.** 2001. Malnutrition, urocanic acid, and sun may interact to suppress immunity in sojourners to high altitude. *Aviat. Space Environ. Med.* **72:** 136–145.

23. **Junkett, G.** 1999. Prevention and treatment of traveler's diarrhea. *Am. Fam. Physician* **60:** 119–124, 135–136.

24. **Leader, R. A., and V. N. Low.** 1995. Tuberculosis of the abdomen. *Radiol. Clin. N. Am.* **33:** 691.

25. **Magill, A. J.** 1998. Fever in the returned traveler. *Infect. Dis. Clin. N. Am.* **12:** 445–469.

26. **Mason, N. P., and P. W. Barry.** 2007. Altitude-related cough. *Pulm. Pharmacol. Ther.* **20:** 388–395.

27. **Maquina, C., and E. Gotuzzo.** 2000. Bartonellosis: new and old. *Infect. Dis. Clin. N. Am.* **14:** 1–22.

28. **McFadden, E. R.** 1987. The lower airway, p. 234–245. *In* J. R. Sutton, C. S. Houston, and G. Coates (ed.), *Hypoxia and Cold.* Praeger, New York, NY.

29. **Meehan, R., U. Duncan, L. Neale, G. Taylor, H. Muchmore, N. Scott, K. Ramsey, E. Smith, P. Rock, R. Goldblum, and C. Houstan.** 1988. Operation Everest II: alterations in the immune system at high altitudes. *J. Clin. Immunol.* **8:** 397–406.

30. **Meehan, R. T.** 1987. Immune suppression at high altitude. *Ann. Emerg. Med.* **16:** 974–979.

31. **Murdoch, D. R.** 1995. Symptoms of infection and altitude illness among hikers in the Mount Everest region of Nepal. *Aviat. Space Environ. Med.* **66:** 148–151.

32. **Murphy, G. S., and E. C. Oldfield III.** 1996. Falciparum malaria. *Infect. Dis. Clin. N. Am.* **10:** 747–775.

33. **Olender, S., S. Mayuko, J. Apgar, K. Gillenwater, C. T. Bautista, A. G. Lescano, P. Moro, L. Caviedes, E. J. Hsieh, and R. H. Gilman.** 2003. Low prevalence and increased household clustering of Mycobacterium tuberculosis infection in high altitude villages in Peru. *Am. J. Trop. Med. Hyg.* **68:** 721–727.

34. **Pandey, M. R., B. Basnayt, and R. P. Neupane.** 1988. Chronic bronchitis and cor pulmonale in Nepal. *J. Inst. Med.* **10:** 263–270.

35. **Sarnquist, F. H.** 1983. Physicians on Mount Everest: a clinical account of the 1981 American medical research expedition to Everest. *West. J. Med.* **139:** 480–485.

36. **Schwartz, E., E. Mendelson, and Y. Sidi.** 1996. Dengue fever among travelers. *Am. J. Med.* **101:** 516–520.

37. **Shlim, D. R., and B. L. Innis.** 2000. Hepatitis E vaccine for travelers. *J. Travel Med.* **7:** 167–169.

38. **Shlim, D. R.** 1999. Traveler's diarrhea. *Wilderness Environ. Med.* **10:** 165–170.

39. **Taylor, R. R., B. Basnyat, and R. M. Scott.** 2008. A diplomatic disease. *J. Travel Med.* **15:** 200–201.

40. **Tiollier, E., L. Schmitt, P. Burnat, J. P. Fouillot, P. Robach, E. Filaire, C. Y. Guezennec, and J. P. Richalet.** 2005. Living high-training low altitude training: effects on mucosal immunity. *Eur. J. Appl. Physiol.* **94:**298–304.

41. **Wainwright, M., N. C. Wickramasinghe, J. V. Narlikar, and P. Rajaratnam.** 2003. Microorganisms cultured from stratospheric air sam-ples obtained at 41km. *FEMS Microbiol. Lett.* **218:**161–165.

42. **West, J. B.** 1998. *High Life: a History of High Altitude Physiology and Medicine,* p. 160. Oxford University Press, Oxford, United Kingdom.

43. **Zafren, K., B. Basnyat, and G. Basnyat.** 2009. Clinical images: a pneumonic confusion. *Wilderness Environ. Med.* **20:**81–82.

INFECTIOUS RISKS OF AIR TRAVEL

Alexandra Mangili and Mark Gendreau

16

Since the inception of commercial air travel, there have been a number of reported outbreaks of serious infectious airborne diseases aboard commercial flights (4, 19), including tuberculosis (TB) (7, 16, 22, 38), severe acute respiratory syndrome (SARS) (28, 42), influenza (21, 25), smallpox (32), and measles (6, 36). Other infections, such as gastroenteritis (23, 34, 44) transmitted by common-vehicle mode, have been reported aboard commercial aircraft, and while less serious outbreaks like the common cold or other viral syndromes have not been reported within the literature, common sense suggests that they can occur and that a lack of reporting and their ubiquitous nature are likely attributable to the difficulties of investigating such outbreaks. In addition, many infections have incubation periods that are longer than the flight, thereby making on-board transmission less recalled. One prospective questionnaire study of air travelers traveling from San Francisco to Denver during the winter months found an upper respiratory tract infection incidence of 3% for

the most restrictive outcome measures to 20% for the least restrictive outcome measure (self-reporting of upper respiratory tract infection by passengers) (46). Indeed, the risk of infectious disease spread by and within commercial aircraft is real and recently gained attention in the spring of 2007, when a man thought to be infected with extremely drug-resistant TB traveled by commercial flights between the United States, Europe, and Canada (30). His actions exposed 27 flight crew members and over 80 fellow passengers on two intercontinental flights and incited a public health scramble to notify all potentially exposed individuals. This chapter focuses on the current knowledge about transmission of infectious diseases in the context of both transmissions within the aircraft passenger cabin and commercial aircraft serving as vehicles of worldwide infection spread.

INFECTION RISK, CABIN ENVIRONMENT, AND CONTROL MEASURES

Individual risk of infection within the aircraft cabin, or generally any enclosed space, involves many factors, including chance, source strength (generation rate of infectious agent), exposure (proximity to the source and duration of the exposure), and ventilation within

Alexandra Mangili, Division of Geographic Medicine and Infectious Disease, Tufts Medical Center, Boston, MA 02111. *Mark Gendreau*, Department of Emergency Medicine, Lahey Clinic, Burlington, MA 01805.

Infections of Leisure, Fourth Edition, Edited by David Schlossberg,
© 2009 ASM Press, Washington, DC

 # 66

 # 67

the enclosed space (17, 18, 19, 39) (Fig. 1). Available evidence suggests that risk is associated with either close contact to the index case or seating within two rows of the index, and current risk assessment protocols used by public health authorities for in-flight infectious disease exposures are typically based upon the proximity of the fellow passenger to the index passenger (seating within two rows of the index passenger) and the duration of the exposure (flight time of >8 h) (19, 40).

This protocol, based upon experiences with previous TB exposures/outbreaks aboard commercial flights, has become conventional wisdom for investigating most aircraft-related infectious disease incidents (40). However, it is fundamentally flawed since it does not consider ventilation—a key component of infection control—particularly for diseases with airborne transmission. In fact, variation in this association has been reported (21, 28). For example, the largest in-flight SARS outbreak (Air China flight 112) involved passengers seated as far as seven rows from the index passenger, and the flight was only 3 h long (28). Ventilation of enclosed spaces is a key determinant of infection spread, and the chain of infection is influenced substantially by the ventilation conditions specific to the aircraft

cabin. Cabin airflow is laminar and side to side, thereby limiting front-to-back cabin contamination (33). Aircraft that recirculate cabin air have no significant differences in self-reported infection rates from aircraft that utilize a single-pass cabin ventilation system (46).

Proper ventilation within any confined space decreases the concentration of airborne organisms in a logarithmic fashion, with one air exchange removing 63% of suspended microorganisms suspended within that particular space (24, 27). In the case of recirculated systems (such as on modern commercial aircraft), where various fractions of air from the passenger cabin are recirculated and mixed with fresh air, this relationship holds only if the recirculated air undergoes filtration through high-efficiency particulate (HEPA) filters (27). Although the practice of removing infectious airborne particles from recirculated air through HEPA filtering is well established as an effective infection control measure, the use of HEPA filters within commercial aircraft is neither required nor regulated by the Federal Aviation Administration or its British (Civil Aviation Authority) and European (Joint Aviation Authority) counterparts. A 2004 survey of major U.S. commercial air carriers by the U.S. Government Accountability Office found that 15% of large commercial aircraft within the U.S. domestic fleet did not routinely use HEPA air filtering and that nearly 50% of smaller regional commercial aircraft did not (35). Incorporating epidemiological data into risk assessment mathematical models may provide insight into how proximity and ventilation influence disease transmission aboard commercial aircraft. For instance, deterministic modeling utilizing data from an in-flight TB investigation revealed that doubling the ventilation rate within the aircraft cabin reduced infection risk by half (17). Clearly, ventilation provides a critical determinant of risk and should therefore be incorporated into the algorithm of whom to notify after an in-flight infectious disease exposure. In addition, efforts to increase ventilation may provide opportunities to reduce the risk of infection, par-

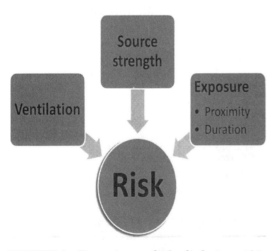

FIGURE 1 Determinants of risk of infection within a confined space.

ticularly at times of a worldwide outbreak such as pandemic influenza. During the 2002–2003 SARS epidemic, screening of airport passengers by visual inspection and thermal scanning was ineffective in identifying infectious individuals (5, 14, 31). Visual screening of arriving passengers typically involves screening for signs of infection, including rash, flushed or pale complexion, jaundice, shivering, sweating, diarrhea, and inability to ambulate without assistance (14). Although flight crews are legally obliged to report potentially infectious passengers, they receive no training on infectious disease control, and anecdotal evidence suggests that in many instances flight crews fail to recognize or report potentially infected passengers.

REPORTED SERIOUS INFECTIOUS IN-FLIGHT OUTBREAKS

Tuberculosis

TB is spread primarily through droplet nuclei (i.e., residua of large droplets containing microorganisms that have evaporated to a size of <5 µm) that are generated and released during talking, coughing, sneezing, vomiting, or aerosolization of feces (24). Unlike large droplets (which travel no further than 1 m), these nuclei become aerosolized, remain suspended in air for indefinite periods, and are capable of dispersing widely, depending upon environmental conditions (27). When inhaled, droplet nuclei are likely to bypass trapping mechanisms of the upper airways and are carried deep into the lungs, where in the case of TB, even a single microorganism has the ability to initiate infection (26). The risk of TB infection (defined as conversion from a negative to a positive tuberculin skin test) ranges from 1 in 100,000 persons for casual social contact to 1 in 5 for dormitory contact to 1 in 3 for home and close work contact (26). Historically, there have been seven incidents of significant TB exposure aboard commercial aircraft—two of which resulted in on-board transmission (7, 16, 22, 38, 40). However, no cases of active disease have been reported as a

result of air travel exposure. The most significant incident involved a passenger with pulmonary TB traveling from Baltimore to Chicago to Honolulu (16). Four of 15 fellow passengers seated within two rows of the index passenger on the Chicago-to-Honolulu flight had a positive tuberculin skin test conversion with no other identifiable risk. A retrospective risk analysis study utilizing epidemiological parameters of that flight suggested an average risk of TB transmission on the order of 1 in 1,000 for all of the passengers on that flight, with the risk decreasing sharply in a stepwise fashion for each row beyond the index passenger (17). Clearly, the risk of transmission is low, and the fact that the sputum smears from the index passenger on the most recent multidrug-resistant TB commercial airline exposure were clear is reassuring, showing that the probability of conversion for even the closest fellow passengers is low. Continued vigilance is warranted, as more aircraft, such as the Airbus A380, are capable of extended flight times of up to 18 h, thereby increasing the potential for increased exposure times.

Influenza

Although there has been no sustained human-to-human spread of influenza aboard commercial flights since the last reported outbreak in 1998 (21), the pandemic potential of highly pathogenic avian influenza H5N1 virus remains a serious global threat, and commercial aircraft will play a major role in rapid spread (29).

SARS

SARS is caused by a coronavirus and was first identified in the southern People's Republic of China in November 2002, with the last known case of person-to-person transmission in July 2003. Close to 800 deaths in 26 countries on five continents occurred during the 2002–2003 SARS outbreak (42). The World Health Organization (WHO) estimates that 6.5 passengers per million traveled on commercial flights originating from regions of active transmission while symptomatic with

#68

probable SARS during the height of the outbreak (42). A total of 40 flights carried 37 probable SARS index cases during the outbreak, resulting in 29 probable on-board secondary cases (42). Air China flight 112 represented the largest on-board transmission event, with 22 individuals developing a probable case of SARS as a consequence of being aboard the flight, and this incident was likely a consequence of the index passenger being a superspreader (28, 37, 44, 45). No vaccine exists for SARS, and prompt identification and isolation remain the most important actions available to prevent in-flight transmission should SARS reemerge.

Measles

Measles transmission during commercial air travel is rare. However, it remains of concern because it is a highly contagious airborne viral infection and can be transmitted during the asymptomatic prodromal phase. Importations from developing countries account for most outbreaks of measles in the United States, and it is estimated that from 1996 to 2000, 30% of all imported cases occurred in people who flew while symptomatic (1). A recent case of measles transmission during a commercial flight in Brazil was reported, resulting in two secondary confirmed cases (6), and two clusters of measles associated with travel by air were described in The Netherlands in 2007 (36). In addition to underreporting of in-flight exposures, the relatively small numbers of cases of aircraft-associated measles transmission may be due to high levels of measles immunity as a result of either vaccination or previous exposure.

Neisseria meningitidis

While in-flight transmission of meningococcal disease has never been reported, it remains a concern, and antimicrobial prophylaxis is recommended for individuals who have had direct contact with an index case or for those seated within two rows of the index passenger. Travelers flying to the hajj pilgrimage or to the sub-Saharan meningitis belt are at particular risk for acquiring meningococcal disease and are included in the current vaccine recommendations to prevent the spread of the illness.

POTENTIAL IN-FLIGHT OUTBREAKS: MULTIDRUG-RESISTANT ORGANISMS

With antibiotic resistance becoming a worldwide concern, the potential risk of transmission of multidrug-resistant bacteria while aboard a commercial aircraft is of concern. In particular, travelers hospitalized during international travel and repatriated by commercial airlines could transmit organisms, such as methicillin-resistant *Staphylococcus aureus,* vancomycin-resistant *Enterococcus,* or multidrug-resistant *Acinetobacter baumannii,* to other passengers or crew members. To date, there have been no published reports of commercial air travel-related outbreaks of these bacteria. Additionally, a recent analysis of patients transported internationally by air ambulance found no increased risk of carriage of multidrug-resistant bacteria compared to that for other hospitalized patients (10).

AIRCRAFT AS VEHICLES OF WORLDWIDE INFECTION SPREAD

Air Travel Restrictions

With over 1.4 million persons crossing international borders on air carriers every day (19), the risk of disease transmission associated with commercial aircraft involves not only the risk to individual passengers and crew within the aircraft but also the public health risk, as commercial aircraft may serve as vehicles of worldwide epidemic spread. The notion of restricting commercial flights to delay an influenza pandemic was recently studied. Several modeling studies concluded that flight restrictions would have little effect on the spread of pandemic influenza (4, 5, 9, 12). One study shows that imposing 90% restriction on all air travel would delay the peak of a pandemic wave by no more than 1 to 2 weeks, whereas halting almost all air travel (99.9%) would delay the pandemic wave up to 2 months (9). Most pan-

#69

demic preparedness plans do not address the issue of commercial air travel (8). Passenger screening measures in airports during the SARS epidemic, such as visual inspection and thermal scanning, were ineffective in identifying infectious individuals (3, 5, 13, 14). This failure was likely due to SARS having low transmissibility (a low basic reproductive number), combined with little presymptomatic transmission and a long incubation period, and to the fact that peak infectivity typically occurred 5 to 10 days after the onset of symptoms, making travel screening ineffective (2, 42). Such screening measures would also be ineffective for pandemic influenza, since shedding of influenza virus typically begins 2 to 5 days after infection (short generation time) and often before the onset of symptoms (high presymptomatic transmission) (2, 5, 11).

Several countries have expanded their quarantine station programs, and the U.S. Centers for Disease Control and Prevention (CDC) has established a centralized electronic passenger database capability (e manifest) to be used during infectious outbreaks for prompt passenger notification and contact tracing (3, 45). The International Air Transport Association, in partnership with the WHO and other stakeholders, recently established guidelines for the aviation industry for operations during pandemic influenza outbreaks in order to minimize commercial air travel spread. These include risk communication to the traveling public, establishment of national passenger exit screening from outbreak regions, and increasing airline preparedness (aircraft cleaning and procedures in case of in-flight illness) (8, 15).

Risk-Based Border Screening

The occurrence of epidemics and pandemics raises many public health questions regarding the application of international law in the context of preventing, protecting against, controlling, and providing a coordinated public health response to the international spread of disease. Many countries plan to use a risk-based approach during the early phase of a

novel-agent pandemic to delay its spread within their borders as well as balancing between societal and economic disruption and public well-being. The goal of risk-based border screening is to identify the likelihood of infection in a traveler, and screening includes a brief interview and travel history. Individuals considered low to no risk for being contagious are given access to the country with no restrictions. Individuals failing the initial screen undergo a more extensive evaluation (Fig. 2). Once a pandemic disease is common in all countries, exit screening and border screening at points of entry will no longer be effective. Further studies on the impacts of such a risk-based approach to screening entering air travelers are needed.

International Health Regulations

In December 2006, the United States formally accepted the revision of the WHO's International Health Regulations, referred to as IHR 2005 (41). IHR 2005 is currently the only international legal instrument that governs the roles of the WHO and its member countries in identifying, responding to, and sharing information about public health emergencies of international concern. Designed to prevent and protect against the international spread of diseases while minimizing interference with world travel and trade, these revised regulations now include influenza virus strains with pandemic potential, and SARS was added to the list of diseases that member states must immediately report to the WHO. Also included in the updated IHR 2005 are expanded routine requirements for disease surveillance and control activities at international airports, seaports, and border crossings and recommendations for the use of nonpharmaceutical interventions to mitigate the community impact of pandemic influenza and other novel infectious agents with pandemic potential.

CLOSING REMARKS

The only way to eliminate virtually any risk of cross-infection within the aircraft cabin and to prevent the aircraft from serving as a vehicle

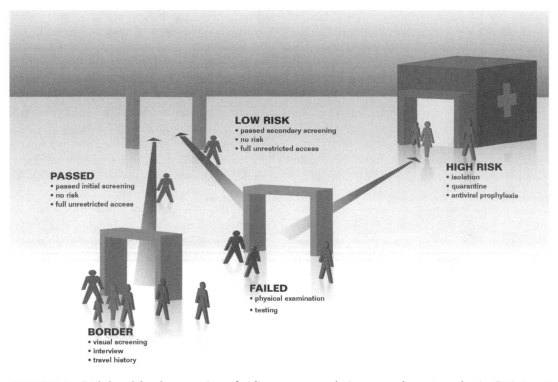

FIGURE 2 Risk-based border screening of airline passengers during a novel-agent pandemic. Risk-based border screening of arriving passengers during a worldwide infectious outbreak involves a visual screening, brief interview, and travel history. Individuals considered to have low or no risk of being contagious are allowed access into the country with no restrictions. Individuals who do not pass the initial screen undergo more extensive evaluation, to include a physical exam and testing. Individuals deemed low risk after being tested are allowed access, whereas high-risk individuals are either isolated or quarantined in addition to receiving antiviral treatment or prophylaxis.

for worldwide epidemic spread is to stop passengers from flying if they either have been exposed substantially to a communicable disease or are contagious. This is neither practical nor possible. Prevention is the most important means of control and requires a proactive approach. For individual air travelers, practicing hand hygiene remains the most effective means of minimizing risk of infection (see "Practical Tips" below). Recently, the CDC and the Air Transport Association established partnerships related to improved communications, and the CDC Division of Global Migration and Quarantine has expanded its quarantine program to 20 stations at major airports and seaports throughout the United States. In response to the SARS experience and pandemic influenza threat, a centralized electronic passenger database capability (e-manifest) has been developed to be used during infectious outbreaks for prompt passenger notification and contact tracing (3). Improved international regulations regarding the inspection, certification, and maintenance of aircraft environmental control systems are warranted. Regulations requiring HEPA filters for any aircraft utilizing recirculated air are needed to minimize the risk of infectious spread on and by commercial aircraft. Governmental, public health, aviation, and medical stakeholders should better educate the general public on health issues related to air travel and infection control.

#70

PRACTICAL TIPS

- Postpone travel if ill. Although it is recommended to postpone travel until one is no longer infectious, in reality this recommendation is not commonly followed by passengers, especially because few travelers purchase travel insurance.
- Minimize exposure while aboard aircraft. Sit near the front. Avoid window seats during the winter. Keep the air-conditioning nozzle on a low setting.
- Good hand hygiene is paramount to reducing the risk of disease transmission. Alcohol-based hand sanitizers are an excellent alternative to hand washing, especially when the hands are not visibly dirty or soap and water are not readily available, such as inside a crowded air cabin. Every traveler should make good hand hygiene part of his or her travel routine.

REFERENCES

1. **Amornkul, P. N., H. Takahashi, A. K. Bogard, M. Nakata, R. Harpaz, and P. V. Effler.** 2004. Low risk of measles transmission after exposure on an international airline flight. *J. Infect. Dis.* **189**(Suppl. 1):S81–S85.
2. **Anderson, R. M., C. Fraser, A. C. Ghani, C. A. Donnelly, S. Riley, N. M. Ferguson, et al.** 2004. Epidemiology, transmission dynamics and control of SARS: the 2002–2003 epidemic. *Philos. Trans. R. Soc. Lond. B* **359**:1091–1105.
3. **Centers for Disease Control and Prevention.** 2006. Exposure to mumps during air travel—United States, April 2006. *MMWR Morb. Mortal. Wkly. Rep.* **55**:401–402.
4. **Colizza, V., A. Barrat, M. Barthelemy, and A. Vespignani.** 2006. The role of the airline transportation network in the prediction and predictability of global epidemics. *Proc. Natl. Acad. Sci. USA* **103**:2015–2020.
5. **Cooper, B. S., R. J. Pitman, W. J. Edmunds, and N. J. Gay.** 2006. Delaying the international spread of pandemic influenza. *PLoS Med.* **3**:e212.
6. **de Barros, F. R., M. C. Danovaro-Holliday, C. Toscano, T. C. Segatto, A. Vicari, and E. Luna.** 2006. Measles transmission during commercial air travel in Brazil. *J. Clin. Virol.* **36**:235–236.
7. **Driver, C. R., S. E. Valway, W. M. Morgan, I. M. Onorato, and K. G. Castro.** 1994. Transmission of Mycobacterium tuberculosis associated with air travel. *JAMA* **272**:1031–1035.
8. **Evans, A., S. Finkelstein, J. Singh, and C. Thibeault.** 2006. Pandemic influenza: a note on international planning to reduce the risk from air transport. *Aviat. Space Environ. Med.* **77**:974–976.
9. **Ferguson, N. M., D. A. Cummings, C. Fraser, J. C. Cajka, P. C. Cooley, and D. S. Burke.** 2006. Strategies for mitigating an influenza pandemic. *Nature* **442**:448–452.
10. **Fischer, D., A. Veldman, V. Schafer, and M. Diefenbach.** 2004. Bacterial colonization of patients undergoing international air transport: a prospective epidemiologic study. *J. Travel Med.* **11**:44–48.
11. **Fraser, C., S. Riley, R. M. Anderson, and N. M. Ferguson.** 2004. Factors that make an infectious disease outbreak controllable. *Proc. Natl. Acad. Sci. USA* **101**:6146–6151.
12. **Germann, T. C., K. Kadau, I. M. Longini, Jr., and C. A. Macken.** 2006. Mitigation strategies for pandemic influenza in the United States. *Proc. Natl. Acad. Sci. USA* **103**:5935–5940.
13. **Hays, G. C., J. D. Houghton, T. Doyle, and J. Davenport.** 2003. Aircraft give a new view of jellyfish behaviour. *Nature* **426**:383.
14. **Institute of Medicine Board on Global Health.** 2005. *Quarantine Stations at Ports of Entry: Protecting the Public's Health.* National Research Foundation, National Academies Press, Washington, DC.
15. **International Civil Aviation Organization.** 2007. *Guidelines for States Concerning the Management of Communicable Disease Posing a Serious Public Health Risk.* International Civil Aviation Organization, Montreal, Canada.
16. **Kenyon, T. A., S. E. Valway, W. W. Ihle, I. M. Onorato, and K. G. Castro.** 1996. Transmission of multidrug-resistant Mycobacterium tuberculosis during a long airplane flight. *N. Engl. J. Med.* **334**:933–938.
17. **Ko, G., K. M. Thompson, and E. A. Nardell.** 2004. Estimation of tuberculosis risk on a commercial airliner. *Risk Anal.* **24**:379–388.
18. **Liao, C. M., C. F. Chang, and H. M. Liang.** 2005. A probabilistic transmission dynamic model to assess indoor airborne infection risks. *Risk Anal.* **25**:1097–1107.
19. **Mangili, A., and M. A. Gendreau.** 2005. Transmission of infectious diseases during commercial air travel. *Lancet* **365**:989–996.
20. Reference deleted.
21. **Marsden, A. G.** 2003. Outbreak of influenza-like illness related to air travel. *Med. J. Aust.* **179**:172–173. (Corrected title.)
22. **McFarland, J. W., C. Hickman, M. Osterholm, and K. L. MacDonald.** 1993. Exposure

to Mycobacterium tuberculosis during air travel. *Lancet* **342:**112–113.

23. **McMullan, R., P. J. Edwards, M. J. Kelly, B. C. Millar, P. J. Rooney, and J. E. Moore.** 2007. Food-poisoning and commercial air travel. *Travel Med. Infect. Dis.* **5:**276–286.

24. **Morawska, L.** 2006. Droplet fate in indoor environments, or can we prevent the spread of infection? *Indoor Air* **16:**335–347.

25. **Moser, M. R., T. R. Bender, H. S. Margolis, G. R. Noble, A. P. Kendal, and D. G. Ritter.** 1979. An outbreak of influenza aboard a commercial airliner. *Am. J. Epidemiol.* **110:**1–6.

26. **Musher, D. M.** 2003. How contagious are common respiratory tract infections? *N. Engl. J. Med.* **348:**1256–1266.

27. **Nardell, E. A.** 2004. Catching droplet nuclei: toward a better understanding of tuberculosis transmission. *Am. J. Respir. Crit. Care Med.* **169:**553–554.

28. **Olsen, S. J., H. L. Chang, T. Y. Cheung, A. F. Tang, T. L. Fisk, S. P. Ooi, et al.** 2003. Transmission of the severe acute respiratory syndrome on aircraft. *N. Engl. J. Med.* **349:**2416–2422.

29. **Ozonoff, D., and L. Pepper.** 2005. Ticket to ride: spreading germs a mile high. *Lancet* **365:**917–919.

30. **Park, A.** 31 May 2007. The TB scare: a broken system? *Time.* http://www.time.com/time/health/article/0,8599,1627159,00.html.

31. **Pitman, R. J., B. S. Cooper, C. L. Trotter, N. J. Gay, and W. J. Edmunds.** 2005. Entry screening for severe acute respiratory syndrome (SARS) or influenza: policy evaluation. *BMJ* **331:**1242–1243.

32. **Ritzinger, F. R.** 1965. Disease transmission by aircraft. *Mil. Med.* **130:**643–647.

33. **Rydock, J. P.** 2004. Tracer study of proximity and recirculation effects on exposure risk in an airliner cabin. *Aviat. Space Environ. Med.* **75:**168–171.

34. **Tauxe, R. V., M. P. Tormey, L. Mascola, N. T. Hargrett-Bean, and P. A. Blake.** 1987. Salmonellosis outbreak on transatlantic flights; foodborne illness on aircraft: 1947–1984. *Am. J. Epidemiol.* **125:**150–157.

35. **U.S. Government Accountability Office.** 2004. *Aviation Safety: More Research Needed in Ef-*

fects of Air Quality on Airliner Cabin Occupants. U.S. Government Accountability Office, Washington, DC.

36. **van Binnendijk, R. S., S. Hahne, A. Timen, G. van Kempen, R. H. Kohl, H. J. Boot, et al.** 2008. Air travel as a risk factor for introduction of measles in a highly vaccinated population. *Vaccine* **26:**5775–5777.

37. **Vogt, T. M., M. A. Guerra, E. W. Flagg, T. G. Ksiazek, S. A. Lowther, and P. M. Arguin.** 2006. Risk of severe acute respiratory syndrome-associated coronavirus transmission aboard commercial aircraft. *J. Travel Med.* **13:**268–272.

38. **Wang, P. D.** 2000. Two-step tuberculin testing of passengers and crew on a commercial airplane. *Am. J. Infect. Control* **28:**233–238.

39. **Wells, W.** 1934. On airborne infection study. II. Droplet nuclei. *Am. J. Hyg.* **20:**611–618.

40. **WHO.** 2006. *Tuberculosis and Air Travel: Guidelines for Prevention and Control,* 2nd ed. WHO/HTM/TB/2006.363. World Health Organization, Geneva, Switzerland.

41. **WHO.** 2005. *Fifty-Eighth World Health Assembly International Health Regulations.* World Health Organization, Geneva, Switzerland.

42. **WHO Department of Communicable Disease Surveillance and Response.** 2003. *Consensus Document on the Epidemiology of Severe Acute Respiratory Distress Syndrome (SARS).* WHO/CDS/CSR/2003.11. World Health Organization, Geneva, Switzerland.

43. **Widdowson, M. A., R. Glass, S. Monroe, R. S. Beard, J. W. Bateman, P. Lurie, and C. Johnson.** 2005. Probable transmission of norovirus on an airplane. *JAMA* **293:**1859–1860.

44. **Wilder-Smith, A., H. N. Leong, and J. S. Villacian.** 2003. In-flight transmission of severe acute respiratory syndrome (SARS): a case report. *J. Travel Med.* **10:**299–300.

45. **Wilder-Smith, A., N. I. Paton, and K. T. Goh.** 2003. Low risk of transmission of severe acute respiratory syndrome on airplanes: the Singapore experience. *Trop. Med. Int. Health* **8:**1035–1037.

46. **Zitter, J. N., P. D. Mazonson, D. P. Miller, S. B. Hulley, and J. R. Balmes.** 2002. Aircraft cabin air recirculation and symptoms of the common cold. *JAMA* **288:**483–486.

PERILS OF THE PETTING ZOO

John R. Dunn and Frederick J. Angulo

17

A wide variety of venues offer petting zoos where public contact with animals is encouraged or permitted. Petting zoos are commonly found at county or state fairs, zoos, and aquariums. In addition to these traditional petting zoo settings, animals are present in many other venues where the public is permitted to contact animals and their environment (2, 32). Thus, humans may have contact with animals in a wide range of settings, and transmission of infectious diseases from animals to humans may occur at any of these venues.

There are many considerations in evaluating perils associated with the wide range of venues where animal contact can occur. First, many venues or events draw large numbers of people; some operate during a short time frame, while others, such as zoos and aquariums, operate year-round. Second, petting zoos and other animal contact venues are particularly popular with children, who are likely to have less stringent hygiene and are more

susceptible to severe disease outcomes. Finally, there is remarkable variability in the physical layout of venues that permit animal contact and in the types of animals that may be contacted. Animal contact areas range from well-designed permanent exhibits targeting risk reduction to various temporary or seasonal exhibits established without detailed planning (4, 7, 12). Many petting zoos house only small ruminant species like sheep and goats, but other venues house a wide variety of mammalian species, exotic animals, poultry and other avian species, reptiles and amphibians, and aquatic animals (4).

Contact with animals can be an enjoyable and beneficial activity. Health benefits have been attributed to animal contact. Reportedly, these benefits include reduced anxiety, lower blood pressure, and other physiologic effects (http://www.cdc.gov/healthypets/health_benefits.htm). In addition to health benefits, petting zoos and animal contact settings provide societal educational opportunities. A growing segment of society in developed countries resides in urban or suburban settings, with limited knowledge of agricultural practices or contact with farm animal species. Petting zoos or agricultural exhibits can provide education regarding food production, agricultural practices, and rural life. Similarly, zoo-

John R. Dunn, Communicable and Environmental Disease Services, Tennessee Department of Health, 425 5th Ave. North, Cordell Hull Building, 1st Floor, Nashville, TN 37047. *Frederick J. Angulo,* Enteric Diseases Epidemiology Branch, Division of Foodborne, Bacterial and Mycotic Diseases, Centers for Disease Control and Prevention, 1600 Clifton Rd., MS A38, Atlanta, GA 30333.

Infections of Leisure, Fourth Edition, Edited by David Schlossberg,
© 2009 ASM Press, Washington, DC

logical parks and aquariums are popular leisure attractions and provide opportunities for education about diverse and nonnative animal species and conservation of natural resources (16). Perils of animal contact include allergies, injury, and zoonotic disease transmission.

ALLERGIES AND INJURY

Many allergens are encountered in petting zoos and animal contact areas. Possible allergens include animal dander, scales, fur, feathers, saliva, and urine (40). In addition, traditional petting zoo settings at fairs include environmental allergens, including dust and hay, which is commonly fed to ruminant animals. While the frequency of persons allergic to various animal allergens is not known, it is likely that the number is substantial. Allergic reactions due to contact with animals and their environment may increase risks for transmission of zoonoses due to more frequent hand-to-face contact.

In addition to allergies, injuries associated with animals in public settings occur. Common injuries include kicks, falls, scratches, and crushing injuries of the hands, feet, or body (4, 40). While any injury can predispose persons to zoonotic disease transmission, animal bites present the greatest peril. Animal bites may also result in transmission of several bacterial and viral pathogens. Bacterial pathogens include *Bartonella henselae*, *Capnocytophaga canimorsus*, *Francisella tularensis*, *Pasteurella multocida*, *Spirillum minor*, *Staphylococcus*, *Streptobacillus moniliformis*, and *Streptococcus*. Viral pathogens include herpes B virus and rabies.

ZOONOTIC DISEASE TRANSMISSION

Zoonotic diseases, infectious diseases transmitted between nonhuman vertebrate animals and humans, are the greatest risk to petting zoo visitors. Table 1 provides a list of potential zoonotic pathogens in petting zoo venues. Among zoonotic disease agents, enteric pathogens are of particular concern in petting zoos.

TABLE 1 Selected zoonotic pathogens in petting zoo and animal contact venues

Bacteria
Aeromonas spp.
Bartonella henselae
Campylobacter spp.
Capnocytophaga canimorsus
Chlamydophila psittaci
Coxiella burnetii
Edwardsiella spp.
Erysipelothrix rhusiopathiae
Francisella tularensis
Mycobacterium spp. (e.g., *M. tuberculosis*, *M. marinum*)
Pasteurella multocida
Salmonella spp.
Shiga toxin–producing *Escherichia coli* (e.g., *E. coli* O157)
Staphylococcus spp.
Streptobacillus moniliformis
Streptococcus spp.
Vibrio spp.

Parasites
Cryptosporidium parvum
Giardia spp.

Viruses
Orf virus
Herpes B virus
Rabies virus

Enteric Pathogens

The most commonly recognized peril of petting zoos and other animal contact settings is transmission of enteric pathogens. Infections with bacterial enteric pathogens, such as Shiga toxin–producing *Escherichia coli* (including *E. coli* O157), *Campylobacter*, and *Salmonella*, and with parasitic enteric pathogens, such as *Cryptosporidium*, typically result in gastrointestinal symptoms of nausea, vomiting, and diarrhea. While most infections with enteric pathogens are self-limited, severe symptoms and outcomes can occur. For example, *E. coli* O157 and other Shiga toxin–producing *E. coli* strains commonly cause hemorrhagic colitis and may result in hemolytic anemia, thrombocytopenia, and acute renal failure (22, 36). This clinical triad is referred to as hemolytic-uremic syndrome (HUS). HUS occurs as a

#72

life-threatening, postdiarrheal complication in 5 to 10% of *E. coli* O157 infections, and the rate is highest among children. HUS survivors may suffer long-term sequelae, including loss of renal function (19).

Fecal-oral transmission is the most common route for transfer of enteric pathogens from animals to humans. Transmission may be due to direct contact with animals or contact with animals through contamination of food and water contaminated with animal feces. Fecal material unavoidably contaminates areas in which animals are housed, and consequently animal fur, hair, skin, and saliva are often contaminated as well (27, 28). Indirect contact with the animal environment or objects (fomites) contaminated while in the animal area can also result in transmission of enteric pathogens. For example, contaminated clothing and shoes, animal bedding, and environmental surfaces in areas used to house animals have been associated with zoonotic disease transmission. Enteric pathogens have previously been isolated from multiple environmental surfaces, including the rafters of a barn which was used to house animals at a fairground (46). Thus, movement of pathogens via air currents and dust is a plausible mechanism that could result in contamination of petting zoo environments and contamination of food or water. Food-borne transmission and waterborne transmission are well-described perils for patrons visiting petting zoos and other animal contact venues (3, 11, 30, 39). Multiple examples of food-borne and waterborne transmission following contamination of food and water at petting zoos and other venues exist. For example, in one report, transmission of *E. coli* O157 was linked to consumption of cotton candy in the animal area (39).

Outbreaks associated with animal contact in petting zoos and other animal contact venues have increasingly been recognized by public health officials (Fig. 1). The Centers for Disease Control and Prevention (CDC) reported over 55 human zoonotic disease outbreaks involving animals in public settings from 1991 to 2005 (44). In addition, international outbreaks and reports of disease transmission have been described (2, 32, 45).

Notable outbreaks have led to a better understanding of transmission risks and to preventive measures in petting zoos. The CDC first published recommendations to reduce perils associated with petting zoos following an outbreak of human *E. coli* O157 infections associated with animal contact in 2000 (6). School trips to a Pennsylvania dairy farm where children could pet and interact with calves resulted in more than 50 children becoming ill; 8 (16%) of the children developed HUS (6, 12). Based on molecular subtyping by pulsed-field gel electrophoresis, human *E. coli* O157 isolates from ill humans were shown to be indistinguishable from *E. coli* O157 isolated from cattle and the environment. Although it was not a traditional petting zoo, direct animal contact was allowed at the dairy farm. Several contributing risk factors were identified, including direct contact with cattle and the farm environment, inadequate hand-washing facilities for children, and the absence of a designated location where visitors could eat and drink outside animal areas.

Outbreaks at some facilities have involved multiple enteric pathogens. Contact with calves and their environment at a children's day camp on a farm in Minnesota resulted in transmission of *Campylobacter jejuni, Cryptosporidium parvum, E. coli* O157, non-O157 Shiga toxin-producing *E. coli,* and *Salmonella enterica* serovar Typhimurium (43). Eighty-four human cases occurred, and all of the above-mentioned pathogens were isolated from the farm day camp calves. An important finding of epidemiological investigations at the farm day camp was the protective effect of hand hygiene. Persons reporting that they washed their hands with soap after touching a calf or before going home were less likely to become ill. Children reporting that they cared for an ill calf or had gotten manure on their

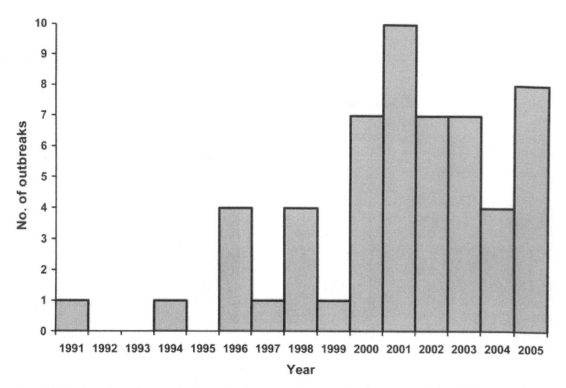

FIGURE 1 Number of reported outbreaks of enteric disease associated with animals in public settings in the United States, by year, from 1991 to 2005. (Reprinted from reference 44 [© 2006 by the Infectious Diseases Society of America], with permission of the publisher.)

hands were at increased risk. Another school farm program in Minnesota experienced recurrent outbreaks of cryptosporidiosis (29). An outbreak of 31 cases resulted in Department of Health recommendations being made to prevent further transmission. However, insufficient implementation of the recommendations resulted in a subsequent outbreak. Thirty-seven additional cryptosporidiosis cases occurred and were attributed to inadequate hand-washing facilities and procedures.

Outbreaks associated with traditional petting zoos, where persons, especially children, are encouraged to pet, feed, and have contact with animals, have been dramatic. A 2005 CDC *Morbidity and Mortality Weekly Report* article described three such petting zoo-associated outbreaks of *E. coli* O157 (7). Outbreaks in Arizona and Florida occurred at a municipal zoo and at agricultural fairs, respec-

tively. At the municipal zoo in Arizona, a temporary exhibit used to attract visitors was implicated. In Florida, 63 persons were infected, including 7 with HUS. Cases occurred at multiple fairs supplied with animals from the same vendor. Risk factors for infection included direct animal contact, contact with sawdust or shavings, and feeding animals. Hand hygiene was demonstrated to have a protective effect if properly performed. Interestingly, knowledge of zoonotic disease risks was a protective factor, indicating that educational efforts may mitigate risks. The third outbreak described in the report occurred in 2004. One hundred eight persons became ill after visiting a petting zoo at the North Carolina State Fair. The petting zoo associated with the outbreak was one of many exhibits where the public could contact animals. It contained numerous livestock species in pens

#73

but also allowed direct interaction and contact with goats and sheep in a large enclosure. The exhibit encouraged direct contact with the animals and facilitated contact with manure and manure-contaminated bedding. Additionally, visitors were permitted to feed the sheep and goats, increasing animal-to-human contact. Figure 2 shows photographs of children in the North Carolina State Fair petting zoo who were infected with *E. coli* O157. Manure and contact with manure-contaminated bedding are evident. The petting zoo was heavily visited by children, 15 of whom developed HUS. Alcohol-based hand sanitizer was available at the exit of the petting zoo, but hand-washing facilities were not. As in the outbreak in Florida, knowledge of zoonotic disease prior to the outbreak had a protective effect. The outbreak strain was isolated from the animal bedding, the animals, and the farm of origin.

Outside the United States, other petting zoo- and animal contact exhibit-associated outbreaks have been described. In Canada, 44 *E. coli* O157 cases occurred after day care and school field trips to a pumpkin patch which had a petting zoo (13). The same molecular subtype of *E. coli* O157 was isolated from patients and from a petting zoo goat. Lack of hand-washing facilities and limited signage were implicated. As was the case at the petting zoo at the 2004 North Carolina State Fair,

alcohol-based hand sanitizer was available; however, it was not optimally placed for use by children.

In addition to recognized outbreaks, studies of human infections not recognized to be part of an outbreak (i.e., sporadic infections) indicate that zoonotic transmission of enteric pathogens likely occurs in petting zoos and other venues where animal contact occurs. For example, risk factors for sporadic human *E. coli* O157 infection included visiting a farm with cows (22, 26, 38). Similar studies of human cryptosporidiosis and campylobacteriosis have described contact with farm animals as a risk factor for infection (17, 23, 41).

From outbreak investigations and studies of enteric pathogen colonization of animals, a number of factors which contribute to the peril posed by petting zoos and other animal contact venues have been noted. Factors associated with the animals and the animal environment, as well as human factors, can increase transmission risks.

It is notable that most animal species harboring human enteric pathogens exhibit no clinical signs. This phenomenon is true for ruminant species such as cattle, sheep, and goats, which are colonized by *Campylobacter*, *Cryptosporidium*, *Salmonella*, and Shiga toxin-producing *E. coli*. Factors associated with animal husbandry and management also contribute to increased risks of disease trans-

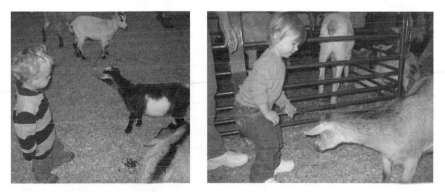

FIGURE 2 Close contact with animals, animal feces, and animal bedding led to a large *E. coli* O157:H7 outbreak at the 2004 North Carolina State Fair. (Photos reproduced with the permission of the North Carolina Division of Public Health.)

mission. For example, enteric pathogen prevalence can be higher in young animals, which are popular in petting zoos (18, 21, 47). Fecal shedding of enteric pathogens is also more likely when animals are stressed. Temporary or seasonal petting zoos subject animals to transportation stress. In general, confinement, crowding, and increased handling by people increase stress and the risk of fecal shedding (10, 24, 25). Some enteric pathogens are also shed more commonly in summer months, when many petting zoos and animal contact exhibits occur (14, 20).

Cattle, sheep, goats, poultry, rodents, and other domestic and wild animals shed enteric pathogens into the environment intermittently. Contamination of the environment can last for months or years, even after attempts to clean or decontaminate it. *E. coli* O157 has been shown experimentally to remain viable in soil for months. Furthermore, viable *E. coli* O157 has been cultured months later from fairgrounds and petting zoos following outbreaks (15, 46). Environmental contamination alone, without direct contact with animals, has been implicated in outbreaks of *E. coli* O157 in Ohio and Oregon (4, 46).

Not surprisingly, the risk of infections or outbreaks is increased by human factors and behaviors, especially in children. These factors include lack of awareness of the risk of disease, inadequate hand washing, a lack of close supervision, and hand-to-mouth behaviors. As mentioned, children are particularly attracted to animal venues and have an increased risk for serious infections. Children younger than 5 years of age are at particularly high risk of serious infections or outcomes. Other groups at increased risk include persons with waning immunity and persons who are mentally impaired, pregnant, or immunocompromised. Recent observational studies have demonstrated that persons visiting petting zoos or other animal contact venues engage in a number of high-risk behaviors and do not commonly wash their hands when leaving. One such study conducted in the United States (35) found that 74% of petting zoo visitors had di-

rect contact with animals, 87% had contact with potentially contaminated surfaces in animal contact areas, 49% had hand-to-face contact, and 22% ate or drank in animal contact areas, but only 38% used hand sanitizer when they exited the petting zoo. A study in Canada showed similar results (48). Despite the availability of hand hygiene facilities, they were infrequently used by visitors. Hand hygiene stations located on an exit route, the presence of hand hygiene reminder signs, and the availability of running water were reported to increase hand hygiene compliance among visitors.

Other Zoonotic Pathogens

There is a broad range of other zoonotic pathogens which pose potential risks in petting zoos and animal contact settings.

Rabies virus (family *Rhabdoviridae,* genus *Lyssavirus*) can infect all mammalian species and is a peril to humans exposed to infected animals in petting zoos and other animal contact venues. Rabid mammals transmit the virus through bites or contamination of mucous membranes, scratches, or other wounds with virus-laden saliva or nervous tissue (5). The Advisory Committee on Immunization Practices provides detailed recommendations for assessment and prophylactic treatment of human rabies (34). The potential for transmission to humans is of concern because infection leads to acute, progressive encephalomyelitis which is almost always fatal. Although no human rabies deaths caused by animal contact in petting zoos or public animal exhibits are documented, the potential for zoonotic transmission of rabies has required extensive public health investigation, medical follow-up, and administration of postexposure prophylaxis to thousands of persons following exposures at fairs, petting zoos, and other animal exhibits. Species to which humans have been exposed include bears, cats, dogs, goats, horses, and sheep (4). Mass rabies exposures occurring at petting zoos present unique challenges for health officials and medical providers. These challenges include identification and notification of potentially exposed persons, proper risk assessment, and provision of timely post-exposure treatment. In 2006, over 150,000 persons attended the Tennessee National Walking Horse Celebration, where a horse was diagnosed with rabies. The rabid horse was accessible to the public visiting the event. State and federal public health officials notified attendees and assessed rabies risk among persons who reported contact with the horse. The Tennessee Department of Health consulted with 53 persons and recommended treatment for 9. In addition, approximately 25 persons in Missouri were advised to receive treatment. In New York, a rabid goat in a petting zoo resulted in 465 persons receiving rabies postexposure prophylaxis (8).

Query fever, or Q fever, is caused by a rickettsia, *Coxiella burnetii*. In humans, infection may be asymptomatic, result in acute influenza-like illness, or progress to life-threatening endocarditis. *C. burnetii* frequently infects cattle, sheep, and goats. Infection can result in abortion but more commonly does not cause a clinical illness. Animal birthing exhibits at fairs or petting zoos have become popular attractions. Despite limited contact by the public during parturition, contact with newborn animals is often encouraged or permitted. Transmission of Q fever is a peril of petting zoos and animal venues that have live-birthing exhibits. Infected animals shed large numbers of organisms at parturition that contaminate the animals and animal environment and can become aerosolized, leading to outbreaks of Q fever. Ninety-five Q fever cases, including 41 hospitalizations, in association with goats and sheep giving birth at petting zoos in indoor shopping malls were described (4). Other, less common perils of petting zoo birthing exhibits include leptospirosis, listeriosis, brucellosis, and chlamydiosis.

Mycobacterium tuberculosis infects humans and animals, notably elephants. Contact with elephants occurs in some petting zoos and animal exhibits. Elephant rides are sometimes incorporated into animal exhibits. Transmission of tuberculosis from elephants to circus elephant handlers at an exotic animal farm was reported in Illinois. Because treatment and cure of *M. tuberculosis* in elephants are difficult, guidelines for removal of infected animals from public contact have been developed (http://www.aphis.usda.gov/animal_welfare/downloads/elephant/tb2003.pdf).

Herpes B virus (cercopithecine herpesvirus 1) is a zoonotic agent found in macaques. In macaques, herpes B virus causes mild oral lesions or no clinical signs. As mentioned above, the virus is transmitted to humans via bites. However, transmission after scratches or splashes to mucous membranes has been reported as well. Human infections most often result in fatal meningoencephalitis. Although not commonly found in petting zoos, macaques are sometimes available in public settings. Internationally, macaques may be present in locations frequented by the public, especially tourists interested in having contact with or feeding them. Recommendations for herpes B assessment and postexposure prophylaxis are available (9).

Chlamydophila psittaci infections cause respiratory disease (commonly called psittacosis) and are usually acquired from psittacine birds. Outbreaks among humans have occurred in public settings. Infection typically causes pneumonia. Walk-through aviaries and interactive avian exhibits have become increasingly popular, especially in zoos. Guidelines for testing and treatment of birds and for diagnosis in humans have been published to address the risks of psittacosis in humans (42).

Orf virus infection in goats and sheep at a children's petting zoo has been described. Infection of humans can result in painful ulcerative lesions (31). Transmission in public settings following contact with infected sheep has occurred. Transmission can be due to direct animal contact or contact with contaminated objects, such as blankets, halters, or brushes.

Zoonoses from aquarium water are of increasing concern (33, 37). Infections with mycobacteria, *Aeromonas* species, *Vibrio* species, *Edwardsiella* species, *Salmonella* species, *Streptococcus iniae*, and *Erysipelothrix rhusiopathiae* can

#74

be encountered in "touch tanks" or aquatic petting zoos. Although few outbreaks have been documented, transmission may occur sporadically, particularly among persons who are immunocompromised.

REDUCING THE PERILS OF THE PETTING ZOO

In the United States, federal oversight of animals in public settings relates to animal care and welfare but not to public health. Some states have developed legislation, usually in response to outbreaks, governing petting zoos and other venues where animals are present in public settings to address zoonotic disease risks. The Association of Zoos and Aquariums includes zoonotic disease risk reduction measures in its accreditation standards. As mentioned previously, the CDC developed guidelines following the above-mentioned outbreak of *E. coli* O157 in Pennsylvania (6). The CDC has also published guidelines for preventing reptile-associated and baby poultry-associated salmonellosis. Other organizations have published guidelines for specific populations (e.g., the immunosuppressed) and settings (e.g., health care settings).

The National Association of State Public Health Veterinarians (NASPHV) and the CDC have published well-recognized, comprehensive recommendations to reduce zoonotic disease perils associated with animals in public settings, including petting zoos (1, 4). Recommendations are designed for use by public health officials, veterinarians, animal venue staff, animal exhibitors, visitors to animal venues, physicians, and others. NASPHV and CDC state that the single most important prevention step for reducing zoonotic disease risks is hand washing. Other recommendations address communication and cooperation among agencies and education for venue operators and staff as well as the visiting public. Management of public and animal contact is also addressed with respect to design of facilities and animal pens, cleaning procedures, and veterinary care and management of animals.

PRACTICAL TIPS

- Hand washing is the single most important preventive measure to minimize infectious disease perils of the petting zoo.
- Educate the public to recognize zoonotic disease perils of the petting zoo.
- Consider contact with animals in public settings, particularly petting zoos, in diagnosing and treating potential zoonotic infections.
- Report possible petting zoo-associated infections and outbreaks to public health officials for further investigation.
- Implement NASPHV and CDC recommendations to reduce zoonotic disease risks associated with animals in public settings.

REFERENCES

1. **Babcock, D. W.** 2006. Legal implications of zoonotic-disease outbreaks at petting zoos and animal exhibits. *J. Environ. Health* **69:**46–47.
2. **Bender, J. B., and S. A. Shulman.** 2004. Reports of zoonotic disease outbreaks associated with animal exhibits and availability of recommendations for preventing zoonotic disease transmission from animals to people in such settings. *J. Am. Vet. Med. Assoc.* **224:**1105–1109.
3. **Bopp, D. J., B. D. Sauders, A. L. Waring, J. Ackelsberg, N. Dumas, E. Braun-Howland, D. Dziewulski, B. J. Wallace, M. Kelly, T. Halse, K. A. Musser, P. F. Smith, D. L. Morse, and R. J. Limberger.** 2003. Detection, isolation, and molecular subtyping of *Escherichia coli* O157:H7 and *Campylobacter jejuni* associated with a large waterborne outbreak. *J. Clin. Microbiol.* **41:**174–180.
4. **Centers for Disease Control and Prevention.** 2007. Compendium of measures to prevent disease associated with animals in public settings. *MMWR Morb. Mortal. Wkly. Rep.* **56**(RR-5):1–14.
5. **Centers for Disease Control and Prevention.** 2007. Compendium of animal rabies prevention and control. *MMWR Morb. Mortal. Wkly. Rep.* **56**(RR-3):1–8.
6. **Centers for Disease Control and Prevention.** 2000. Outbreaks of *Escherichia coli* O157:H7 infections among children associated with farm visits—Pennsylvania and Washington. *MMWR Morb. Mortal. Wkly. Rep.* **50:**293–297.
7. **Centers for Disease Control and Prevention.** 2005. Outbreaks of *Escherichia coli* O157:H7 associated with petting zoos—North Carolina,

Florida, and Arizona, 2004 and 2005. *MMWR Morb. Mortal. Wkly. Rep.* **54:**1277–1280.

8. **Chang, H. G. H., M. Eidson, C. Noonan-Toly, C. V. Trimarchi, R. Rudd, B. J. Wallace, P. F. Smith, and D. L. Morse.** 2002. Public health impact of reemergence of rabies, New York. *Emerg. Infect. Dis.* **8:**909–912.

9. **Cohen, J. I., D. S. Davenport, J. A. Stewart, S. Deitchman, J. K. Hilliard, and L. E. Chapman.** 2002. Recommendations for prevention of and therapy for exposure to B virus (cercopithecine herpesvirus 1). *Clin. Infect. Dis.* **35:**1191–1203.

10. **Corrier, D. E., C. W. Purdy, and J. R. DeLoach, Jr.** 1990. Effects of marketing stress on fecal excretion of *Salmonella spp* in feeder calves. *Am. J. Vet. Res.* **51:**866–869.

11. **Crump, J. A., C. R. Braden, M. E. Dey, R. M. Hoekstra, J. M. Rickelman-Apisa, D. A. Baldwin, S. J. De Fijter, S. F. Nowicki, E. M. Koch, T. L. Bannerman, F. W. Smith, J. P. Sarisky, N. Hochberg, and P. S. Mead.** 2003. Outbreaks of *Escherichia coli* O157 infections at multiple county agricultural fairs. a hazard of mixing cattle, concession stands and children. *Epidemiol. Infect.* **131:**1055–1062.

12. **Crump, J. A., A. C. Sulka, A. J. Langer, C. Schaben, A. S. Crielly, R. Gage, M. Baysinger, M. Moll, G. Withers, D. M. Toney, S. B. Hunter, R. M. Hoekstra, S. K. Wong, P. M. Griffin, and T. J. Van Gilder.** 2002. An outbreak of *Escherichia coli* O157:H7 infections among visitors to a dairy farm. *N. Engl. J. Med.* **347:**555–560.

13. **David, S. T., L. MacDougall, K. Louie, L. McIntyre, A. M. Paccagnella, S. Schleicher, and A. Hamade.** 2004. Petting zoo-associated *Escherichia coli* O157:H7—secondary transmission, asymptomatic infection, and prolonged shedding in the classroom. *Can. Commun. Dis. Rep.* **30:**173–180.

14. **Dunn, J. R., J. E. Keen, and R. A. Thompson.** 2004. Prevalence of Shiga-toxigenic *Escherichia coli* O157:H7 in adult dairy cattle. *J. Am. Vet. Med. Assoc.* **224:**1151–1158.

15. **Durso, L. M., K. Reynolds, N. Bauer, Jr., and J. E. Keen.** 2005. Shiga-toxigenic *Escherichia coli* O157:H7 infections among livestock exhibitors and visitors at a Texas County Fair. *Vector Borne Zoonotic Dis.* **5:**193–201.

16. **Falk, J. H., E. M. Reinhard, C. L. Vernon, K. Bronnenkant, N. L. Deans, and J. E. Heimlich.** 2007. *Why Zoos & Aquariums Matter: Assessing the Impact of a Visit.* Association of Zoos & Aquariums, Silver Spring, MD.

17. **Friedman, C. R., R. M. Hoekstra, M. Samuel, R. Marcus, J. Bender, B. Shiferaw, S.**

Reddy, S. D. Ahuja, D. L. Helfrick, F. Hardnett, M. Carter, B. Anderson, and R. V. Tauxe. 2004. Risk factors for sporadic *Campylobacter* infection in the United States: a case-control study in FoodNet sites. *Clin. Infect. Dis.* **38**(Suppl. 3)**:**S285–S296.

18. **Garber, L. P., S. J. Wells, D. D. Hancock, M. P. Doyle, J. Tuttle, J. A. Shere, and T. Zhao.** 1995. Risk factors for fecal shedding of *Escherichia coli* O157:H7 in dairy calves. *J. Am. Vet. Med. Assoc.* **207:**46–49.

19. **Garg, A. X., R. S. Suri, N. Barrowman, F. Rehman, D. Matsell, M. P. Rosas-Arellano, M. Salvadori, R. B. Haynes, and W. F. Clark.** 2003. Long-term renal prognosis of diarrhea-associated hemolytic uremic syndrome: a systematic review, meta-analysis, and meta-regression. *JAMA* **290:**1360–1370.

20. **Hancock, D. D., T. E. Besser, D. H. Rice, D. E. Herriott, and P. I. Tarr.** 1997. A longitudinal study of *Escherichia coli* O157 in fourteen cattle herds. *Epidemiol. Infect.* **118:**193–195.

21. **Hancock, D. D., T. E. Besser, M. L. Kinsel, P. I. Tarr, D. H. Rice, and M. G. Paros.** 1994. The prevalence of *Escherichia coli* O157:H7 in dairy and beef cattle in Washington state. *Epidemiol. Infect.* **113:**199–207.

22. **Henderson, H.** 2008. Direct and indirect zoonotic transmission of Shiga toxin-producing *Escherichia coli*. *J. Am. Vet. Med. Assoc.* **232:**848–859.

23. **Hunter, P. R., S. Hughes, S. Woodhouse, Q. Syed, N. Q. Verlander, R. M. Chalmers, K. Morgan, G. Nichols, N. Beeching, and K. Osborn.** 2004. Sporadic cryptosporidiosis case-control study with genotyping. *Emerg. Infect. Dis.* **10:**1241–1249.

24. **Hurd, H. S., J. D. McKean, R. W. Griffith, I. V. Wesley, and M. H. Rostagno.** 2002. *Salmonella enterica* infections in market swine with and without transport and holding. *Appl. Environ. Microbiol.* **68:**2376–2381.

25. **Hurd, H. S., J. D. McKean, I. V. Wesley, and L. A. Karriker.** 2001. The effect of lairage on *Salmonella* isolation from market swine. *J. Food Prot.* **64:**939–944.

26. **Kassenborg, H. D., C. W. Hedberg, M. Hoekstra, M. C. Evans, A. E. Chin, R. Marcus, D. J. Vugia, K. Smith, S. D. Ahuja, L. Slutsker, and P. M. Griffin.** 2004. Farm visits and undercooked hamburgers as major risk factors for sporadic *Escherichia coli* O157:H7 infection: data from a case-control study in 5 FoodNet sites. *Clin. Infect. Dis.* **38**(Suppl. 3)**:**S271–S278.

27. **Keen, J. E., T. E. Wittum, J. R. Dunn, J. L. Bono, and L. M. Durso.** 2006. Shiga-toxigenic *Escherichia coli* O157 in agricultural fair livestock, United States. *Emerg. Infect. Dis.* **12:**780–786.

28. **Keen, J. E., and R. O. Elder.** Isolation of Shiga-toxigenic *Escherichia coli* O157 from hide surfaces and the oral cavity of finished beef feedlot cattle. 2002. *J. Am. Vet. Med. Assoc.* **220:**756–763.

29. **Kiang, K. M., J. M. Scheftel, F. T. Leano, C. M. Taylor, P. A. Belle-Isle, E. A. Cebelinski, R. Danila, and K. E. Smith.** 2006. Recurrent outbreaks of cryptosporidiosis associated with calves among students at an educational farm program, Minnesota, 2003. *Epidemiol. Infect.* **134:**878–886.

30. **Korlath, J. A., M. T. Osterholm, L. A. Judy, J. C. Forfang, and R. A. Robinson.** 1985. A point-source outbreak of campylobacteriosis associated with consumption of raw milk. *J. Infect. Dis.* **152:**592–596.

31. **Lederman, E. R., C. Austin, I. Trevino, M. G. Reynolds, H. Swanson, B. Cherry, J. Ragsdale, J. Dunn, S. Meidi, H. Zhao, Y. Li, H. Pue, and I. K. Damon.** 2007. ORF virus infection in children: clinical characteristics, transmission, diagnostic methods, and future therapeutics. *Pediatr. Infect. Dis. J.* **26:**740-744.

32. **LeJeune, J. T., and M. A. Davis.** 2004. Outbreaks of zoonotic enteric disease associated with animal exhibits. *J. Am. Vet. Med. Assoc.* **224:**1440–1445.

33. **Lewis, F. M., B. J. Marsh, and C. F. von Reyn.** 2003. Fish tank exposure and cutaneous infections due to *Mycobacterium marinum:* tuberculin skin testing, treatment, and prevention. *Clin. Infect. Dis.* **37:**390–397.

34. **Manning, S. E., C. E. Rupprecht, D. Fishbein, C. A. Hanlon, B. Lumlertdacha, M. Guerra, M. I. Meltzer, P. Dhankhar, S. A. Vaidya, S. R. Jenkins, B. Sun, and H. F. Hull.** 2008. Human rabies prevention: United States, 2008—recommendations of the Advisory Committee on Immunization Practices. *MMWR Recomm. Rep.* **57**(RR-3):1–28.

35. **McMillian, M., J. R. Dunn, J. E. Keen, K. L. Brady, and T. F. Jones.** 2007. Risk behaviors for disease transmission among petting zoo attendees. *J. Am. Vet. Med. Assoc.* **231:**1036–1038.

36. **Mead, P. S., and P. M. Griffin.** 1998. *Escherichia coli* O157:H7. *Lancet* **352:**1207–1212.

37. **Nemetz, T. G., and J. R. Shotts.** 1993. Zoonotic diseases, p. 214–220. *In* M. K. Stoskopf (ed.), *Fish Medicine*. W. B. Saunders Company, Philadelphia, PA.

38. **O'Brien, S. J., G. K. Adak, and C. Gilham.** 2001. Contact with farming environment as a major risk factor for Shiga toxin (Vero cytotoxin)-producing *Escherichia coli* O157 infection in humans. *Emerg. Infect. Dis.* **7:**1049–1051.

39. **Payne, C. J., M. Petrovic, R. J. Roberts, A. Paul, E. Linnane, M. Walker, D. Kirby, A.** Burgess, R. M. Smith, T. Cheasty, G. Willshaw, and R. L. Salmon. 2003. Vero cytotoxin-producing *Escherichia coli* O157 gastroenteritis in farm visitors, North Wales. *Emerg. Infect. Dis.* **9:**526–530.

40. **Pickering, L. K., N. Marano, J. A. Bocchini, F. J. Angulo, et al.** 2008. Exposure to nontraditional pets at home and to animals in public settings: risks to children. *Pediatrics* **122:**876–886.

41. **Roy, S. L., S. M. DeLong, S. A. Stenzel, B. Shiferaw, J. M. Roberts, A. Khalakdina, R. Marcus, S. D. Segler, D. D. Shah, S. Thomas, D. J. Vugia, S. M. Zansky, V. Dietz, and M. J. Beach.** 2004. Risk factors for sporadic cryptosporidiosis among immunocompetent persons in the United States from 1999 to 2001. *J. Clin. Microbiol.* **42:**2944–2951.

42. **Smith, K. A., K. K. Bradley, M. G. Stobierski, and L. A. Tengelsen.** 2005. Compendium of measures to control *Chlamydophila psittaci* (formerly *Chlamydia psittaci*) infection among humans (psittacosis) and pet birds, 2005. *J. Am. Vet. Med. Assoc.* **226:**532–539.

43. **Smith, K. E., S. A. Stenzel, J. B. Bender, E. Wagstrom, D. Soderlund, F. T. Leano, C. M. Taylor, P. A. Belle-Isle, and R. Danila.** 2004. Outbreaks of enteric infections caused by multiple pathogens associated with calves at a farm day camp. *Pediatr. Infect. Dis. J.* **23:**1098–1104.

44. **Steinmuller, N., L. Demma, J. B. Bender, M. Eidson, and F. J. Angulo.** 2006. Outbreaks of enteric disease associated with animal contact: not just a foodborne problem anymore. *Clin. Infect. Dis.* **43:**1596–1602.

45. **Stirling, J., M. Griffith, J. S. Dooley, C. E. Goldsmith, A. Loughrey, C. J. Lowery, R. McClurg, K. McCorry, D. McDowell, A. McMahon, B. C. Millar, J. Rao, P. J. Rooney, W. J. Snelling, M. Matsuda, and J. E. Moore.** 2008. Zoonoses associated with petting farms and open zoos. *Vector Borne Zoonotic Dis.* **8:**85–92.

46. **Varma, J. K., K. D. Greene, M. E. Reller, S. M. DeLong, J. Trottier, S. F. Nowicki, M. DiOrio, E. M. Koch, T. L. Bannerman, S. T. York, M. A. Lambert-Fair, J. G. Wells, and P. S. Mead.** 2003. An outbreak of *Escherichia coli* O157 infection following exposure to a contaminated building. *JAMA* **290:**2709–2712.

47. **Webb, C. R.** 2006. Investigating the potential spread of infectious diseases of sheep via agricultural shows in Great Britain. *Epidemiol. Infect.* **134:**31–40.

48. **Weese, J. S., L. McCarthy, M. Mossop, H. Martin, and S. Lefebvre.** 2007. Observation of practices at petting zoos and the potential impact on zoonotic disease transmission. *Clin. Infect. Dis.* **45:**10–15.

INFECTIONS ON CRUISE SHIPS

Vivek Kak

18

Until the advent of air travel, ships were the only way to travel across the high seas. The presence of large groups of people on ships, with limited sanitation as well as poor food supplies, led to an increased risk of infectious diseases such as typhus as well as diseases of deficiency such as scurvy. The spread of new diseases into nonimmune populations often involved the introduction of pathogenic organisms or their vectors into these populations from ships and their crew. With the advent of air travel, the number of persons traveling by sea decreased until the recent resurgence of the cruise ship industry. The popularity of cruise ships for vacation travel has grown rapidly in recent years. It was estimated by the Passenger Shipping Association that 10 million people traveled on cruise ships in 2000 and that this number will reach 20 million by 2010 (35). The cruise industry has responded to these increasing passenger loads by increasing the size and capacity of cruise ships, as exemplified by the recent launch of the liner *Queen Mary 2,* which has a guest capacity of over 3,000 passengers. At the same time,

cruise ships are expanding their areas of operation and reaching shores which are often inaccessible by other means of travel. A modern cruise ship is a traveling city with its common food and water supply, shared sanitation and air-conditioning systems, and a large number of individuals traveling together. The individuals are often from different cultures, with different immunization backgrounds and health statuses. The proximity between passengers as well as crew members in semienclosed spaces, with interactions in the dining halls and recreational rooms, increases the possibility of organisms being transmitted among them. At the same time, an infecting agent has the potential to enter the food or water supply or the sanitation systems in these ships, to be distributed widely across the ship, and to cause significant morbidity. The typical cruise passenger is often an elderly individual and may have chronic illnesses, which can make him or her more susceptible to infection and its complications. It is thus vital to the safety of passengers that any potential for the introduction of an infecting agent as well as its transmission be minimized on cruise ships.

THE VESSEL SANITATION PROGRAM
The occurrence of typhoid fever and shigellosis on cruise liners in the early 1970s led to the establishment of the Vessel Sanitation Pro-

Vivek Kak, W. A. Foote Hospital, 1100 E. Michigan Ave., #305, Jackson, MI 49201.

Infections of Leisure, Fourth Edition, Edited by David Schlossberg, © 2009 ASM Press, Washington, DC

#76

gram (VSP) by the Centers for Disease Control and Prevention (CDC) in 1975 (15, 25). The aim of this cooperative program is to minimize the risk of gastrointestinal disease on cruise ships by maintaining a high degree of sanitation. The program conducts random unannounced twice-yearly inspections of cruise ships carrying 13 or more passengers docking at U.S. ports. The ships are rated on various items that can impact the occurrence as well as spread of infections aboard cruise ships, such as (i) water sanitation, (ii) food handling and preparation, (iii) personal hygiene and sanitation practices by the ship staff, (iv) pool and spa sanitation, (v) potential for food and water contamination and disinfection, and (vi) general cleanliness. The ships are given a score, which is published and is also available on the Internet at www.cdc.gov/nceh/vsp/default.htm. A score of 86 or higher (out of 100) implies an acceptable level of sanitation. A review of recent scores shows more than 25 cruise ships having the maximum score attainable (7).

U.S. regulations also require that cruise vessels notify public health authorities about cases of diarrhea as well as onboard deaths. The VSP thus receives notification of significant illnesses on board cruise ships and often leads epidemiological as well as environmental investigations of significant diarrheal diseases on cruise ships.

GASTROINTESTINAL INFECTIONS

#75

Acute diarrheal illnesses are the most notorious of cruise ship infections. There have been numerous outbreaks of gastroenteritis on cruise ships. A World Health Organization review of sanitation on ships listed over 100 different outbreaks of gastroenteritis on cruise ships from 1970 to 2000, affecting over 16,000 individuals (35). The CDC's VSP web page lists over 150 more outbreaks of gastroenteritis since then, suggesting that this is a continuing problem (6). The presence of a common food and water supply, along with the semienclosed setting of the ships, easily lends itself to the development of outbreaks of diarrheal dis-

eases. The presentation of the illness generally involves a sudden onset of diarrhea, with persistent loose bowel movements accompanied with vomiting. There may be associated symptoms of abdominal cramps, headache, myalgia, or fever. Patients occasionally may also complain of tenesmus and/or blood with their bowel movements, suggesting dysentery, though these symptoms are generally rare.

The vast majority of outbreaks of gastroenteritis acquired on cruise ships are due to noroviruses, formerly known as Norwalk-like viruses (Fig. 1). This group of viruses is notorious for causing diarrheal diseases in closed settings such as nursing homes (29). There have been multiple outbreaks of these infections on multiple cruise ships over the past years (6, 34, 35). These infections are often facilitated by the close living quarters, common food supplies, and intermingling of individuals that occur on cruise ships. Several routes, including fecal-oral transmission, aerosolization during vomiting, food and water as vehicles, and environmental contamination by symptomatic patients or asymptomatic carriers, can spread these viruses (13). The reports in the literature have implicated water supplies, various food items, and poor food-handling techniques, along with person-to-

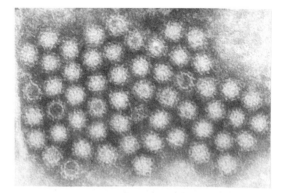

FIGURE 1 Transmission electron micrograph of norovirus virions. Noroviruses are nonenveloped, single-stranded RNA viruses that belong to the genus *Norovirus* and the family *Caliciviridae*. Source: Charles D. Humphrey, CDC (http://phil.cdc.gov/phil/quicksearch.asp).

person spread, as methods of transmission of the virus to passengers on cruise ships (35). The incubation period for noroviral gastroenteritis in humans is usually less than 2 days, though cases can occur within 12 h after exposure. Noroviral gastroenteritis presents as an acute onset of vomiting, with watery nonbloody diarrhea accompanied by nausea and abdominal cramps. Among children, vomiting tends to be more pronounced, but high-grade fever is usually not a feature of this condition and should suggest an alternative etiology. This is a self-limiting condition and usually requires medical attention only for dehydration. The widespread use of reverse transcription-PCR techniques has led to an improvement in the diagnosis of this infection and an increased appreciation of the role of this virus in causing widespread epidemics of diarrhea on cruise ships (34). The control of an outbreak is often very difficult and should involve aggressive infection control, with active disinfection, isolation of sick individuals, strict hand-washing techniques, and training of food handlers in proper food-handling procedures. A recent study of the behaviors of passengers on cruise ships during noroviral diarrheal outbreaks suggested that passengers often had diarrhea before embarking on a cruise and, once on the cruise, often did not report their symptoms to the ship's infirmary. They also were less likely to wash their hands or to isolate themselves if they were sick (28). These behaviors often perpetuate and amplify an illness in the ship's closed environment.

Though less common than noroviral outbreaks, bacterial gastroenteritis outbreaks have occurred on cruise ships. The bacterial pathogens implicated in cruise ship outbreaks of gastroenteritis reported include enterotoxigenic *Escherichia coli*, *Salmonella* species, including *Salmonella enterica* serovar Typhi, *Shigella* species, *Vibrio* species, *Clostridium perfringens*, *Campylobacter jejuni*, and *Staphylococcus aureus* (11, 14, 21–25, 27, 32, 35). These infections often tend to be more severe than those caused by noroviruses and have led to sporadic deaths of cruise ship passengers. The majority

of these outbreaks were caused by contamination of the ship water supply by sewage.

The parasitic causes of diarrhea reported on cruise ships include *Cyclospora* species, which were implicated in a large outbreak on a cruise ship where the passengers acquired the infection by eating raspberries (12). There have been sporadic outbreaks of diarrhea on ships due to *Cryptosporidium* species and *Trichinella spiralis* (31, 35).

According to one study, the probability of contracting a diarrheal disease on a 7-day cruise is less than 1% (13). The majority of the diarrheal outbreaks on cruise ships involve the introduction of the pathogen into the food and water supply, with the subsequent breakdown of the food and water sanitation chain. The factors implicated in various studies include the use of contaminated food or water, inadequate food storage, cross-contamination of food, and infected food handlers (35). The prevention of gastrointestinal infections on cruise ships involves controlling potential deficiencies in food and water handling as well as in cooking and catering, preventing sewage contamination of the water supply, and isolating sick persons. In the absence of effective vaccines for the prevention of infections by the majority of the above organisms, with the exception of *Salmonella* serovar Typhi, these efforts are the primary preventive methods to decrease the burden of gastrointestinal illnesses on cruise ships. The prevention of these diseases may also be enhanced by routine screening of embarking passengers, especially if they are sick; education of passengers and staff about gastrointestinal illness; and an enhanced focus on improving hand-washing practices on cruise ships.

RESPIRATORY INFECTIONS

The presence of an isolated environment on a cruise ship, with close interaction between a vast cohort of individuals, increases the risk of a passenger's being exposed to various respiratory secretions and, potentially, to infectious respiratory viruses. The presentation of these infections is nonspecific and can vary from an

78

upper respiratory tract infection to a life-threatening pneumonia. A study of the epidemiology of injuries and illnesses among passengers on cruise ships revealed that respiratory tract infections were the most common cause for seeking medical attention by passengers and crew members aboard the ship (30).

There have been well-documented reports of both influenza A and influenza B outbreaks on cruise ships (2, 9, 10, 18, 26). These infections tend to have a high attack rate, with a large number of individuals being infected before the epidemic is contained. These outbreaks can occur even in summertime, in regions where influenza virus is not in seasonal circulation. The virus can be introduced into the cruise ship population by either the passengers or the crew members. Thus, it is recommended that passengers at high risk for complications of influenza (e.g., persons aged ≥50 years, immunocompromised persons, and persons with chronic disorders of the pulmonary or cardiovascular systems) who were not vaccinated with influenza vaccine during the preceding fall or winter should consider receiving influenza vaccine before traveling (i) with large organized tourist groups at any time of year, (ii) to the tropics, or (iii) to the Southern Hemisphere from April through September (the time of increased influenza activity in that hemisphere) (8). It is also recommended that cruise lines should attempt to achieve at least an 80% vaccination rate among crew members on each ship each year (4). To limit the potential of cruise ships to import the pathogenic organism to the United States, these recommendations may be modified if the next pandemic influenza outbreak occurs initially outside the United States. The other respiratory viruses that have caused outbreaks among cruise ships include cases of rubella, though the list is probably underreported, as most respiratory viruses can be transmitted efficiently in the close environments of a cruise ship (5).

Among the bacterial pathogens causing respiratory infections on cruise ships, the most common infections reported have been due to *Legionella* species. There have been over 50 different incidents of Legionnaires' disease associated with cruise ships (27, 35). The largest confirmed cluster involved 50 cases spread over nine different cruises of a single ship (20). The factors involved in these outbreaks often involve contamination of the ship's water supply, the spas or pools, or the air-conditioning system. The prevention of *Legionella* infections on cruise ships involves treatment of contaminated water by using proper disinfection and filtration as well as properly cleaning and disinfecting spas and other devices which can disseminate bacteria (17).

There have also been reported cases of vaccine-preventable infections, such as diphtheria and rubella, acquired on cruise ships (3, 4). The presence of individuals, especially crew members and passengers from different countries, with differing immunization statuses can lead to transmission of vaccine-preventable diseases such as measles and rubella on cruise ships. It is thus of utmost importance that prior to a cruise, passengers update their immunization status and get appropriate vaccinations.

SKIN INFECTIONS

The presence of hot tubs and spas and the proximity of individuals on cruise ships can lead to the spread of skin infections among the passengers. I have seen a case of necrotizing soft tissue infection caused by community-acquired methicillin-resistant *Staphylococcus aureus* that presented soon after the patient's return from a cruise trip. With the widespread dissemination of community-acquired methicillin-resistant *S. aureus* isolates across the country and the proximity of individuals who may be carriers of this organism on cruise ships, it is inevitable that more cases of these infections acquired on cruise ships will be reported. The other organisms that may be seen include *Pseudomonas aeruginosa* presenting as hot tub folliculitis (19). The symptoms of most of these infections tend to be painful, pustular lesions on the body. The vast majority of these

#77

infections can be, and often are, prevented by meticulous care and disinfection of the hot tubs and spas on cruise ships.

OTHER INFECTIONS

Cruise passengers are also at risk for infections that they may acquire while on land excursions that are part of the cruise. They can also become symptomatic with infections that may have been incubating before the start of the cruise. Thus, infections that are endemic in the ports of call, such as malaria, may appear on board or after return from the cruise. There have been isolated cases of meningitis acquired aboard cruise ships, though these are uncommon (16).

The health care workers on board cruise ships, as well as physicians seeing passengers after they return from cruises, need to be aware of infections that may be acquired on board or from the ports of call. The American College of Emergency Physicians has published guidelines for the health care facilities on cruise ships (1). These guidelines give recommendations on appropriate health care facilities on board as well as on staff numbers and qualifications for these facilities. A good cruise ship medical facility, in general, is similar to an urgent care center and can take care of an estimated 95% of cruise ship illnesses; however, for passengers with serious medical problems or those traveling on smaller cruise ships, the facilities may be inadequate for comprehensive medical care (33).

SUMMARY

Cruise ships are an ever more popular mechanism of travel and leisure. These ships, which vary in size from small vessels to huge behemoths, carry a large population of travelers and crew in close proximity, often for an extended duration. There is a potential infectious risk in these travels (Table 1). This risk may be from introduction of a pathogen in the food and water supply or in the ship's sanitation system or spas. Passengers and crew may also transmit respiratory or gastrointestinal pathogens because of close contact. Oc-

TABLE 1 Infectious pathogens and diseases of potential risk on cruise ships

Gastrointestinal infections
Noroviral infections
Enterotoxigenic *Escherichia coli*
Salmonella gastroenteritis
Shigella species
Vibrio species
Clostridium perfringens
Campylobacter jejuni
Staphylococcus aureus enteritis
Cyclospora species
Cryptosporidium species
Trichinella spiralis

Respiratory infections
Influenza (A and B)
Rubella
Measles
Legionella species
Diphtheria

Skin infections
Hot tub folliculitis
Community-acquired methicillin-resistant *Staphylococcus aureus* folliculitis

Infections that may be acquired at ports of call
Malaria
Meningitis
Yellow fever

casionally, individuals may get sick from acquiring an infection while on shore. The prevention of these infections involves meticulous care of the ship's sanitary conditions, receiving appropriate vaccinations as necessary, and following basic infection control mechanisms, especially hand washing.

PRACTICAL TIPS

- Before booking a vacation on a particular cruise ship, passengers should visit the website www.cdc.gov/nceh/vsp/default.htm and check the inspection score of that ship. A score of 85 or lower is unacceptable.
- Passengers should update their immunization status and get appropriate vaccinations, including influenza vaccinations, vaccinations against food-borne diseases such as ty-

phoid and hepatitis A, and vaccinations based on the area of the cruise.

• Passengers should be counseled about gastrointestinal illnesses and asked to report their symptoms to the ship's infirmary. They should remain in their cabins if sick to prevent spreading the illness to the rest of the ship.

• The importance of standard infection control measures, especially hand washing, should be emphasized.

REFERENCES

1. **American College of Emergency Physicians.** 1998. Health care guidelines for cruise ship medical facilities. *Ann. Emerg. Med.* **35:**535.

2. **Anonymous.** 1999. Influenza on a cruise ship in the Mediterranean. *Commun. Dis. Rep. CDR Wkly.* **9:**209–212.

3. **Anonymous.** 1997. Diphtheria acquired during a cruise in the Baltic Sea. *Commun. Dis. Rep. CDR Wkly.* **7:**207.

4. **Bodnar, U. R., S. M. Maloney, and K. L. Fielding.** 1999. *Preliminary Guidelines for the Prevention and Control of Influenza-Like Illness among Passengers and Crew Members on Cruise Ships.* U.S. Department of Health and Human Services, CDC, National Center for Infectious Diseases, Atlanta, GA.

5. **Centers for Disease Control and Prevention.** 1998. Rubella among crew members of commercial cruise ships—Florida, 1997. *MMWR Morb. Mortal. Wkly. Rep.* **46:**1247–1250.

6. **Centers for Disease Control and Prevention.** 20 October 2008, accession date. *Outbreak Updates for International Cruise Ships.* CDC, Atlanta, GA. http://www.cdc.gov/nceh/vsp/surv/GIlist.htm.

7. **Centers for Disease Control and Prevention.** 20 October 2008, accession date. *Cruise Ship with Inspections with Score of 100.* CDC, Atlanta, GA. http://wwwn.cdc.gov/vsp/InspectionQueryTool/Forms/InspectionWith100Score.aspx.

8. **Centers for Disease Control and Prevention.** 2000. Prevention and control of influenza: recommendations of the Advisory Committee on Immunization Practices (ACIP). *MMWR Morb. Mortal. Wkly. Rep.* **49**(RR-3):1–38.

9. **Centers for Disease Control and Prevention.** 1998. Outbreak of influenza A infection—Alaska and the Yukon Territory, June–July 1998. *MMWR Morb. Mortal. Wkly. Rep.* **47:**638.

10. **Centers for Disease Control and Prevention.** 1998. Update: outbreak of influenza A infection—Alaska and the Yukon Territory, July–August 1998. *MMWR Morb. Mortal. Wkly. Rep.* **47:**685–688.

11. **Centers for Disease Control and Prevention.** 1994. Outbreak of *Shigella flexneri* 2a infections on a cruise ship. *MMWR Morb. Mortal. Wkly. Rep.* **43:**657.

12. **Centers for Disease Control and Prevention.** 1997. Update: outbreaks of cyclosporiasis—United States and Canada. *MMWR Morb. Mortal. Wkly. Rep.* **46:**521–523.

13. **Cramer, E. H., C. J. Blanton, L. H. Blanton, G. H. Vaughan, C. A. Bopp, and D. L. Forney.** 2006. Epidemiology of gastroenteritis on cruise ships, 2001–2004. *Am. J. Prevent. Med.* **30:** 252–257.

14. **Daniels, N. A., J. Neimann, A. Karpati, U. D. Parashar, K. D. Greene, J. G. Wells, A. Srivastava, R. V. Tauxe, E. D. Mintz, and R. Quick.** 2000. Traveler's diarrhea at sea: three outbreaks of waterborne enterotoxigenic *Escherichia coli* on cruise ships. *J. Infect. Dis.* **181:** 1491–1495.

15. **Davies, J. W., W. R. Simon, E. J. Bowmer, A. Mallory, and K. G. Cox.** 1972. Typhoid at sea: epidemic aboard an ocean liner. *Can. Med. Assoc. J.* **106:**877–883.

16. **DiGiovanna, T., T. Rosen, R. Forsett, K. Sivertson, and G. D. Kelen.** 1992. Shipboard medicine: a new niche for emergency medicine. *Ann. Emerg. Med.* **21:**1476–1479.

17. **Edelstein, P. H., and M. S. Cetron.** 1999. Sea, wind and pneumonia. *Clin. Infect. Dis.* **28:** 39–41.

18. **Ferson, M. J., and K. A. Ressler.** 2005. Bound for Sydney town: health surveillance on international cruise vessels visiting the Port of Sydney. *Med. J. Aust.* **182:**391–394.

19. **Gregory, D. W., and W. Schaffner.** 1987. Pseudomonas infections associated with hot tubs and other environments. *Infect. Dis. Clin. N. Am.* **1:**635–648.

20. **Jernigan, D. B., J. Hofman, M. S. Cetron, C. A. Genese, J. P. Nuorti, B. S. Fields, R. F. Benson, R. J. Carter, P. H. Edelstein, I. C. Guerrero, S. M. Paul, H. B. Lipman, and R. Breiman.** 1996. Outbreak of Legionnaires' disease among cruise ship passengers exposed to a contaminated whirlpool spa. *Lancet* **347:**494–499.

21. **Koo, D., K. Maloney, and R. Tauxe.** 1996. Epidemiology of diarrhoeal disease outbreaks on cruise ships, 1986 through 1993. *JAMA* **275:** 545–547.

22. **Lawrence, D. N., P. A. Blake, J. C. Yashuk, J. G. Wells, W. B. Creech, and J. H. Hughes.** 1979. *Vibrio parahaemolyticus* gastroen-

teritis outbreaks aboard two cruise ships. *Am. J. Epidemiol.* **109:**71–80.

23. **Lew, J. F., D. L. Swerdlow, M. E. Dance, P. M. Griffin, C. A. Bopp, M. J. Gillenwater, T. Mercatante, and R. I. Glass.** 1991. An outbreak of shigellosis aboard a cruise ship caused by a multiple-antibiotic-resistant strain of *Shigella flexneri. Am. J. Epidemiol.* **134:**413–420.

24. **Lumish, R. M., R. W. Ryder, D. C. Anderson, J. G. Wells, and N. D. Puhr.** 1980. Heat-labile enterotoxigenic *Escherichia coli* induced diarrhea aboard a Miami based cruise ship. *Am. J. Trop. Med. Hyg.* **111:**432–436.

25. **Merson, M. H., J. H. Tenney, J. D. Meyers, B. T. Wood, J. G. Wells, W. Rymzo, B. Cline, W. E. DeWitt, P. Skaliy, and F. Mallison.** 1975. Shigellosis at sea: an outbreak aboard a passenger cruise ship. *Am. J. Epidemiol.* **101:**165–175.

26. **Miller, J. M., T. W. S. Tam, S. Maloney, K. Fukuda, N. Cox, J. Hockin, D. Kertesz, A. Klimov, and M. Cetron.** 2000. Cruise ships: high-risk passengers and the global spread of new influenza viruses. *Clin. Infect. Dis.* **31:**433–438.

27. **Minooee, A., and L. S. Rickman.** 1999. Infectious diseases on cruise ships. *Clin. Infect. Dis.* **29:**737–743.

28. **Neri, A. J., E. H. Cramer, G. H. Vaughan, J. Vinjé, and H. M. Mainzer.** 2008. Passenger behaviors during norovirus outbreaks on cruise ships. *J. Travel Med.* **15:**172–176.

29. **Noel, J. S., R. L. Fankhauser, T. Ando, S. S. Monroe, and R. I. Glass.** 1999. Identification of a distinct common strain of "Norwalk-like viruses" having a global distribution. *J. Infect. Dis.* **179:**1334–1344.

30. **Peake, D. E., C. L. Gary, M. R. Ludwig, and C. D. Hill.** 1999. Descriptive epidemiology of injury and illness among crew members of commercial cruise ship passengers. *Ann. Emerg. Med.* **33:**67–72.

31. **Singal, M., P. M. Schanta, and S. B. Werner.** 1976. Trichinosis acquired at sea—report of an outbreak. *Am. J. Trop. Med. Hyg.* **25:**675–681.

32. **Waterman, S. H., T. A. Demarcus, J. G. Wells, and P. A. Blake.** 1987. Staphylococcal food poisoning on a cruise ship. *Epidemiol. Infect.* **99:**349–353.

33. **Wheeler, R. E.** 2001. Travel health at sea: cruise ship medicine, p. 275–287. *In* J. N. Zuckerman (ed.), *Principles and Practices of Travel Medicine.* John Wiley and Sons, New York, NY.

34. **Widdowson, M. A., E. H. Cramer, L. Hadley, et al.** 2004. Outbreaks of acute gastroenteritis on cruise ships and on land: identification of a predominant circulating strain of norovirus—United States, 2002. *J. Infect. Dis.* **190:**27–36.

35. **World Health Organization.** 2001. *Sanitation on Ships: Compendium of Outbreaks of Food Borne and Waterborne Disease and Legionnaires' Diseases Associated with Ships, 1997–2000.* WHO, Geneva, Switzerland.

EXOTIC AND TRENDY CUISINE

Jeffrey K. Griffiths

19

Fashions in food have always carried the cachet of class and trendiness, and sometimes the cost of fashion is illness. As travel has expanded the locales that the traveler may visit, it has also expanded the range of food-related illnesses that may be acquired by the individual on vacation or on a business trip. Moreover, one need not be traveling to suffer these maladies, as sometimes they are imported to one's home given the globalization of food production. As the consumption of novel foods and the pleasures of international travel spread from the trendiest groups to society at large, the pool of people at risk for these illnesses increases. Indeed, as our societies and diets become more diverse, the opportunities for exotic, weird, and otherwise fascinating diseases multiply.

Many foods, such as seafood or dairy products, are preferentially eaten raw or unpasteurized in their most fresh and tasty form. This maximizes their potential to act as vectors for bacteria, viruses, and parasites. Some of these pathogens are well known to clinicians; others cause rare zoonoses that do not normally infect humans and may escape early recognition, and some may in fact cause newly emerging diseases. In recognition of this potential, the food industry has made some changes in how it processes foods. For example, fish destined to be eaten raw for sushi is now often frozen before consumption to kill *Anisakis* parasites. Alas, even cooked food can transmit prions, leading to diseases such as kuru, but since the ingestion of human brains is now rare, in this chapter I focus on more likely or exotic diseases.

With the current trends towards freshness and purity, there has also been a trend towards home or artisanal production of foods. Some of these, such as yogurt and mayonnaise, are wonderful culture media for specific bacteria, such as *Staphylococcus aureus* and *Salmonella* species. For toxin-mediated diseases, cooking or heating the food (culture media) may kill the bacterium but leave the bacterial toxin to do its damage. Patterns of food storage can also predispose to disease. In some parts of the world, such as Africa and Asia, uneaten rice is stored overnight and eaten for breakfast. Unfortunately, *Vibrio cholerae*, the etiologic agent of cholera, has been shown (131) to be capable of increasing in number in cooked rice from 10^2/g to over 10^{10}/g during storage. The ad-

Jeffrey K. Griffiths, Graduate Programs in Public Health, Department of Public Health and Family Medicine, and Department of Medicine, Tufts University School of Medicine, 136 Harrison Ave., Boston, MA 02111.

Infections of Leisure, Fourth Edition, Edited by David Schlossberg,
© 2009 ASM Press, Washington, DC

venturous yet fastidious traveler who partakes of leftover rice for breakfast may be greatly surprised, to say the least, when this leads to cholera!

The capture or slaughter of some animals for food can also be risky. The recent pandemic of severe acute respiratory syndrome (SARS) caused by a coronavirus is illustrative. Molecular analysis of the SARS coronavirus has shown that it resembles a coronavirus found in civets, animals most closely related to the mongoose (38a). Civets are a delicacy in Chinese cuisine, and they are commonly kept alive at restaurants in anticipation of a gourmet's meal. SARS may have been introduced into a human population seeking the thrill of an exotic dinner. Outbreaks of Ebola virus in hunters have been linked to "bush meat" (monkeys or other primates) in Africa, and some have conjectured that human immunodeficiency virus (HIV) may have entered the human population through the same route (22a). This only goes to show that the simple pursuit of a delicious dinner can result in both personal illness and worldwide pandemics! Below, I discuss the risks of eating but not catching these foods.

RAW FISH AND SEAFOOD: WORMS IN THE TIME OF CHOLERA

Perhaps no food has been trendier in the United States than sushi, in which the freshest of seafood is matched with rice, pickled vegetables, and other condiments. Sushi is now a global mainstream food item. Originally from Japan and Korea, it has become commonly available throughout the world (several years ago I had excellent sushi in Nairobi, Kenya). In many cultures, raw seafood, such as herring, anchovies, and oysters in Europe and sea urchins in the Mediterranean and Far East, has been popular. The Latin American and Caribbean dishes of raw seafood marinated in acidic fruit juices, such as ceviche, have also become widely favored. Through this spread of once regional cuisines, a number of pathogens have been brought to the naïve consumer.

Anisakiasis is a potentially catastrophic disease caused by the larval stages of marine nematodes of the family Anisakidae (82), sometimes called "herring worms." The adult forms of these parasites are typically found in the stomachs of large sea mammals, and humans are only infected by the larvae as dead-end hosts. *Pseudoterranova decipiens,* a common offender, is a pathogen of seals, sea lions, and walruses, while *Anisakis simplex* is a parasite of porpoises and whales. The larvae develop first in small crustaceans and then in fish and squid, which serve as transport hosts until the larvae are eaten by the definitive host. These transport larvae may be harbored in cod, sole, flounder, fluke, salmon, mackerel, herring, yellow corbina, sea eel, ling, yellowtail, octopus, and squid (55, 63); more than 200 species of fish have had anisakid larvae detected in them. Alas, many of these make delicate sushi and sashimi, and new aquatic hosts are described frequently. For example, American shad *(Alosa sapidissima)* from Oregon, a springtime delicacy for many, were shown to harbor *A. simplex* (124). Live larval forms are ingested when raw fish is eaten. Humans may be vulnerable to raw, lightly pickled, salted, insufficiently microwaved, or undercooked fish. The prevalence of this group of parasites is higher in the Pacific than in the Atlantic Ocean, perhaps reflecting the larger number of Pacific sea mammals. A survey from Okhotsk Sea basin fish in Russia showed that 58.8% of 9,223 examined fish had larvae of the Anisakidae (141).

The hallmark of acute anisakiasis, or anisakidosis, is sudden abdominal pain, either intermittent or constant, beginning 1 to 24 h after consumption of raw fish. Nausea, vomiting, fever, and epigastric pain are common. Not infrequently, the worm is regurgitated, ending the episode (70). Many people have gone to surgery after a presumptive diagnosis of a perforated viscus, appendicitis, or tumor. The most severe cases are apparently caused by *A. simplex,* with milder disease often caused by *P. decipiens.* If endoscopy is performed early, it is possible to retrieve the slender, 1- to 4-cm-long larval worm in about half the

#79

cases, with immediate resolution of pain (53). A little more than half the time, the larvae are found in the greater curvature, with severe mucosal edema (60). The parasite attempts to burrow into the stomach, expecting it to be the thick one of a sea mammal, and may perforate it. Eventually the parasite will perish in the inappropriate human host, leaving a granulomatous reaction in the stomach wall or wherever else it may have come to rest. A case series from Italy described the finding of anisakids in the gastric wall, the intestinal wall, the omentum, the spleen, the mesentery, and even the appendix (98). Freezing fish for 24 to 72 h at −20°C kills the larvae, and in fact most salmon served as sushi in the United States are now frozen after being harvested to decrease this risk.

With increased awareness, other syndromes associated with anisakiasis have emerged. First, there is a set of unusual syndromes, such as intestinal obstruction (134), esophageal disease in the setting of reflux esophagitis (139), tonsillar anisakiasis (9), continuous ambulatory peritoneal dialysis peritonitis (94), and pulmonary disease (80). Respiratory anisakiasis can be accompanied by high fever and pleural effusions; curiously, in one case report, eosinophilia did not accompany the extraordinarily high anti-*Anisakis* immunoglobulin E (IgE) levels found during the disease. Small intestinal anisakiasis can be evaluated with ultrasonography, which typically reveals ascites, small bowel dilatation, and focal edema of Kerckring's folds. Giant gastric folds may be seen (95). The ascites is typically eosinophilic. In the clinical setting of an acute abdomen after the recent ingestion of seafood, eosinophilic ascites, and ultrasonographic findings as noted above, conservative management without laparotomy may be considered (52); in one study, symptoms resolved in 18 patients by the eighth day after onset when treated conservatively (125). Chronic infestation, marked by feelings of chronic ill health and abdominal pain, has been described (14). In such a case, serologic testing is often positive, and surgery is necessary for the resection of the eosino-

philic lesion that (diagnostically) contains a larva with Y-shaped lateral cords. In contrast, an incidental detection of an *Anisakis* larva in continuous ambulatory peritoneal dialysis effluent (147) was reported, suggesting that not everyone with anisakiasis is clinically "ill" (84a, 96a).

Another emerging syndrome associated with anisakiasis is allergy and IgE-mediated anaphylaxis (5a, 15a, 28, 33, 40). Anaphylaxis can occur in those who ingest cooked, killed *Anisakis* larvae—presumably after an earlier intimate exposure to the parasite, e.g., after an episode of anisakiasis (6). The overall prevalence of allergy to anisakid larvae is unknown. In one study from Spain, 14 (1.4%) of 1,008 serum samples from individuals with no clinical suspicion of anisakiasis (43) showed high levels, and 47 (4.7%) showed intermediate levels, of antibody to *Anisakis*. It is thus not surprising that rheumatological complaints have now been identified following anisakiasis (23). Surveys of commercially important wild marine fish have frequently found that infection rates are high. One survey from Norway found that 99.6, 97.8, and 88.0% of saithe, cod, and redfish (respectively) contained *A. simplex* in the viscera or muscles (132). Another survey from the Bohai Sea, China, revealed that 5,992 third-stage larvae of *A. simplex* were found in 121 of 156 assorted fish (15 of 19 species) and in 15% of one species of squid (75). Thus, exposure to anisakid larvae must be common in those who consume these fishes. Commercial salmon farming has become common. Deardorff and Kent (29) found that all 50 wild sockeye salmon caught during their spawning migration were infected with *A. simplex* larvae, whereas none of 237 Atlantic, coho, and chinook salmon raised in commercial pens carried the parasite. Thus, for those who eat raw salmon, and especially for those with allergy to *Anisakis,* farmed fish may be safer than wild fish, no matter the potential compromise in taste that some claim only wild fish has.

Anisakiasis may be more prevalent than commonly recognized. Spanish workers have found that dyspeptic individuals undergoing

#80

upper digestive tract endoscopy have a higher seroprevalence of antibody to anisakid antigens, and this correlates well with the consumption of fish in vinegar, raw fish, or smoked fish (138). One series of 25 cases from Spain noted that all identified patients had eaten raw herring (107).

Another group of truly horrible parasites transmitted by raw freshwater fish and other creatures are the *Gnathostoma* species of worms. Adult worms live attached to the stomach walls of mammals, such as felines, boars, weasels, and dogs. The eggs are passed in the feces of the definitive host, and water-living *Cyclops* species are the host for the first- and second-stage larvae. Fish, frogs, and snakes are the usual next hosts for the third-stage larvae. These animals, when eaten raw, are the usual vectors for transmission to humans, in whom the parasite cannot develop. Instead, larvae unable to complete development wander through the unfortunate person's tissues, sometimes for years, causing mayhem and pain as they search for the unattainable (e.g., a dog's stomach) (3). It is hard to believe that the unfulfilled aspirations of a lost worm can cause such human misery (49a, 69a).

Gnathostomiasis is a major problem in Thailand and Southeast Asia, where it is considered the most common symptomatic tissue helminth infection. It has also been described to occur in Japan, India, Latin America (including Mexico), the Middle East (25, 96), and Africa (48). Worms recovered from humans are 2 to 3 mm long and <0.5 mm wide; adults in the definitive host are up to 5 cm in length. Soon after ingestion of the raw fish or other paratenic host, nausea, vomiting, diarrhea, and abdominal cramps are followed by malaise, chest discomfort, cough, myalgias, weakness, and migratory swellings. Most chronic clinical manifestations are related to the restless, relentless, and clinically cruel migration of the parasite through the host, and cutaneous migrations are accompanied by intensely pruritic swelling and eruptions. Concurrent marked eosinophilia, high IgE levels, and parasite-specific antibody are usually

found. Most worrisome are invasions of the central nervous system (CNS) and ocular system, which may be fatal. Gnathostomiasis can cause an eosinophilic meningitis in association with painful radiculopathy, subarachnoid hemorrhage, and the cutaneous symptoms and signs already mentioned. The latter help to differentiate it from eosinophilic meningitis caused by *Angiostrongylus cantonensis,* the rat lungworm, in which the associated symptoms of *Gnathostoma* infection are not found (104, 122). *Angiostrongylus* eosinophilic meningitis is usually manifested by headache, paresthesias, generalized weakness, and occasionally, visual difficulties and extraocular muscle palsies (64).

Concerning this disease, regions of interest to travelers or their health care providers include Mexico (93), Japan (56, 87), and most of Southeast Asia. The first recorded case of North American gnathostomiasis was in Mexico in 1970, and reporting of this disease is on the increase (45, 93). Most Thai cases of the disease are believed to be caused by *Gnathostoma spinigerum*. Both *Gnathostoma doloresi* and *Gnathostoma nipponicum* are well established in Japan, where wild boars and pigs can act as the final host, and fish, frogs, and snakes can act as the intermediate hosts of the former. Interestingly, a study has suggested that small rodents and insectivores can also serve as paratenic intermediate hosts for *G. nipponicum* (97). Throughout Asia, raw carp, kokanee, ice fish, and loach are savored meals and excellent vectors for *Gnathostoma* parasites (136), and loach imported into Korea from China have been found to be infected with *Gnathostoma hispidum* (128). Thus, the indiscriminate individual who consumes the odd raw snake, frog, fish, mouse, or rat in East or Southeast Asia risks infection with the apparently equally indiscriminate and cosmopolitan *Gnathostoma*.

In 1988, 8 of 12 diplomats attending a dinner in Dhaka, Bangladesh (8a) developed *G. spinigerum* infection after eating a fish pâté that had been frozen and then marinated (pH 5.0). Six of the eight developed intermittent, migratory subcutaneous swellings, and two had systemic symptoms, including diarrhea, weight loss, and abdominal and thoracic pain. Sero-logic studies performed at Mahidol University in Bangkok, Thailand, documented anti-*Gnathostoma* antibody titers of >1:1,600 in the symptomatic diplomats and <1:25 in the asymptomatic diplomats. Despite multiple courses of thiabendazole and mebendazole, symptoms and migratory swellings persisted beyond 10 months in five of the six affected individuals. In a *Gnathostoma* outbreak in Mexico, everyone who ate a ceviche made from freshwater perch developed acute throat pain, chest and joint pains, headache, and fe-ver, with edematous migrating skin lesions (34). These outbreak reports prove the point that the attack rate can be very high when infected fish are consumed. It is clear that freezing of the fish and subsequent marination in a mildly acidic lime juice solution were not sufficient to kill the parasite, although it is not known whether a temperature of −20°C was reached and sustained. Two studies (59, 65) have reported that albendazole has an efficacy rate of >90%, and similar efficacy has been reported for ivermectin (90), yet in a case se-ries from London, England, 3 of 16 (19%) pa-tients treated with these agents required sec-ond courses of treatment (84).

The prevalence of gnathostomiasis is not well understood. The outbreak in Mexico mentioned above led to a seroepidemiological investigation. In the affected agricultural and fishing community of Sinaloa, 36% of house-holds reported the consumption of raw fish, 35% of individuals were seropositive for *Gnathostoma,* and 12 additional individuals who had a history of migrating skin lesions were identified. Five fish species and four fish-eating bird species were infected with *Gnathostoma binucleatum,* a species found in Mexico and Ecuador. Gnathostomiasis may be a true emerging disease, with far more affected people than heretofore recognized.

One may expect that with time, other par-asites will be added to the list of those causing sushi-related (raw fish) diseases. Several groups have reported cases of *Eustrongylides* infection presenting as appendicitis (86, 146). This nematode is a parasite of fish-eating birds, and people have been infected by eating raw fresh-water fish. Larvae are also found in reptiles and amphibians, which may serve as paratenic (transport) hosts (71, 99). Presenting with se-vere right lower quadrant pain and peritoneal signs, thought to be acute appendicitis, the af-flicted individuals have undergone surgery and had small (~4-cm) pink-red worms recovered from the peritoneum. Three patients who swallowed live minnows in Maryland had a similar disease; in one the disease resolved spontaneously, but the other two underwent laparotomy and *Eustrongylides* larvae were found to have perforated their ceca (20). Probably even sushi devotees can be per-suaded not to eat live minnows; one wonders whether, in the era of eating live goldfish, these infections were more common.

Diphyllobothrium latum is a tapeworm ac-quired by eating the raw or undercooked muscle of fish. It is a big problem, primarily in the sense that it grows to a length of 20 to 30 ft. The adult worm is found in humans, cats, dogs, foxes, bears, wolves, and pigs, an-imals that eat freshwater and marine fish. Eggs passed in human or animal feces embryonate in water and are ingested by freshwater crus-taceans. When a crustacean is eaten by a fish, the parasite penetrates the intestinal wall, where it develops into a plerocercoid, which is infectious to carnivores that subsequently eat the infected fish. These plerocercoids are 1 to 5 cm long and visible to the naked eye. Of note is the potential for worms such as *Di-phyllobothrium* to cause sparganosis, a disease in which the undifferentiated plerocercoid is found in humans, instead of the usual hosts. The usual route of acquisition of sparganosis is the ingestion of raw frogs or snakes (21) or the direct application of raw snake flesh to the skin (66). Other reports have included de-scriptions of ocular (12) and testicular (116) sparganosis, attesting to the variety of places where people put raw foods.

Fish species that have been found to be in-fected include salmon, whitefish, rainbow trout, pike, perch, turbot, and ruff (142). Areas of endemicity include subarctic and temperate Asia and Europe, the lake regions of the European Alps, the Danube River basin, and many parts of North and South America where human immigration has carried the parasite. About 10% of people in Scandinavia are infected with *Diphyllobothrium*. Salmon spend a portion of their lives in freshwater, and fresh salmon from Alaska were implicated in an outbreak of fish tapeworm disease along the west coast of the United States in 1979 and 1980 (19). It is presumed that young salmon are infected after hatching in spawning rivers contaminated by infected bears as they are fishing. In a fascinating discovery, the existence of neolithic yuppies has now been confirmed: the analysis of human coprolites (feces) from the neolithic site of Chalain, France, has revealed eggs of *Diphyllobothrium* species (as well as the more mundane helminths *Trichuris* spp. and *Fasciola hepatica*) (13). Thus, the human association is an ancient one.

Like other physicians trained in New York City, I was taught to suspect *D. latum* infection in any vitamin B-deficient Jewish immigrant from eastern Europe who prepares gefilte fish in the traditional way. This ethnic delicacy is made with chopped freshwater fish, and the proper balance of spices can only be made as the (still uncooked) fish dish is being made. Indeed, pernicious megaloblastic anemia is sometimes caused by the special ability of the tapeworm to absorb vitamin B$_{12}$ in the proximal small intestine. For reasons that are unclear, this complication of infection is more common in Europe than in the United States, where the worm can be found in Great Lake fish (117). Other nonspecific symptoms include abdominal pain and weight loss. Diagnosis is made by examination of the stool for proglottids and the oval eggs, which have a characteristic operculum (121). Several agents, including the time-tested niclosamide and praziquantel, are curative with single-dose treatment.

Other *Diphyllobothrium* species may well be involved in human infection. Curtis and Bylund have discussed the other species thought to infect humans in the circumpolar Arctic region (24), including *Diphyllobothrium dendriticum, Diphyllobothrium ursi, Diphyllobothrium dalliae,* and *Diphyllobothrium klebanovskii*. Interestingly, there are no reports of anemia in individuals infected with one of the abovementioned non-*D. latum* species. It is not possible to distinguish infections with different *Diphyllobothrium* species by stool exam, as the eggs are very similar and the proglottids of the non-*D. latum* species are easily confused with those of *D. latum*. There is some evidence that the fish reservoirs for the different *Diphyllobothrium* species are separable; for example, *D. dendriticum* is usually found in salmonid fish such as salmon, trout, whitefish, and Arctic char and has never been reported to occur in perch and pike. Perch and pike are the usual intermediate hosts for *D. latum,* and salmonids rarely harbor *D. latum*.

Of note is the intestinal fluke *Nanophyetus salmincola,* which has been reported to cause disease in people who have eaten raw salmon, Pacific steelhead trout, or steelhead roe that was undercooked or smoked (38, 41). Unlike with many other flatworm infections, the majority of reported cases (13 of 20 cases) involved abdominal pain, diarrhea, bloating, nausea and vomiting, weight loss, and fatigue. One individual reported fever. Ten of 18 individuals examined had eosinophilia of >500 eosinophils per ml. One individual has been reported to have acquired the infection after handling a naturally infected coho salmon (49), reminiscent of the direct invasion of the human host from the raw flesh of frogs and snakes that leads to sparganosis. Diagnosis is made by examining stools for the oval, operculated eggs, using concentrated fecal specimens or trichrome-stained stools. Most cases have been reported from the Pacific Northwest region, and praziquantel appears to be an effective therapy. Nanophyetiasis may be the most commonly encountered naturally occurring trematode infection in North America. Other trematodes, such as *Fasciola buski, Heterophyes heterophyes, Metagonimus yokogawai,* and *Echinostoma ilocanum*—endemic to Southeast Asia and the Nile Delta—may increasingly be found in North America after the ingestion of imported raw snails, freshwater plants, or fish and are on the increase (35).

Many lovers of sushi are aware that the puffer fish (species of *Fugu* or *Takifugu*) is highly poisonous, with high concentrations of tetrodotoxin found in the liver, ovaries, intestines, and skin of the fish (54). The toxin causes respiratory failure, paralysis, paresthesias, numbness, nausea, and ataxia. Paresthesia is the usual early-presenting complaint, consisting of either numbness or tingling of the lips, tongue, mouth, hands, and feet, rapidly followed by flaccid paralysis and respiratory failure. Most individuals requiring respirator support recover in 12 to 48 h without sequelae (61). Even the dried fillets of the puffer fish, perhaps contaminated during preparation, can contain high levels of toxin and cause neurotoxic food poisoning (51). *Vibrio* species have been found to produce tetrodotoxin, and a theory has arisen that tetrodotoxin-containing fish and animals (puffer fish, the California newt, gobies, *Atelopus* frogs, gastropod mollusks, the blue-ringed octopus, etc.) bioaccumulate the toxin made by these symbiotic bacteria (69).

Unpleasant fish toxins probably are more widely extant than previously suspected. Sohn et al. reported a case of *Stellantchasmus falcatus* infection in a 33-year-old man in Seoul, Republic of Korea, who had eaten raw brackish-water fish; after a single dose of praziquantel and a magnesium-salt purge, 17 adult worms were found (127). The patient had had vague abdominal pain and discomfort. This mild illness pales in comparison to the acute renal failure and hepatitis suffered by 13 Koreans who ate raw carp bile (100). All of the individuals initially reported gut upset after ingestion of the raw carp, followed by oliguria in 7, jaundice in 8, and hematuria in 10. The severity of the symptoms was related to the amount of bile ingested; all recovered with supportive therapy, including dialysis. Biopsy samples of the kidney and liver revealed changes consistent with an acute tubular necrosis produced by nephrotoxins, and those of

the liver revealed changes of acute toxic hepatitis. Clearly, even lovers of sushi may wish to reconsider the ingestion of raw bile!

As already noted, ceviche is the generic name for raw fish dishes prepared in South and Central America. Depending upon the locale, the fish may be steeped in lime or lemon juice (and other condiments) for 24 h before being eaten or may be briefly rinsed in acidic fruit juice on its way to the mouth of the impatient diner. This dish is extremely popular with indigenous populations, and increasingly so with the adventurous tourist or business traveler from abroad. Citrus juices are added to many foodstuffs around the world, and they clearly have a protective effect against bacterial pathogens. Lime juice was found to be a protective factor during the 1994 cholera epidemic in Guinea-Bissau, decreasing the risk of infection by about 80% (109). A follow-up study during the 1996 epidemic of cholera in the same locale similarly found that lime juice in the sauce eaten with rice was strongly protective against infection (decrease of 69%) (110). Cranberry, lemon, and lime juices demonstrate at least a 5-log-unit inactivation of *Salmonella, Listeria,* and *Escherichia coli* O157: H7 in laboratory studies (89). My advice is to drown your ceviche with lime, and add plenty of lemon or lime juice when eating risky food!

Cholera

Epidemic cholera emerged throughout South and Central America in the 1990s, and it is endemic along the U.S. Gulf Coast. The world has suffered from seven pandemics since the first pandemic began in India in 1817. Cholera has been epidemiologically associated with the ingestion of raw seafood (74). It is difficult to convey how important this disease is and how many people can be affected or even killed by it. For example, the Pan American Health Organization estimated that during the onset of the Western Hemisphere epidemic in 1991, 322,562 cases of cholera occurred in Peru in that year alone; indeed, nearly a million cases were reported and over 9,000 people died (47). In a well-publicized outbreak of interest to travelers, 75 cases of acute cholera in 1991 were linked to the ingestion of a cold seafood salad aboard an airliner that flew from Peru to California. Presumably the salad was contaminated with *V. cholerae,* either by a handler or from the start, perhaps because preparation was inadequate to kill the bacterium. Similarly, 11 cases of cholera were associated with eating crab smuggled from Colombia into New Jersey. Episodic cases have been reported for U.S. citizens and foreigners returning from South and Central America after eating raw seafood (108). Gulf Coast raw shellfish and crabs have historically been the reservoir for a few cases per year in the United States; the risk of cholera from eating raw seafood in the more southern Americas has now become far greater and deserving of a cautionary word to those departing to those areas. With the transport of raw seafood delicacies across continents to appease the appetites of trendy epicureans, cholera may appear anywhere.

In an illustrative report, Swaddiwudhipong et al. described several sporadic outbreaks of El Tor cholera in the northern Chiang Mai region of Thailand (133). Two of the three outbreaks were associated with infected food handlers (one was a butcher and one was a food packer); in the other, six young men ate raw fish from a canal contaminated with *V. cholerae.* Thus, both marine and freshwater fish may carry and transmit cholera.

Cholera is the prototypical dehydrating diarrheal disease. It can lead to death in as little as 6 h after the onset of diarrhea. The key to treatment (and survival) is rehydration with fluids that contain the salts lost in the diarrheal flux. In the majority of cases, vigorous oral rehydration prevents death and restores euvolemia. Antimicrobials play a secondary role in the treatment of cholera, shortening the duration of illness and stopping further contamination of the environment with viable vibrios (62, 114). It is an error of management and judgment to focus on drug therapy and not on the fluid replacement needs in this disease, which can be prodigious.

For better or for worse, the profile of the modern traveler has changed: he or she is more likely to be obese. With corpulence come gastrointestinal reflux and the use of agents to neutralize stomach acid; use of such agents has been shown to decrease the infectious dose of *V. cholerae* 10,000-fold in volunteer studies (17). Individuals taking such agents should be warned about these increased risks, and the use of alternative agents may be prudent. Cannabis or marijuana smokers are at increased risk of cholera as well (85), since heavy cannabis users have lower mean and histamine-induced concentrations of gastric acid than do nonsmokers. Marijuana-smoking overweight travelers with reflux and adventurous tastes may run special risks!

RAW BEEF, RAW PORK, AND DYSENTERY

Raw beef and pork are famous for transmission of the beef and pork tapeworms, *Taenia saginata* and *Taenia solium,* respectively. Those epicureans who favor dishes such as steak tartare are protected in some countries by strict public health measures, but in some regions, such as Africa and the Middle East, the estimated prevalence of bovine cysticercosis exceeds 10%. In some parts of Europe, eastern and Southeast Asia, and Latin America, the rates are 0.1 to 5%. *T. saginata* infections are usually asymptomatic, though mild epigastric discomfort, nausea, vomiting, weight loss, and diarrhea may be reported. The most common complaint is the passage per the anus of motile, muscular proglottids, which seems rarely to occur at a discreet time or location, but rather during public speeches, dinner parties, or similarly inconvenient events. Rarely, acute appendicitis, pancreatitis, bowel obstruction, or cholangitis may occur with an obstructing bolus of worm. Tissue invasion with larval forms of *T. saginata* is rare, and cysticercosis with this parasite is reportable.

In contrast, the pork tapeworm, *T. solium,* has a far higher potential to cause invasive disease. Though infection of humans with the mature tapeworm form is clinically indistin-

#83

guishable from infection with *T. saginata*, infection with the larval form (cysticercoid), or cysticercosis, can be extremely unpleasant. This infection has been controlled in many countries by the mandatory freezing of pork before sale is allowed and by rigidly excluding potentially infected foodstuffs from swine feed. The larval stages of the parasite can be hematogenously spread from the gut to the liver, brain, long muscles, subcutaneous tissues, and eye, among other tissues. The cysticerci become surrounded by a connective tissue membrane and can live for up to 10 years after the acute infection. When the cysticerci die, antigens may leak into the surroundings and cause inflammation. In Mexico, cerebral cysticerci are found in 10 to 30% of patients undergoing craniotomies and in about 3% of individuals autopsied. In one series from Mexico City, neurocysticercosis was the main identified cause of adult-onset epilepsy (83). Fully half of the 100 patients studied had evidence of cysticercal disease, as documented by computed tomography, electroencephalography, cerebrospinal fluid (CSF) analysis, serologic testing, and (in some cases) angiography and surgical extirpation. Thirty-six of the 50 individuals had seizures, 41 had parenchymal calcifications, and 15 had two or more lesions.

Seizures, motor deficits, and visual impairment are common in this disease. About 5% of CNS cysticercosis cases involve the spinal cord. Peripheral eosinophilia is usually absent or low grade, and the CSF may be normal or show nonspecific increases in protein concentration or cell counts, including those of eosinophils and plasma cells. Computed tomography often shows parenchymal, subarachnoid, or intraventricular cysts, hydrocephalus, and punctate calcifications. Enhancement of the lesions with contrast agents is variable. Serologic studies are positive for only about 80% of individuals.

The therapy of cerebral cysticercosis has been filled with controversy; praziquantel and albendazole have been the two most frequently used agents (144). Steroids may be required to decrease the inflammatory sequelae after killing the parasites with antiparasitic agents, and seizures often warrant the use of anticonvulsants. Shunting procedures may be indicated when ventricular obstruction is present (31, 37, 129, 135). Vasquez and Sotelo reviewed the course of seizures after treatment for cerebral cysticercosis (140) and found that treatment was usually associated with a remission or marked improvement in the associated seizure disorder, correlating with a marked decrease in the number of cysts. While a proportion of cysts are destroyed by the host's immune response, scarring at the focus can lead to persistent seizures; in this study, drug therapy was least likely to lead to persistent seizures. In contrast, others have found that treatment may not alter the course of neurocysticercosis and have been more cautious as to the benefits of therapy (143). A consensus guideline published in 2002 recognized that clinical manifestations of this disease are highly variable and depend on the number, stage, and size of the lesions, as well as the host response. Principles of therapy include individual therapeutic decisions based on the number, location, and viability of the parasites; the need to manage growing cysticerci with either drug therapy or surgical excision; prioritizing the management of intracerebral hypertension before any other form of therapy; and the management of seizures (42). Criteria for the diagnosis of cysticercosis have also been published (30).

While there does not appear to be an increased incidence of cerebral cysticercosis in people with HIV, the lack of cellular immunity may change the expression of the disease. Giant cysts and racemose forms of the infection may be more frequent in HIV-infected persons. Delobel et al. reported a case of epidural spinal racemose cysticercosis causing a cauda equina syndrome (32).

A patient's abstinence from pork should not prevent the clever physician from considering *T. solium* infection in the proper clinical setting. Schantz and colleagues investigated an outbreak of neurocysticercosis in an Orthodox

Jewish community in New York City (118). Seven of 17 immediate family members were seropositive for the parasite, and two children had cystic CNS lesions. Of note, the afflicted families had employed housekeepers who were seropositive for the parasite or for whom stool exams were positive for *Taenia* eggs. The housekeepers were recent immigrants from Latin America and were the presumed sources of infection for the Orthodox Jewish families. Even the vegetarian gourmet is at risk of neurocysticercosis!

Eating raw pork is well associated with infection by *Trichinella spiralis,* the cause of trichinosis. This disease is found everywhere in the world except for Australia and Puerto Rico. When undercooked meat is eaten, the larvae are released from cysts in the muscle tissue. The larvae move to the intestine, where they mature. Following copulation, the adult female worms burrow into the gut, and the released larvae enter the systemic circulation and are distributed among the tissues, primarily skeletal muscle. Female worms are thought to be capable of producing about 1,500 larvae during their lifetime. Larvae enter single cells and encyst within them, remaining viable for months to years. The symptoms of trichinosis relate to both the intestinal stage and the dissemination of the new larvae into the tissues. When only a few larvae infect the host, symptoms may be absent. With heavy infections, diarrhea, cramps, and sometimes constipation result from the original infection of the small bowel. Secondary larval spread causes severe myositis and neurological, pulmonary, and cardiovascular manifestations, including inflammatory myocarditis, that can lead to death (101). In addition to the pig, larvae are found in bears, wild boars, walruses, and other carnivorous mammals. Data also suggest that a number of *Trichinella* species can infect humans (10). Interestingly, species or genotypes from the Arctic survive the freezing of their rat hosts better than tropical isolates, suggesting a degree of adaptation to the environment (78). This means that even meat that has been frozen through the wintertime may still be infectious.

Many of the hosts for *Trichinella* are game animals, a particular delight of gourmets, especially when only lightly cooked. The Centers for Disease Control and Prevention reviewed its experience with trichinosis reported in the United States from 1997 to 2001. Wild game meat is now the most common source of infection, with transmission from bears, cougars, and boars being well documented (113). Only 12 cases, 4 of them traced to a foreign source, could be traced to commercial pork products. For example, an epidemic of trichinosis in Ohio was linked to inadequately cooked meat from a bear shot in Ontario, Canada. The index patient "had eaten two bear burgers that were cooked rare in a microwave oven" (88). In another epidemic in Canada, patients with confirmed cases were more likely to have eaten dried bear meat than boiled meat (120). Dried prosciutto and other dried pork products from Europe (only recently allowed into the United States by the Department of Agriculture) are also salted. Satisfyingly, Smith and coworkers in Canada have shown that the appropriate salt curing process of these raw meat delicacies destroys *T. spiralis,* as demonstrated by rat bioassay and pepsin digestion methods (126). Outbreaks associated with eating wild boar meat and pig have been reported in Spain (111). In Italy, wild boar meat has been implicated in 9.4% of the 584 cases diagnosed since 1961, but it is not believed to play a major role in the sylvatic cycle of *Trichinella* in Piedmont and Liguria; none of 1,518 samples of wild boar muscle were found to be infected during the period from 1987 to 1990, whereas 14 of 608 wild foxes were infected (112).

In some countries, the incidence of trichinellosis remains high, with substantial mortality related to the migration of the parasites through the tissues. These cases represent the tip of the iceberg. For example, in Thailand, many thousands of people are estimated to have been infected with *Trichinella* in the last 30 years, and 85 of them have died. Pigs raised by hill tribes are thought to be the main source of human infections (102). The number of infected humans surely exceeds this figure by several orders of magnitude. To give some historical perspective to this study, epidemics in Germany during the 1800s were associated with mortality rates as high as 30% (46). In contrast, with the implementation of public health measures, the increasing use of frozen pork, and a trend away from home preparation of fresh pork sausage, the incidence has fallen dramatically in some countries. The number of reported cases in the United States fell from around 400 per year in the late 1940s, with 10 to 15 deaths yearly, to 57 per year, with 3 deaths, in the 5 years from 1982 to 1986 (7). One to two percent of human autopsy examinations of the diaphragm muscle are still positive for larvae, however. Pork products are responsible for about two-thirds of U.S. cases, with the rest associated with ground beef and wild animal meat. Cattle are not naturally infected with the parasite, and it is believed that ground beef products are accidentally contaminated with infected pork products. The number of cases attributable to commercial pork sources continues to fall, whereas the number of cases attributed to wild game (bear, wild boar, etc.) has remained relatively constant. There are marked variations in the incidence of infected porcine populations in the United States: no infected animals were found in the 3,245 sampled in 1983 to 1985 from the Midwest, whereas 0.73% of 5,315 hogs slaughtered in New England were infected. In contrast, colleagues in China have reported that the rate of pig trichinellosis is as high as 4% in some Chinese provinces (72). Many Eastern European countries have had major increases in trichinellosis related to their difficult political and economic circumstances, and the breakdown of veterinary services, since 1990 (44). Alas, some French gourmets were the victims of *Trichinella*-infected horsemeat imported from the United States, reinforcing the point that trendy foods that gourmets must fear need not originate in the developing world (68).

Special mention should be made of trichinosis in the Arctic regions, where among Inuit populations the ingestion of raw walrus and polar bear meat is common. Trichinosis in the Arctic is caused by a nematode biologically and genetically distinct from the temperate and tropical *Trichinella* organism, and it has been proposed that the northern variant is a distinct species, *Trichinella nativa* (15). In a variety of surveys, the prevalence of *Trichinella* in polar bears was 45%, that in wolves was 22.3%, that in Arctic foxes was 4%, and that in walruses was 2.6% (77), demonstrating the ubiquitous nature of the parasite in Arctic carnivores. Many cases have been linked to the ingestion of walrus meat, which is preferentially eaten raw among the Inuit, in contrast to polar bear meat, which is most often eaten cooked. A new syndrome has been described in the Arctic, marked by prolonged diarrhea, that is distinct from the classic myopathic form. The group that described this new entity has presented evidence that it represents a secondary infection in previously sensitized individuals (76). Diarrhea is prominent, with >10 stools a day at the onset, and persistent diarrhea with two to five loose motions and prominent abdominal pain are common, accompanied by high-level eosinophilia.

The classic myopathic disease may begin with abdominal pain and diarrhea, thought to reflect the invasion of the gut by the adult nematode females. This intestinal stage usually begins within 7 days of ingestion of the cysts, and nausea, vomiting, diarrhea, constipation, malaise, epigastric or right lower abdominal pain, and low-grade fever are common. It is followed by a visceral stage, which is manifested by fever, edema, muscle weakness, and myalgias; the last is the cardinal symptom that has been used in survey work. Chills, cough, diaphoresis, diarrhea or constipation, and pruritus may also be seen. Skin rashes, petechiae, and conjunctivitis may also be noted. Muscle pain and swelling are striking features, with the most commonly affected muscles being the diaphragm, extraocular, masseter, tongue, laryngeal, intercostal, neck, back, and deltoid muscles. Symptoms are related to the specific muscle groups affected; dyspnea is associated with the diaphragmatic and intercostal muscles, dysphagia is associated with the pharyngeal and tongue muscles, etc. CNS involvement results in generalized seizures, focal motor deficits, deafness, and encephalopathy. These neurological symptoms are seen in 10 to 24% of hospitalized patients. Cardiac involvement can lead to myocarditis, arrhythmias, congestive heart failure, and death. Eosinophilia is prominent, and elevated levels of muscle enzymes (creatine phosphokinase and serum glutamic oxalacetic transaminase) in serum are found, sometimes being extraordinarily high in severe cases. Other findings include decreased serum proteins, hypokalemia, leukocytosis, and mild elevations of hepatocellular enzymes. Muscle biopsy is diagnostic, as it shows the larvae within muscle cells. These are observed live and instantaneously by crushing the sample on a slide and viewing it under low-power light microscopy. However, given the life cycle, muscle biopsy may not be positive until the third or fourth week of illness. The deltoid and gastrocnemius muscles are preferred tissue sites to sample. Stool examination is usually not helpful, as eggs are not produced by this viviparous worm, and larval or adult worms are rarely seen. Albendazole has been shown to be superior to thiabendazole for treatment, and the administration of steroids may be prudent in severe cases

(119). Mebendazole appears to be ineffective (103). The convalescent stage is marked by the resolution of fever and myalgias, usually during the third or fourth week of illness. Treatment for this parasite, as well as the others, is summarized in Table 1.

An underappreciated consequence of eating poorly cooked beef may be exposure to bacterial pathogens that cause diarrhea and other intestinal complaints. E. coli O157:H7 is an enteric pathogen that causes hemorrhagic colitis and is strongly linked with hemolytic-uremic syndrome (HUS) and thrombotic thrombocytopenic purpura. In a classic study published by the Mayo Clinic in Rochester, MN, it was the fourth most common bacterial pathogen isolated during a 6-month period (79). This organism produces toxins structurally and functionally similar to the prototypical Shiga toxin of Shigella dysenteriae type 1 (91); however, it is not enteroinvasive and does not produce the heat-labile or heat-stable enterotoxins associated with enterotoxigenic E. coli. Wells and colleagues investigated several outbreaks of HUS associated with raw-milk consumption in the United States and found that enterohemorrhagic E. coli (EHEC) organisms such as O157:H7 could be isolated from local

TABLE 1 Worms in gourmet delights

Parasite	Therapy[a]
Anisakidae	Removal
D. latum	Niclosamide[b] or praziquantel[c]
Eustrongylides	Removal
Gnathostoma species	Albendazole[a,d]
N. salmincola	Praziquantel[d]
S. falcatus	Praziquantel[d]
T. saginata	Niclosamide or praziquantel
T. solium	Niclosamide or praziquantel for gut forms
Cysticerci	Praziquantel[e] or albendazole[f] for CNS disease, often with steroids and/or antiseizure medications, as indicated; surgery may be required
T. spiralis	Albendazole[g] or thiabendazole[h]; steroids if symptoms are severe

[a] For some infections, only scanty data are available.
[b] 2 g orally once in adults; for body weights of 11 to 34 kg, 1 g orally once; for body weights of >34 kg, 1.5 g once.
[c] 10 to 20 mg/kg orally once.
[d] Unclear which regimen to use.
[e] Total of 50 mg/kg/day in three divided doses for 2 weeks.
[f] Total of 15 mg/kg/day for 1 month; some investigators believe that a 3-day course is sufficient.
[g] 400 mg orally twice per day for 14 days; for some persons with AIDS, repeat treatment may be required.
[h] Total of 25 mg/kg twice daily (maximum, 3 g/day) for 5 days; for some people with AIDS, repeat treatment may be required.

dairy cattle (heifers and calves), milk samples, and raw beef samples (142a). Similar results have been obtained in Canada (105), where 10.4% of 225 beef samples were culture positive and where 26.4% of the samples harbored bacteria producing the cytotoxin, based upon cytotoxicity assays. Thus, EHEC is present in the food chain (specifically in cattle and dairy products) in areas where HUS occurs.

The direct association between HUS and infection with *E. coli* O157:H7 has been illuminated by several studies. Chart and colleagues found serologic evidence for infection in 44 of 60 patients with HUS and in none of 16 controls (22). Tarr and coworkers have published clear-cut evidence that the timing of initial stool cultures in cases of postdysenteric HUS in the United States directly affects the likelihood of isolating *E. coli* O157:H7 from the stool, with the highest success rate in the first 6 days of diarrheal illness (137). Thus, the pathogen that is linked epidemiologically with HUS is present in dairy cattle and in raw or undercooked meat. The magnitude of the problem is not yet known, as it is now recognized that children with hemorrhagic colitis routinely develop a spectrum of coagulation disorders related to the infection, and only a fraction develop overt HUS (92). HUS due to *E. coli* O157:H7 remains the most common cause of acute renal failure in children in the United States. The bloody hamburger enjoyed by many is, unhappily, ubiquitously at risk of containing *E. coli* O157:H7 (2).

Treatment of *E. coli* O157:H7 infections with antibiotics is controversial. Experimental evidence suggests that antibiotic treatment increases the release of the miscreant toxin from *E. coli* O157:H7 and leads to death in mice (118). No studies have shown that antibiotic treatment alters the course of the disease. A meta-analysis suggesting that treatment may not cause adverse events has been the subject of no little controversy (115). I do not treat *E. coli* O157:H7 infections with antibiotics (122a, 137a).

Salmonella, which is ubiquitously present in animals of commercial food importance, such as fowl and cattle, and in some household pets, such as turtles, is discussed in chapters 7 and 8.

STEAK TARTARE AND TOXOPLASMOSIS

While McDonald's, Burger King, and Wendy's hamburgers have unintentionally been vehicles for EHEC, *Salmonella*, and other organisms and are the essence of Americana, they are not the trendiest of foodstuffs. Hence, I turn to steak tartare, a flavorful concoction of raw chopped beef, raw egg, onion, capers, and a vinaigrette. Unfortunately, other things get into steak tartare, including *Toxoplasma gondii*, the etiologic agent of toxoplasmosis. *T. gondii* is an obligate intracellular parasite found throughout the world. Infection with the parasite is followed by dissemination into the tissues, most often including the brain, heart, and skeletal muscle. Encysted *Toxoplasma* is usually asymptomatic, and chronic silent infection is the rule. The acute symptomatic infection is less common, accounting for 10 to 20% of infections in adults. Though symptomatic infection is usually benign and self-limiting and often resembles an infectious mononucleosis-like syndrome, the severe end of the spectrum of clinical manifestations includes myocarditis, pneumonitis, and meningoencephalitis.

The definitive hosts for *Toxoplasma* are felines, in which both an enteroepithelial cycle and an extraintestinal cycle occur; in contrast, only the extraintestinal cycle occurs in other mammalian, avian, and saurian hosts. Tachyzoites are the form found in tissues during acute infection and invade all mammalian cells except red cells. Tissue cysts developing within host muscle cells are the infectious form eaten by epicureans ingesting raw meat. The intestinal digestive juices (peptic and tryptic) disrupt the cyst wall, liberating the tachyzoites, which invade gut enterocytes. From this focus, the parasites disseminate systemically using lymphatic or hematogenous routes, usually setting up new foci in the brain, heart, and skeletal muscle, although all tissues can be affected. Once new tissue cysts develop in the newly infected host, these persistent forms may serve as a source of recrudescent disseminated disease, especially in the immunosuppressed. In felines (members of the family Felidae), parasites which infect gut cells go through both an asexual cycle (schizogony) and a sexual cycle (gametogony), leading to the development of oocysts, which are excreted in feces. The intestinal cycle in cats occurs primarily in young animals and for a limited period, with eventual resolution. Oocysts are hardy, environmentally resistant forms that can survive in warm, moist soil for months to a year. Ingestion of oocysts also causes infection in humans.

Infection is usually acquired by eating food with infectious tissue cysts, by ingesting infectious oocysts, or transplacentally. Rare cases have been reported of infection via contaminated water, transfusion, and transplantation and through laboratory accidents. The prevalence of cysts in raw beef is not well studied; according to Remington and McLeod (106), approximately 10% of lamb and 25% of pork are infected. In one study, viable *T. gondii* was isolated from 51 of 55 Massachusetts pigs destined for human consumption; 2 of the infected pigs were seronegative by the Sabin-Feldman dye test, the modified agglutination test, and Western blotting (36)! In the United States and Europe, the highest rates of seropositivity in humans are in young adults, which is thought to be secondary to eating undercooked pork, lamb, or beef. In contrast, in countries such as Burundi, Panama, and Somalia, undercooked meat is rarely eaten (especially pork), and there is widespread environmental contamination with oocysts. Infection is often acquired in early childhood, and children have the highest seropositivity rates (5, 39, 130).

Toxoplasmosis has always been of major public health importance because of the congenital disease that can occur (see below). This concern has increased considerably in the AIDS era. In countries such as Finland and Slovenia, where the prevalence of *Toxoplasma* antibody in adults is relatively low, the incidence of infection during pregnancy is around 3 per 1,000 pregnancies (67, 73), comparable to the range of 2.5 to 5.5 cases per 1,000 pregnancies in studies conducted in the United Kingdom (4). In contrast, in countries where raw meat is favored—such as France (58), Germany, Pakistan (8), Turkey (18), and Sudan (1)—the *Toxoplasma* antibody seropositivity rate is high, as is the seroconversion rate during pregnancy, and it poses more of a public health problem. In screening studies in Paris conducted between October 1981 and September 1983, the standardized prevalence rate in pregnant French women was 71% ± 4%, compared to 51% ± 5% in immigrant women, and the incidence of seroconversion in nonimmune pregnant women was estimated to be 1.6% (123)!

The rate of congenital toxoplasmosis infection is ~1 in 12,000 live births, based on 14 years of newborn screening data in Massachusetts. Interestingly, the odds ratio for infection is increased if the mother's educational level is that of a college graduate or higher (57). Since education is linked to income, this may be an indication that people who ingest expensive, trendy foods really are at elevated risk of this disease!

The usual infection in a child or adult results in a mononucleosis-like syndrome, with the most frequent manifestation being lymphadenopathy. Any and all lymph nodes can be involved; with involvement of the abdominal group, abdominal pain and fever can be dominant. The lymph nodes become enlarged and firm but do not suppurate. Other manifestations include hepatitis and hepatosplenomegaly, myalgias and arthralgias, urticaria and a maculopapular rash that spares the palms and soles, confusion, headache, and meningismus. These symptoms and signs usually resolve without specific therapy—and indeed are rarely recognized as being toxoplasmosis—in the healthy host. Unhappily, in some individuals more severe disease may be seen, including hepatitis, pneumonitis, meningoencephalitis or encephalitis, pericarditis or myocarditis, and polymyositis.

#91

Special mention of ocular and CNS disease should be made. Acute chorioretinitis can produce epiphora, photophobia, scotomata, pain, and blurred vision; if the macula is involved, central vision may be lost. In congenital disease, strabismus, nystagmus, anisometropia, cataracts, small cornea, and microophthalmia may result. In infants, the only site of clinically overt infection may be the eyes, and examination by an ophthalmologist is important; chronic infection and inflammation can cause scarring, vision loss, and optic nerve atrophy. In contrast, in AIDS patients, significant inflammatory changes are less common, and necrotic eye disease is caused by the direct effects of the parasite.

CNS disease mainly occurs in two groups, the congenitally infected and those with HIV infection. Women who become infected while pregnant have an increased risk of transmitting the parasite to the fetus the nearer they are to term; however, the disease is most severe in the first trimester, less so in the second trimester, and rarely problematic in the third trimester. The parasites cause irremediable CNS and ocular disease in the still-developing early fetus, whereas damage to other organs and tissues can often be compensated. Congenital infection can cause protean manifestations in newborns, affecting all organ systems. In those with signs of active infection at birth, deafness, mental retardation, epilepsy, spasticity, palsies, and blindness may occur. Chorioretinitis occurs in about half of congenitally infected children, including the asymptomatic, and less commonly, mental or physical retardation, epilepsy, blindness, and strabismus may result. In a study of 23,000 pregnancies (123), children born to highly seropositive (antibody titer of 256 to 512) mothers had a 60% increase in microcephaly, a 30% increase in low intelligence quotient (<70), and a doubling in the rate of deafness. In a subgroup of women with high indirect-hemagglutination antibody levels or seroconversions with IgM, there were 15 pregnancies: two children had congenital toxoplasmosis, and three were stillborn.

In individuals with AIDS, the most common manifestation of toxoplasmosis is recrudescent disease of the brain from old, formerly silent cysts. Acute infection does occur in regions of high prevalence and can result in a protean disseminated disease. The latter is often fulminant and rapidly fatal, but it is less common than the typical CNS presentation. In these patients, symptoms and signs of CNS toxoplasmosis are related to the mass lesions, meningoencephalitis, and encephalopathy that occur; thus, seizures, fever, focal neurological deficits, and headache are common. The basal ganglia are most often affected, followed by the frontal, parietal, and occipital lobes; the cerebellum is not often involved. Magnetic resonance imaging is even more sensitive than contrast-enhanced computed tomography for the detection of lesions. The CSF is usually abnormal, although a lumbar puncture may be contraindicated if cerebral edema exists. CNS toxoplasmosis is the most common CNS opportunistic infection in AIDS patients in the developed world (81). It is uniformly fatal if not treated.

There is evidence that treatment of pregnant women with acute toxoplasmosis leads to reduced risk of disease in the fetus. Daffos and colleagues (26) in Paris reported their experience using pyrimethamine and sulfa drugs in 15 women, in a cohort of 746, who developed acute toxoplasmosis in pregnancy and carried their infants to term. Of the 15 infants, 2 had chorioretinitis and the others remained clinically well during follow-up. Members of this group published another study in which 52 women with Toxoplasma infection acquired during pregnancy were treated with spiramycin and monitored to term; 54 live infants were born. Forty-three of the 52 women were also treated with pyrimethamine and sulfonamides. Only one infant had severe congenital toxoplasmosis, and this child was the result of one of the nine pregnancies not additionally treated with pyrimethamine and sulfa. The researchers recommended that spiramycin be started as soon as the diagnosis of maternal Toxoplasma infection during pregnancy is proven or strongly suspected (50). It is less clear whether postnatal treatment of the congenitally infected infant is as helpful. Wilson and Remington have published suggested treatment regimens for toxoplasmosis in pregnant women and congenitally infected infants which incorporate their own experience with that of Jacques Couvreur at the Institut de Puériculture in Paris (145). It is recommended that sulfa drugs be avoided in the first trimester of pregnancy and at term, with the latter related to the risk of kernicterus. Prenatal diagnosis of congenital toxoplasmosis using PCR tests of amniotic fluid may prove helpful (106); European workers have now reported that PCR diagnosis using amniotic fluid is as reliable as amniocentesis and fetal blood sampling (40a).

For persons with AIDS, a number of treatment regimens have been recognized as efficacious. The standard of treatment is pyrimethamine plus either sulfadiazine or clindamycin. Trimethoprim-sulfamethoxazole and pyrimethamine plus either clarithromycin, azithromycin, atovaquone, or dapsone are also efficacious in human trials or in in vitro and in vivo experiments (27, 106). In individuals who are seropositive for both *Toxoplasma* and HIV, regimens such as trimethoprim-sulfamethoxazole, pyrimethamine-dapsone, and sulfadoxine-pyrimethamine provide prophylaxis against the development of clinical disease (76). Studies have also shown pyrimethamine plus azithromycin to be an acceptable alternative to pyrimethamine plus sulfadiazine for ocular disease (11). Treatment regimens are summarized in Table 2.

There is no evidence that treatment is appropriate for the healthy individual with asymptomatic or mildly symptomatic toxoplasmosis.

UNPASTEURIZED MILK PRODUCTS

Unpasteurized milk products have always enjoyed a reputation for having a slightly fresher taste and aroma than their pasteurized cousins. Although unpasteurized milk has previously been used chiefly by the poor, many of the famous local cheeses of Europe can only be made, in the opinion of the local artisans, with unpasteurized milk, and this belief has been accepted on the far side of the Atlantic. Indeed, I often enjoy a glass of wine with locally produced, no doubt disease-ridden cheese of artisanal production. Pathogens that can be acquired from eating unpasteurized food products include *Mycobacterium bovis, Mycobacterium tuberculosis, Listeria monocytogenes, Salmonella* species, *Campylobacter jejuni, Yersinia enterocolitica, Brucella abortus,* and *Streptococcus equi* subsp. *zooepidemicus;* the toxin-mediated diseases caused by *E. coli* and *S. aureus* can also be acquired this way (2).

TURISTA

Travel expands the mind, and loosens the bowels.
Anonymous

"Turista" is a term that can be used to describe an affliction of the traveler, i.e., diarrhea. It is instructive to reflect upon the fact that foreigners who visit developed countries such as the United States also suffer from diarrhea; in other words, one needs to adapt to the indigenous bacterial and viral flora and fauna wherever one might travel (15b, 123a).

In some studies, up to 98% of travelers, many of whom indulge in eating delicious but unhealthfully raw foods, developed diarrhea during a lengthy trip abroad. In addition to the usual viral offenders, a number of bacteria can wreak havoc with the traveler's bowels: in most studies, enterotoxigenic *E. coli* is high on the list, followed by *Salmonella, Campylobacter,* and *Shigella* species. Avoidance of raw salads, food that is cold or has cooled, and ice cubes when in a hot and tropical clime is indeed difficult but is important nonetheless in avoiding diarrhea. Cholera has thankfully been rare among healthy, well-nourished travelers. However, as the world pandemic spreads and involves regions frequented by pleasure seekers, more malignant and profuse turista can be expected to occur.

Many of the foodstuffs discussed in this chapter can act as vectors of a diarrheal disease; I only wish to make a few personal sugges-

TABLE 2 Therapy for toxoplasmosis

Host characteristics	Therapy
Pregnant women	
Acute disease, first 18 wk of pregnancy, or at any time if fetal infection is excluded[a]	Spiramycin, 1 g orally 3 times daily. If fetal infection is documented at 18–20 wk by amniocentesis and PCR, begin pyrimethamine, sulfadiazine, and folinic acid (leucovorin) as outlined below. If infection is excluded, spiramycin may be continued to term.
Fetal infection confirmed after 17th wk of gestation of maternal infection acquired late in pregnancy	Pyrimethamine[b] + sulfadiazine[c] + folinic acid[d]
Congenital infection	
Infants without AIDS	Pyrimethamine[e] + sulfadiazine[f] + folinic acid[g] for 1 yr; some treat with this combination for 6 mo and then alternate monthly with spiramycin. If active chorioretinitis is present or CSF protein level is ≥1 g/dl, use steroids.[h]
Infants with AIDS	As for infants without AIDS; duration of therapy is unknown
Chorioretinitis in healthy older children or adults	Pyrimethamine, sulfadiazine, and folinic acid as for pregnant women until 1–2 wk after resolution, + steroids[h]
Life-threatening organ damage in healthy children or adults	Pyrimethamine, sulfadiazine, and folinic acid as for pregnant women, with duration of 4–6 wk or until 1–2 wk after symptoms and signs of infection are resolved. No indication for steroids unless chorioretinitis or CSF inflammation is present.
Immunocompromised children or adults (e.g., transplantation patients)	Pyrimethamine, sulfadiazine, and folinic acid as for chorioretinitis in healthy older children or adults, with a duration of 4–6 wk beyond resolution of symptoms and signs of infection; no steroids
AIDS patients (active treatment)	Pyrimethamine, sulfadiazine, and folinic acid as for chorioretinitis in healthy children and adults, to be continued indefinitely. Clindamycin[i] may replace sulfadiazine for adults (unclear for children). Other agents that may be useful and replace sulfadiazine in this regimen include azithromycin, atovaquone, dapsone, and clarithromycin. Steroids should be used only if there is evidence of cerebral edema. Another alternative regimen is trimethoprim-sulfamethoxazole[j]

[a] Avoid sulfa drugs in first trimester; avoid them just before birth of infant, unless in combination with pyrimethamine and folinic acid for treatment of congenital infection.

[b] 50 mg twice daily for 2 days and then once daily thereafter; for adult patients with AIDS, 50 to 75 mg/day.

[c] 100 mg/kg/day in two to four divided doses (maximum, 4 g/day).

[d] 5 to 20 mg/day, adjusted for anemia, thrombocytopenia, or granulocytopenia; blood counts must be monitored.

[e] 2 mg/kg/day for 2 days and then 1 mg/kg/day.

[f] 100 mg/kg/day in two to four divided doses daily.

[g] 5 to 10 mg/day, adjusted for anemia, thrombocytopenia, or granulocytopenia; blood counts must be monitored

[h] 1 mg of prednisone per kg per day, or equivalent. Steroids should be used until high CSF protein level or chorioretinitis has subsided and should then be tapered and discontinued; use only with pyrimethamine sulfadiazine-folinic acid regimens.

[i] 600 to 1,200 mg every 6 h, orally or intravenously.

[j] 5-mg/kg trimethoprim portion every 6 h, orally or intravenously.

tions. First, I do not recommend prophylactic drug treatment in the absence of diarrhea but do suggest the avoidance of risky foods, the use of only boiled or bottled beverages (preferably fine wines, of course, but carbonated water will do in a pinch), and when appropriate, the use of prophylactic bismuth subsalicylate. When diarrhea is persistent, bloody, or associated with fever, I currently use empirical therapy with ciprofloxacin or azithromycin. I suggest these drugs because many of the pathogens around the world are resistant to drugs such as trimethoprim-sulfamethoxazole, ampicillin, and tetracycline, and untreated or mistreated shigellosis is not a mild disease.

The importance of turista should not be underestimated; through the ages, nasty tourists have died from turista—the Visigoths at the gates of Rome and the Imperial French army in Haiti after the slave revolt immediately come to mind. Great literature, such as *Love in the Time of Cholera* and *The Horseman on the Roof* (also about a cholera epidemic), may have been conceived by fertile writers after particularly bad cases of turista.

SUMMARY
You can get an unbelievable number of gross and unpleasant diseases by eating raw or contaminated foods, most of which are delicious and delightful. Enjoy!

PRACTICAL TIPS
- Cannabis users may be at increased risk for gastrointestinal infections, particularly cholera.
- Treatment of traveler's diarrhea acquired in Southeast Asia with azithromycin may be optimal, in view of the increasing resistance of *Campylobacter* to fluoroquinolones.
- It is possible that antibiotic treatment of *E. coli* O157:H7 gastroenteritis facilitates development of hemolytic-uremic syndrome, especially in children. Many clinicians prefer to treat such patients with supportive care only.
- Although the lime or lemon juice in ceviche is partially protective against some ingested pathogens, the protection is not complete, and severe infections have been transmitted via ceviche that was well-soaked in lime juice.

REFERENCES
1. **Abdel-Hameed, A. A.** 1991. Sero-epidemiology of toxoplasmosis in Gezira. *Sudan J. Trop. Med. Hyg.* **94:**329–332.
2. **Acheson, D. W. K., and R. K. Levinson.** 1998. *Safe Eating: Protect Yourself against E. coli, Salmonella, and Other Deadly Food-Borne Pathogens.* Dell Publishing Co., New York, NY.
3. **Adame, J., and P. R. Cohen.** 1996. Eosinophilic panniculitis: diagnostic considerations and evaluation. *J. Am. Acad. Dermatol.* **34:**229–234.
4. **Ades, A. E.** 1992. Methods for estimating the incidence of primary infection in pregnancy: a reappraisal of toxoplasmosis and cytomegalovirus data. *Epidemiol. Infect.* **108:**367–375.
5. **Ahmed, H. J., H. H. Mohammed, M. W. Yusus, S. F. Ahmed, and G. Huldt.** 1988. Human toxoplasmosis in Somalia. Prevalence of Toxoplasma antibodies in a village in the lower Scebelli region and in Mogadishu. *Trans. R. Soc. Trop. Med. Hyg.* **82:**330–332.
5a.**Alonso, A. A. Daschner, and A. Moreno-Ancillo.** 1997. Letter. *N. Engl. J. Med.* **337:**350–351.
6. **Audicana, M. T., I. J. Ansotegui, L. F. de Corres, and M. W. Kennedy.** 2002. Anisakis simplex: dangerous—dead and alive? *Trends Parasitol.* **18:**20–25.
7. **Bailey, T. M., and P. M. Schantz.** 1990. Trends in the incidence and transmission patterns of trichinosis in humans in the United States: comparisons of the periods 1975–1981 and 1982–1986. *Rev. Infect. Dis.* **12:**5–11.
8. **Bari, A., and G. A. Khan.** 1990. Toxoplasmosis among pregnant women in northern parts of Pakistan. *J. Pakistani Med. Assoc.* **40:**288–289.
8a.**Bennish, M. L., C. Sullivan, and S. Michelson.** 1988. *Program Abstr. 28th Intersci. Conf. Antimicrob. Agents Chemother.,* abstr. 1098.
9. **Bhargava, D., R. Raman, M. Z. El Azzouni, K. Bhargava, and B. Bhusnurmath.** 1996. Anisakiasis of the tonsils. *J. Laryngol. Otol.* **110:**387–388.
10. **Bolas-Fernandez, F.** 2003. Biological variation in Trichinella species and genotypes. *J. Helminthol.* **77:**111–118.
11. **Bosch-Driessen, L. H., F. D. Verbraak, M. S. Suttorp-Schulten, R. L. van Ruyven, A. M. Klok, C. B. Hoyng, and A. Rothova.** 2002. A prospective, randomized trial of pyrimethamine and azithromycin vs. pyrimethamine and sulfadiazine for the treatment of ocular toxoplasmosis. *Am. J. Ophthalmol.* **134:**34–40.

12. **Botterel, F., and P. Bouree.** 2003. Ocular sparganosis: a case report. *J. Travel Med.* **10:**245–246.

13. **Bouchet, F., P. Petrequin, J. C. Paicheler, and S. Dommelier.** 1995. First paleoparasitologic approach of the neolithic site in Chalain (Jura, France). *Bull. Soc. Pathol. Exot.* **88:**265–268. (In French.)

14. **Bouree, P., A. Paugam, and J. C. Petithory.** 1995. Anisakidosis: report of 25 cases and review of the literature. *Comp. Immunol. Microbiol. Infect. Dis.* **18:**75–84.

15. **Britov, V. A., and S. N. Boev.** 1972. Taxonomic rank of various strains of Trichinella and their circulation in nature. *Vestn. Akad. Med. Nauk SSSR* **28:**27–32.

15a.**Buendia, E.** 1997. Editorial. *Allergy* **52:**481–482.

15b.**Cabada, M. M., and A. C. White, Jr.** 2008. Travelers' diarrhea: an update on susceptibility, prevention, and treatment. *Curr. Gastroenterol. Rep.* **10:**473–479.

16. **Carr, A., B. Tindall, B. J. Brew, D. J. Marriott, J. L. Harkness, R. Penny, and D. A. Cooper.** 1992. Low-dose trimethoprim-sulfamethoxazole prophylaxis for toxoplasmic encephalitis in patients with AIDS. *Ann. Intern. Med.* **117:**106–111.

17. **Cash, R. A., S. I. Music, J. P. Libonati, M. J. Snyder, R. P. Wenzel, and R. P. Hornick.** 1974. Response of man to infection with Vibrio cholerae. I. Clinical, serologic, and bacteriologic responses to a known inoculum. *J. Infect. Dis.* **129:**45–52.

18. **Cengir, S. D., F. Ortac, and F. Soylemez.** 1992. Treatment and results of chronic toxoplasmosis. Analysis of 33 cases. *Gynecol. Obstet. Investig.* **33:**105–108.

19. **Centers for Disease Control.** 1981. Diphyllobothriasis associated with salmon—United States. *MMWR Morb. Mortal. Wkly. Rep.* **30:**331–332, 337–338.

20. **Centers for Disease Control.** 1982. Intestinal perforation caused by larval Eustrongylides—Maryland. *MMWR Morb. Mortal. Wkly. Rep.* **31:**383–384, 389.

21. **Chang, K. H., J. G. Chi, S. Y. Cho, M. H. Han, D. H. Han, and M. C. Han.** 1992. Cerebral sparganosis: analysis of 34 cases with emphasis on CT features. *Neuroradiology* **34:**1–8.

22. **Chart, H., H. R. Smith, S. M. Scotland, B. Rowe, D. V. Milford, and C. M. Taylor.** 1991. Serological identification of Escherichia coli O157:H7 infection in haemolytic uraemic syndrome. *Lancet* **337:**138–140.

22a.**Courgnaud, V., S. Van Dooren, F. Liegeois, X. Pourrut, B. Abela, S. Loul, E. Mpoudi-Ngole, A. Vandamme, E. Delaporte, and M. Peeters.** 2004. Simian T-cell leukemia virus (STLV) infection in wild primate populations in Cameroon: evidence for dual STLV type 1 and type 3 infection in agile mangabeys *(Cercocebus agilis)*. *J. Virol.* **78:**4700–4709.

23. **Cuende, E., M. T. Audicana, M. Garcia, M. Anda, L. Fernandez Corres, C. Jimenez, and J. C. Vesga.** 1998. Rheumatic manifestations in the course of anaphylaxis caused by Anisakis simplex. *Clin. Exp. Rheumatol.* **16:**303–304.

24. **Curtis, M., and G. Bylund.** 1991. Diphyllobothriasis: fish tapeworm disease in the circumpolar north. *Arct. Med. Res.* **50:**18–24.

25. **Daengsvang, S.** 1981. Gnathostomiasis in Southeast Asia. *Southeast Asian J. Trop. Med. Public Health* **12:**319–332.

26. **Daffos, F., F. Forestier, M. Capella-Pavlovsky, P. Thulliez, C. Aufrant, D. Valenti, and W. L. Cox.** 1988. Prenatal management of 746 pregnancies at risk for congenital toxoplasmosis. *N. Engl. J. Med.* **318:**271–275.

27. **Dannemann, B., J. A. McCutchan, D. Israelski, D. Antoniskis, C. Leport, B. Luft, J. Nussbaum, N. Clumeck, P. Morlat, and J. Chiu.** 1992. Treatment of toxoplasmic encephalitis in patients with AIDS. A randomized trial comparing pyrimethamine plus clindamycin to pyramethamine plus sulfadiazine. *Ann. Intern. Med.* **116:**33–43.

28. **Daschner, A., C. Cuellar, S. Sanchez-Pastor, C. Y. Pascual, and M. Martin-Esteban.** 2002. Gastro-allergic anisakiasis as a consequence of simultaneous primary and secondary immune response. *Parasite Immunol.* **24:**243–251.

29. **Deardorff, T. L., and M. L. Kent.** 1989. Prevalence of larval Anisakis simplex in pen-reared and wild-caught salmon (Salmonidae) from Puget Sound, Washington. *J. Wildl. Dis.* **25:**416–419.

30. **Del Brutto, O. H., V. Rajshekhar, A. C. White, Jr., V. C. Tsang, T. E. Nash, O. M. Takayanagui, R. M. Schantz, C. A. Evans, A. Flisser, D. Correa, D. Botero, J. C. Allan, E. Sarti, A. E. Gonzalez, R. H. Gilman, and H. H. Garcia.** 2001. Proposed diagnostic criteria for neurocysticercosis. *Neurology* **57:**177–183.

31. **Del Brutto, O. H., and J. Sotelo.** 1988. Neurocysticercosis: an update. *Rev. Infect. Dis.* **10:**1075–1087.

32. **Delobel, P., A. Signate, M. El Guedj, P. Couppie, M. Gueye, D. Smadja, and R. Pradinaud.** 2004. Unusual form of neurocysticercosis associated with HIV infection. *Eur. J. Neurol.* **11:**55–58.

33. **del Pozo, M. D., I. Moneo, L. F. de Corres, M. T. Audicana, D. Munoz, E. Fernandez, J. A. Navarro, and M. Garcia.** 1996. Laboratory determinations in Anisakis simplex allergy. *J. Allergy Clin. Immunol.* **97:**977–984.

34. **Diaz Camacho, S. P., K. Willms, M. D. C. de la Cruz Otero, M. L. Zazueta Ramos, S. Bayliss Gaxiola, R. Castro Velazquez, I. Osuna Ramirez, A. Bojorquez Contreras, E. H. Torres Montoya, and S. Sanchez Gonzales.** 2003. Acute outbreak of gnathostomiasis in a fishing community in Sinaloa, Mexico. *Parasitol. Int.* **52:**133–140.

35. **Dixon, B. R., and R. B. Flohr.** 1997. Fish- and shellfish-borne trematode infections in Canada. *Southeast Asian J. Trop. Med. Public Health* **28**(Suppl. 1)**:**58–64.

36. **Dubey, J. P., H. R. Gamble, D. Hill, C. Sreekumar, S. Romand, and P. Thuilliez.** 2002. High prevalence of viable Toxoplasma gondii infection in market weight pigs from a farm in Massachusetts. *J. Parasitol.* **88:**1234–1238.

37. **Earnest, M. P., L. B. Reller, C. M. Filley, and A. J. Grek.** 1987. Neurocysticercosis in the United States; 35 cases and a review. *Rev. Infect. Dis.* **9:**961–979.

38. **Easthurn, R. L., T. R. Fritsche, and C. A. Terhune, Jr.** 1987. Human intestinal infection with Nanophyetus salmincola from salmonid fishes. *Am. J. Trop. Med. Hyg.* **36:**586–591.

38a. **Enserink, M.** 2004. Infectious diseases: one year after outbreak, SARS virus reveals some secrets. *Science* **304:**1097.

39. **Excler, J. L., E. Pretat, B. Pozzetto, B. Charpin, and J. P. Garin.** 1988. Seroepidemiological survey for toxoplasmosis in Burundi. *Trop. Med. Parasitol.* **39:**139–141.

40. **Fernandez de Corres, L., M. Audicana, M. D. Del Pozo, D. Munoz, E. Fernandez, J. A. Navarro, M. Garcia, and J. Diez.** 1996. Anisakis simplex induces not only anisakiasis: report on 28 cases of allergy caused by this nematode. *J. Investig. Allergol. Clin. Immunol.* **6:**315–319.

40a. **Forestier, F., P. Hohlfeld, Y. Sole, and F. Daffos.** 1998. Letter. *Prenatal Diagn.* **18:**407–409.

41. **Fritsche, T. R., R. L. Easthurn, L. H. Wiggins, and C. A. Terhune, Jr.** 1989. Praziquantel for treatment of human Nanophyetus salmincola (Troglotrema salmincola) infection. *J. Infect. Dis.* **160:**896–899.

42. **Garcia, H. H., C. A. Evans, T. E. Nash, O. M. Takayanagui, A. C. White, Jr., D. Botero, V. Rajshekhar, V. C. Tsang, P. M. Schantz, J. C. Allan, A. Flisser, D. Correa, E. Sarti, J. S. Friedland, S. M. Martinez, A. E. Gonzalez, R. H. Gilman, and O. H. Del Brutto.** 2002. Current consensus guidelines for treatment of neurocysticercosis. *Clin. Microbiol. Rev.* **15:**747–756.

43. **Garcia-Palacios, L., M. L. Gonzalez, M. I. Esteban, E. Mirabent, M. J. Perteguer, and C. Cuellar.** 1996. Enzyme-linked immunosorbent assay, immunoblot analysis and RAST fluoroimmunoassay analysis of serum responses against crude larval antigens of Anisakis simplex in a Spanish random population. *J. Helminthol.* **70:**281–289.

44. **Geerts, S., J. de Borchgrave, P. Dorny, and J. Brandt.** 2002. Trichinellosis: old facts and new developments. *Verh. K. Acad. Geneeskd. Belg.* **64**(4)**:**233–248.

45. **Gorgolas, M., F. Santos-O'Connor, A. L. Unzu, M. L. Fernandez-Guerrero, T. Garate, R. M. Troyas Guarch, and M. P. Grobusch.** 2003. Cutaneous and medullar gnathostomiasis in travelers to Mexico and Thailand. *J. Travel Med.* **10:**358–361.

46. **Gould, S. E.** 1970. *Trichinosis in Man and Animals.* Charles C Thomas, Springfield, IL.

47. **Guthmann, J. P.** 1995. Epidemic cholera in Latin America: spread and routes of transmission. *J. Trop. Med. Hyg.* **98:**419–427.

48. **Hale, D. C., L. Blumberg, and J. Frean.** 2003. Case report: gnathostomiasis in two travelers to Zambia. *Am. J. Trop. Med. Hyg.* **68:**707–709.

49. **Harrell, L. W., and T. L. Deardorff.** 1990. Human nanophyetiasis: transmission by handling naturally infected coho salmon (Oncorhynchus kisutch). *J. Infect. Dis.* **161:**146–148.

49a. **Herman, J. S., E. C. Wall, C. van Tulleken, P. Godfrey-Faussett, R. L. Bailey, and P. L. Chiodini.** 2009. Gnathostomiasis acquired by British tourists in Botswana. *Emerg. Infect. Dis.* **15:**594–597.

50. **Hohlfeld, P., F. Daffos, P. Thulliez, C. Aufrant, J. Couvreur, J. MacAleese, D. Descombey, and F. Forestier.** 1989. Fetal toxoplasmosis: outcome of pregnancy and infant follow-up after in utero treatment. *J. Pediatr.* **115:**765–769.

51. **Hwang, D. F., Y. W. Hsieh, Y. C. Shiu, S. K. Chen, and C. A. Cheng.** 2002. Identification of tetrodotoxin and fish species in a dried dressed fish fillet implicated in food poisoning. *J. Food Prot.* **65:**389–392.

52. **Ido, K., H. Yuasa, M. Ide, K. Kimura, K. Toshimitsu, and T. Suzuki.** 1998. Sonographic diagnosis of small intestinal anisakiasis. *J. Clin. Ultrasound* **26:**125–130.

53. **Ikeda, K., R. Kumashiro, and T. Kifune.** 1989. Nine cases of acute gastric anisakiasis. *Gastrointest. Endosc.* **35:**304–308.

54. **Isbister, G. K., J. Son, F. Wang, C. J. Maclean, C. S. Lin, J. Ujma, C. R. Balit, B. Smith, D. G. Milder, and M. C. Kiernan.** 2002. Puffer fish poisoning: a potentially life-threatening condition. *Med. J. Aust.* **177:**650–653.

55. Ishikura, H., K. Kikuchi, K. Nagasawa, T. Ooiwa, H. Takamiya, N. Sato, and K. Sugane. 1993. Anisakidae and anisakidosis. *Prog. Clin. Parasitol.* **3:**43–102.

56. Ishiwata, K., S. P. Diaz Camacho, K. Amrozi, Y. Horii, N. Nawa, and Y. Nawa. 1998. Gnathostomiasis in wild boars from Japan. *J. Wildl. Dis.* **34:**155–157.

57. Jara, M., H. W. Hsu, R. B. Eaton, and A. Demaria, Jr. 2001. Epidemiology of congenital toxoplasmosis identified by population-based newborn screening in Massachusetts. *Pediatr. Infect. Dis. J.* **20:**1132–1135.

58. Jeannel, D., G. Niel, D. Costagliola, M. Danis, B. M. Traore, and M. Gentilini. 1988. Epidemiology of toxoplasmosis among pregnant women in the Paris area. *Int. J. Epidemiol.* **17:**595–602.

59. Jelinek, T., M. Ziegler, and T. Loscher. 1994. Gnathostomiasis nach Aufenthalt in Thailand. *Dtsch. Med. Wochenschr.* **119:**1618–1622.

60. Kakizoe, S., H. Kakizoe, K. Kakizoe, Y. Kakizoe, M. Maruta, T. Kakizoe, and S. Kakizoe. 1995. Endoscopic findings and clinical manifestation of gastric anisakiasis. *Am. J. Gastroenterol.* **90:**761–763.

61. Kanchanapongkul, J. 2001. Puffer fish poisoning: clinical features and management experience in 25 cases. *J. Med. Assoc. Thailand* **84:**385–389.

62. Keusch, G. T., and J. K. Griffiths. 1993. Cholera, p. 634–636. *In* F. D. Burg (ed.), *Gellis and Kagan's Current Pediatric Therapy,* 14th ed. W. B. Saunders Company, Philadelphia, PA.

63. Kliks, M. M. 1986. Human anisakiasis: an update. *JAMA* **255:**2605.

64. Koo, J., F. Pien, and M. M. Kliks. 1988. Angiostrongylus (Parastrongylus) eosinophilic meningitis. *Rev. Infect. Dis.* **10:**1155–1162.

65. Kraivichian, P., M. Kulkumthorn, P. Yingyourd, P. Akarbovorn, and C. C. Paireepai. 1992. Albendazole for the treatment of human gnathostomiasis. *Trans. R. Soc. Trop. Med. Hyg.* **86:**418–421.

66. Kron, M. A., R. Guderian, A. Guevara, and A. Hidalgo. 1991. Abdominal sparganosis in Ecuador: a case report. *Am. J. Trop. Med. Hyg.* **44:**146–150.

67. Lappalainen, M., P. Koskela, K. Hedman, K. Teramo, P. Ammala, V. Hiilesmaa, and M. Koskiniemi. 1992. Incidence of primary toxoplasma infections during pregnancy in southern Finland: a prospective cohort study. *Scand. J. Infect. Dis.* **24:**97–104.

68. Laurichesse, H., M. Cambon, D. Perre, T. Ancelle, M. Mora, B. Hubert, J. Beytout, and M. Rey. 1997. Outbreak of trichinosis in France associated with eating horse meat. *Commun. Dis. Rep. CDR Rev.* **7:**R69–R73.

69. Lee, M.-J., D.-Y. Jeong, W.-S. Kim, H.-D. Kim, C.-H. Kim, W.-W. Park, Y.-H. Park, K.-S. Kim, H.-M. Kim, and D.-S. Kim. 2000. A tetrodotoxin-producing *Vibrio* strain, LM-1, from the puffer fish *Fugu vermicularis radiatus. Appl. Environ. Microbiol.* **66:**1698–1701.

69a.Li, D. M., X. R. Chen, J. S. Zhou, Z. B. Xu, Y. Nawa, and P. Dekumyoy. 2009. Case of gnathostomiasis in Beijing, China. *Am. J. Trop. Med. Hyg.* **80:**185–187.

70. Lichtenfels, J. R., and F. P. Brancato. 1976. Anisakid larva from the throat of an Alaskan Eskimo. *Am. J. Trop. Med. Hyg.* **25:**691–693.

71. Lichtenfels, J. R., and B. Lavies. 1976. Mortality in red-sided garter snakes, *Thamnophis sirtalis parietalis,* due to larval nematode, *Eustrongylides* sp. *Lab. Anim. Sci.* **26:**465–467.

72. Liu, M., and P. Boireau. 2002. Trichinellosis in China: epidemiology and control. *Trends Parasitol.* **18:**553–556.

73. Logar, I., Z. Novak-Antolic, A. Zore, V. Cerar, and M. Likar. 1992. Incidence of congenital toxoplasmosis in the Republic of Slovenia. *Scand. J. Infect. Dis.* **24:**105–108.

74. Loury, P. W., A. T. Pavia, L. M. McFarland, B. H. Peltier, T. J. Barrett, H. B. Bradford, J. M. Quan, J. Lynch, J. B. Mathison, R. A. Gunn, and P. A. Blacke. 1989. Cholera in Louisiana. Widening spectrum of seafood vehicles. *Arch. Intern. Med.* **149:**2079–2084.

75. Ma, H. W., T. J. Jiang, F. S. Quan, X. G. Chen, H. D. Wang, Y. S. Zhang, M. S. Cui, W. Y. Zhi, and D. C. Jiang. 1997. The infection status of anisakid larvae in marine fish and cephalopods from the Bohai Sea, China and their taxonomical consideration. *Korean J. Parasitol.* **35:**19–24.

76. MacLean, J. D., L. Poirier, T. W. Gyorkos, J. F. Proulx, J. Bourgeault, A. Corriveau, S. Illisituk, and M. Staudt. 1992. Epidemiologic and serologic definition of primary and secondary trichinosis in the Arctic. *J. Infect. Dis.* **165:**908–912.

77. MacLean, J. D., I. Viallet, C. Law, and M. Staudt. 1989. Trichinosis in the Canadian Arctic: report of five outbreaks and a new clinical syndrome. *J. Infect. Dis.* **160:**513–520.

78. Malakauskas, A., and C. M. Kapel. 2003. Tolerance to low temperatures of domestic and sylvatic Trichinella spp. in rat muscle tissue. *J. Parasitol.* **89:**744–748.

79. Marshall, W. F., C. A. McLimans, P. K. W. Yu, F. J. Allerberger, R. E. Van Scoy, and J. P. Anhalt. 1990. Results of a 6-month survey of stool cultures for Escherichia coli O157:H7. *Mayo Clin. Proc.* **65:**787–792.

80. Matsuoka, H., T. Nakama, H. Kisanuki, H. Uno, N. Tachibana, H. Tsubouchi, Y.

Horii, and Y. Nawa. 1994. A case report of serologically diagnosed pulmonary anisakiasis with pleural effusion and multiple lesions. *Am. J. Trop. Med. Hyg.* **51:**819–822.

81. McArthur, J. C. 1998. Neurologic complications of human immunodeficiency virus infection, p. 956–973. *In* S. L. Gorbach, J. G. Bartlett, and N. R. Blacklow (ed.), *Infectious Diseases.* W. B. Saunders, Philadelphia, PA.

82. McKerrow, J., J. Sakanari, and T. L. Deardorff. 1988. Revenge of the sushi parasite. *N. Engl. J. Med.* **319:**1228–1229.

83. Medina, M. T., E. Rosas, F. Rubio-Donnadieu, and J. Sotelo. 1990. Neurocysticercosis as the main cause of late-onset epilepsy in Mexico. *Arch. Intern. Med.* **150:**325–327.

84. Moore, D. A., J. McCroddan, P. Dekumyoy, and P. L. Chiodini. 2003. Gnathostomiasis: an emerging imported disease. *Emerg. Infect. Dis.* **9:**647–650.

84a.Nakaji, K. 2009. Enteric anisakiasis which improved with conservative treatment. *Intern. Med.* **48:**573.

85. Nalin, D. R., M. M. Levine, J. Rhead, E. Bergquist, M. Rennls, T. Hughes, S. O'Donnell, and R. B. Hornick. 1978. Cannabis, hypochlorhydria, and cholera. *Lancet* **ii:**859–862.

86. Narr, L. L., J. G. O'Donnell, B. Lister, P. Alessi, and D. Abraham. 1996. Eustrongylidiasis—a parasitic infection acquired by eating live minnows. *J. Am. Osteopath. Assoc.* **96:**400–402.

87. Nawa, Y., H. Maruyama, and K. Ogata. 1997. Current status of gnathostomiasis dorolesi [sic] in Miyazaki Prefecture, Japan. *Southeast Asian J. Trop. Med. Public Health* **28**(Suppl. 1):11–13.

88. Nelson, M., T. L. Wright, A. Pierce, and R. A. Krogwold. 2003. A common-source outbreak of trichinosis from consumption of bear meat. *J. Environ. Health* **65:**16–19, 24.

89. Nogueira, M. C., O. A. Oyarzabal, and D. E. Gombas. 2003. Inactivation of Escherichia coli O157:H7, Listeria monocytogenes, and Salmonella in cranberry, lemon, and lime juice concentrates. *J. Food Prot.* **66:**1637–1641.

90. Nontasut, P., V. Bussaratid, S. Chullawichit, N. Charoensook, and K. Visetsuk. 2000. Comparison of ivermectin and albendazole treatment for gnathostomiasis. *Southeast Asian J. Trop. Med. Public Health* **31:**374–377.

91. O'Brien, A. D., G. D. LaVeck, M. R. Thompson, and S. B. Formal. 1982. Production of Shigella dysenteriae type 1-like cytotoxin by Escherichia coli. *J. Infect. Dis.* **146:**763–769.

92. Ochoa, T. J., and T. G. Cleary. 2003. Epidemiology and spectrum of disease of Escherichia coli O157. *Curr. Opin. Infect. Dis.* **16:**259–263.

93. Ogata, K., Y. Nawa, H. Akahane, S. P. Diaz Camacho, R. Lamothe-Argumedo, and A. Cruz-Reyes. 1988. Short report: gnathostomiasis in Mexico. *Am. J. Trop. Med. Hyg.* **58:**316–318.

94. Ohta, M. K. Ikeda, H. Miyakoshi, K. Nishide, T. Horigami, T. Akao, S. Yamagishi, and S. Hirano. 1995. Letter. *Am. J. Gastroenterol.* **90:**1902–1903,

95. Okanobu, H., J. Hata, K. Haruma, M. Hara, K. Nakamura, S. Tanaka, and K. Chayama. 2003. Giant gastric folds: differential diagnosis at US. *Radiology* **226:**686–690. (Erratum, **228:**904.)

96. Ollague, W., J. Ollague, A. Guevara de Veliz, and S. Penaherrera. 1984. Human gnathostomiasis in Ecuador (nodular migratory eosinophilic panniculitis). First finding of the parasite in South America. *Int. J. Dermatol.* **23:**647–651.

96a.Oomori, S., S. Kikuiri, and S. Ono. 2008. Gastric anisakiasis associated with bleeding gastric ulcer. *Indian J. Gastroenterol.* **27**(3):129.

97. Oyamada, N. T., H. Kobayashi, T. Kindou, N. Kudo, H. Yoshikawa, and T. Yoshikawa. 1996. Discovery of mammalian hosts to Gnasthostoma nipponicum larvae and prevalence of the larvae in rodents and insectivores. *J. Vet. Med. Sci.* **58:**839–843.

98. Pampiglione, S., F. Rivasi, M. Criscuolo, A. De Benedittis, A. Gentile, S. Russo, M. Testini, and M. Villan. 2002. Human anisakiasis in Italy: a report of eleven new cases. *Pathol. Res. Pract.* **198:**429–434.

99. Panesar, T. S., and P. C. Beaver. 1979. Morphology of the advanced-stage larva of Eustrongylides wenrichi Canavan 1929, occurring encapsulated in the tissues of Amphiuma in Louisiana. *J. Parasitol.* **65:**96–104.

100. Park, S. K., D. G. Kim, S. K. Kang, J. S. Han, S. G. Kim, J. S. Lee, and M. C. Kim. 1990. Toxic acute renal failure and hepatitis after ingestion of raw carp bile. *Nephron* **56:**188–193.

101. Pawlowski, Z. S. 1983. Clinical aspects in man, p. 367–401. *In* W. C. Campbell (ed.), *Trichinella and Trichinosis.* Plenum Press, New York, NY.

102. Pozio, E., and C. Khamboonruang. 1989. Trichinellosis in Thailand: epidemiology and biochemical identification of the aetiological agent. *Trop. Med. Parasitol.* **40:**73–74.

103. Pozio, E., D. Sacchini, L. Sacchi, A. Tamburrini, and F. Alberici. 2001. Failure of mebendazole in the treatment of humans with

Trichinella spiralis infection at the stage of encapsulating larvae. *Clin. Infect. Dis.* **32**:638–642.

104. **Punyagupta, S., T. Bunnag, and P. Juttijudata.** 1990. Eosinophilic meningitis in Thailand. Clinical and epidemiological characteristics of 162 patients with myeloencephalitis probably caused by Gnathostoma spinigerum. *J. Neurol. Sci.* **96**:241–256.

105. **Read, S. C., C. L. Gyles, R. C. Clarke, H. Lior, and S. McEwen.** 1990. Prevalence of verocytotoxigenic Escherichia coli in ground beef, pork, and chicken in southwestern Ontario. *Epidemiol. Infect.* **105**:11–20.

106. **Remington, J. S., and R. McLeod.** 1998. Toxoplasmosis, p. 1620–1640. *In* S. L. Gorbach, J. G. Bartlett, and N. R. Blacklow (ed.), *Infectious Diseases*. W. B. Saunders, Philadelphia, PA.

107. **Repiso Ortega, A., M. Alcantara Torres, C. Gonzalez de Frutos, T. de Artaza Varasa, R. Rodriguez Merlo, J. Valle Munoz, and J. L. Martinez Potenciano.** 2003. Gastrointestinal anisakiasis. Study of a series of 25 patients. *Gastroenterol. Hepatol.* **26**:341–346. (In Spanish.)

108. **Ries, A. A.** 22 July 1992. *Cholera Epidemic in the Americas—Update 92-13. Revised Memorandum.* Centers for Disease Control, Atlanta, GA.

109. **Rodrigues, A., H. Brun, and A. Sandstrom.** 1997. Risk factors for cholera infection in the initial phase of an epidemic in Guinea-Bissau: protection by lime juice. *Am. J. Trop. Med. Hyg.* **57**:601–604.

110. **Rodrigues, A., A. Sandstrom, T. Ca, H. Steinsland, H. Jensen, and P. Aaby.** 2000. Protection from cholera by adding lime juice to food—results from community and laboratory studies in Guinea Bissau, West Africa. *Trop. Med. Int. Health* **5**:418–422.

111. **Rodrigues-Osorio, M., V. Gomez-Garcia, J. Rodriguez-Perez, and M. A. Gomez Morales.** 1990. Seroepidemiological studies of five outbreaks of trichinellosis in southern Spain. *Ann. Trop. Med. Parasitol.* **84**:181–184.

112. **Rossi, L., and V. Dini.** 1990. Importance of the wild boar in the epidemiology of wild trichinellosis in Piedmont and Liguria. *Parassitologia* **32**:321–326. (In Italian.)

113. **Roy, S. L., A. S. Lopez, and P. M. Schantz.** 2003. Trichinellosis surveillance—United States, 1997–2001. *Morb. Mortal. Wkly. Rep.* **52**(SS-6):1–8.

114. **Sack, D. A.** 1998. Cholera and related illnesses caused by Vibrio species and Aeromonas, p. 738–748. *In* S. L. Gorbach, J. G. Bartlett, and N. R. Blacklow (ed.), *Infectious Diseases*. W. B. Saunders, Philadelphia, PA.

115. **Safdar, N., A. Said, R. E. Gangnon, and D. G. Maki.** 2002. Risk of hemolytic uremic syndrome after antibiotic treatment of Escherichia coli O157:H7 enteritis: a meta-analysis. *JAMA* **288**:996–1001.

116. **Sakamoto, T., C. Gutierrez, A. Rodriguez, and S. Sauto.** 2003. Testicular sparganosis in a child from Uruguay. *Acta Trop.* **88**:83–86.

117. **Salokannel, J.** 1970. Intrinsic factor in tapeworm anaemia. *Acta Med. Scand.* **517**(Suppl.):1–51.

118. **Schantz, P. M., A. C. Moore, J. L. Munoz, B. J. Hartman, J. A. Schaefer, A. M. Aron, D. Persaud, E. Sarti, M. Wilson, and A. Flisser.** 1992. Neurocysticercosis in an Orthodox Jewish community in New York City. *N. Engl. J. Med.* **327**:692–695.

119. **Schantz, P. M., and M. K. Michelson.** 1998. Trichinosis, p. 1616–1620. *In* S. L. Gorbach, J. G. Bartlett, and N. R. Blacklow (ed.), *Infectious Diseases*. W. B. Saunders, Philadelphia, PA.

120. **Schellenberg, R. S., B. J. Tan, J. D. Irvine, R. Stockdale, A. A. Gajadhar, B. Serhir, J. Botha, C. A. Armstrong, S. A. Woods, J. M. Blondeau, and T. L. McNab.** 2003. An outbreak of trichinellosis due to consumption of bear meat infected with Trichinella nativa, in 2 northern Saskatchewan communities. *J. Infect. Dis.* **188**:835–843.

121. **Schmidt, G. D.** 1986. *Handbook of Tapeworm Identification. Key to the Genera Taeniidae*, p. 221–227. CRC Press, Boca Raton, FL.

122. **Schmutzhard, E., P. Boongird, and A. Vejjajiva.** 1988. Eosinophilic meningitis and radiculomyelitis in Thailand, caused by CNS invasion of Gnathostoma spinigerum and Angiostrongylus cantonensis. *J. Neurol. Neurosurg. Psychiatry* **51**:80–87.

122a.**Serna, A., IV, and E. C. Boedeker.** 2008. Pathogenesis and treatment of Shiga toxin-producing Escherichia coli infections. *Curr. Opin. Gastroenterol.* **24**:38–47.

123. **Sever, J. L., J. H. Ellenberg, A. C. Ley, D. L. Madden, D. A. Fuccillo, N. R. Tzan, and D. M. Edmonds.** 1988. Toxoplasmosis. Maternal and pediatric findings in 23,000 pregnancies. *Pediatrics* **82**:181–192.

123a.**Shah, N., H. L. DuPont, and D. J. Ramsey.** 2009. Global etiology of travelers' diarrhea: systematic review from 1973 to the present. *Am. J. Trop. Med. Hyg.* **80**:609–614.

124. **Shields, B. A., P. Bird, W. J. Liss, K. L. Groves, R. Olson, and P. A. Rossignol.** 2002. The nematode Anisakis simplex in American shad (Alosa sapidissima) in two Oregon rivers. *J. Parasitol.* **88**:1033–1035.

125. **Shirahama, M., T. Koga, H. Ishibashi, S. Uchida, Y. Ohta, and Y. Shimoda.** 1992. Intestinal anisakiasis: US in diagnosis. *Radiology* **185**:789–793.

126. **Smith, H. J., S. Messier, and F. Tittinger.** 1989. Destruction of Trichinella spiralis spiralis during the preparation of the "dry cured" pork products prosciutto, prosciuttini and Genoa salami. *Can. J. Vet. Res.* **53:**80–83.

127. **Sohn, W. M., J. Y. Chai, and S. H. Lee.** 1989. A human case of Stellantchasmus falcatus infection. *Kisaengch'ung Hak Chapchi* **27:**277–279.

128. **Sohn, W. M., and S. H. Lee.** 1996. Identification of larval Gnathostoma obtained from imported Chinese loaches. *Korean J. Parasitol.* **34:**161–167.

129. **Sotelo, J., F. Escobedo, J. Rodriguez-Carbajal, B. Torres, and F. Rubio-Donnadieu.** 1984. Therapy of parenchymal brain cysticercosis with praziquantel. *N. Engl. J. Med.* **310:**1001–1007.

130. **Sousa, O. E., R. E. Saenz, and J. K. Frenkel.** 1988. Toxoplasmosis in Panama: a 10-year study. *Am. J. Trop. Med. Hyg.* **38:**315–322.

131. **St. Louis, M. E., J. D. Porter, A. Helal, K. Drame, N. Hargrett-Bean, J. G. Wells, and R. V. Tauxe.** 1990. Epidemic cholera in West Africa: the role of food handling and high-risk foods. *Am. J. Epidemiol.* **131:**719–727.

132. **Stromnes, E., and K. Andersen.** 1998. Distribution of whaleworm (Anisakis simplex, Nematoda, Ascaridoidea) L3 larvae in three species of marine fish: saithe (Pollachius virens (L.)), cod (Gadus morhua L.) and redfish (Sebastes marinus (L.)) from Norwegian waters. *Parasitol. Res.* **84:**281–285.

133. **Swaddiwudhipong, W., P. Akarasewi, T. Chayaniyayodhin, P. Kunasol, and H. M. Foy.** 1989. Several sporadic outbreaks of El Tor cholera in Sunpathong, Chiang Mai, September-October, 1987. *J. Med. Assoc. Thailand* **72:**583–588.

134. **Takabe, K., S. Ohki, O. Kunihiro, T. Sakashita, I. Endo, Y. Ichikawa, H. Sekdo, T. Amano, Y. Nakatani, K. Suzuki, and H. Shimada.** 1998. Anisakidosis: a cause of intestinal obstruction from eating sushi. *Am. J. Gastroenterol.* **93:**1172–1173.

135. **Takayanagui, O. M., and E. Jardim.** 1992. Therapy for neurocysticercosis. Comparison between albendazole and praziquantel. *Arch. Neurol.* **49:**290–294.

136. **Taniguchi, Y., K. Hashimoto, S. Ichikawa, M. Shimizu, K. Ando, and Y. Kotani.** 1991. Human gnathostomiasis. *J. Cutan. Pathol.* **18:**112–115.

137. **Tarr, P. I., M. A. Neill, C. R. Clausen, S. L. Watkins, D. L. Christie, and R. O. Hickman.** 1990. Escherichia coli O157:H7 and the hemolytic uremic syndrome: importance of early cultures in establishing the etiology. *J. Infect. Dis.* **162:**553–556.

137a.**Taylor, C. M.** 2008. Enterohaemorrhagic *Escherichia coli* and *Shigella dysenteriae* type 1-induced haemolytic uraemic syndrome. *Pediatr. Nephrol.* **23:**1425–1431.

138. **Toro, C., M. L. Caballero, M. Baquero, J. García-Samaniego, I. Casado, M. Rubio, and I. Moneo.** 2004. High prevalence of seropositivity to a major allergen of *Anisakis simplex,* Ani s 1, in dyspeptic patients. *Clin. Diagn. Lab. Immunol.* **11:**115–118.

139. **Urita, Y., M. Nishino, H. Koyama, E. Kondo, Y. Naruki, and S. Otsuka.** 1997. Esophageal anisakiasis accompanied by reflux esophagitis. *Intern. Med.* **36:**890–893.

140. **Vazquez, V., and J. Sotelo.** 1992. The course of seizures after treatment for cerebral cysticercosis. *N. Engl. J. Med.* **327:**696–701.

141. **Vitomskova, E. A., and A. S. Dovgalev.** 2001. Rates of infection of fishes from Okhotsk sea with human Anisakidae. *Med. Parazitol. Parazit. Bolezni* **2001:**31–34. (In Russian.)

142. **von Bonsdorff, B., and G. Bylund.** 1982. The ecology of Diphyllobothrium latum. *Ecol. Dis.* **1:**21–26.

142a.**Wells, J. G., L. D. Shipman, K. D. Greene, E. G. Sowers, J. H. Green, D. N. Cameron, F. P. Downes, M. L. Martin, S. M. Ostroff, M. E. Potter, R. V. Tauxe, and I. K. Wachsmuth.** 1991. Isolation of *Escherichia coli* serotype O157:H7 and other Shiga-like-toxin-producing *E. coli* from dairy cattle. *J. Clin. Microbiol.* **29:**985–989.

143. **White, A. C.** 1997. Neurocysticercosis. *Clin. Infect. Dis.* **24:**101–115.

144. **White, A. C., Jr.** 2000. Neurocysticercosis: updates on epidemiology, pathogenesis, diagnosis, and management. *Annu. Rev. Med.* **51:**187–206.

145. **Wilson, C. B., and J. S. Remington.** 1992. Toxoplasmosis, p. 2057–2069. *In* R. D. Feigin and J. D. Cherry (ed.), *Pediatric Infectious Diseases,* 3rd ed. W. B. Saunders, Philadelphia, PA.

146. **Wittner, M., J. W. Turner, G. Jacquette, L. R. Ash, M. P. Salgo, and H. B. Tanowitz.** 1989. Eustrongylidiasis—a parasitic infection acquired by eating sushi. *N. Engl. J. Med.* **320:**1124–1126.

147. **Yeum, C. H., S. K. Ma, S. W. Kim, N. H. Kim, J. Kim, and K. C. Choi.** 2002. Incidental detection of an Anisakis larva in continuous ambulatory peritoneal dialysis effluent. *Nephrol. Dial. Transplant.* **17:**1522–1523.

148. **Zhang, X., A. D. McDaniel, L. E. Wolf, G. T. Keusch, M. K. Waldor, and D. W. Acheson.** 2000. Quinolone antibiotics induce Shiga toxin-encoding bacteriophages, toxin production, and death in mice. *J. Infect. Dis.* **181:**664–670.

INDEX